ADVANCES IN
Chiropractic

VOLUME 2

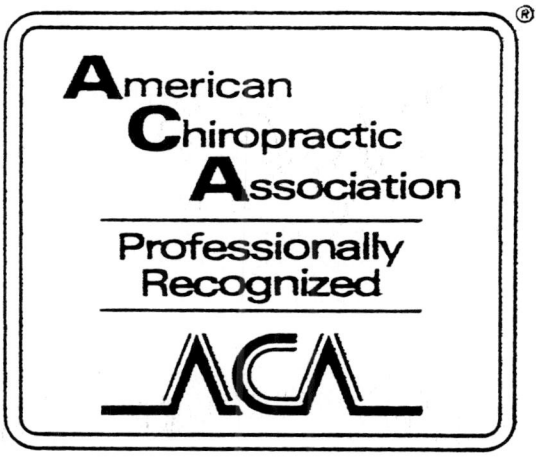

ADVANCES IN Chiropractic

VOLUME 1

Imaging Decisions in the Management of Low Back Pain, *by John A.M. Taylor and Donald Resnick*

Clinical Electromyographic and Related Neurophysiologic Responses, *by John J. Meyer*

Headache Diagnosis, *by Craig F. Nelson*

Which Orthopedic Tests Are Really Necessary? *by Thomas Souza*

On the Field Evaluation of Athletic Injuries of the Head and Neck, *by William T. Roth*

The Domino Theory of Ligamentous Failure in the Lower Cervical Spine, *by Stephen M. Foreman and Michael J. Stahl*

Informed Consent to Chiropractic Treatment, *by David A. Chapman-Smith and Ronald J. Paterson*

The Conservative Management of Lumbar Spinal Stenosis, *by Dale Mierau and William H. Kirkaldy-Willis*

Exercises in the Treatment of Chronic Low Back Pain: A Community-Based Approach for Private Practitioners, *by Stephen H. Burns*

Chiropractic Rehabilitation in the Small Clinic Setting, *by Craig S. Liebenson*

Dispelling the Myths About Therapeutic Ultrasound, *by Edward Feinberg*

Spinal Manipulation Under Anesthesia, *by Randall H. Beckett and Robert Francis*

Specific-Contact, Short Lever-Arm Articular Procedures: Advances in the Gonstead Technique, *by Gregory Plaugher*

Findings on the Relationship Between Spinal Manipulation and Cervical Passive End-Range Capability, *by Dale Nansel and Mark Szlazak*

Prospects for the Future of Chiropractic Guidelines, *by Daniel T. Hansen*

Neurovascular Assessment for Risk Management in Chiropractic Practice, *by Joseph S. Ferezy*

ADVANCES IN Chiropractic

VOLUME 2

Editor-in-Chief
Dana J. Lawrence, D.C., F.I.C.C.
Professor, Department of Chiropractic Practice, Director, Department of Editorial Review and Publication, National College of Chiropractic, Lombard, Illinois

Associate Editors
J. David Cassidy, D.C., M.Sc. (orth), F.C.C.S.(C.), Ph.D.
Director of Research, Department of Orthopaedics, Royal University Hospital, Saskatoon, Saskatchewan, Canada

Marion McGregor, B.Sc., D.C., F.C.C.S.(C.), M.Sc.
Associate Researcher, Canadian Memorial Chiropractic College; Private Consultant, Richardson, Texas

William C. Meeker, D.C., M.P.H.
Dean of Research, Palmer College of Chiropractic-West, President, Consortium for Chiropractic Research, San Jose, California

Howard T. Vernon, D.C., F.C.C.S.
Associate Dean, Research Director, Canadian Memorial Chiropractic College, Toronto, Ontario

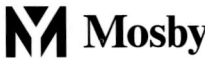

St. Louis Baltimore Berlin Boston Carlsbad Chicago London Madrid
Naples New York Philadelphia Sydney Tokyo Toronto

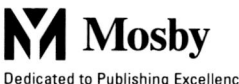
Dedicated to Publishing Excellence

Vice President and Publisher, Continuity Publishing: Kenneth H. Killion
Director, Editorial Development: Gretchen C. Murphy
Acquisitions Editor: Linda M. Steiner
Manager, Continuity—EDP: Maria Nevinger
Project Manager: Jill C. Waite
Assistant Project Supervisor: Sandra Rogers
Proofreading Supervisor: Barbara M. Kelly
Vice President, Professional Sales and Marketing: George M. Parker
Senior Marketing Manager: Eileen M. Lynch
Marketing Specialist: Lynn D. Stevenson

Copyright © 1995 by Mosby–Year Book, Inc.

All rights reserved. No part of this publication may be reproduced, stored in a retrieval system, or transmitted, in any form or by any means, electronic, mechanical, photocopying, recording, or otherwise, without prior written permission from the publisher.

Permission to photocopy or reproduce solely for internal or personal use is permitted for libraries or other users registered with the Copyright Clearance Center, provided that the base fee of $4.00 per chapter plus $.10 per page is paid directly to the Copyright Clearance Center, 27 Congress Street, Salem, MA 01970. This consent does not extend to other kinds of copying, such as copying for general distribution, for advertising or promotional purposes, for creating new collected works, or for resale.

Printed in the United States of America
Composition by The Clarinda Company
Printing/binding by The Maple-Vail Book Manufacturing Group

Mosby–Year Book, Inc.
11830 Westline Industrial Drive
St. Louis, Missouri 63146

Editorial Office:
Mosby–Year Book, Inc.
200 North LaSalle Street
Chicago, Illinois 60601

International Standard Serial Number: 1074-7990
International Standard Book Number: 0-8151-5307-4

Contributors

Cynthia A. Baum, D.C., D.A.C.B.R.
Radiological Consulting Practice, Chatsworth, California; Postgraduate Faculty, Los Angeles College of Chiropractic, Whittier, California

Thomas F. Bergmann, D.C., F.I.C.C.
Professor, Department of Chiropractic Methods, Faculty Clinician, Center for Clinical Studies, Northwestern College of Chiropractic, Bloomington, Minnesota

Robert Cooperstein, M.A., D.C.
Associate Professor, Palmer College of Chiropractic West, San Jose, California

Arthur C. Croft, M.S., D.C., F.A.C.O.
Director, Spine Research Institute, San Diego, California; Assistant Adjunct Professor, Los Angeles College of Chiropractic, Los Angeles, California; Assistant Adjunct Professor, New York Chiropractic College, Seneca Falls, New York

Darryl D. Curl, D.D.S., D.C.
Director, Pacific Coast Faculty Resource Group, Whittier, California; Associate Professor, Department of Diagnosis, Los Angeles College of Chiropractic, Whittier, California

John Danchik, D.C., C.C.S.P.
Private Practice, Belmont, Massachusetts

Neil Fried, D.C., D.P.M.
Instructor and Senior Staff Clinician, National College of Chiropractic, Lombard, Illinois; Attending, Department of Surgery, Doctor's Hospital of Hyde Park, Chicago, Illinois

Arlan W. Fuhr, D.C.
President, Activator Methods, Inc., Phoenix, Arizona

Meridel I. Gatterman, M.A., D.C.
Research Department, New York Chiropractic College, Seneca Falls, New York

Daniel T. Hansen, D.C.
Private Practice, Olympia, Washington; Medical Director, Chiropractic Network Services, Lynnwood, Washington

Tom Hyde, D.A.C.B.S.P.
Executive Director, American Chiropractic Association Council on Sports Injuries and Physical Fitness, Miami, Florida

Grant C. Iannelli, B.S., D.C., D.A.A.P.M., C.P.H.O.
Associate Professor of Clinics; Quality Assurance Coordinator, National College of Chiropractic, Lombard, Illinois

Sharon A. Jaeger, D.C., D.A.C.B.R., F.I.C.C.
Secretary/Treasurer, Foundation on Chiropractic Education and Research; Board of Regents, Los Angeles College of Chiropractic, Whittier, California; Consulting Practice, Chatsworth, California; Private practice, North Hollywood, California

Jennifer R. Jamison, Ph.D., M.B., B.Ch., Ed.D.
Professor of Diagnostic Sciences, School of Chiropractic and Osteopathy, Faculty of Biomedical and Health Sciences, Royal Melbourne Institute of Technology, Bundoora, Australia

Margaret Karg, D.C., C.C.S.P.
Private Practice, Belmont, Massachusetts

Tony S. Keller, Ph.D.
Assistant Professor of Mechanical Engineering, University of Vermont, Burlington, Vermont

Alan B. Korbett, D.C., D.O., D.A.B.C.O., C.C.S.P., D.A.C.A.N.
PGYI Psychiatry Resident/House Staff, Department of Psychiatry, University of Iowa Hospitals and Clinics, Iowa City, Iowa

Gary R. Lindquist, D.C., D.A.C.B.R.
Radiological Consulting Practice, Chatsworth, California; Postgraduate Faculty, Los Angeles College of Chiropractic, Whittier, California

Edward L. Maurer, D.C., D.A.C.B.R.
Postgraduate Faculty in Radiology, National College of Chiropractic, Lombard, Illinois

Marion McGregor, B.Sc., D.C., F.C.C.S.(C.), M.Sc.
Research Consultant, Private Practice, Richardson, Texas

Paul J. Osterbauer, D.C., M.P.H.
Director of Research, Activator Methods, Inc., Phoenix, Arizona

Bill Russell, M.A., M.F.A., D.C., C.C.S.P.
Post Doctoral Faculty, Logan College, Dance/Sports Injuries, St. Louis, Missouri

Robert C. Shiel, Ph.D.
Associate Professor, National College of Chiropractic, Lombard, Illinois

Paula J. Stern, B.Sc., D.C., F.C.C.S.C.
Private Practice, Saskatoon, Saskatchewan, Canada

William C. Toth, D.C., D.A.C.B.S.P.
Instructor, Post Graduate Division, National College of Chiropractic, Lombard, Illinois

John J. Triano, D.C., M.A.
Private Practice, Texas Back Institute, Plano, Texas; Board of Advisors, Institute of Spine and Biomedical Research, Plano, Texas

Howard T. Vernon, D.C., F.C.C.S.(C.)
Associate Dean of Research, Canadia Memorial Chiropractic College, Toronto, Ontario, Canada

Walter I. Wardwell, Ph.D.
Professor Emeritus of Sociology, University of Connecticut, Storrs, Connecticut

Preface

This past year saw the publication of federal guidelines relating to the treatment of low back pain (Bigos S, Bowyer O, Braen G, et al: *Acute Low Back Problems in Adults*. Clinical Practice Guideline No. 14. Rockville, Md, Agency for Health Care Policy and Research, U.S. Department of Health and Human Services, December 1994), under the auspices of the Agency for Health Care Policy and Research (AHCPR). These guidelines recommended, in part, the use of spinal manipulation for managing various types of low back pain. While many within the chiropractic profession saw this event as a substantial measure of vindication, some within the profession viewed this as perhaps another nail in the coffin of medical co-optation of the chiropractic profession. While I certainly cannot agree with this latter view, I cannot totally agree with the former either.

There is an important point in all this. The AHCPR guidelines were developed through a process that started with the examination of over 11,000 literature citations, which then winnowed that body of evidence down to nearly 2,000 pieces of literature, and which ultimately ended finding far fewer that could meet rigorous methodological criteria for inclusion. Why mention this? Because it is important to realize that all health care professions must move toward evidence-based practice. This does not mean, as so many seem to think, that without rigorous scientific evidence one cannot practice or deliver various forms of care. If that were so, none of us in health care could do very much at all. But we do need to have rational reasons for what we do; they need to be grounded in the available evidence.

Evidence is not just scientific research reports, though those are of critical importance to the evidence process. It will always be best to have research supporting what we do, but the reality is that there is simply not enough money to fund everything that we would like. In fact, within chiropractic, there is precious little funding at all. Thus, books such as this also have an important role to play.

This *Advances* series attempts to publish new and interesting information related to the developing interests of the chiropractic profession. Last year saw the release of the first volume in the series, and I am pleased to note here the publication of the second. This publication provides an overview of the profession's interests; it helps to give us a sense of where we are going, and also where we might go.

I once again thank Drs. Cassidy, McGregor, Meeker, and Vernon for their continual support and help in managing this project. I thank as well the many people at Mosby–Year Book who provide support of a different kind—in particular, Gretchen Murphy, Rona Taylor, Linda Steiner, and Ken Killion. On behalf of them all, I hope that you find this material informative and useful, and I invite you to write with your comments.

Dana J. Lawrence, D.C.

Contents

Contributors — v
Preface — vii

Advances in the Clinical Understanding of Acceleration/Deceleration Injuries to the Cervical Spine.
By Arthur C. Croft — 3

- Biomechanics — 3
  - Early Research — 3
  - Recent Research — 5
- Sequence of Events in CAD Injury — 10
  - Phase One — 10
  - Phase Two — 11
  - Phase Three — 13
  - Phase Four — 13
- Physical Factors Affecting the Injury — 15
  - Head Restraints — 15
  - Seat Belts and Shoulder Harnesses — 15
  - Shock-Attenuating Bumper Systems — 17
- Human Factors Affecting the Injury — 18
  - Age — 18
  - Preparedness — 18
  - Gender — 18
  - Stature — 18
  - Occupant Position — 21
- Soft Tissue Injuries — 21
  - Experimental Studies — 21
  - Neck Pain — 23
  - Neck Stiffness — 23
  - Shoulder Pain — 24
  - Headaches — 24
  - Interscapular Pain — 24
  - Back Pain — 24
  - Paresthesiae — 26
  - Extremity Pain and Weakness — 26
  - Dizziness and Lightheadedness — 26
  - Auditory Disturbances — 27
  - Vertigo — 27
  - Short Duration Vertigo — 27
  - Ocular Dysfunction — 27

       Dysphagia and Hoarseness   27
       Facial Pain   28
       Hypothyroidism   28
   Conclusion   28

Spinal Stenosis.
By Edward L. Maurer   39

   Etiology and Pathogenesis   40
       Congenital and Developmental Stenosis   40
       Acquired Stenosis   44
       Postoperative Spinal Stenosis   53
       Posttraumatic Spinal Stenosis   55
       Metabolic and Endocrine Disorders with Stenosis   56
       Miscellaneous Disorders with Spinal Stenosis   56
   Clinical Considerations   58
   Differential Diagnosis   59
   Diagnosis   63
       Electrodiagnosis   63
       Diagnostic Imaging   64
   Treatment   72
   Discussion   74

Low Back Pain and Pregnancy.
By Paula J. Stern   97

   Physiology   97
   Epidemiology   98
   Etiology   99
   History and Physical Examination   100
   Differential Diagnosis   103
       Disk Herniation   103
       Pubic Pain   104
       Leg Cramps   104
       Osteoporosis   105
       Other Causes   105
   Neurological Conditions   105
       Meralgia Paresthetica   105
       Multiple Sclerosis   105
       Tarsal Tunnel Syndrome   106
   Complications of Pregnancy   106
       Spontaneous Abortion (Miscarriage)   106
       Ectopic Pregnancy   106
       Preterm Labor   106
       Preeclampsia-Eclampsia   107
       Placenta Previa   107

Abruptio Placentae	107
Deep Venous Thrombosis and Pulmonary Embolism	107
Management	108
Spinal Manipulation	108
Education	108
Exercise	113
Postpartum	116

Running Injuries: A Fresh Perspective.
By William C. Toth — 121

Biomechanics of Running	122
Gait Cycle	122
Heel Strike	122
Stance Phase	122
Swing Phase	123
Muscular Control of the Ankle While Running	123
Categories of Runners	124
Categories of Running Injuries	124
Training Errors	124
Shoe Fit	127
Evaluation of Running Injuries	128
Diagnosis	128
History	129
Physical Examination	129
Radiographic Examination	132
Biomechanical Evaluation	132
Shoe Evaluation	132
Anatomical Faults and Conditions	134
Patellofemoral Arthralgia	134
Iliotibial Band Syndrome	135
Posterior Tibial Syndrome	135
Popliteal Tendinitis	136
Achilles Tendinitis	136
Plantar Fasciitis	136
General Foot Ankle Rehabilitation	137
RICE	137
Proprioceptive Rehabilitation	137
Strengthening	138
Return to Running	140
Conclusion	141

The Temporomandibular Joint.
By Darryl D. Curl — 143

Screening Procedures for TM Disorders	146
Distant Sources of Pain	146
Head Posture	146

Mandibular Postural Rest Position	150
Screening Questionnaire	152
Examination of the TM Apparatus	153
Patient History	153
Inspection	153
Palpation	155
Percussion	158
Auscultation	159
Instrumentation	160
Range of Motion	161
Provocative Tests	162
Neurological Tests	165
Common TM Disorders and How to Recognize Them	166
Disorders Involving TMJ	167
Disorders Involving the Muscles of Mastication	168
Disorders of Mandibular Mobility	168
Treatment: Should the TMJ Be Adjusted?	171
Indications	171
Contraindications	172
Injuries Resulting from Delayed Diagnoses	172
Fibrous Ankylosis of the Disk	172
Capsular Contracture	173
Myofibrotic Contracture	174
Common Questions	174

Reflex Sympathetic Dystrophy and Chiropractic.
By Howard T. Vernon   183

Definitions	183
Epidemiological and Clinical Features of RSD and SMP	184
Clinical Course of RSD	186
Diagnostic Methods	187
Clinical Methods	187
Neural Blockade Testing	187
Mechanisms	188
Peripheral Mechanisms	188
Central Mechanisms	190
Treatment	192
Chiropractic Implications	192

Pronation and Associated Disorders.
By Neil Fried   195

What Is Pronation?	195
Associated Disorders	198
Flexible Flatfoot	198
Tarsal Coalition	199
Tibialis Posterior Rupture and Tenosynovitis	200

    Plantar Fasciitis   202
    Sinus Tarsitis   203
    Hallux Valgus   204
    Hallux Limitus and Hallux Rigidus   205
    Hammertoes   207
    Adducto Varus of Fourth and Fifth Toes   208

Chiropractic Medicine for Dance.
By Bill Russell   211

  Cause of Injury   212
  Dance Screening Examination   213
    Personal Information   214
    Young Dancers   214
    Medical History   215
    Dance Injury History   215
    Dance History   215
    Technique Factors   215
    Occupational Factors   221
    Screening   223
    Postural Examination   223
    Specific Area Evaluation   225
    Screening Conclusion   230
  Psoas Insufficiency Syndrome   230
  Treatment of Dance Injuries   233
  Rehabilitation of the Injured Dancer   234
    Stretches   235
  Proprioceptive Rehabilitation   235
    Structure and Function   236
    Common Causes of Injury   236
    Dance-Specific Movement   237
    Proprioceptive Testing   237
    Special Maneuvers   239
    Proprioceptive Rehabilitation Equipment   240
    Motor Development Skills Exercises   243
    Body Therapies   243
  Video and Dance Injuries   246
  Conclusion   249

Depressive Disorders, Prevalence, Assessment in, and Impact on the Primary Care Setting.
By Alan B. Korbett   255

  Historical Perspective of Mental Illness   255
  Development of the Diagnostic and Statistical Manuals of Mental Disorders   256
  Use of DSM-IV   257
    Defining Axes I to V   257
    Diagnostic Coding   259

Mood Disorders	260
Depression	260
Detecting and Diagnosing Mood Disorders	264
Conclusion	276

Conservative Management of Shoulder Injuries in Athletes.
By Tom Hyde, Margaret Karg, and John Danchik   279

History	279
Anatomy	280
Sternoclavicular Joint	280
Acromioclavicular Joint	280
Glenohumeral Joint	280
Scapulothoracic Articulation	281
Shoulder Bursae	281
Rotator Cuff	281
Vascular Supply to the Shoulder	282
Venous Supply	283
Biomechanics	283
Elevation	283
Internal and External Rotation	283
Horizontal Flexion and Extension	283
Orthopedic Examination	283
Anterior Shoulder Instability Test	285
Posterior Shoulder Instability Tests	287
Other Tests	289
Acromioclavicular Joint Injuries	298
Radiographic Studies	300
Treatment	300
Rotator Cuff Injuries	302
Throwing Injuries	304
Examination	304
Biomechanics of Throwing	306
Other Considerations	308
Treatment	308
Shoulder Instability	309
Treatment	310
Neurovascular Injuries	311
Cervical Burners	311
Treatment	312
Additional Shoulder Disorders	312
Osteochondritis Dissecans	312
Osteolysis of the Distal Clavicle	313
Levator Scapula Syndrome	313
Injuries of the Distal Clavicular Physis in Children	313
Latissimus Dorsi Tendinitis	313

Disorders of the Infraspinatus Muscle ... 314
Shoulder Pain in the Wheelchair Athlete ... 315
Synoviochondrometaplasia ... 315
Fractures ... 315
Conservative Treatment and Rehabilitation Considerations ... 319
Diagnostic Imaging ... 320

The Many Faces of the Facets.
By Sharon A. Jaeger, Cynthia A. Baum, and Gary R. Lindquist ... 331
    Plane Film ... 331
    Imaging ... 332
    Anatomy ... 332
    Nerve Supply ... 333
    Plane of Orientation ... 333
    Developmental Variations ... 334
    Facet Notching: Gouge Defect ... 337
    Tropism ... 338
    Congenital Blocking ... 341
    Agenesis ... 341
    Hypoplasia or Hyperplasia ... 341
    Ununited Apophyseal Growth Centers: Ossicles of Oppenheimer ... 342
    Trauma to the Cervical Spine ... 343
        Locked Facets ... 343
        Unilateral Facet Dislocation: Stable Injury ... 343
        Bilateral Facet Dislocation: Unstable Injury ... 347
        Perched Facets ... 349
        Delayed Dislocation ... 349
        Distracted Facets ... 350
        Facet Fracture ... 350
    Trauma to the Thoracic and Lumbar Spine ... 350
        Thoracolumbar Junction ... 350
        Burst Fractures ... 351
    Inflammatory Spondyloarthropathy ... 352
        Ankylosing Spondylitis and Its Variants ... 352
    Rheumatoid Arthritis ... 353
        Juvenile Rheumatoid Arthritis (Juvenile Chronic Arthritis) ... 353
        Crystal Deposition Disease ... 353
        Gout ... 353
    Osteoarthritis (Facetal Arthrosis) ... 353
    Five Sequential Stages of Facetal Degeneration ... 354
        1. Synovitis ... 354
        2. Laxity of Joint Capsule ... 354
        3. Articular Cartilage Breakdown ... 355

4. Subarticular Bone Erosion	355
5. Hyperostosis	356
Less Commonly Manifested Radiographic Findings	358
Degenerative Ossicles	358
Synovial Hyperplasia	358
Segmental Instability	358
Vacuum Phenomenon	358
Degenerative Synovial Cysts	358
Tarlov Cyst	358
Intra-Articular Fusion	359
Chondromalacia Facetae	360
Degenerative Pseudospondylolisthesis	360
Joint Instability	360
Facetal Imbrication (Shakelike, Overlapping, or Telescoping)	362
Spinographic Measurements Related to the Facets	365
Hadley's Curve	365
MacNab's Line (Posterior Joint Body Line)	366
Lumbosacral Disk Angle	367
Sacral Base Angle (Ferguson's Sacral Base Angle)	367
Weight Bearing: Gravitational Line of L-3	367

Chiropractic Today.
By Walter I. Wardwell

	373
Media Acceptance	373
Legal and Legislative Acceptance	373
Acceptance by the Public	376
Professional Acceptance	377
Third-Party Reimbursements	380
Major Problems in the 1990s	380
Conclusion	384

Educational Issues in Chiropractic.
By Jennifer R. Jamison

	387
General Implications of Paradigm Assumptions on Teaching and Learning	389
Competency-Based Education: A Forum for Paradigm Interaction	391
Problem Solving	392
Problem-Based Learning	393
Teaching Strategies	394
Learning Preferences	397
Assessment Options	399
Staff Appraisal	402

Education in the Interstices of Paradigms ... 403
Conclusion ... 405

Chiropractic Technique: An Overview.
By Thomas F. Bergmann ... 413
  Forms of Manual Therapy ... 417
  Adjustive Mechanics ... 420
    Adjustive Localization ... 421
    Patient Positioning ... 421
    Assisted and Resisted Positioning ... 422
  Effects of Adjustive Therapy ... 423
    Mechanical Effects ... 425
    Soft Tissue Effects ... 426
    Neurological Effects ... 427
    Psychological Effects ... 427
  Teaching of Chiropractic Technique ... 428
  Summary ... 432

Contemporary Approach to Understanding Chiropractic Technique.
By Robert Cooperstein ... 437
  Chiropractic as Art, Science, and Philosophy—But Especially Art ... 437
  Chiropractic Technique Qua Technique ... 438
  Proliferation of Chiropractic Technique Systems ... 439
  Why There Are So Many Technique Systems ... 440
    Development at the Margin ... 440
    Lack of Market Penetration ... 441
    The Economic Advantage of Retaining Several Techniques ... 441
    The Chiropractor as a Generalist ... 443
    Mercantile Bent of the Founders ... 443
    Lack of Knowledge ... 443
    The Quest for "Nerve Interference" ... 444
    The Allure of Brand Name Techniques ... 444
    The Glass House Effect ... 445
  The Spectacle of Pseudoscientific Technique ... 446
  Chiropractic Technique and the Colleges ... 447
  Taxonomy of Chiropractic Technique ... 448
    Segmentalism Vs. Posturalism ... 449
    Misalignment Vs. Fixation ... 449
    Structure Vs. Function ... 450
    Anatomicophysiological Vs. Reflex Techniques ... 450
    Forceful Vs. Light-Force (and Even Non-Force) Techniques ... 451
    Characterization of Technique Procedures ... 452
    Practice Parameters ... 452

The Consensus Process	455
Practice Guidelines and Standards of Care	455
Managed Health Care: The "Black Box" of Treatment	455
Conclusion	456

Advances in Subluxation Terminology and Usage.
By Meridel I. Gatterman

	461
Subluxation Field of Terms	462
Historical Perspective	463
Subluxation-Related Dysfunction	464
Clinical Manifestations of Subluxation	465
Metaphorical Use of Subluxation	465
Operationally Defining Subluxation	465
Terminology Related to the Treatment of Subluxation	466
Conclusion	468

Description and Analysis of Activator Methods Chiropractic Technique.
By Paul J. Osterbauer, Arlan W. Fuhr, and Tony S. Keller

	471
History	471
Diagnostic Procedures	475
Background of the Chiropractic Subluxation	475
Treatment Procedures	484
Clinical Studies of MFMA Procedures	486
Case Series	487
Case Reports	493
Role of Kinematics in Chiropractic Manipulation/Adjustment	493
Vertebral Forces and Movements During Spinal Manipulation and Mobilization	494
New Methods of Characterization of the Dynamic Mechanical Properties of the Spine	495
Mechanical Impulse for Spinal Diagnosis and Therapy	498
Future Perspective: Computer-Assisted Manipulation	500
Conclusion	501
Appendix 1: Activator Methods Chiropractic Technique Summary	513
Appendix 2: Kinematic and Biomechanical Behavior of the Normal and Pathological Spine	517

Principles of Quality Management in Chiropractic Practice.
By Grant C. Iannelli

	521
History of Quality Management in Health Care	521
Definitions	521
Quality in Health Care: 1860s–1990s	522

Quality Management in Ambulatory Health Care	525
Chiropractic Attempts	525
Other Ambulatory Quality Management Attempts	526
Ambuqual Quality Management System	527
Quality Management Activities	528
Ambuqual Implementation	528
Physician Performance Audit	532
Patient Satisfaction Audit	536
Ambuqual System Scoring	542
Implementation Issues	543
Conclusion	543
Appendix 1: National College Chiropractic Clinics Quality Assurance Plan	549
Appendix 2: Procedure: Physician Performance Audit	557
Appendix 3: "Give Us A Grade": Patient Satisfaction Audit Questions	561

Assessing Clinical Research Material: The Clinician's Role and Responsibility.
By Marion McGregor

	565
The Case	565
The Past	566
Colleagues	567
Product Information	568
Textbooks	569
The Present	570
Defining the Reading Purpose and Finding a Source	570
Separating Fact from Opinion	572
Appraising the Applicability of the Information from the Facts	573
IME Literature Support for the Decision on Mrs. B.T.	579
Generalizing from the Sample to Mrs. B.T.	580
Initial Assessment	581
Time and Treatment	583
Final Assessment	584
Analysis	584
Summary	585
Preponderance of Evidence	585

Physician-Patient Interactions.
By Robert C. Shiel

	595
Patient's Context	597
Models of Physician Behavior	601
Narration: The Patient in Personal Context	604
Physician and Patient in Relationship	607
Structures in the Relationship Between Physician and Patient	612

Modeling Cooperative Interactions: Prisoner's Dilemma ... 618
Conclusions: Dimensions of Caregiving ... 624
    Acknowledgment Vs. Disqualification ... 625
    Acceptance Vs. Approval or Disapproval ... 626
    Understanding Vs. Probing ... 628
    Empathy Vs. Reassuring ... 629
    Respect Vs. Advice ... 630
    Flexibility Vs. Defensiveness ... 631

Applications of Quality Assurance in Chiropractic Practice.
By Daniel T. Hanson and John J. Triano ... 635
    Historical and Social Perspectives ... 636
    Defining Quality ... 640
    National Standards in QA ... 644
        NCQA ... 645
        JCAHO ... 646
        HEDIS-2.0 ... 646
        Council on Chiropractic Education ... 647
    Typical Applications of QA for the Chiropractic Office ... 649
    Credentialing of Chiropractic Doctors ... 649
    Economic Credentialing ... 649
    Facility and Staff Credentialing ... 650
    Accessibility ... 651
    Utilization Management ... 652
    Continuity of Care ... 652
    Record Keeping ... 653
    QA Staff Position ... 654
    Informed Consent ... 655
    Other Applications in the Chiropractic Office ... 655
        QA in Chiropractic Diagnosis ... 655
        QA in Chiropractic Treatment ... 656
    QA and Outcomes ... 662
        Practice Monitoring of Outcomes ... 664
    Health Status and Health Policy ... 664
    Future Considerations ... 665
Index ... 671

Mosby Document Express

Copies of the full text of journal articles referenced in this book are available by calling Mosby Document Express, toll-free, at 1-800-55-MOSBY.

With Mosby Document Express, you have convenient 24-hour-a-day access to literally every journal reference within this book. In fact, through Mosby Document Express, virtually any medical or scientific article can be located and delivered by FAX, overnight delivery service, international airmail, electronic transmission of bit-mapped images (via Internet), or regular mail. The average cost of a complete delivered copy of an article, including copyright clearance charges and first-class mail delivery, is $12.

For inquiries and pricing information, please call the toll-free number shown above.

Advances in the Clinical Understanding of Acceleration/Deceleration Injuries to the Cervical Spine

Arthur C. Croft, M.S., D.C., F.A.C.O.
Director, Spine Research Institute, San Diego, California; Assistant Adjunct Professor, Los Angeles College of Chiropractic, Los Angeles, California; Assistant Adjunct Professor, New York Chiropractic College, Seneca Falls, New York

This chapter is about whiplash injuries to the neck. More precisely, it is about the cervical acceleration/deceleration, or CAD, injuries engendered by rear impact motor vehicle accidents. After reading this chapter, the reader should be convinced that such accidents are sufficiently unlike lateral or frontal collisions to justify my suggestion that we phase out the older, less specific term "whiplash," even though it has been recognized in both lay and medical dictionaries. Having done that, of course, we will need terms for the injuries arising out of lateral and frontal accidents. "Lateral CAD injury" and "cervical deceleration injury" are sufficiently unambiguous terms for this purpose. I have proposed a classification system that considers the vector of collision along with the grade of severity and stage of recovery in CAD trauma. This system is outlined in Table 1.

Although the title of this chapter promises new insight from a clinical perspective, I would be inexcusably remiss if I failed to provide an ample discussion of biomechanics because "clinical understanding" has historically foundered on the shoals of ignorance of these very issues. Earlier workers have often misgauged the magnitude of energy delivered to the spine and soft tissues, particularly in low-speed impacts, and their resulting hypotheses have had more foundation in intuition than in rigorous scientific analysis. Experiments designed to test such heuristic hypotheses have often provided misleading truths as is so common in science. Benefitting from almost 30 years of further research and with the acuity of hindsight, I can provide an excellent example of this phenomenon. Based on his clinical observations, Macnab[1] correctly observed that patients exposed to CAD trauma were often left with permanent conditions. He hypothesized that most of the blame could be attached to an abrupt hyperextension of the neck. To test this hypothesis, he[2] designed an experimental apparatus that subjected primates to cervical hyperextension injury and observed a number of resulting lesions that correlated

TABLE 1.
Classification of Cervical Acceleration/Deceleration Trauma from Motor Vehicle Accidents (SRISD)*†

Classification	Description
Type of Collision:	(Occupant may be driver or passenger, vehicle struck may be moving or stationary.)
Type I	primary rear impact.
Type II	primary side impact.
Type III	primary frontal impact.
Grade of Injury Severity	
Grade I	minimal; no limitation of motion; no ligamentous injury; no neurological findings.
Grade II	slight; limitation of motion; no ligamentous injury; no neurological findings.
Grade III	moderate; limitation of motion; some ligamentous injury; neurological findings may be present.
Grade IV	moderate to severe; limitation of motion; ligamentous instability; neurological findings present; fracture or disc derangement.
Grade V	severe; requires surgical management/stabilization.
Stages of Injury:	
Stage I	acute; inflammatory phase; up to seventy-two hours
Stages II	subacute; repair phase; seventy-two hours to fourteen weeks
Stage III	remodeling phase; fourteen weeks to twelve months or more
Stage IV	chronic; permanent

*From Croft AC: *Palmer J Research* 1:10–21, 1994. Used by permission.
†SRISD = Spine Research Institute of San Diego. These criteria do not consider loss of consciousness, the use of seatbelts or shoulder harnesses, nor other factors that will be accounted for in a forthcoming revised prognostic index.

with many of those he had observed in his own patients at surgery, thus seemingly validating his hypothesis. Because Macnab did not consider the flexion phase of the injury to be as severe as the extension phase, his experimental apparatus did not produce flexion, and because his writings were seminal in the CAD arena, this hyperextension theory has been most influential and is still widely accepted. In fairness to Macnab, who

I revere as a pioneer, however, his hypothesis, tendered as it was in the early 1960s, was much less problematic then than it has since become with the addition of head restraints and shoulder harnesses to automobiles—safety devices that have been shown to magnify rather than mollify neck and spine injuries in such collisions. Many authors since that time have clouded the water with less than scholarly musings based on their own personal observations and bias and so have served only to obfuscate and till the fertile garden of controversy. The farrago of literature available today is itself a lesson in epistemology concerning how a knowledge base should not develop.

More recent scientific installments to our pool of knowledge concerning the kinematics of CAD trauma will be followed in this chapter by a discussion of the physical (i.e., vehicular) and human variables that affect the nature and complexity of these injuries. The more erudite of clinicians will carefully dissect each case as a unique event, taking into account all of these factors. Because of the almost occult nature of these soft tissue injuries, they are among the most challenging conditions to treat effectively in all of chiropractic or medicine. And successful management depends on an accurate diagnosis. Superficial examinations often result in dilatory and unsuccessful case management and probably explain, at least in part, the rather dismal outcome for many patients. This chapter is about understanding rather than managing the condition. Although I[3] have recently dealt with management in some detail, practitioners trained in the treatment of musculoskeletal conditions will no doubt find useful clinical application of the material in this chapter.

An appreciation of the resulting biomechanics is prerequisite for the understanding of the nature and broad range of clinical conditions that the practitioner must address. The last part of this chapter concerns itself (in brief detail) with a discussion of the clinical pastiche of CAD trauma aftermath. Although the acronym CAD implies a primary cervical injury, lesions both above and below the neck (e.g., brain and low back) are commonplace.

BIOMECHANICS

Since the invention of the automobile, we have known about whiplash. For the most part it has been held suspect, vilified, scorned, and generally disowned by the medical establishment, perhaps understandably so. After all, patients claim to have all manner of neuromusculoskeletal and even cognitive complaints after sometimes trivial trauma. Often there are few firm objective findings that might substantiate such claims. Moreover, these patients are frequently litigating, and the drivers and occupants of the striking car are rarely injured. Besides, most of us have been involved in minor collisions without being injured. Even today such reductionist reasoning forms the capstone for legal defense arguments in such cases. The logic is simply too seductive for most jurors unless it can be properly disabused with the facts.

EARLY RESEARCH

In the 1950s, before the time that Macnab conducted his pioneering work, a team headed by Severy[4] set out to test a new hypothesis—that the occupant of a vehicle that was struck from the rear by another vehicle would experience acceleration forces greater than the vehicle itself. Using both humans and anthropometric dummies as subjects (occupants), they conducted crash tests at speeds of up to about 10 mph. The first test vehicles were World War II vintage cars equipped with mechanical accelerometers. The occupants were fitted with electronic accelerometers. In tests of 8 mph, a human volunteer experienced acceleration forces two and one-half times that of the car he was sitting in. This ratio, however, is not fixed. At higher-speed collisions the head and neck may be exposed to 4 to 10 times the car's acceleration. In this ground-breaking research the authors made a number of other discoveries that enhanced our fundamental understanding of CAD trauma and, in particular, our understanding of the pathomechanics of low-speed rear impact collisions. Their work marked a watershed event in CAD research and has become the most cited literature in this area.[4]

Figure 1 depicts an exemplar graph of the Severy et al.[4] findings. It was the authors' intentions to simulate a crash involving a real world, unsuspecting motorist so the volunteer was instructed not to brace for the impact. In a 10-mph collision the volunteer was similarly instructed, but high-speed film of the event revealed that he was, in fact, tensed at the time of impact. The interesting observation, which has subsequently been observed by States et al.,[5] was that when tensed, the occupant's acceleration was similar in magnitude (rather than a multiple of it) to that of the car, thus providing one clue as to why struck vehicle occupants might be injured to a greater degree than those in the striking car who are presumably aware of the impending collision in most cases.

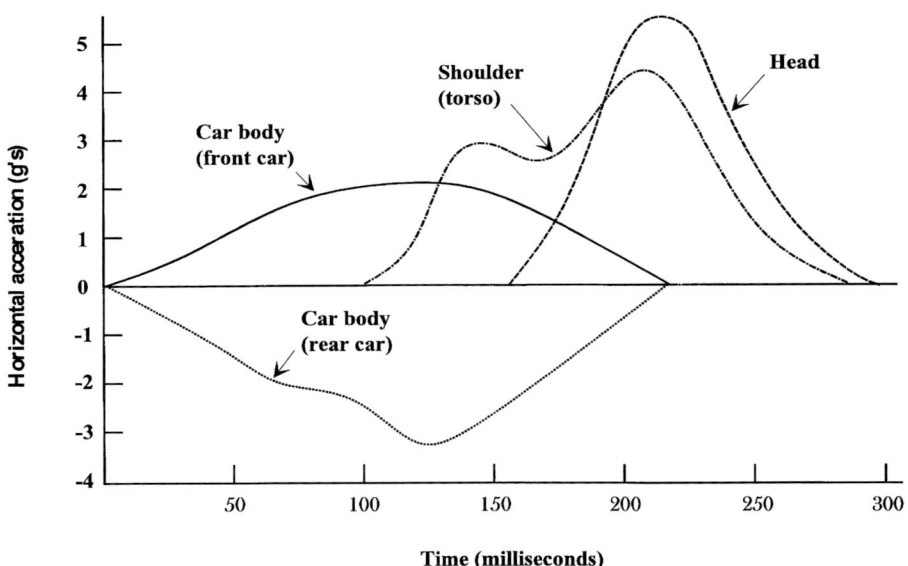

FIGURE 1.
Effects of full-scale rear impact crash testing using a human volunteer. Impact speed was 8 mph. No brakes were applied. The head is exposed to acceleration forces two and one half times that of the vehicle. (Adapted from Severy DM, Mathewson JH, Bechtol CO: *Can Services Med J* 11:727–758, 1955.)

Severy et al.[4] also observed that the occupant loaded the seat back as the car accelerated below him. As the head began to extend over the neck, the torso began its forward excursion, amplified by the seat back's forward spring, resulting in significant shear and axial stretching of the cervical spine. These and other complex phenomena resulting from the interface of a human and a machine are described in more detail elsewhere[6] and provide exculpatory understanding of this otherwise maligned condition. However, critics have more recently repudiated this early research, arguing that it fails to account for the smaller, lighter cars on the road today—cars equipped with head restraints, three-point seat belt restraints, and shock-attenuating rear bumpers. Such arguments have prima facie merit and have served as the grist for successful defense-based rhetoric in many soft tissue injury cases.

Unfortunately, none of these arguments has a factual basis. For example, cars on the road today are frequently as heavy or heavier than those tested by Severy et al.[4] On the other hand, there is a greater disparity in the sizes of cars on the road today, leaving drivers of subcompacts in considerable relative jeopardy. It is a simple fact of physics, for example, that the relative masses of two colliding vehicles will play a significant role in determining the forces incurred by the occupants[7-9]; the occupants of a smaller car will be injured to a greater degree when struck by a larger car (i.e., one with greater mass), whereas the occupants of a larger car will suffer fewer or less severe injuries when struck by a smaller car. Head restraints have not proved to provide much protection against CAD trauma and may actually increase the likelihood of injury. Similarly, seat belts and shoulder harnesses, although they reduce morbidity and mortality significantly in high-speed collisions, have been shown in several studies to intensify minor neck and back injuries in lower-speed collisions. Shock-attenuating bumper systems have been shown to raise the threshold of property damage to the vehicle but provide little or no injury-sparing benefit to the occupant. Predictably, rhetorical medicolegal arguments, such as those condemning the Severy et al.[4] work, develop pari passu with scientific research, with the only requirement being their credibility with jurors—a phenomenon all too often aided and abetted by expert witnesses who obediently condone this form of pseudoscience.

RECENT RESEARCH

Researchers[10-16] at the University of British Columbia (UBC) and elsewhere have conducted crash testing similar to that of Severy et al.[4] using late-model Volkswagens, Toyotas, and Nissans. In contrast to earlier tests, these cars were equipped with both seat belts and shoulder harnesses. They were also fitted with head restraints and shock-attenuating bumpers. Most of this work involved Volkswagen Rabbits, which were fitted with bumper isolators—fluid- and gas-filled shock absorbers that mount between the bumper and frame. Thomson et al.[12] measured the resulting forces from rear-impact collision simulations conducted at UBC (Fig 2). A 927-kg pendulum struck the rear of Volkswagen Rabbits at speeds comparable with those of earlier studies. Inside the cars were placed Hybrid II anthropometric dummies. Acceleration forces for both car and dummy were measured. Occupant braking was simulated with the parking brake.

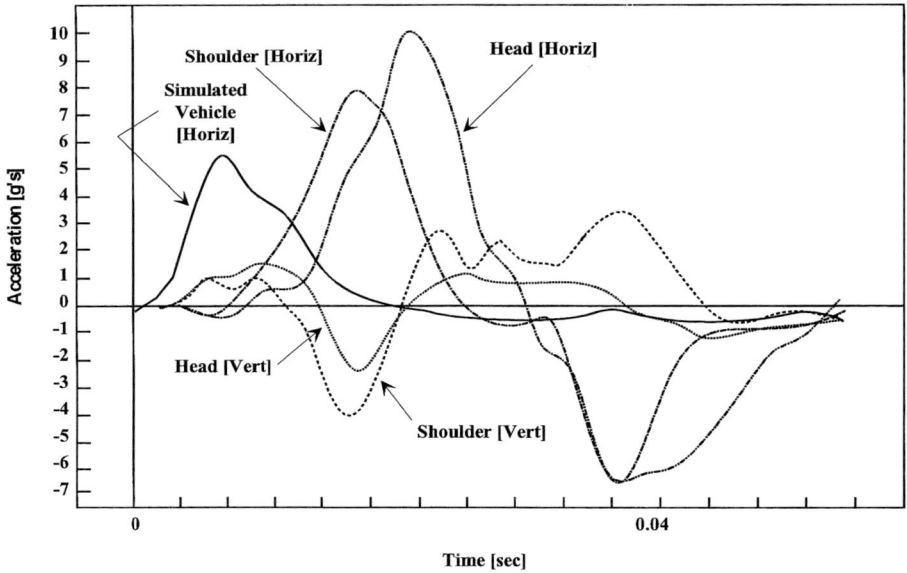

FIGURE 2.
Results of rear impact crash testing using late-model Volkswagen Rabbits and Hybrid II antromometric dummies. The parking brake was set to simulate driver braking. Compare the resulting deceleration curves to those of Figure 1. (Adapted from Thomson RW, Romilly DP, Navin FPD, et al: Energy attenuation within the vehicle during low speed collisions. Report to Transport Canada, Vancouver, University of British Columbia, August 1989.)

Like their predecessors (Severy et al.[4]), the UBC group found that the acceleration pulse of the shoulder began just after that of the vehicle and was followed in turn by that of the head. The same relationship between peak acceleration amplitudes was found (i.e., head greater than shoulder; shoulder greater than car). In contrast to earlier studies, however, the UBC group produced greater deceleration forces due to the contribution of braking.

Severy et al.[4] observed a slight flexion of the hips and knees of their human test subjects at the moment of impact that would suggest that the foot, resting on the brake pedal with only enough pressure applied to prevent forward movement of a car stopped in traffic, could easily be pulled away from the pedal at impact, thereby allowing the car to accelerate further. Indeed, it has been shown that the center of mass of the thigh is above the hip joint in a seated vehicle occupant. The inertia of the thigh, coupled with the corresponding moment, will result in hip flexion.[17] This phenomenon has been observed in experiments with cadavers.[18] Release of brake pressure would magnify the resulting acceleration of the occupant, quite possibly at the precise moment that it would have the most detrimental effect, and would also increase the likelihood of a second collision with a vehicle in front of the occupant's vehicle. Moreover, as the occupant decelerates and is thrust forward in the seat, the foot would most likely renew its contact with the brake pedal at a time that would closely correspond to the car's deceleration phase, thereby intensifying the deceleration phase and the final deceleration of the occupant as well. In other words, release of the brake pedal would intensify the extension injury, and reapplication of the brake would intensify the flexion component. It is perhaps noteworthy that the researchers who have simulated brake resistance have done so statically by setting the parking brake. Therefore, the effect of this hypothetical dynamic braking model has yet to be observed experimentally. However, it is conceivable that the measured decelerations of Severy et al.[4] and the measured accelerations and decelerations of Romilly et al.[11] underestimate the forces that might be experienced by real world motorists.

The UBC group used Hybrid II anthropometric dummies, which, although state of the art several years ago, have been subsequently improved in the newer Hybrid III dummies. Nevertheless, both types have been criticized on the grounds of less than perfect biofidelity. In particular, the motion and stiffness characteristics of the neck do not precisely simulate those of an unsuspecting or relaxed motorist. And although some authors[16] have demonstrated that the Hybrid neck can be detuned to better simulate the human neck under such conditions, the Navin et al.[10] group did not detune the necks of their dummies. Accordingly, we can anticipate that excursions of cervical range of motion, and perhaps also amplitudes of peak acceleration and deceleration, might have been underestimated in these experiments to some degree.

A significant crush of the vehicle indicates that the collision has a greater degree of plasticity, and some of the energy of the impact will consequently be absorbed by the deforming vehicle. The trend in the Thomson et al.[12] study was that of increasing head and shoulder acceleration in a relatively linear pattern with increasing impact speed. When the impact speed reached about 9 mph, these upward sloping lines flattened out. Not coincidentally, visible damage to the vehicle occurred at about 8.7 mph. In other words, the greatest increases in occupant acceleration occur before visible damage to the vehicle occurs, within the elastic range. This observation is consistent with the comments of the Severy et al.[4] group concerning plastic and elastic collisions. This finding of Thomson et al.[12] is illustrated in Figure 3.

The most recent contribution to our understanding of the dynamics of low-speed CAD trauma is provided by McConnell et al.,[19] who subjected four volunteers to full-scale crash testing at speeds ranging from less than 2 mph to speeds just under 5 mph. All volunteers were healthy male adults. The vehicles used in the testing included a late-model Dodge convertible, a Buick coupe, a Ford van, and a GMC pickup truck. The volunteers were exposed to multiple tests over several days. Three out of four subjects did complain of transient neck pain after these tests, but no long-term pain was reported. The authors recorded these collisions on high-speed videotape and also recorded the complex accelerations and decelerations occurring throughout the sequences of crashes. Using an exemplar test run of 4.87 mph, the following observations were described by the authors:

1. *Initial phase (≤ 100 msec)*. The vehicle moved forward beneath the test subject, compressing the seat back cushion. This caused an ini-

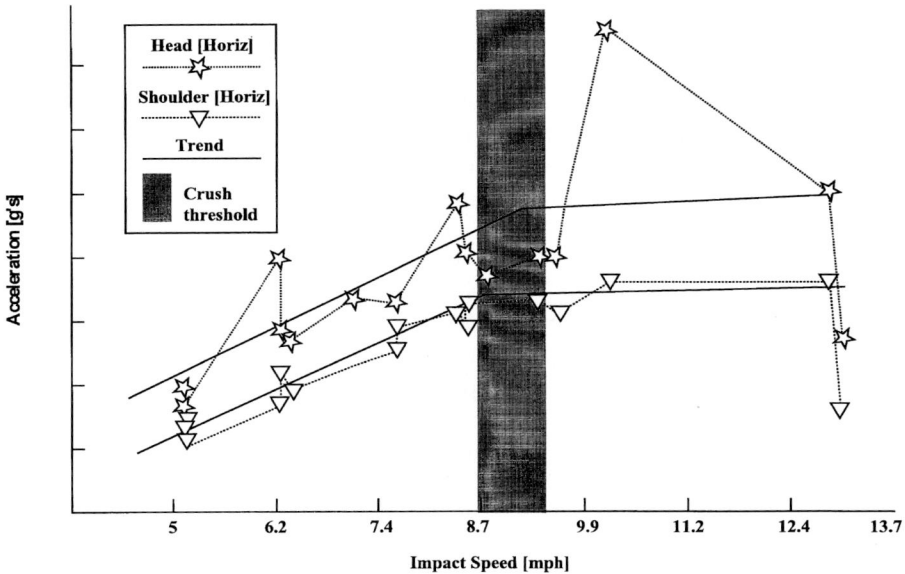

FIGURE 3.
Discrete measurements of head *(stars)* and shoulder *(inverted triangles)* accelerations are plotted for the corresponding impact speed, with trends described by solid lines. Upward sloping trends flatten out at the point vehicle crush occurs *(gray bar)* demonstrating how elastic collisions convey a greater transference of energy to vehicle occupants than plastic collisions. (Adapted from Thomson RW, Romilly DP, Navin FPD, et al: Energy attenuation within the vehicle during low speed collisions. Report to Transport Canada, Vancouver, University of British Columbia, August 1989.)

tial forward and vertical motion of the hips and low back. Simultaneously, the upper part of the seat back began to flex rearward under the load of the torso, which remained nearly stationary at this stage.

2. *Principal forward acceleration (100–200 msec).* At 100 msec the seat back had reached its maximal rearward excursion of about 10 degrees, and the test subject had started to move upward and forward. The neck appeared to be compressed axially at this point. The cervical spine appeared straightened and moved upward and rearward. At about that time the head began to rotate rearward (i.e., chin-up position). By 160 msec the vertical motion of the torso began to pull the neck forward into apparent tension as the head continued into extension. This event probably coincides with the release of elastic energy of the flexed seat back and was also observed by Severy et al.[4] and Severy and Mathewson[20] (see Fig 1). Significant shear forces are likely during this phase.

3. *Head overspeed/torso recovery (200–300 msec).* At 200 msec maximal extension of the head and neck had occurred (in this case to 45 degrees), and maximal vertical motion had also taken place (a total of 3.5 in.). At 250 msec the head had started its forward motion, and the trunk was descending back down the seat back. The seat back had returned to its original position. It was estimated that the torso was

being restrained at this point by the restraint system. The authors noted that the seat belt retractors spooled in the slack seat belt produced by the initial loading of the seat back. However, it is noteworthy that in other crash test research investigators[11] have found that seat belt retractors did not operate quickly enough to spool in slack created by the rearward movement of the occupant.

4. *Head deceleration/torso rest (300–400 msec).* By 300 msec the descent of the trunk was complete, and the torso was moving at the same velocity as the vehicle. Active deceleration of the neck was noted at about 400 msec. This was accomplished through voluntary action. The volunteer's head began to return to its original position.

5. *Restitution phase (400–600 msec).* At 450 msec all body parts were moving at the vehicle's velocity, and impact-related motions had been nearly completed. The authors further commented that the apparent upward motion of the test subjects was probably related to an initial straightening of the cervical, thoracic, and perhaps also lumbar curvatures. The sudden and "surprisingly vigorous" descent of the trunk was conjectured to be the result of a combination of a "rubberband" effect—a response to a stretched and straightened spine and trunk—and the restriction imposed by the lap belt. In light of other research into this phenomenon, we might also assume that some of this movement was caused by ramping.

The authors concluded that the 5-mph runs appeared to be at the threshold of a mild cervical strain injury for the repetitively exposed test subjects. None of the test subjects was exposed to a single run, so it is impossible to tell whether a single run could have resulted in cervical injury at this speed.

This latest installment on our knowledge base related to CAD trauma is most interesting, coming as it did at a time when misconceptions about low-speed rear impacts were rife within the medicolegal community. The authors have provided important additional information related to the kinematics of the whiplash phenomenon. There are, however, several limitations to the extrapolation of their data to real world crash victims, particularly as the data relate to the incidence and severity of injuries sustained in these tests. Most investigators have found that women are more frequently and more chronically affected by CAD trauma than men.[21-26] Because there were no women included in this study, no reasonable conclusions can be drawn regarding injury thresholds for women, although the authors did not make any distinction regarding gender in their statement concerning this threshold.

Severy et al.[4] and Severy and Mathewson[20] clearly demonstrated a profound difference in subject acceleration exposures between relaxed subjects and tensed subjects anticipating the impact. This variance is nearly impossible to control for, particularly in subjects exposed to multiple runs. It became apparent that the subjects of the McConnell et al.[19] test were actively decelerating their necks within less than 0.5 second after impact. And because one of the accelerometers was attached to a bite plate that required active contraction of the masticatory muscles (which are intimately associated with cervical spine muscular tone), it is unlikely that these test subjects were in a state of relaxation comparable to unsuspecting motorists. Moreover, CAD trauma affects the very young and the very old. Many victims have concomitant or preexisting conditions that predispose them to more significant injury. In contrast, all of the subjects of this experiment were men described as "robustly healthy."

As in the testing conducted by earlier investigators, no brakes were applied in these tests. Conceivably, with brakes applied and without anticipation of the impact, greater deceleration measurements and forward excursions of the head would have been observed, a difference that probably would have resulted in greater injury. These collision tests involved relatively like-sized vehicles. They do not account for collisions between vehicles with greatly disparate masses. Yet collisions between large pickup or utility trucks and small passenger cars, where the car is struck by the truck, are not uncommon on the roadway. In such cases the potential for injury is greatly increased.

Observation of the relatively severe degree of extension (45 degrees, close to the full extent of the range of extension for a man of this age) measured in a robust adult male volunteer who was, to one degree or another, anticipating the impact and visibly and actively decelerating, in a relatively low-speed collision (<5 mph), provides compelling evidence for the potential for significant soft tissue injury in these low-speed impacts. McConnell et al.[19] proposed mechanisms that might be responsible for these injuries. Their findings that symptoms were of a transient nature only should not be interpreted to imply that real world motorists are unlikely to suffer longer-term or even permanent injury from these types of collisions.

To summarize, the pioneering research and observations of Severy et al.[4] have been further validated by recent research by several research groups[10-16] using late-model cars, who employed Hybrid anthropometric dummies, and by McConnell et al.[19] who used adult male human volunteers. These latter studies have further enhanced our understanding of the mechanical and biomechanical phenomena of CAD trauma.

SEQUENCE OF EVENTS IN CAD INJURY

The whiplash phenomenon results in high rotational and translational accelerations of the victim's head that are much greater than those of the vehicle itself. Examination of the sequence of events after the rear impact collision facilitates a better understanding of the complex dynamics involved. The following paradigm is a synthesis of existing research[4, 5, 7-20] and can be easily described in four separate phases.

PHASE ONE

Initially, as the vehicle in front is struck from the rear by another vehicle, the two quickly attain a common velocity, as is typical for a nonelastic collision. The greater the impact speed, the greater the deformation of the vehicles and therefore the more plastic the collision. The torso, which is the first part of the victim's body to be affected by whiplash in a rear impact collision, moves backward into the seat back. The head and neck initially remain fixed while the vehicle moves forward underneath. Because of the abrupt upward movement of the torso during this phase and due to the straightening of the cervical, thoracic, and possibly lumbar spines, the cervical spine becomes compressed (Fig 4). At the end of this rearward translation, the head and neck begin to extend. At this time, the neck is subjected to very high tensile forces, which equates essentially to axial stretching. These are the same forces that Clemens and Burow[27] observed in experimental acceleration/deceleration whiplash simulations using cadavers.

PHASE TWO

It is during the second phase of the CAD injury (Fig 5) that the temporomandibular joint (TMS) can be injured.[28] The subject of TMJ injury is explored in some detail elsewhere.[29, 30] However, the link between CAD trauma and TMJ injury and its corresponding clinical condition, usually referred to as TMJ disorder or dysfunction (TMD), is well established,[31-35] although the precise mechanism of injury remains a subject

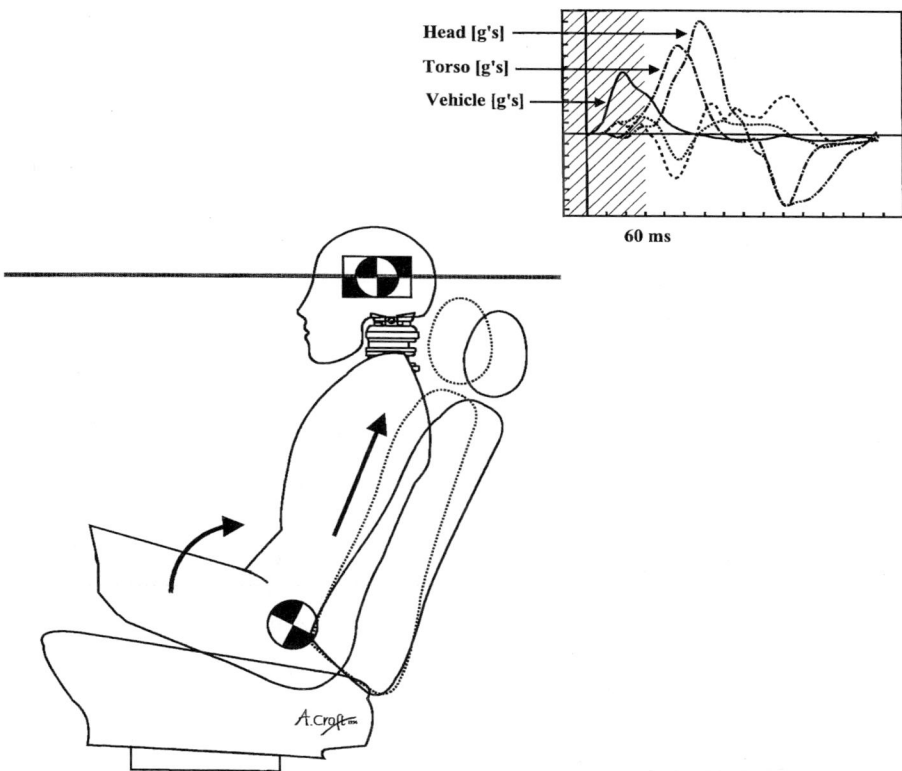

FIGURE 4.
Phase one of a typical rear impact collision. Inset graph at upper right corner is that of Figure 2. Cross-hatched region of the graph corresponds to the time that has elapsed by this phase. The seat back has been loaded and the occupant's cervical spine is straightened and compressed. (From Croft AC: Biomechanics, in Foreman SM, Croft AC [eds]: *The Cervical Acceleration/Deceleration Syndrome*, ed 2. Baltimore, Williams & Wilkins, 1995, p 67. Used by permission.)

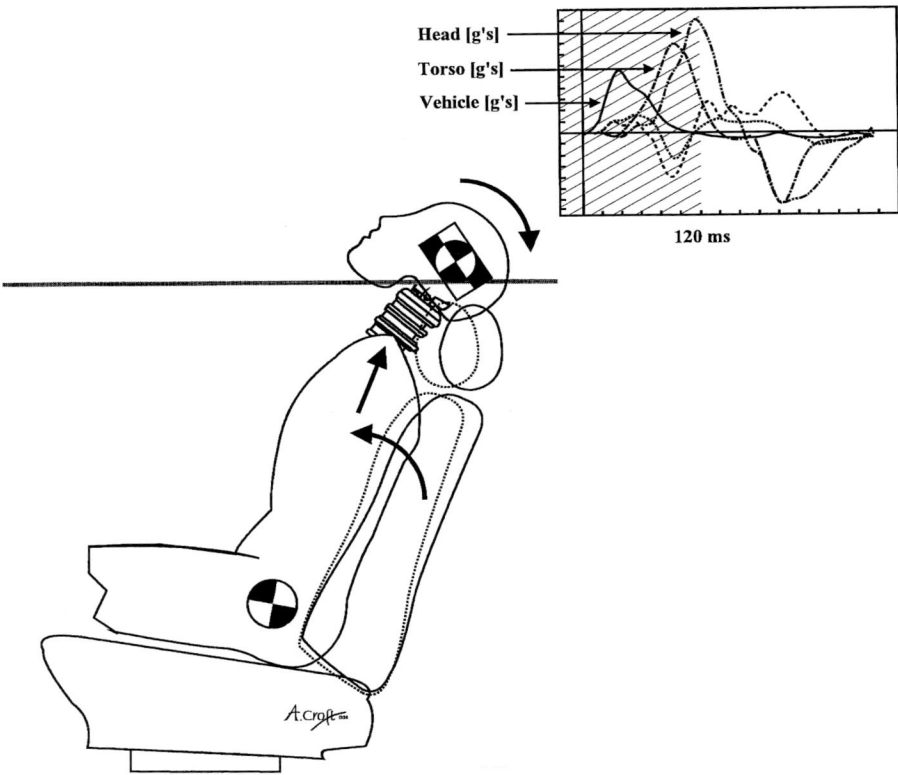

FIGURE 5.
Phase two of a typical rear impact collision. Inset graph at upper right corner is that of Figure 2. Cross-hatched region of the graph corresponds to the time that has elapsed by this phase. The vehicle, torso, and head are at peak acceleration, although the head continues to extend as the torso moves forward. Vertical motion of the torso continues. This ramping effect allows the head to rise above the head restraint. (From Croft AC: Biomechanics, in Foreman SM, Croft AC [eds]: *The Cervical Acceleration/Deceleration Syndrome*, ed 2. Baltimore, Williams & Wilkins, 1995, p 67. Used by permission.)

of some debate. The seat back, which has been loaded with elastic energy, will begin to return to its previous position at a time coinciding with the change of direction of the torso, so that as the torso begins its forward excursion, the seat back may add an additional impulse of acceleration. At the same time, however, the head is still moving in the opposite direction (i.e., into extension), and the vehicle remains at or near its peak acceleration. This divergence of motion imparts significant shear strain to the cervicothoracic and lower cervical spine.

Because the torso tends to rise up in the seat after rear impact, and because the torso moves rearward in the seat, some degree of slack is created in the lap belt and shoulder restraint system. As noted earlier in this chapter, the foot may be drawn away from the brake pedal, thereby allowing the vehicle to accelerate further. At the end of this phase both torso and vehicle will be at or near their peak acceleration while the head is just beginning its acceleration pulse.

PHASE THREE

During the third phase of the injury (Fig 6), both head and torso reach peak acceleration while the vehicle's acceleration pulse is tapering off. Any slack left in the restraint system will allow added forward movement of the pelvis, torso, and head and will enhance the potential for injury in phase four of the CAD phenomenon. It is during this third phase that the brake pedal pressure will probably be reapplied (if it was lost during phase two), and this will result in a more robust deceleration. In both cases this enhanced deceleration potential will result in greater flexion rotational forces in the neck and cervical spine.

PHASE FOUR

In the fourth and final phase of the injury (Fig 7), the vehicle is no longer accelerating and the head and torso are at full deceleration. The shoulder harness may abruptly restrain the torso, but the head will continue to decelerate unrestrained in a forward arc, carried by its own inertia. A very

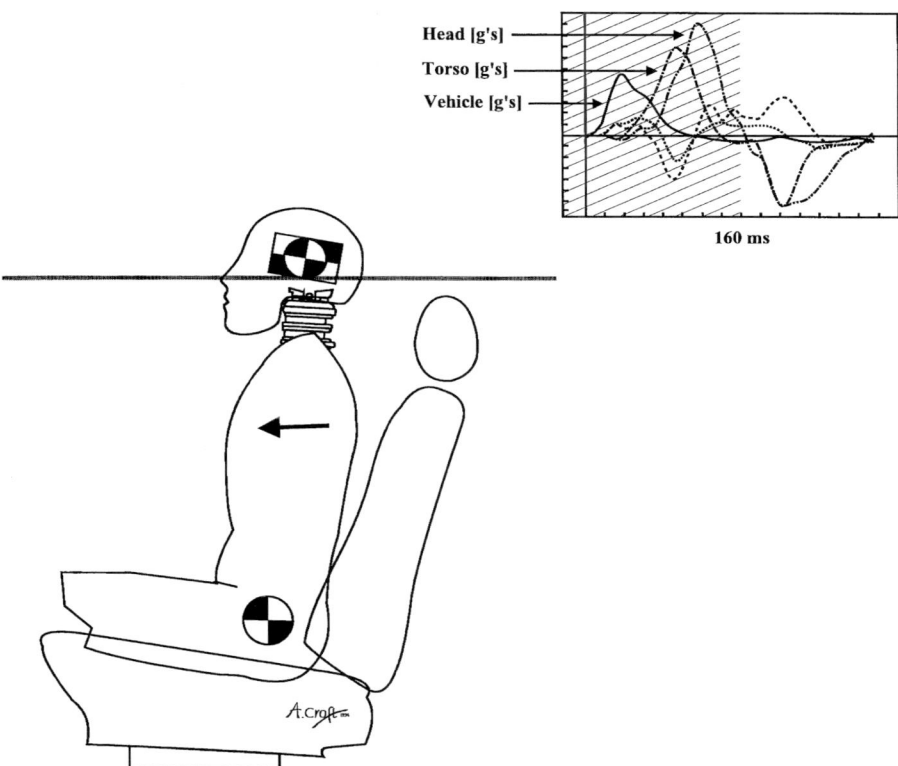

FIGURE 6.
Phase three of a typical rear impact collision. Inset graph at upper right corner is that of Figure 2. Cross-hatched region of the graph corresponds to the time that has elapsed by this phase. The vehicle's acceleration has tapered off while both head and torso are thrust forward, approaching maximum deceleration. (From Croft AC: Biomechanics, in Foreman SM, Croft AC [eds]: *The Cervical Acceleration/Deceleration Syndrome*, ed 2. Baltimore, Williams & Wilkins, 1995, p 68. Used by permission.)

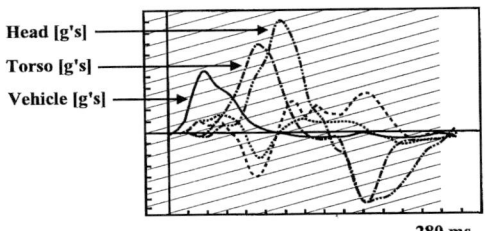

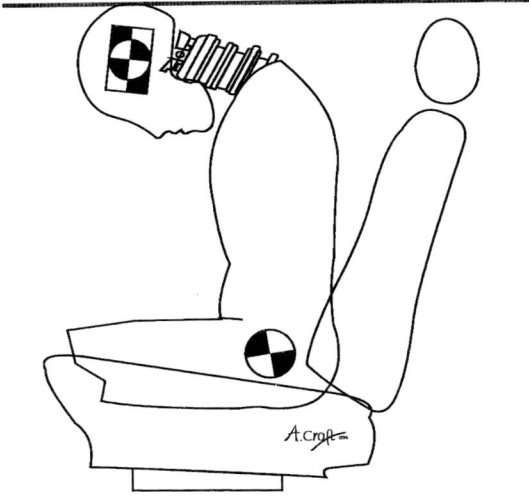

FIGURE 7.
Phase four of a typical rear impact collision. Inset graph at upper right corner is that of Figure 2. Cross-hatched region of the graph corresponds to the time that has elapsed by this phase. The head and torso decelerate abruptly. The shoulder harness will restrain the torso while the head's inertia carries it forward. (From Croft AC: Biomechanics, in Foreman SM, Croft AC [eds]: *The Cervical Acceleration/Deceleration Syndrome*, ed 2. Baltimore, Williams & Wilkins, 1995, p 68. Used by permission.)

acute and violent bending moment will occur at the lower cervical and cervicothoracic spine. This mechanism is probably responsible for the majority of cervical ligamentous and muscular soft tissue injury seen in CAD trauma.

The foregoing description is relatively consistent with the existing pool of literature on the subject. However, it is important to remember that a number of variables will affect the relative timing of these acceleration and deceleration curves, as well as their relative amplitudes. For example, Severy et al.[4] conducted full-scale crash testing with no brakes applied, as did McConnell et al.[19] The corresponding decelerations measured by Severy et al.[4] and the flexion motions of the head and neck observed by McConnell et al.[19] would no doubt have been more pronounced if brakes had been applied. In contrast, the research conducted at UBC,[11] where the parking brake was used to simulate braking, produced much greater deceleration pulses. Discussion of other important mechanical and human factors affecting the CAD phenomenon follows.

PHYSICAL FACTORS AFFECTING THE INJURY

In addition to factors already mentioned, such as the relative sizes of colliding vehicles, clinicians should consider the effect of second collisions. When cars are struck with sufficient force to propel them into other cars in front, the flexion phase of the injury is usually compounded. Such second collisions can also result when occupants strike parts of the car's interior, such as the steering wheel. Some safety devices, such as air bags and seat belt/shoulder harness pretensioners, are not activated in rear impact collisions. Others, such as seat belts and shoulder harnesses, are not universally effective in preventing injury, and still others, such as head restraints and bumper isolators, are only marginally effective, if at all. Facts such as these render many currently popular legal arguments fallacious.

HEAD RESTRAINTS

Studies have shown that fewer than 39% of us properly position our head restraints.[36, 37] Yet the effectiveness of the restraint is largely dependent on proper positioning.[38] At best, integral restraints have been shown to reduce injuries by 24.5%, whereas adjustable restraints reduce injury by only 14.8%.[24] Other reports have been consistent with these figures, suggesting an injury reduction of 11% to 24%.[39-41] As dismal as these figures are, one recent study[42] has suggested that head restraints do not appear to influence the incidence of neck injury at all, whereas Romilly et al.[11] observed that heads may actually rebound off the restraints, resulting in magnified acceleration. I have hypothesized that upper cervical flexion/compression injuries can result from head restraints that fail to support the neck (Fig 8).[43]

SEAT BELTS AND SHOULDER HARNESSES

Seat belt and shoulder harness use has decreased the number of fatalities and serious facial and chest trauma but have significantly increased the number of minor and sometimes disabling cervical, thoracic, and lumbar injuries, as well as numerous types of abdominal injuries.[24, 25, 44-67] Children are particularly prone to seat belt injury because neither the car seat nor the seat belt/shoulder harness was designed to fit them optimally. Numerous pediatric injuries related to restraint system use have been reported. Usually the most serious are spinal injuries.[55, 56, 68-77] A recent study by Wolf et al.[78] provides reassurance to pregnant women, however, that the use of seat belts does not place them or their fetuses at significantly greater risk in the event of an accident. In one of the largest studies of its kind (N = 13,000), Nygren[24] noted that minor neck injuries were three times more likely to occur in belted drivers than in unbelted drivers. Deans et al.[45] found that of the patients who had been wearing restraints, 34% continued to be symptomatic at 1 year, whereas of the patients who were not wearing restraints, only 20% remained symptomatic after 1 year. Galasko et al.[62] reported an increase in all forms of "neck sprain" after the introduction of seat belts. Yoganandan et al.[79] found that seat belts were effective in reducing the incidence of serious cervical spine injuries yet increased the incidence of minor (whiplash) injuries.

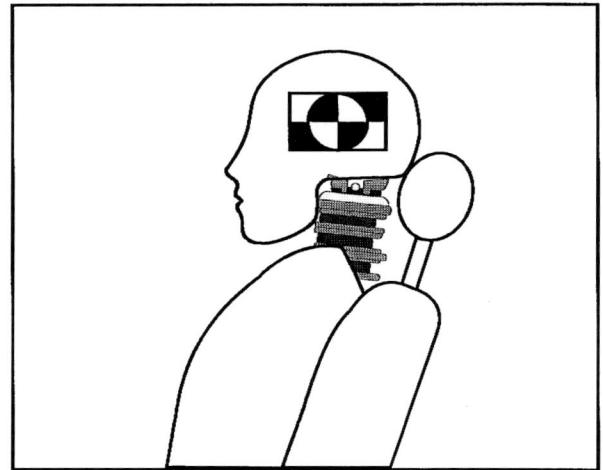

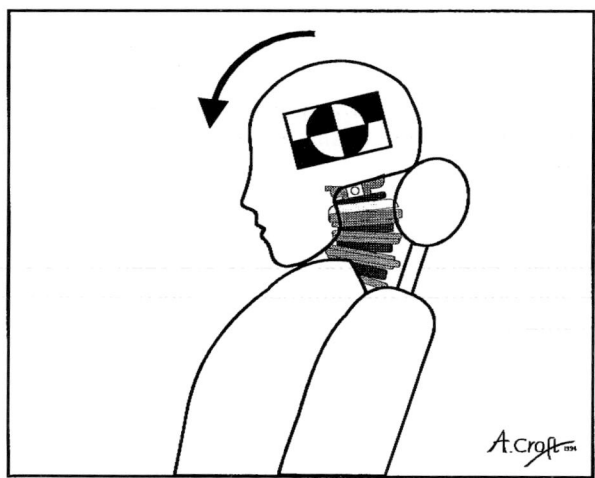

FIGURE 8.
When the head is in contact with the head restraint at the moment of rear impact, a significant flexion and compression of the neck may occur if the neck is not firmly supported. (From Croft AC: Biomechanics, in Foreman SM, Croft AC [eds]: *The Cervical Acceleration/Deceleration Syndrome*, ed 2. Baltimore, Williams & Wilkins, 1995, p 80. Used by permission.)

The primary reason that neck injuries are accentuated by restraint systems is that the shoulder harness abruptly restrains the decelerating trunk of the occupant while the head's inertia carries it forward unrestrained. This results in a tremendous bending moment at the cervicothoracic region and is one of the primary reasons why today the flexion injury is often more significant than the extension injury. Another reason is because the head restraint usually limits extension of the neck. Slack between the torso and the shoulder harness will accentuate this deceleration impact phenomenon. In rear impacts, where occupants load the seat back with their own inertia and cause the seat back to deflect several degrees, the problem may be compounded because it has been observed that standard seat belt retractors cannot spool the slack fast enough in rear impact accidents.[11] Some newer cars are equipped with seat belt pretensioners, which, like air bags, detect crash-level decelerations and cinch down the restraint systems before loading, thereby effectively reducing the seat belt loads by as much as 10%.[80] In their crash testing research at collision speeds less than 5 mph, McConnell et al.[19] reported that belt retractors were able to spool in slack webbing before the occupant deceleration phase.

SHOCK-ATTENUATING BUMPER SYSTEMS

Current basic bumper systems typically include a fascia and bumper beam and some type of impact absorber. Materials used in the construction of the fascia include aluminum, steel, and RIM urethane or other thermoplastics. Bumper beams may be constructed of aluminum, steel, or fiber-reinforced thermoplastics and thermosets. Isolators (gas- and fluid-filled units resembling standard shock absorbers), polyurethane and polystyrene foam cores, deformable steel struts, rubber shear blocks, and leaf springs are examples of common impact absorbers.[14] Research has shown that bumper isolators, designed to prevent vehicle damage from collisions with barriers or other vehicles, can set the threshold of visible vehicular damage at 8 to 9 mph in some modern cars.[11] Yet below this threshold, the occupant can be exposed to significant acceleration pulses through transference of impact energy. Similar effects are seen in cars equipped with polystyrene and polyurethane bumpers.[14] These physical factors are summarized in Table 2.

TABLE 2.
Physical Factors Affecting the Injury

Factor	Effect*
Head restraint	+/−
Seat belt system	+
Shock attenuating bumper	Negligible
Second collision	+
Larger striking vehicle	+
Smaller striking vehicle	−
Off center collision	+
Release of brake at impact	+

* + = exacerbates injury; − = mitigates injury.

HUMAN FACTORS AFFECTING THE INJURY

AGE

With increasing age, the elasticity of tissues decreases. Range of motion in the cervical spine also decreases.[81, 82] In both cases, the potential for injury is increased because the neck is less resilient. In addition, the strength of the neck musculature diminishes with age. Over the adult life span, cervical range of motion is reduced by an average of nearly 40% (Fig 9), cervical muscle reflexes slow by 23%, and voluntary strength capability diminishes by 25%.[83] The largest age group of CAD patients is the 20- to 40-year group, which coincides, of course, with the largest group of licensed drivers. Young children are less frequently injured because they are more resistant to injury and because their heads usually are protected by the relatively high seat back. In fact, children up to 10 years of age are said to be at one-sixth the risk of neck injury from motor vehicle accidents of adults.[25]

PREPAREDNESS

For reasons outlined earlier there will usually be a larger number of and more serious injuries in surprise rear collisions (i.e., those in which an occupant is unaware of the impending crash) than in those rear collisions in which the occupant is braced for the impending crash. It has been suggested that in a surprise rear collision, neuromuscular reflexes might come into play and perhaps help to mitigate some of the injury.[4, 38] However, Foust et al.[83] have shown that the average reflex time for muscles of the cervical spine is slightly more than 60 msec. Full activation of muscles requires about another 60 msec. If the head does not reach full extension until about 200 msec, it is possible that activation of muscles could attenuate some of the damaging acceleration forces. In older persons, however, even at low-speed impacts, this is unlikely. In moderate- to high-speed impacts, even in young people, this attenuation is also unlikely.[83, 84] It is quite possible, in fact, that activation of a stretch reflex in the anterior cervical musculature may be manifest at the time the head and neck are reaching maximum flexion. In such a scenario the response might compound the injury rather than mitigate it.

GENDER

Gender plays a pronounced part in the outcome of this injury, in that women seem to be injured more seriously or suffer more prolonged symptoms or disability than men.[21, 24-26, 86] Other physiological variances that may have a negative effect on acceleration/deceleration injury outcome include congenital anomalies of the spine, previous surgeries of the spine, osteoporosis, osteoarthritis, rheumatic disorders, metabolic disorders affecting bone, primary or metastatic neoplasia, infection of bone, and previous CAD or other significant cervical spine or neck injury.

STATURE

Stature is also an important consideration. Ommaya et al.[25] found that persons less than 152 cm tall have a 40% lower risk of neck injury than

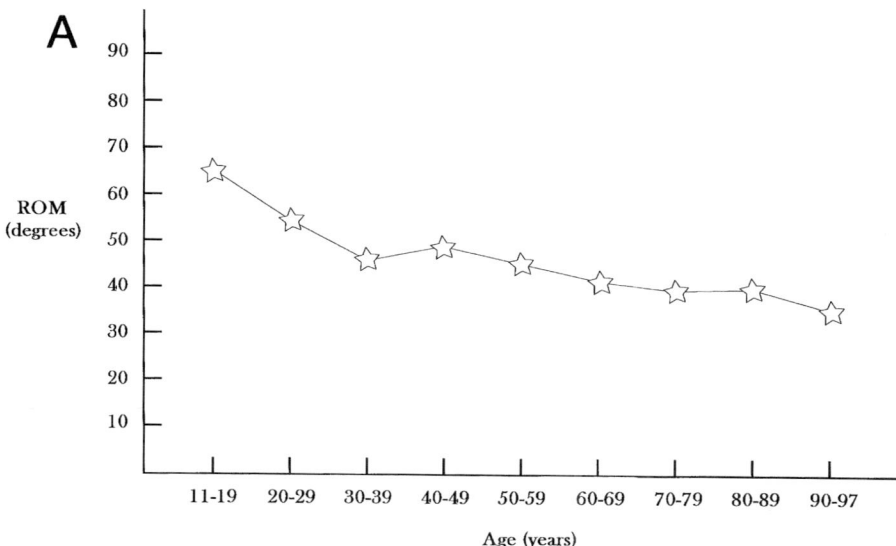

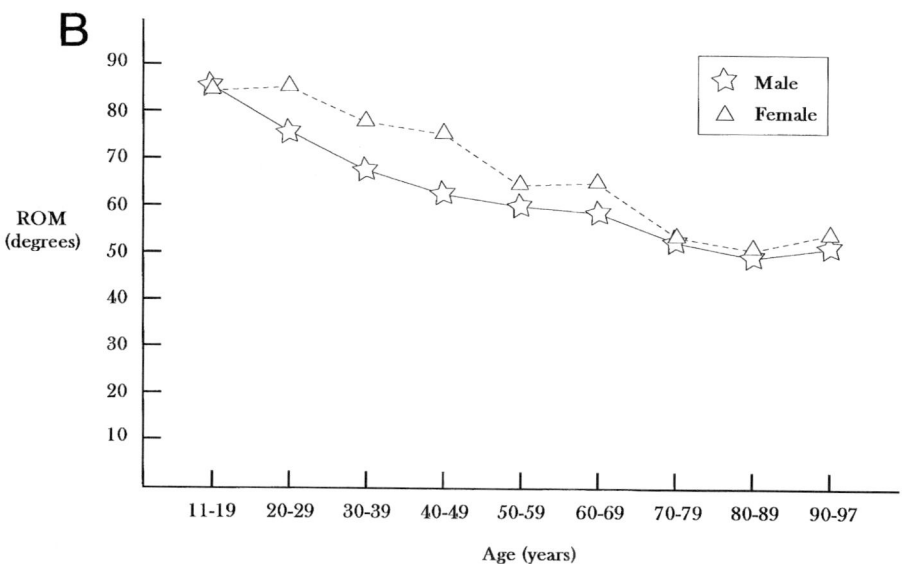

FIGURE 9.
A, mean range of motion *(ROM)* for the cervical spine in flexion. No gender effect was found. **B,** mean ROM for the cervical spine in extension. *(Continued.)*

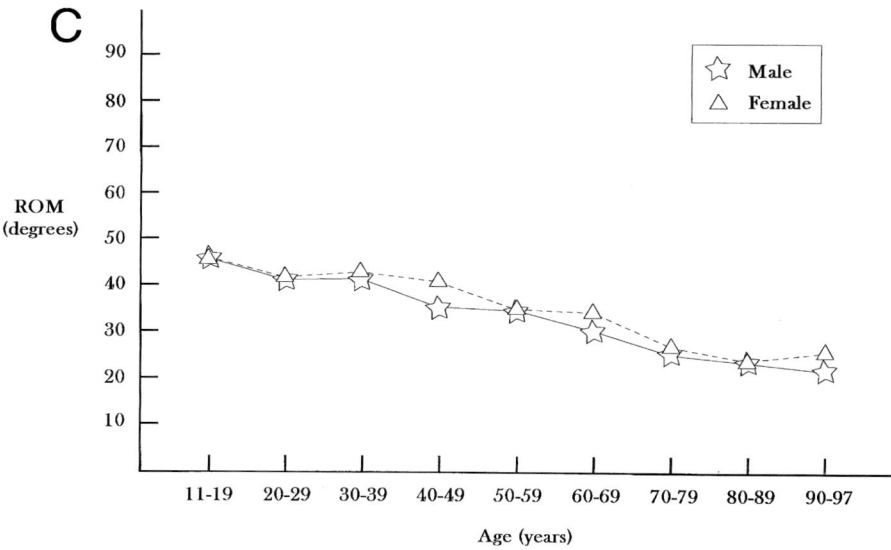

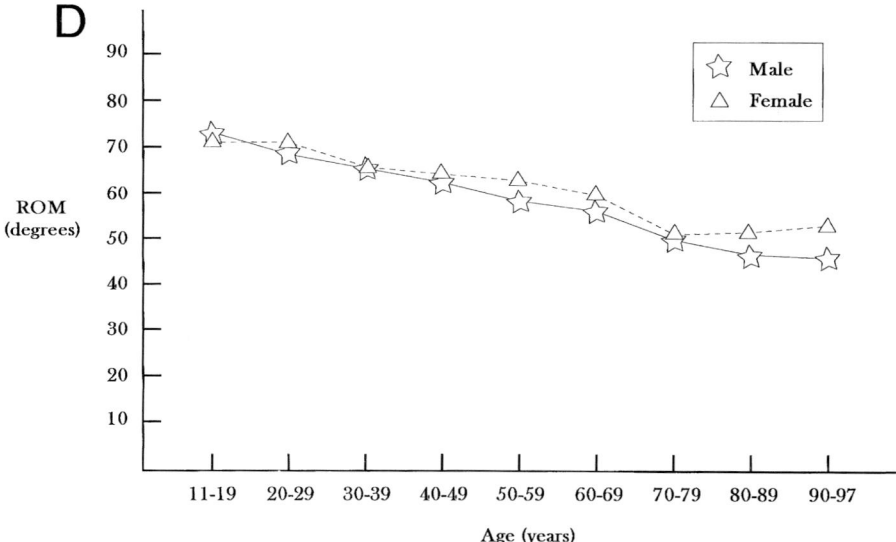

FIGURE 9 (cont.).
C, mean ROM for the cervical spine in left lateral flexion. (Right lateral flexion is similar.) **D,** mean ROM for the cervical spine in left rotation. (Right rotation is similar.) (Adapted from data of Youdas JW, Garrett, TR, Suman VJ, et al: *Phys Ther* 72:770–780, 1992.)

taller persons. Presumably this effect can be attributed to greater protection of the neck from the head restraint. However, shorter persons are at greater risk of vascular injury in the neck from their shoulder harnesses.[47] Because car seats are usually designed for 50th percentile males (178 cm) one might presume that drivers taller than this are at greater risk, especially because a longer neck allows a greater bending moment and is less protected by ill-adjusted head restraints.

OCCUPANT POSITION

It has been demonstrated in cadaver sled tests that out-of-position occupants are subjected to significantly greater forces during collisions. When occupants are rotated in their seats, leaning forward, or slumped, the resulting acceleration and deceleration forces may be magnified greatly.[86, 87] Slack restraint systems allow for greater ramping effects because the pelvis is poorly anchored and because greater excursions within the seat are possible. With greater degrees of ramping, occupants' heads will rise above even adequately positioned head restraints. Moreover, the human spine and supporting structures are more vulnerable to oblique forces than to anterior/posterior forces.[88] These factors are summarized in Table 3.

SOFT TISSUE INJURIES

With the ever-increasing number of automobiles on the road, whiplash injuries have become more and more prevalent in our society. With an increase in this type of injury, of course, has come an increase in the number of personal injury liability suits. Those on the defense side in these suits generally have held that the plaintiff was fabricating or exaggerating his or her symptoms to attain a larger settlement, suggesting that once the case was over, the symptoms would miraculously clear up. This myth, sometimes referred to as "litigation neurosis" or "accident neurosis," has been largely disabused[89] as a chimera, although some authors continue to exhort us to harbor some doubt in all litigated cases.[90, 91] Livingston[92] describes a delay in the emergence of whiplash in Great Britain and attributes this to a form of "social copying," indicating that the condition was more a learned behavior than a physical disorder.

EXPERIMENTAL STUDIES

To many observers, however, it soon became clear that the constellation of symptoms complained of by these patients was relatively typical, con-

TABLE 3.
Human Factors Affecting the Injury

Factor	Effect*†
Increasing age	+
Surprise collision	+
Male gender	−
Female gender	+
Tall stature	+
Short stature	−
Preexisting disease	+
Out-of-position occupant	+

*See text.
†+ = exacerbates injury; − = mitigates injury.

sistent, and somewhat predictable. Such would not likely have been the case had these people truly been malingering. Investigators began to experiment with anthropometric dummies, laboratory animals, cadavers, and human volunteers. The findings were sometimes surprising. Macnab[2] secured anesthetized animals to a chair mounted on vertical rails. The animals were dropped from heights ranging from 0.6 to 12 m. At the end of the rail the chair would stop abruptly, thereby jerking the animal's head backward, simulating an acceleration injury. Depending on the height of the drop, and hence the magnitude of hyperextension injury produced, various types and severities of lesions resulted. These ranged from minor tears in the sternocleidomastoid muscle to tears of the longus colli muscle. This latter injury was usually associated with a retropharyngeal hematoma and occasionally with damage to the cervical sympathetic nervous system. Also noted were hemorrhages in the muscular coats of the esophagus. In some cases, the anterior longitudinal ligament was torn and the disk avulsed from the vertebra. These lesions were not detectable with standard radiographic procedures but have been clearly seen on magnetic resonance imaging.[93]

Extensive animal research has also been carried out by Wickstrom et al.,[94] Wickstrom,[95] Martinez et al.,[96] Unterharnscheidt et al.,[97] Katayama,[98] Ommaya and Hirsch,[99] Ommaya and Gennarelli,[100]

TABLE 4.
Postconcussion Syndrome

Lightheadedness
Vertigo/dizziness
Neck pain
Headache
Photophobia
Phonophobia
Tinnitus
Impaired memory
Easy distractibility
Impaired comprehension
Forgetfulness
Impaired logical thought
Difficulty with new or abstract concepts
Insomnia
Irritability
Easy fatigability
Apathy
Outbursts of anger
Mood swings
Depression
Loss of libido
Personality change
Intolerance to alcohol

TABLE 5.
Cervical Acceleration/Deceleration Syndrome

1. Neck pain and stiffness
2. Shoulder pain
3. Upper back pain
4. Suboccipital (or frontal) headache
5. Diffuse pain in upper extremities
6. Mild non-dermatomal sensory abnormalities in the upper and lower extremities
7. Scapular and interscapular pain
8. Development of trigger points in neck/upper back
9. Lower back pain

Gennarelli et al.,[101] Thibault et al.,[102] Margulies et al.,[103] and Liu et al.[104, 105] The range of experimental lesions produced in these CAD simulations correlates well with those seen clinically. The literature is also replete with clinical reports of similar conditions seen in humans, including single and multiple cranial nerve palsies,[106, 107] carpal tunnel syndrome,[108] perilymphatic labyrinthine fistula (with its accompanying clinical manifestation of benign paroxysmal positional vertigo,[109] cervical vertigo,[109] thoracic outlet syndrome (TOS),[110–114] oculomotor dysfunction,[115, 116] posttraumatic stress disorder,[117–119] cervical ligamentous and disk disruption,[44, 93, 98, 108, 120–133] ulnar neuropathy,[108] spinal cord injury,[93, 134, 135] retropharyngeal hematoma,[136] damage to the subarachnoid space,[134, 137] mediastinitis,[110] TMJ disorder,[31–35, 44, 108, 111, 138–145] hypopharyngeal, tracheal, or esophageal perforation,[108, 146–149] brain injury,[108, 114, 134, 150–161] hypothalamic-pituitary-thyroid axis disorder,[162] damage to the posterior cervical sympathetic nerves,[121, 163–166] and low back disorders.[21, 167–169]

Under the rubric of CADS, a number of related conditions may reside, sometimes lending an almost inscrutable nature to the injury. These allied conditions include the postconcussion syndrome (Table 4), myofascial pain disorders (MPDs), TMD, and TOS. Most of the symptoms associated with CADS, including those that are delayed in onset, can be easily explained on a physiological basis.[170] The more common constellations of these symptoms are listed in Table 5. Although space does not permit a lengthy dissertation of these topics, the following is a brief discussion of the more common symptoms of CADS.

NECK PAIN

Tearing of any soft tissue (including nerve), fracture of bone, or disk disruption may be responsible for neck pain. Immediate pain indicates more severe injury.[26, 93]

NECK STIFFNESS

Protective muscle spasm secondary to most injuries of the neck will result in stiffness. Chronic stiffness may indicate myofascial fibrosis or contraction, ligamentous contraction (particularly of joint capsules), disk degeneration, or secondary osteoarthritic change.

SHOULDER PAIN

Pain may result from direct injury to the shoulder, such as from a shoulder harness or impact with car's interior, or from referred pain from the neck or disk lesion. Other causes of shoulder pain, such as impingement syndromes and rotator cuff inflammation, may develop secondary to CAD trauma, either as a result of muscular disuse or paresis of muscles or muscle groups. Imbalance between agonist and antagonist muscles can precipitate shoulder disorders or convert subclinical conditions to clinical conditions.

HEADACHES

Headaches arise from injury to the upper cervical spine or from reflex or protected muscle spasm in the neck. Trauma can also play an important role in converting postural faults into clinical headaches.[171] Headaches also may be a clinical manifestation of TMD or may result from direct brain injury (i.e., posttraumatic headaches).

INTERSCAPULAR PAIN

This upper back pain results from either direct injury to paraspinal muscles or referred (scleratogenous) pain from the neck. It also may be seen with disk lesions. In the chronic stage, one of the most common causes of this type of pain is MPD.

BACK PAIN

Foreman and Croft[167] found low back pain in 57% of their CAD cases (71% in broadside collisions). Braaf and Rosner[168] found LBP in 42% of their cases. Hohl[21] found low back pain in 35% of his cases. In their recent follow-up of 35 patients, followed for an average of 10.8 years, Watkinson et al.[172] found that initially 24% of the group complained of low back pain. Of these, 5% resolved later. However, at follow-up, 34% complained of low back pain.

The exact mechanism of low back injury, although not entirely clear, is probably multifactorial. Factors affecting the incidence, nature, and severity of low back injury in automobile accidents include the following:

1. Position of the occupant in the vehicle
2. The use or nonuse of seat belts and shoulder harnesses
3. Deployment of an air bag system
4. Type of restraint system (i.e., conventional restraints vs. restraints with pretensioners)
5. Stiffness of the seat back
6. Inclination of the seat back
7. Properties of the seat back padding
8. Degree of ramping
9. Vector and severity of the collision
10. Second collisions inside or outside the occupant's vehicle
11. Snugness of the restraint system

12. Positioning of the restraint system on the occupant
13. Positioning of the restraint system anchors within the vehicle
14. Physical makeup of the occupant, including stature, build, age and level of fitness
15. Preparedness for the collision

Frontal impacts are the most frequent type of accident and are also responsible for the most severe injuries. However, when the magnitude of the accident is controlled for (i.e., the actual amount of force involved), injuries are much more frequent in rear impact collisions. As mentioned earlier, one of the prime reasons for this is that drivers who hit other cars are typically aware of the impending collision in time to brace for the impact. Steering wheels, brake pedals, and floorboards, in combination with the ride-down of vehicle crush, provide adequate additional support to prevent many injuries.

In side impacts, the occupants of most production car seats are offered little protection to lateral acceleration forces by either the seat back or restraint system. This probably explains why Dr. Foreman and I found such a high incidence of low back pain in this type of collision. The initial response to impact is lateral flexion toward the striking vehicle, with compression of spinal structures on the concave side and stretching of myofascial and other structures on the convex side. The lap belt will serve as an anchor for the pelvis, thus preventing serious injury, but may intensify bending moments in the lumbosacral or thoracolumbar spine, thus increasing the likelihood of soft tissue injury. Intervertebral disk injuries, as well as ligamentous and muscular injuries, are common.

Broadside collisions should be analyzed carefully. Forces incurred by striking and struck vehicles are rarely fully perpendicular. For example, if a broadside collision occurs between two cars in an intersection and both are traveling at similar speeds, the actual resulting vectors of deceleration for the occupants will be oblique: In the case of the car that is struck on the driver's side, the occupant will decelerate in a vector that is forward and toward the striking car; in the case of the striking car, the occupant will decelerate forward and toward the direction the other car came from. Such oblique collisions are particularly difficult to describe both kinetically and kinematically. However, it is clear from studies conducted by Viano[87] that oblique rear impact collisions hold much greater potential for injury than the pure rear impact variety.

Occupants wearing only a lap belt are more vulnerable to lumbar injury than those wearing a three-point system due to the tendency to rebound forward immediately after loading the seat back in the acceleration phase of a rear impact collision. Shoulder straps will mitigate some of the inertia of the decelerating trunk. Research has demonstrated the potential to ramp up the seat back after rear impact collision. This tendency is even greater in out-of-position occupants.[86] The initial effect of ramping will be abrupt violent axial stretch of the lumbar spine, especially if the pelvis is firmly anchored by the lap belt. Many occupants slouch or lean forward in their car seats. In this case, the first area of the body to be accelerated by the seat back will be the pelvis, resulting in a bending movement that will effectively flex the lumbosacral spine until the thorax comes into full contact with the seat back. As the seat back is loaded with elastic energy from the inertia of the occupant, it extends backward in proportion to these forces—a movement that can exceed 30 degrees. At this time significant slack can develop in the restraint belts. Then, as the head and torso accelerate in the forward direction, carried along by a combination of their own inertia and the released elastic energy from the seat back, this slack is encountered suddenly, resulting in acute peaks in deceleration forces and subjecting the lumbar spine to its second flexion injury, this time in combination with the shear force provided by the restraining lap belt. In this case the inertia of the pelvis and lower extremities are unrestrained and carry the lower half of the body against the belt. If the occupant is fully braced against the brake or floorboards, this effect will be significantly minimized. I refer to this mechanism as the "double-flexion" injury.

It is well to consider the physics of this deceleration to get a true appreciation of the forces at work. Even in an 8.5-mph collision, the torso can decelerate at up to 6 g.[173] For an 80-kg man, this would be roughly the equivalent of simultaneously loading all weight-bearing areas (lap and shoulder belts, hands on the steering wheel, buttocks on the seat pan, feet against the floorboards) with a force of ½ ton within a span of only about 50 msec. In an unprepared driver, this loading will be concentrated over the restraint belts.

PARESTHESIAE

Altered sensations commonly occur because of a temporary TOS created in large part by swelling and spasm of cervical musculature. Paresthesiae are also known to occur as part of the scleratogenous referred pain phenomenon, a mode of sensory aberration that should be familiar to clinicians who treat musculoskeletal disorders.[174–180] Other explanations include cord injury, disk protrusion, cervical root contusion or stretch injury, injury to the brachial plexus or peripheral nerves, and abnormal sympathetic activity.

EXTREMITY PAIN AND WEAKNESS

All of the previously mentioned may apply. Braaf and Rosner[168] found sciatica in 15% of their cases. MPD and TOS also can result in extremity weakness.

DIZZINESS AND LIGHTHEADEDNESS

Injection of saline solution into the sternocleidomastoidens (SCM) can produce dizziness.[121] Accordingly, any muscular injury here may also have this effect. More likely is the explanation of vascular compromise secondary to injury to the sympathetic nervous system in the neck. A clear link has been established between dysautonomia and dizziness and vertigo.[181, 182] The influence of the sympathetic nervous system on the vestibular apparatus may be mediated by cochlear blood flow.[183, 184] One of the prominent symptoms associated with Chiari's malformation is dizziness.[185, 186] Dizziness and vertigo may also be the result of slowed blood flow through the vertebrobasilar system.[187] In some cases it may result from inner ear damage such as a perilymphatic labyrinthine fistula[188–190] or labyrinthine concussion, or it may be seen in mild traumatic brain injury. It can also be a manifestation of TMD. Migraine headaches are often accompanied by dizziness as well.[191] Vascular compromise, although less likely, also may result from compression of vertebral arteries secondary to muscle spasm or even disk herniation.[192]

AUDITORY DISTURBANCES

Tinnitus is seen in the Barré-Liéou syndrome and may also be seen (along with a sense of fullness in the ear) with TMD.[193, 194] In one unusual report, a woman described the sound of paper crumpling in her ear. Examination revealed a herniation of the TMJ contents into the external ear canal.[195] Phonophobia is a common complaint after minor head injury, and hearing loss is often experienced after inner ear injury.

VERTIGO

Vertigo is an extreme sensation and should not be confused with simple dizziness. It usually indicates a labyrinthine pathological condition, vascular insufficiency, or brain stem disorder. Acute onset of vertigo, nausea, and vomiting, without tinnitus or hearing loss, may be the result of vestibular neuronitis rather than physical injury.[196-198] It should also be pointed out that vertigo immediately after cervical spine manipulation may be a harbinger of brain stem injury.[199, 200]

SHORT DURATION VERTIGO

Vertigo lasting only 5 to 10 seconds may result from "cupolithiasis," an injury to the otolithic membrane resulting in detachment of otoconia, which then settle into the ampulla of the posterior semicircular canal. With changes of head position, these otoconia may cause displacement of the cupola, causing, in turn, benign paroxysmal positional vertigo.[201, 202]

OCULAR DYSFUNCTION

Pupillary dilatation is usually the result of injury to the sympathetic nervous system. (Note: Interruption of sympathetic fibers results in miosis of the pupil, e.g., Horner's syndrome. Irritation of these fibers may have the opposite effect.) Nystagmus often indicates a disturbance of the vestibular apparatus, and photophobia is common in mild head trauma. Hildingsson et al.[115] had proposed disturbance of the proprioceptive system of the cervicocranial region as an explanation for visual tracking (smooth pursuit) abnormalities. Radanov et al.[203] have described the "cervicoencephalic syndrome," a condition arising out of soft tissue injuries to the neck. Most of their cases were the result of CAD injury. Patients complained of headache, fatigue, dizziness, poor concentration, disturbed visual accommodation, and impaired adaptation to light intensity.

DYSPHAGIA AND HOARSENESS

Difficulty swallowing usually indicates swelling or spasm of the longus colli muscle. In some cases it may be caused by retropharyngeal or retrotracheal hematoma or esophageal perforation and should prompt further investigation.[148, 204] In extreme cases, dysphagia may be caused by large anterior osteophytes.[205] Hoarseness has also been reported in direct injuries to cranial nerves (and brain stem lesions) or injuries to the larynx or recurrent laryngeal nerve.

FACIAL PAIN

Facial pain is usually the result of TMD or related MPD. Associated symptoms include clicking, popping, and crepitus at the joint, along with palpable pain of masticatory muscles, pain on chewing, limited mouth opening (closed lock), and biomechanical deviations of the normal dynamics of that joint.

HYPOTHYROIDISM

Wickstrom et al.[94] reported hemorrhage or inflammation in the thyroid glands of 50% of the animals they subjected to acceleration/deceleration testing. However, there have been no subsequent reports in the literature of thyroid injury or dysfunction in humans as a result of CAD trauma. We have, however, noticed a trend for patients injured in this way to subsequently develop hypothyroid conditions. Most recently our research has yielded interesting new findings and correlations in this regard.[162] In particular, it seems there may be some justification for the diagnosis of "posttraumatic hypothyroidism."

CONCLUSION

Understanding the mechanics of CAD trauma is prerequisite to understanding the protean and sometimes bewildering array of soft tissue lesions resulting from it. This trauma is entirely unique and is therefore not comparable with other forms, such as low back strains from lifting. That it is otherwise perceived stands as a tribute to those who have not resisted the temptation to bestow on us their incongruous logic constructed of tenuous extrapolations and theories based on intuition rather than fact. From such works at the hairy edge of science spring the prosaic instructions to clinicians that CAD patients should be treated for 6 to 10 weeks and no more regardless of the patient's condition. These precepts, besides lacking validity, cast the hippocratic oath into the wind because most of us swore an oath to respect the patient's welfare as the supreme law.

Such are the issues facing bioethicists today who will help to shape the future of the health delivery system in the United States. In the meantime, the degree of solicitude offered to these patients by clinicians should be guided by traditional paradigms that concern themselves more with clinical results and patients' needs than actuarial tables and statistics.

REFERENCES

1. Macnab I: Acceleration injuries of the cervical spine. *J Bone Joint Surg* 46A:1797–1799, 1964.
2. Macnab I: Acceleration extension injuries of the cervical spine, in Rothman RH, Simeone FA (eds): *The Spine*, ed 2. Philadelphia, WB Saunders, 1982, p 650.

3. Croft AC: Management of soft tissue injuries, in Foreman SM, Croft AC (eds): *The Cervical Acceleration/Deceleration Syndrome*, ed 2. Baltimore, Williams & Wilkins, 1995.
4. Severy DM, Mathewson JH, Bechtol CO: Controlled automobile rear-end collisions, an investigation of related engineering and mechanical phenomenon. *Can Services Med J* 11:727–758, 1955.
5. States JD, Balcerak JD, Williams JS, et al: Injury frequency and head restraint effectiveness in rear end impact accidents, in *Proceedings of the 16th Stapp Car Crash Conference*. Detroit, Society of Automotive Engineers, 1972, pp 228–257.
6. Croft AC: Biomechanics, in Foreman SM, Croft AC (eds): *The Cervical Acceleration/Deceleration Syndrome*, ed 2. Baltimore, Williams & Wilkins, 1995, pp 1–92.
7. Evans L, Frick MC: Car mass and fatal risk—has the relationship changed? *Am J Public Health,* in press.
8. Evans L, Frick MC: Mass ratio and relative driver fatality risk in two-vehicle crashes. *Accid Anal Prev* 25:213–224, 1993.
9. Evans L, Frick MC: Car size or car mass: Which has greater influence on fatality risk? *Am J Public Health* 82:1105–1112, 1992.
10. Navin FPD, Romilly DP: An investigation into vehicle and occupant response subjected to low-speed rear impacts. Proceedings of the Multidisciplinary Road Safety Conference VI. Fredericton, New Brunswick, June 5–7, 1989.
11. Romilly DP, Thomson RW, Navin FPD, et al: Low speed rear impacts and the elastic properties of automobiles. Proceedings: 12th International Conference of Experimental Safety Vehicles. Gothenburg, May–June 1989.
12. Thomson RW, Romilly DP, Navin FPD, et al: Energy attenuation within the vehicle during low speed collisions. Report to Transport Canada, Vancouver, University of British Columbia. August 1989.
13. Thomson RW, Romilly DP, Navin FPD, et al: Dynamic requirements of automobile seat backs. *SAE Technical Paper Series 930349*, Detroit, March 1993, pp 193–198.
14. Bailey MN, King DJ, Romilly DP, et al: Characterization of automobile bumper components for low speed impacts. Proceedings Canadian Multidisciplinary Road Safety Conference VII. Vancouver, British Columbia, June 1991, pp 190–203.
15. Thomson RW, Romilly DP: Simulation of bumpers during low speed impacts. Proceedings: Canadian Multidisciplinary Road Safety Conference VIII. Saskatoon, Saskatchewan, June 1993, pp 237–247.
16. Emori RI, Horiguchi J: Whiplash in low speed vehicle collisions. *SAE Paper 900542*, Detroit, 1990, pp 103–108.
17. James MB, Strother CE, Warner CY, et al: Occupant protection in rear end collisions: I. Safety priorities and seat belt effectivenesses, SAE 912913, in *Proceedings of the 35th Stapp Car Crash Conference*. Detroit, Society of Automotive Engineers, 1991, pp 369–378.
18. Hu AA, Bean SP, Zimmerman RM: Response of belted dummy and cadaver to rear impact. SAE 770929. *Proceedings of the Twenty-First Stapp Car Crash Conference*, Detroit, Society of Automobile Engineers, 1977, pp 587–635.
19. McConnell WH, Howard RP, Guzman HM, et al: Analysis of human test subject kinematic responses to low velocity rear end impacts. *SAE Technical Paper Series 9308889*. Detroit, Society of Automotive Engineers, 1993, pp 21–31.
20. Severy DM, Mathewson JH: Automobile barrier and rear-end collision per-

formance. Presented at the Society of Automotive Engineers summer meeting, Atlantic City, NJ, June 8–13, 1958.
21. Hohl M: Soft tissue injuries of the neck in automobile accidents: Factors influencing prognosis. *J Bone Joint Surg* 56A:1675–1682, 1974.
22. Pearce JMS: Whiplash injury: A reappraisal. *J Neurol Neurosurg Psychiatr* 52:1329–1331, 1989.
23. Balla JI: The late whiplash syndrome. *Aust NZ J Surg* 50:610–614, 1980.
24. Nygren A: Injuries to car occupants—some aspects of interior safety of cars. *Acta Otolaryngol* 1(suppl 394), 1984.
25. Ommaya A, Backaitis S, Fan W, et al: Automotive neck injuries. Ninth International Technical Conference on Experimental Safety Vehicles, US Department of Transportation, National Highway Traffic Safety Administration. Kyoto, Japan, Nov 1–4, 1982, pp 274–278.
26. Parmar HV, Raymakers R: Neck injuries from rear impact road traffic accidents: Prognosis in persons seeking compensation. *Injury* 24:75–78, 1993.
27. Clemens HJ, Burow K: Experimental investigation on injury mechanisms of cervical spine at frontal and rear-front vehicle impacts. SAE 720960. *Proceedings of the Sixteenth Stapp Car Crash Conference*. Detroit, Society of Automotive Engineers, 1972, pp 76–104.
28. Croft AC: The cervical acceleration/deceleration syndrome, in Steigerwald DP, Croft AC (eds): *Whiplash and Temporomandibular Joint Dysfunction: An Interdisciplinary Approach to Case Management*. Encinitas, Keiser, Calif, 1992, pp 35–39.
29. Curl D: Whiplash and temporomandibular joint injury: Principles of detection and management, in Foreman SM, Croft AC (eds): *The Cervical Acceleration/Deceleration Syndrome*, ed 2. Baltimore, Williams & Wilkins, 1995.
30. Steigerwald DP, Croft AC: *Whiplash and Temporomandibular Disorders: An Interdisciplinary Approach to Case Management*. Encinitas, Keiser, Calif, 1992.
31. Steigerwald D: Acceleration-deceleration injury as a precipitating cause of temporomandibular joint dysfunction. *Am Chiropractic Assoc J Chiropr* 26(11):61–64, 1989.
32. Weinberg S, Lapoint H: Cervical extension-flexion injury (whiplash) and internal derangement of the temporomandibular joint. *J Oral Maxillofac Surg* 45:653–656, 1987.
33. Roydhouse RH: Whiplash and temporomandibular dysfunction. *Lancet* 1:1394–1395, 1973.
34. Lader E: Cervical trauma as a factor in the development of TMJ dysfunction and facial pain. *Craniomandibular Pract* 1:85, 1983.
35. Schneider K, Zernicke RF, Clark G: Modeling of jaw-head-neck dynamics during whiplash. *J Dent Res* 68:1360-1365, 1989.
36. Kahane CJ: An evaluation of head restraints: Federal motor vehicle safety standard 202. Natl Highway Traffic Safety Administration Tech Report DOT HS-806-108, February 1982.
37. Lubin S, Sehmer J: Safety—are automobile head restraints used effectively? Survey of parked and moving cars in Vancouver. *Can Fam Phys* 39:1584–1588, 1993.
38. Mertz HJ Jr, Patrick LM: Investigation of the kinematics and kinetics of whiplash, SAE 670919, in Proceedings, 11th Stapp Car Crash Conference. Detroit Society of Automotive Engineers, 1967.
39. Hohl M: Soft tissue injuries to the neck. *Clin Orthop* 109:42, 1975.
40. Thomas C, Faverjou G, Hartemann F, et al: Protection against rear-end accidents. Proceedings of the 7th International IRCOBI Conference on Biomechanics of Impacts. Brou, France, 1982.
41. Larder DR, Twiss MK, Mackay GM: Neck injury to car occupants using seat

belts. 29th Annual Proceedings of the American Association of Automotive Medicine, 1985.
42. Bradbury A, Robertson C: Prospective audit of the pattern, severity and circumstances of injuries sustained by vehicle occupants as a result of road traffic accidents. *Arch Emerg Med* 10:15–23, 1993.
43. Croft AC: Biomechanics. In Foreman SM, Croft AC (eds): *The Cervical Acceleration/Deceleration Syndrome*, ed 2. Baltimore, Williams & Wilkins, 1995, p 80.
44. Dunn EJ, Blazar S: Soft-tissue injuries of the lower cervical spine. Instructional course lectures, American Academy Orthopaedic Surgeons, 1987, vol 36, pp 499–512.
45. Deans GT, Magalliard JN, Kerr M, et al: Neck sprain—a major cause of disability following car accidents. *Injury* 18:10–12, 1987.
46. Allen MJ, Barnes MR, Bodivala GG: The effect of seatbelt legislation on injuries sustained by car occupants. *Injury* 16:471, 1985.
47. Hayes CW, Conway WF, Walsh JW, et al: Seat belt injuries: Radiological and clinical correlation. *Radiographics* 11:23–36, 1991.
48. Rutledge R, Thomason M, Oller D, et al: The spectrum of abdominal injuries associated with the use of seat belts. *J Trauma* 31:820–826, 1991.
49. Conry BG, Hall CM: Cervical spine fractures and rear seat car restraints. *Arch Dis Child* 62:1267–1268, 1987.
50. Reddy K, Furer M, West M, et al: Carotid artery dissection secondary to seatbelt trauma: Case report. *J Trauma* 30:630–633, 1990.
51. Gogler H, Athanasiadis S: Fatal cervical dislocation related to wearing a seatbelt: A case report. *Injury* 10:196–200, 1979.
52. Huelke D, Kaufer H: Vertebral column injuries and seatbelts. *J Trauma* 15:304–318, 1975.
53. Sumchai A, Eliastam M, Werner P: Seatbelt cervical injury in an intersection type vehicular accident. *J Trauma* 28:1384–1388, 1988.
54. Hart RG, Easton JD: Dissections of cervical and cerebral arteries. *Neurol Clin* 1:155–182, 1983.
55. Johnson DL, Falci S: The diagnosis and treatment of pediatric lumbar spine injuries caused by rear seat lap belts. *Neurosurgery* 26:434–440, 1990.
56. Reid AB, Letts RM, Black GB: Pediatric chance fractures: Association with intra-abdominal injuries and seatbelt use. *J Trauma* 30:384–391, 1990.
57. Holt BW: Spines and seatbelts: Mechanisms of spinal injury in motor vehicle crashes. *Med J Aust* 2:411–413, 1976.
58. Hudson I, Kavanagh TG: Duodenal transection and vertebral injury occurring in combination in a patient wearing a seatbelt. *Injury* 15:6–9, 1983.
59. Asbun HJ, Irani H, Roe EJ, et al: Intra-abdominal seatbelt injury. *J Trauma* 30:189–193, 1990.
60. Taylor TKF, Nade S, Bannister JH: Seat belt fractures of the cervical spine. *J Bone Joint Surg* 58B:328–331, 1976.
61. Jeffry RS, Cook PL: Seatbelts and reclining seats. *Injury* 22:416–417, 1991.
62. Galasko CSB, Murray PM, Pitcher M, et al: Neck sprains after road traffic accidents: A modern epidemic. *Injury* 24:155–157, 1993.
63. Mackay M: Mechanisms of injury and biomechanics—a vehicle design and crash performance. *World J Surg* 163:420–427, 1992.
64. Williams N, Ratcliff DA: Gastrointestinal disruption and vertebral fracture associated with the use of seat belts. *Ann R Coll Surg Engl* 75:129–132, 1993.
65. Triantafyllou SJ, Gertzbein SD: Flexion distraction injuries of the thoracolumbar spine—a review. *Orthopedics* 15:357–364, 1992.
66. Howdieshell TR, Delaurier G: An unusual injury of the sigmoid colon produced by seatbelt trauma. *Am Surg* 59:355–358, 1993.

67. Roh LS, Fazzalaro W: Transection of the trachea due to improper application of automatic seatbelt (submarine effect). *J Forensic Sci* 38:972–977, 1993.
68. Williams N, Rose GK, Goodman AM: Lap-style seat belt associated with high cervical cord injury in a child. *Injury* 24:209–210, 1993.
69. Hoy GA, Cole WG: The pediatric cervical seat belt syndrome. *Int J Care Injured* 24:297–299, 1993.
70. Brennan FJ, Goff WB: Seat belt injury to a pelvic kidney as demonstrated by CT. *J Comp Assist Tomogr* 17:664–665, 1993.
71. Taiwo B, Sloan J: Hand injury in a child—a rare adverse effect of rear seat belt use. *Arch Emerg Med* 8:147–149, 1991.
72. Ruta D, Beattie T, Narayan V: A prospective study of non-fatal childhood road traffic accidents: what can seat restraint achieve? *J Public Health Med* 15:88–92, 1993.
73. Statter MB, Coran AG: Appendiceal transection in a child associated with a lap belt restraint: case report. *J Trauma* 33:765–766, 1992.
74. Glassman SD, Johnson JR, Holt RT: Seat belt injuries in children. *J Trauma* 33:882–886, 1992.
75. Osberg JS, Di Scala C: Morbidity among pediatric motor vehicle crash victims: The effectiveness of seat belts. *Am J Pub Health* 82:422–425, 1992.
76. Rumball K, Jarvis J: Seat belt injuries of the spine in young children. *J Bone Joint Surg* 74B:571–574, 1992.
77. Ebraheim NA, Savolaine ER, Southworth SR, et al: Pediatric lumbar seat belt injuries. *Orthopedics* 14:1010–1013, 1991.
78. Wolf ME, Alexander BH, Rivara FP, et al: A retrospective cohort study of seat belt use and pregnancy outcome after a motor vehicle crash. *J Trauma* 34:116–119, 1993.
79. Yoganadan N, Haffner M, Maiman DJ, et al: Epidemiology and injury biomechanics of motor vehicle related trauma to the human spine, SAE 892438, in Proceedings of the 33rd Stapp Car Crash Conference. Detroit, Society of Automotive Engineers, 1989, pp 223–242.
80. Mitzkus JE, Eyrainer H: Three-point belt improvements for increasing occupant protection. *SAE Tech Paper* 141:245, 1984.
81. Ferlic D: The range of motion of the "normal" cervical spine. *Johns Hopkins Hosp Bull* 110:59–65, 1962.
82. Youdas JW, Garrett TR, Suman VJ, et al: Normal range of motion of the cervical spine: An initial goniometric study. *Phys Ther* 72:770–780, 1992.
83. Foust DR, Chaffin DB, Snyder RF, et al: Cervical range of motion and dynamic response and strength of cervical muscles, SAE 730975, in *Proceedings, 17th Stapp Car Crash Conference*. Detroit Society of Automotive Engineers, 1973.
84. Soechtling JF, Paslay PR: A model for the human spine during impact including muscular influence. *J Biomech* 6:195–203, 1973.
85. Schutt CH, Dohan FC: Neck injury to women in auto accidents. *JAMA* 206:2689–2692, 1968.
86. Warner CY, Strother CE, James MB, et al: Occupant protection in rear end collisions: II. The role of seat back deformation in injury reduction, SAE 912914, in *Proceedings of the 35th Stapp Car Crash Conference*, Detroit, Society of Automotive Engineers, 1991, pp 379–389.
87. Viano DC: Restraint of a belted or unbelted occupant by the seat in rear end impacts, SAE 922522, in *Proceedings of the 36th Stapp Car Crash Conference*, Detroit, Society of Automotive Engineers, 1992, pp 165–177.
88. Dvorak J, Panjabi MM: Functional anatomy of the alar ligaments. *Spine* 12:186–189, 1987.

89. Croft AC: The case against litigation neurosis in mild brain injuries and cervical acceleration/deceleration trauma. *J Neuromusculoskeletal System* 1:149–155, 1993.
90. Tarola GA: Whiplash: General considerations in assessment, treatment, management and prognosis (part I). *Am Chiropractic Assoc J Chiropr* 30:63–70, 1993.
91. Tarola GA: Whiplash: general considerations in assessment, treatment, management and prognosis (part II). *Am Chiropractic Assoc J Chiropr* 30:47–67, 1993.
92. Livingston M: Whiplash injury: Misconceptions and remedies. *Aust Fam Phys* 21:1642–1643, 1992.
93. Davis SJ, Teresi LM, Bradley WG Jr, et al: Cervical spine hyperextension injuries. MR findings. *Radiology* 180:245–251, 1991.
94. Wickstrom J, Martinez J, Rodriguez R: Cervical strain syndrome: Experimental acceleration injuries of the head and neck, in *Proceedings Prevention of Highway Injury*. Ann Arbor, Mich, Highway Safety Research Institute, University of Michigan, 1967, pp 182–187.
95. Wickstrom J: Effects of whiplash injury. *JAMA* 194:40, 1965.
96. Martinez JL, Wickstrom JK, Barcelo BT: The whiplash injury—a study of head-neck action and injuries in animals. ASME paper 65-WA/HVF-6. New York, American Society of Mechanical Engineers, 1965.
97. Unterharnscheidt F: Pathological and neuropathological findings in rhesus monkeys subjected to −Gx and +Gx indirect impact acceleration, in Sances A, Thomas DJ, Ewing CL, et al (eds): *Mechanisms of Head and Spine Trauma*. Goshen, NY, Aloray, 1986, pp 565–663.
98. Katayama K: Histopathological study of the whiplash injury. *J Jpn Orthop Assoc* 44:439–453, 1970.
99. Ommaya AK, Hirsch AE: Tolerances for cerebral concussion from head impact and whiplash in primates. *J Biomech* 4:13–21, 1971.
100. Ommaya AK, Gennarelli TA: Cerebral concussion and traumatic unconsciousness. *Brain* 97:633–654, 1974.
101. Gennarelli TA, Thibault LE, Tomei G, et al: Directional dependence of axonal brain injury due to centroidal and noncentroidal acceleration, SAE 872197 in *Proceedings of the Thirty-First Stapp Car Crash Conference*. Detroit, Society of Automotive Engineers, 1987, pp 49–53.
102. Thibault LE, Margulies SS, Gennarelli TA: The temporal and spacial deformation response of a brain model in inertial loading, SAE 87, in *Proceedings of the 31st Stapp Car Crash Conference*. Detroit, Society of Automotive Engineers, 1987, pp 267–272.
103. Margulies SS, Thibault LE, Gennarelli TA: Physical model simulations of brain injury in the primate. *Biomechanics* 23:823–836, 1990.
104. Liu YK, Wickstrom JK, Saltzberg B, et al: Subcortical EEG changes in rhesus monkeys following experimental whiplash: *26th ACEMB* 1973, p 404.
105. Liu YK, Chandran KB, Heath RG, et al: Subcortical EEG changes in rhesus monkeys following experimental hyperextension-hyperflexion (whiplash). *Spine* 9:329–338, 1984.
106. Rosa L, Carol M, Bellegarrigne R, et al: Multiple cranial nerve palsies due to a hyperextension injury to the cervical spine. *J Neurosurg* 61:172–173, 1984.
107. Dukes IK, Bannerjee SK: Hypoglossal nerve palsy following hyperextension neck injury. *Br J Accid Surg* 24:133–134, 1993.
108. Evans RW: Some observations on whiplash injuries. *Neurol Clin* 10:975–997, 1992.
109. Chester JB Jr: Whiplash, postural control, and the inner ear. *Spine* 16:716–720, 1991.

110. Rotstein OD, Rhame FS, Molina E, et al: Mediastinitis after whiplash injury. *Can J Surg* 29:54–56, 1986.
111. Razi DM, Wassel HD: Traffic accident induced thoracic outlet syndrome: Decompression without rib resection, correction of associated recurrent thoracic aneurysm. *Int Surg* 78:25–27, 1993.
112. Leffert RD: Thoracic outlet syndromes. *Hand Clin* 8:285–297, 1992.
113. Sanders RJ, Pearce WH: The treatment of thoracic outlet syndrome: A comparison of different operations. *J Vasc Surg* 10:626–634, 1989.
114. Pennie B, Agambar L: Patterns of injury and recovery in whiplash. *Injury* 22:57–59, 1991.
115. Hildingsson C, Wenngren B-I, Bring G, et al: Oculomotor problems after cervical spine injury. *Acta Orthop Scand* 60:513–516, 1989.
116. Burke JP, Orton HP, West J, et al: Whiplash and its effects on the visual system. *Graefes Arch Clin Exp Ophthalmol* 230:335–339, 1992.
117. Jones RW, Peterson LW: Posttraumatic stress disorder in a child following automobile accident. *J Fam Pract* 36:223–225, 1993.
118. Green MM, McFarlane AC, Hunter CE, et al: Undiagnosed posttraumatic stress disorder following motor vehicle accidents. *Med J Aust* 159:529, 1993.
119. Mayou R, Bryant B, Duthie R: Psychiatric consequences of road traffic accidents. *BMJ* 307:647–651, 1993.
120. Goldberg AC, Rothfus WE, Deeb ZL, et al: Hyperextension injuries of the cervical spine. *Skeletal Radiol* 18:283–288, 1989.
121. Macnab I: The "whiplash syndrome." *Orth Clin North Am* 2:389–403, 1971.
122. Lewis LM, Docherty M, Ruoff BE, et al: Flexion-extension views in the evaluation of cervical-spine injuries. *Ann Emerg Med* 20:117–121, 1991.
123. Webb JK, Broughton RBK, McSweeney T, et al: Hidden flexion injury of the cervical spine. *J Bone Joint Surg* 58B:322–327, 1976.
124. Herkowitz HN, Rothman RH: Subacute instability of the cervical spine. *Spine* 9:348–357, 1984.
125. Clark WM, Gehweiler JA, Laib R: Twelve significant signs of cervical spine trauma. *Skeletal Radiol* 3:201–205, 1979.
126. Cintron E, Gigula LA, Murphy WA, et al: The widened disc space: A sign of cervical hyperextension injury. *Radiology* 141:639–644, 1981.
127. Gehweiler JA, Clark WM, Schaaf RE, et al: Cervical spine trauma: The common combined conditions. *Radiology* 130:77–86, 1979.
128. Paakkala T: Prevertebral soft tissue changes in cervical spine injury. *CRC Crit Rev Diagn Imag* 24:201–236, 1985.
129. Harris WH, Hamblen DL, Ojemann RG: Traumatic disruption of cervical intervertebral disk from hyperextension injury. *Clin Orthop* 60:163–167, 1968.
130. Gotten N: Survey of one hundred cases of whiplash injury after settlement of litigation. *JAMA* 162:865–867, 1956.
131. Green JD, Harle TS, Harris JH Jr: Anterior subluxation of the cervical spine: Hyperflexion sprain *AJNR* 2:243–250, 1981.
132. Evans DK: Anterior cervical subluxation. *J Bone Joint Surg* 58B:318–321, 1976.
133. Saternus KS: Zur mechanik des schleuder-traumas der halswirbelsäule. *Uebersichitsreferat Z Rechtsmed* 88:1–11, 1982.
134. Hadley MN, Sonntag VKH, Rekate HL, et al: Infant whiplash-shake injury syndrome: A clinical and pathological study. *Neurosurgery* 24:536–540, 1989.
135. Marar BC: Hyperextension injuries of the cervical spine. *J Bone Joint Surg* 56A:1655–1662, 1974.
136. Myssiorek D, Shalmi C: Traumatic retropharyngeal hematoma. *Arch Otolaryngol Head Neck Surg* 115:1130–1132, 1989.

137. Ellertsson AB, Sigurjóusson K, Thorsteinsson T: Clinical and radiographic study of 100 cases of whiplash injury. *Acth Neurol Scand* 67(suppl):269, 1978.
138. Frankel VH: Temporomandibular pain syndrome following deceleration injury to the cervical spine. *Bull Hosp Joint Dis* 26:47, 1969.
139. Heise AP, Laskin DM, Gervin AS: Incidence of temporomandibular joint symptoms following whiplash injury. *J Oral Maxillofac Surg* 50:825–828, 1992.
140. Romanelli GG, Mock D, Tenenbaum HC: Characteristics and response to treatment of posttraumatic temporomandibular disorder: A retrospective study. *Clin J Pain* 8:6–17, 1992.
141. Moses AJ: Legal perspectives on TMJ/whiplash. *J Craniomandibular Pract* 11:237–240, 1993.
142. Braun BL, DiGiovanna A, Schiffman E, et al: A cross-sectional study of temporomandibular joint dysfunction in post-cervical trauma patients. *J Craniomandibular Dis Fac Oral Pain* 6:24–30, 1992.
143. Gibilisco JA: Dental perspective on face pain. *Postgrad Med* 76:121–132, 1984.
144. Harness DM, Donlon WC, Eversole LR: Comparison of clinical characteristics in myogenic, TMJ internal derangement and atypical facial pain patients. *Clin J Pain* 6:4–17, 1990.
145. Bogduk N: The anatomy and pathophysiology of whiplash. *Clin Biomech* 1:92–101, 1986.
146. Pollock RA, Apple DF, Purvis JM, et al: Esophageal and hypopharyngeal injuries in patients with cervical spine trauma. *Ann Otol Rhinol Laryngol* 90:323–327, 1981.
147. Stringer WL, Kelly DL, Johnson FR, et al: Hyperextension injury of the cervical spine with oesophageal perforation. *J Neurosurg* 53:541–543, 1980.
148. Reddin A, Mirvis SE, Diaconis JN: Rupture of the cervical esophagus and trachea associated with cervical spine fracture. *J Trauma* 27:564–566, 1987.
149. Hulse M: The functional voice disorder after an injury to the cervical spine. *Laryngorhinootologie* 70:599–603, 1991.
150. Gibbs FA: Objective evidence of brain disorder in cases of whiplash injury. *Clin Electroencephalogr* 2:107–110, 1971.
151. Torres F, Shapiro SK: Electroencephalograms in whiplash injury. *Arch Neurol* 5:28–35, 1961.
152. Goldstein J: Posttraumatic headache and the postconcussion syndrome. *Med Clin North Am* 75:641–651, 1991.
153. Pennie B, Agambar L: Patterns of injury and recovery in whiplash. *Injury Br J Accid Surg* 22:57–59, 1991.
154. Aubrey JB, Dobbs AR, Rule BQ: Layperson's knowledge about the sequelae of minor head injury and whiplash. *J Neurol Neurosurg Psychiatry* 52:842–846, 1989.
155. Payne-Johnson JC: Evaluation of communication competence in patients with closed head injury. *J Commun Disord* 19:237–249, 1986.
156. Fischer RP, Carlson J, Perry JF: Postconcussive hospital observation of alert patients in a primary trauma center. *J Trauma* 21:920–924, 1981.
157. Taylor AR: Post-concussional sequelae. *BMJ* 3:67–71, 1967.
158. Guthkelch AN: Posttraumatic amnesia, post-concussional symptoms and accident neurosis. *Eur Neurol* 19:91–102, 1980.
159. Kraus JG, Nourjah P: The epidemiology of mild, uncomplicated brain injury. *J Trauma* 28:12, 1988.
160. Elkind AH: Headache and head trauma. *Clin J Pain* 5:77–87, 1989.
161. Hildingsson C, Wenngren B-I, Toolanen G: Eye motility after soft tissue injury of the cervical spine. *Acta Orthop Scand* 64:129–132, 1993.

162. Sehnert KW, Croft AC: Basal metabolic temperature vs. laboratory assessment in "posttraumatic hypothyroidism." Accepted for publication. *J Manip Physiol Ther*, 1995.
163. Gay JR, Abbott KG: Common whiplash injuries of the neck. *JAMA* 152:1698, 1953.
164. Tamura T: Cranial symptoms after cervical injury. *J Bone Joint Surg* 71B:283–287, 1989.
165. Barré M: Sur un syndrome sympathetique cervical pastericur et sa cause fréquent: l'arthrite cervicale. *Reu Neurol Strasbourg* 33:1246–1248, 1926.
166. Golding DN: Whiplash injuries. *Br J Rheum* 32:174, 1992.
167. Foreman SM, Croft AC: Whiplash Injuries, in *The Cervical Acceleration/Deceleration Syndrome*. Baltimore, Williams & Wilkins, 1988, p 293.
168. Braaf MM, Rosner S: Symptomatology and treatment of injuries of the neck. *NY State J Med* 55:237–242, 1955.
169. Dies S, Strapp JW: Chiropractic treatment of patients in motor vehicle accidents: A statistical analysis. *J Can Chiropra Assoc* 36:139–145, 1992.
170. Croft AC: Whiplash: The Masters' Program, *Module 1: Whiplash, an Overview*, ed 2. Coronado, Calif, Spine Research Institute of San Diego, 1994.
171. Watson DH, Trott PH: Cervical headache—an investigation of natural head posture and upper cervical flexor muscle performance. *Cephalalgia* 13:272–284, 1993.
172. Watkinson A, Gargan MG, Bannister GC: Prognostic factors in soft tissue injuries of the cervical spine. *Injury* 22:307–309, 1991.
173. Lindgren K-A, Leino E: Subluxation of the 1st rib: A possible thoracic outlet syndrome mechanism. *Arch Phys Med Rehabil* 68:692–695, 1988.
174. Kellgren JH: On distribution of pain arising from deep somatic structures with charts of segmental pain areas. *Clin Sci* 4:35–46, 1939.
175. Inman VT, Saunders JBdeCM: Referred pain from skeletal structures. *J Nerv Ment Dis* 99:660–667, 1944.
176. Feinstein B, Langton JNK, Jameson RM, et al: Experiments of pain referred from deep somatic tissues. *J Bone Joint Surg* 36A:981–997, 1954.
177. Hockaday JM, Whitty CWM: Patterns of referred pain in the normal subject. *Brain* 90:481–496, 1967.
178. Bogduk N, Marsland A: The cervical zygapophyseal joints as a source of neck pain. *Spine* 13:610–617, 1988.
179. Dwyer A, Aprill C, Bogduk N: Cervical zygapophyseal joint pain patterns: I. A study in normal volunteers. *Spine* 15:453–457, 1990.
180. Aprill C, Dwyer A, Bogduk N: Cervical zygapophyseal joint pain patterns: II. A clinical evaluation. *Spine* 15:458–461, 1990.
181. Nakagawa H, Ohashi N, Kanda K, et al: Autonomic nervous system disturbance as etiological background of vertigo and dizziness. *Acta Otolaryngol* 113(suppl 504):130–133, 1993.
182. Vanlieshout JJ, Tenharkel ADJ, Wieling W: Physical maneuvers for combatting orthostatic dizziness in autonomic failure. *Lancet* 339:897–898, 1992.
183. Ren TY, Laurikainen E, Quirk WS, et al: Effects of electrical stimulation of the superior cervical ganglion on cochlear blood flow in guinea pig. *Acta Otolaryngol* 113:146–151, 1993.
184. Ren TY, Laurikainen E, Miller JM, et al: Effects of stellate ganglion stimulation on bilateral cochlear blood flow. *Ann Otol Rhinol Laryngol* 102:378–384, 1993.
185. Stovner LJ: Headache associated with the Chiari type-1 malformation. *Headache* 33:175–181, 1993.
186. Hendrix RA, Bacon CK, Scalfani AP: Chiari-I malformation associated with asymptomatic sensorineural hearing loss. *J Otolaryngol* 21:102–107, 1992.

187. Kikuchi S, Kaga K, Yamasoba T, et al: Slow blood flow of the vertebrobasilar system in patients with dizziness and vertigo. *Acta Otolaryngol* 113:257–260, 1993.
188. Kubo T, Kohno M, Naramura H, et al: Clinical characteristics of hearing recovery in perilymphatic fistulas of different etiologies. *Acta Otolaryngol* 113:307–311, 1993.
189. Nomura Y, Okuno T, Hara M, et al: Floating labyrinth—pathophysiology and treamtent of perilymph fistula. *Act Otolaryngol* 113:186–191, 1992.
190. Herdman SJ, Tusa RJ, Zee DS, et al: Single treatment approaches to benign paroxysmal positional vertigo. *Arch Otolaryngol Head Neck Surg* 119:450–454, 1993.
191. Gobel H, Krapat S: Psychological status during migraine attack and interval before and after treatment with a selective 5-HT(1)-agonist. *Headache* 33:118–120, 1993.
192. Radanov BP, Distefano GD, Schnidrig A, et al: Cognitive functioning after common whiplash: A controlled follow-up study. *Arch Neurol* 50:87–91, 1993.
193. Chole RA, Parker WS: Tinnitus and vertigo in patients with temporomandibular disorder. *Arch Otolaryngol Head Neck Surg* 118:817–821, 1992.
194. Morgan DH: The great impostor: Diseases of the temporomandibular joint. *JAMA* 235:2395, 1976.
195. Kryzer TC, Lambert PR: Herniation of temporomandibular joint contents into the external ear canal. *Otolaryngol Head Neck Surg* 23:607–608, 1992.
196. Cooper CW: Vestibular neuronitis—a review of a common cause of vertigo in general practice. *Br J Gen Pract* 43(369):164–167, 1993.
197. Baggersjoback D, Perols O, Bergenius J: Audiovestibular findings in patients with vestibular neuronitis—a long-term follow-up study. *Acta Otolaryngol* 113(suppl 503):16–17, 1993.
198. Ryu JH: Vestibular neuronitis—an overview using a classical case. *Acta Otolaryngol* 113(suppl 503):25–30, 1993.
199. Sacco RL, Freddo L, Bello JA, et al: Wallenberg's lateral medullary syndrome—clinical magnetic resonance imaging correlations. *Arch Neurol* 50:609–614, 1993.
200. Vibert D, Rohrlefloch J, Gauthier G: Vertigo as manifestation of vertebral artery dissection after chiropractic neck manipulations. *ORL* 55:140–142, 1993.
201. Schuknecht H: Cupolithiasis. *Arch Otolaryngol* 90:113–126, 1969.
202. Eviatar L, Bergtraum M, Randel RM: Post-traumatic vertigo in children: A diagnostic approach. *Pediatr Neurol* 2:61–66, 1986.
203. Radanov BP, Dvorak J, Valach L: Cognitive deficits in patients after soft tissue injury of the cervical spine. *Spine* 17:127–131, 1992.
204. McLauchlan CAJ, Pidsley R, Vandenberk PJM: Minor trauma—major problem. Neck injuries, retropharyngeal hematoma and emergency airway management. *Arch Emerg Med* 8:135–139, 1991.
205. Kissel P, Youmans JR: Posttraumatic anterior cervical osteophyte and dysphagia—surgical report and literature review. *J Spinal Dis* 5:104–107, 1992.

Spinal Stenosis

Edward L. Maurer, D.C., D.A.C.B.R.
Postgraduate Faculty in Radiology, National College of Chiropractic, Lombard, Illinois

Although no population-based studies have been conducted to determine the exact prevalence of spinal stenosis,[1] little question remains of its clinical significance. As a clinical entity it has taken a prominent position in the understanding, diagnosis, and treatment of numerous neurological and neuromusculoskeletal patient complaints. Historically this clinical importance was frequently overlooked or misunderstood because of inadequate diagnostic technology.

The initial concept of spinal stenosis dates back to 1803 when Portal[2] proposed that stenotic vertebral canals could cause low back pain. The idea was somewhat ignored save by anatomists until 1911 when compression of the lumbosacral spinal cord and nerve roots—the result of osteoarthritis was recognized.[3] In 1931, compression, a result of spondylitic ridges with thickening of the ligamenta flava was described.[4] It was not until 1954, when Verbiest[5] described a radicular syndrome from developmental narrowing of the vertebral canal, that the term spinal stenosis and its clinical importance became a part of biomedical parlance. With the use of myelography, and more recently computed tomography (CT) and magnetic resonance imaging (MRI), the frequency of spinal canal stenosis and the attending explanation of concurrent biomechanical manifestations has brought the topic into focus.

Stenosis is defined as an occlusion (narrowing or stricture) of ducts or canals, caused, among other things, by narrowing of their walls. This narrowing of the space available for the cauda equina and the spinal nerve roots may lead to physical and chemical alterations responsible for various symptoms, including pain, weakness, reflex alterations, and paresthesia.[6] The term spinal stenosis is used to describe in rather broad brush strokes a narrowing of various anatomical structures within the spine but usually refers to the spinal canal, neural canal (neuroforamen), and lateral recesses. Just as the cause of stenosis is multifactorial, so are its clinical manifestations. Some have referred to the presenting symptoms as protean or exceedingly variable,[7,8] and for this reason the presenting complaints of the patient are often misunderstood by the clinician. It is only with a thorough knowledge and recognition of the signs and symptoms of spinal stenosis that early recognition is possible.

ETIOLOGY AND PATHOGENESIS

Spinal stenosis may be local, segmental, or generalized and may be secondary to soft tissue or bony enlargement.[9-15] It represents an abnormal quantitative relationship between the spinal canal and the neural structures it contains.[16] The amount of space available for the spinal cord and nerve roots within the spinal canal and intervertebral foramen is determined by architectural or developmental variations and by degenerative changes of the articular structures. Although stenosis is demonstrated at all levels of the spine, it is most frequently encountered in the cervical and lumbar spines.

CONGENITAL AND DEVELOPMENTAL STENOSIS

Morphologically the lumbar vertebrae begin formation after the seventh week of gestation, when a pair of chondrification centers form in each vertebral arch.[17,18] Ossification and bony union of the centrum with its neural arch define the dimensions of the neural canal and foramina and are not completed until several years after birth.[19] Should the paired dorsolateral ossification centers of one or more lumbar vertebrae cease growth prematurely, the spinal canal may become stenotic, even in an otherwise normally developed individual.[20] The congenital or developmental stenosis was originally described in children[21] and later in adults[22] as most frequently caused by an idiopathic reduction in the normal spinal canal dimensions or by achondroplastic dwarfism. The vertebrae of patients with congenital lumbar stenosis are characterized by short and thick pedicles, and there is diminished interpedicular distance.[23-25] This results in both anteroposterior and lateral stenosis of the canal.

The vertebral canal typically reaches maturity in its cross-sectional area and sagittal diameter by 4 years of age. Thereafter the pedicular diameter widens and the shape changes but not the overall size. Factors that impair growth before age 4 that may result in developmental stenosis include various interuterine disorders resulting from toxins, drugs, alcohol, bacterial or viral infections, and placental insufficiency. These can leave a permanently stunted canal with no capacity for catch-up growth. The entire spinal canal from cervical to lumbar levels is small.

Various types of congenital or developmental stenosis are identified (Table 1). These can be subdivided into chondrodystrophic[20,24,26-37] and idiopathic.[4,38-73] The *idiopathic* form manifests with stenosis the result of anatomical variation in the absence of a concurrent, clinically identifiable condition such as achondroplasia. Patients are usually asymptomatic until between the ages of 35 and 65 years and are most frequently male. The presenting complaint is typical for other forms of spinal stenosis. The vertebral column is normal in height, but the pedicles tend to be short and the articular pillars massive.[40,42,43,46,52] The trefoil shape of the spinal canal is frequently found. The typical nearly round spinal canal considered as normal is capacious both centrally and laterally with an average anteroposterior diameter of 12 mm (Fig 1). The minimal cross-sectional area that accommodates the neural elements is at least 77 ($\pm$13) mm.[6] The trefoil configuration associated with congenital stenosis mani-

TABLE 1.
Major Causes of Spinal Stenosis

Congenital-developmental stenosis
   Idiopathic
   Achondroplasia or hypochondroplasia
   Hypophosphatemia vitamin D–resistant rickets
   Morquio's mucopolysaccharidosis
   Spinal dysraphism
   Down syndrome
   Scoliosis
Acquired stenosis
   Degenerative
     Spondylosis
     Spondylolisthesis
     Scoliosis
     Calcification or ossification of the posterior longitudinal ligament
     Calcification or ossification of the ligamentum flavum
     Intraspinal synovial cysts
   Postoperative
     Laminectomy
     Fusion
     Chemonucleolysis/discectomy
   Posttraumatic (late)
   Metabolic or endocrine
     Epidural lipomatosis (Cushing's disease)
     Osteoporosis
     Acromegaly
     Calcium pyrophosphate dihydrate deposition disease (CPPD)
     Renal osteodystrophy
     Hypoparathyroidism
   Miscellaneous
     Paget's disease of bone
     Rheumatoid arthritis
     Ankylosing spondylitis
     Diffuse idiopathic skeletal hyperostosis (DISH)
     Fluorosis
     Conjoined origin of lumbosacral nerve roots

fests with sometimes severe narrowing, particularly of the lateral recesses. This is unfavorable because little room for accommodation to changes that occur as a result of aging or degenerative alteration is possible. Similar neurocompressive alteration is found in vertebral segments with anatomically shortened pedicles (i.e., pedicogenic stenosis) (Fig 2).[74]

    Familial development of lumbar stenosis has been documented and suggests that the anatomical dimensions of the spinal canal may, in some patients, be regulated by genetic factors.[64, 75] Postacchini[75] and Moreland et al.[1] have suggested that this predisposition toward familial stenosis

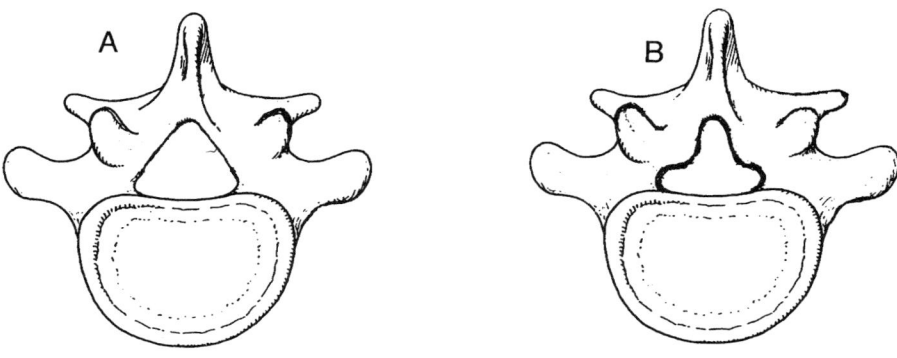

FIGURE 1.
A, normal shape of the spinal canal is either round or ovoid. **B,** the trefoil or fleur-de-lis appearance.

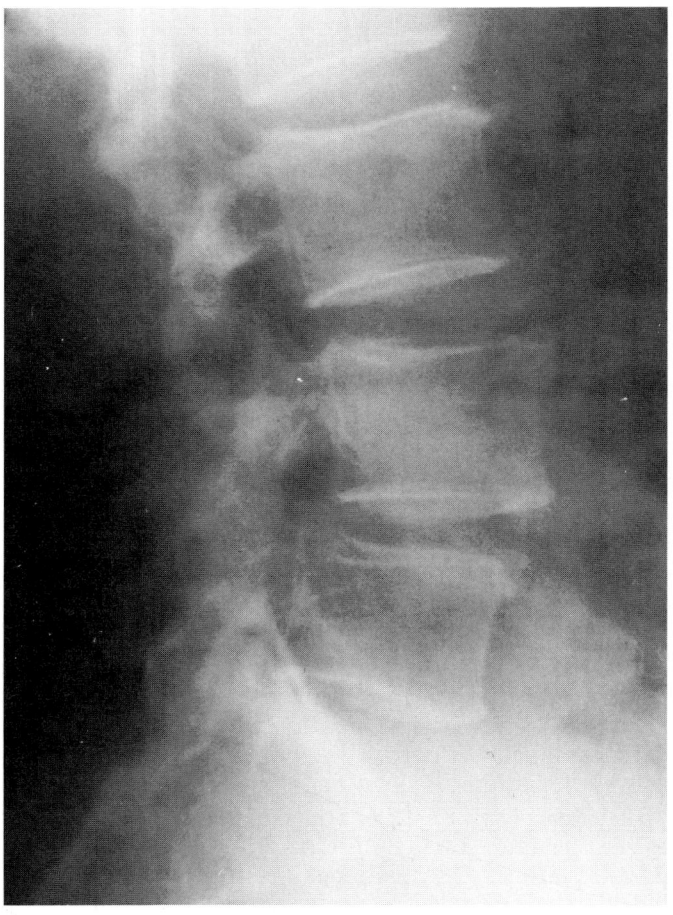

FIGURE 2.
Anatomical short pedicles at L-5. Pedicogenic stenosis with spinal canal narrowing is probable. Anterolisthesis of L-4.

may be helpful in identifying patients at risk. By measuring the spinal canal by noninvasive methods, one could advise an individual at risk against occupations that predispose to degenerative vertebral changes. Given the near constant presence of spinal stenosis in achondroplasia and other congenital disorders, a genetic factor seems likely in these disorders and idiopathic stenosis as well.

The importance of nutrition in developmental idiopathic spinal stenosis has been documented relating to an episode of malnutrition encountered many years ago. Its importance today is problematical. Prehistoric North American Indians underwent a dietary change from a hunting-gathering, protein-rich diet to a maize-agricultural, protein-deficient diet between 940 and 1300 A.D. Lumbar and thoracic vertebral canal dimensions, intervertebral foramen widths, vertebral heights, and vertebral osteophytosis were measured in Indian skeletons from the Dickson Mounds archaeological excavation in Illinois, and the spinal canal was found to be significantly smaller in the protein-deficient Indians. This finding suggests that developmental idiopathic spinal stenosis may be related to prenatal and infant malnutrition.[68]

The *chondrodystrophic* forms of congenital-developmental stenosis (see Table 1) all manifest with various alterations in size or shape of the spinal canal. Each condition has individual characteristics clinically and radiologically. Achondroplasia or achondroplastic dwarfism is an autosomal dominant condition that manifests with short limbs, abnormal enchondral bone formation, and premature fusion of the cartilaginous synchondroses.[24, 25, 36, 37, 76] The vertebrae are broad, somewhat wedge shaped, with short, thick pedicles and are noted for their decrease in interpedicular distance. This combination results in stenosis of both the anteroposterior and lateral measurement of the spinal canal. All components of the central canal are small. Clinically the most common site of compressive myeloradiculopathy is the lumbar spine or thoracolumbar junction.* As adults these patients often develop syndromes involving progressive compression of the spinal cord or cauda equina.[79] *Hypochondroplasia* is closely related to achondroplasia but is less likely to develop into spinal stenosis, and when it does, it is much less severe. In its most severe form it may be indistinguishable from the severe forms of achondroplasia.[36]

In adult *hypophosphatemia vitamin D–resistant rickets* both the anteroposterior and transverse diameters of the lumbar spine were found to be significantly narrower than those of a control group. These patients form excessive osteoid, and when it occurs in the spinal canal, it tends to increase the development of spinal cord compression.[80-84] *Morquio's mucopolysaccharidosis* is characterized as dwarfism with a short spine but relatively normal extremity length. Radiographically the vertebral bodies appear hypoplastic, flattened, or oval. Atlantoaxial instability secondary to odontoid hypoplasia or aplasia is common, and spinal cord compression may occur secondary to thoracolumbar kyphosis with posterior displacement of a vertebral body.[77]

In numerous *other congenital disorders* such as metatrophic dwarf-

---

*References 24, 25, 36, 37, 39, 77, 78.

ism, spondyloepiphyseal dysplasia, multiple epiphyseal dysplasia, chondrodysplasia punctata, and Down syndrome, one of the primary findings in each is laxity of the atlantoaxial articulation. A few cases of associated spinal stenosis have been reported.[77, 78] In *congenital spondylolisthesis* the degree of forward displacement of one vertebra on another tends to accelerate during the adolescent growth spurt. It is at this time that the patient seeks consultation regarding symptoms. Common findings may include paresthesia, restricted straight leg raising, weak ankle reflexes, and other signs associated with spinal stenosis.[67, 85-87]

Both *idiopathic thoracolumbar and lumbar scoliosis* in adults may cause spinal stenosis. Age at manifestation varies from 20 to 70 years and both commonly present findings of foraminal narrowing, facet subluxation, and pedicular kinking of the nerve roots. Root entrapments of sciatic distribution are common and are found on the side opposite the major curve, coming from the concavity of the compensatory lumbosacral curves. Regardless of the type of curve, neurological entrapment usually arises on the side of concavity.[88-90]

ACQUIRED STENOSIS

Acquired stenosis is most commonly the result of degenerative processes of the spine. Spontaneous or posttraumatic tears, degeneration, fibrosis, and collapse of the disk lead to the failure of mechanical function and then to subperiosteal osteogenesis (i.e., spondylosis), where the herniating or bulging annulus is attached to the cartilaginous plates with the epiphyseal ring of the vertebral body.[91, 92] As patients grow older, biomechanical failure of the disk increases the stress on facet joints and ligamentous attachments, resulting in hypertrophy of the facets and ligaments, particularly in the lumbar spine.[93] Bone tends to thicken at the pedicles, laminae, and facets as a result of chronic stress or repeated minor trauma.[94-98] A loss of disk height further narrows the neural foramina and permits the superior facet from the vertebra below to migrate upward (i.e., imbrication of the articular facets). Collapse of the disk reduces the interlaminar space, causing marked narrowing of the spinal canal (Fig 3).[94] Posterior protrusion of the annulus and disk contribute to stenosis and nerve root entrapment in the midline (Fig 4), lateral recesses (Fig 5), and foramina.[99]

In addition to degenerative spondylosis or discogenic spondylosis just described, other commonly encountered conditions often produce spinal or neural canal stenosis. Degenerative spondylolisthesis, lateral recess stenosis, ligamentous hypertrophy, ossification and calcification (Fig 6), and scoliosis all may contribute to clinically significant signs and symptoms of stenosis.[53-58, 100-130] The most common levels involved are L-4 and L-5 in the lumbar region and C-3 and C-4 in the cervical spine.[62]

Spondylosis

The pathogenesis of spondylosis is currently believed to be the result of recurrent rotational strains in cyclic axial loading that result in disk resorption, loss of disk height, and ensuing facet hypertrophy.[131] Repeated synovial reactions and circumferential tears cause cartilage destruction

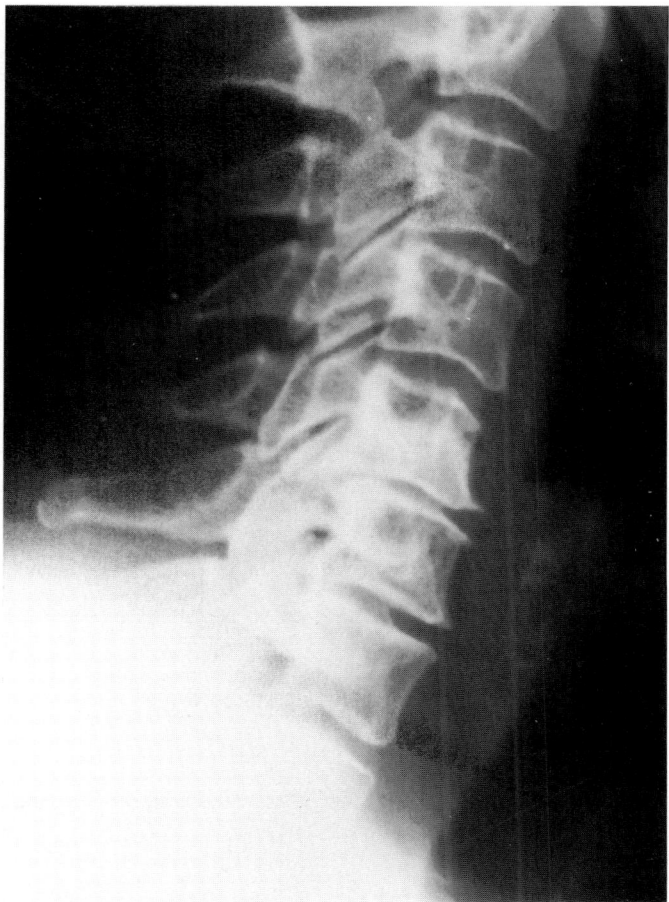

FIGURE 3.
Discogenic spondylosis at C5-6 with large osteophytic posterolateral spur. Combined with discal thinning, neural canal stenosis is likely. Clinical radiculopathy is present.

and internal disruption, leading to osteophyte formation, disk height loss, subluxation, and disk resorption with resultant lateral nerve root entrapment (Fig 7) and spinal stenosis.[132–137] Progressive change due to recurrent strains occurs, often leading to multilevel spinal stenosis. The final stage is severe osteoarthropathy, often with some degree of scoliosis in the area affected, and in some instances both central and lateral canal stenosis.[131, 132, 135] Interarticular facet degeneration (i.e., posterior vertebral joint arthrosis) may result in the backward displacement of one or more vertebrae (retrolisthesis).[138]

Numerous authors[78, 105, 117, 139, 140] have described an *isolated intervertebral disk resorption*, which, in contrast to the usual manifestation of spondylosis, is typically an isolated process in an otherwise normal spine.[139–143] This isolated disk resorption usually occurs at the L-5 to S-1 intervertebral disk space and develops over several years. Its clinical

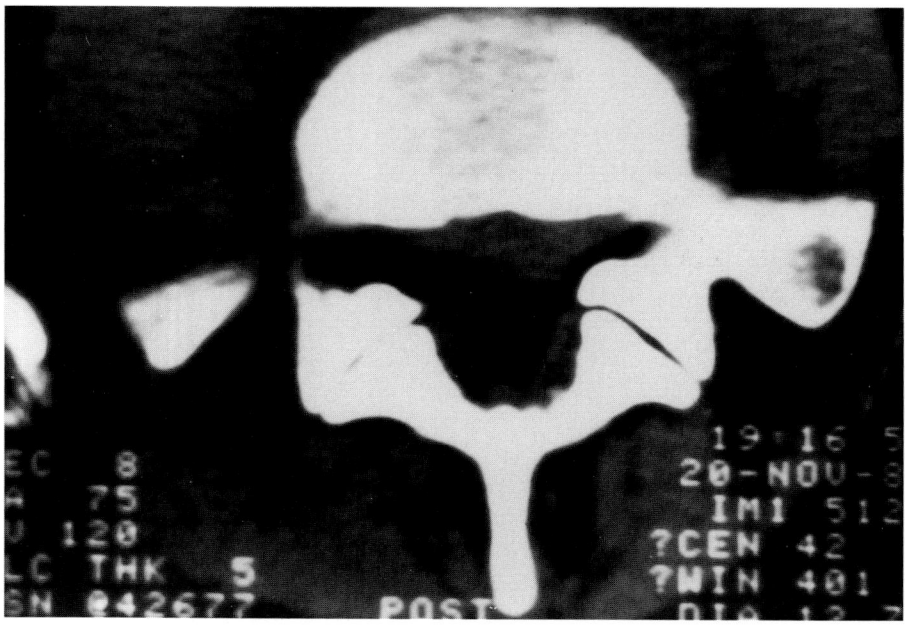

FIGURE 4.
Left paracentral herniation. Compression of the cord and nerve root. Hypertrophy of the left ligamentum flavum.

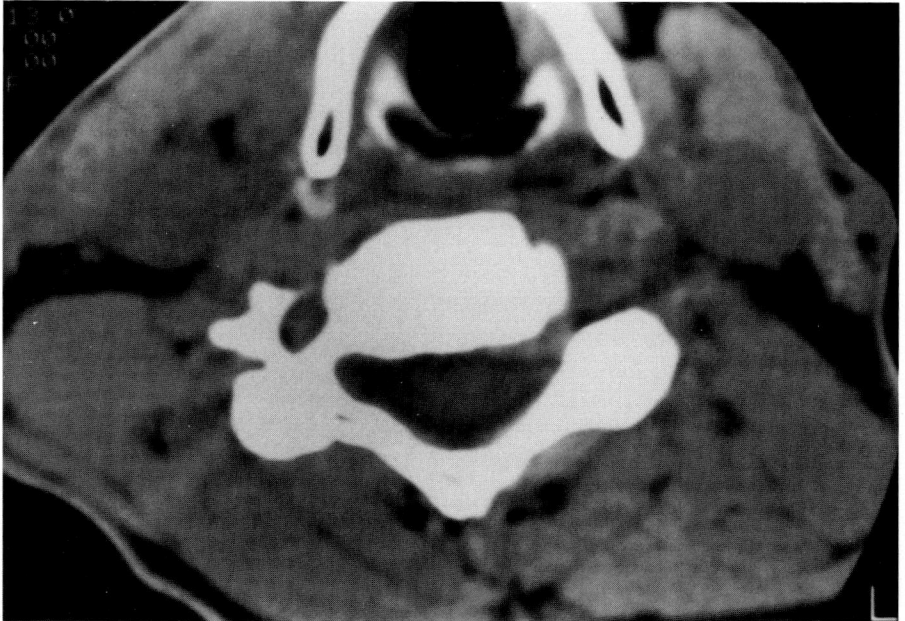

FIGURE 5.
Neural canal stenosis caused by herniated cervical disk on the left. Neurovascular compressive defect with clinical radiculopathy.

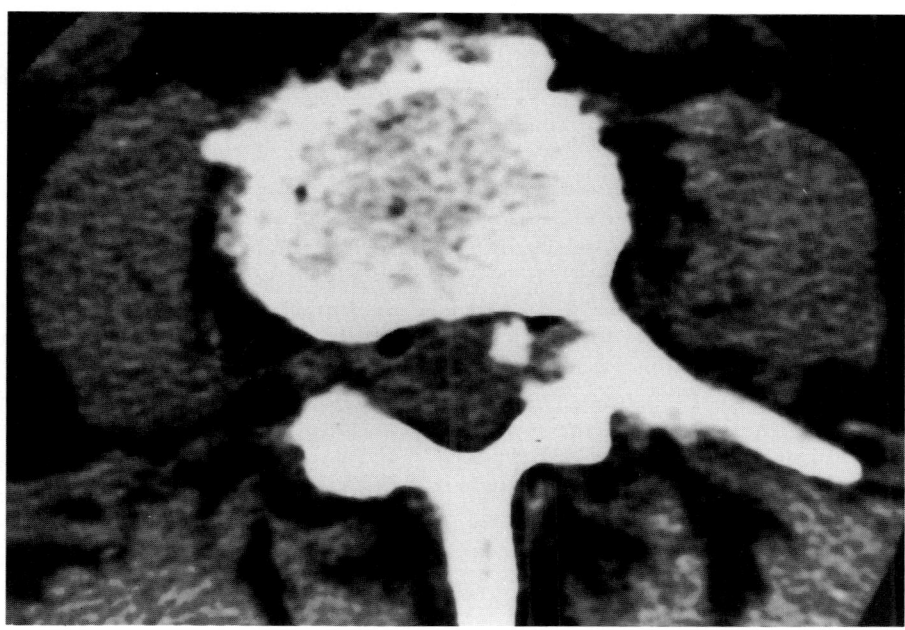

FIGURE 6.
Calcified discal fragment causing moderate stenosis of the lateral recess. Marked vertebral end-plate spondylosis.

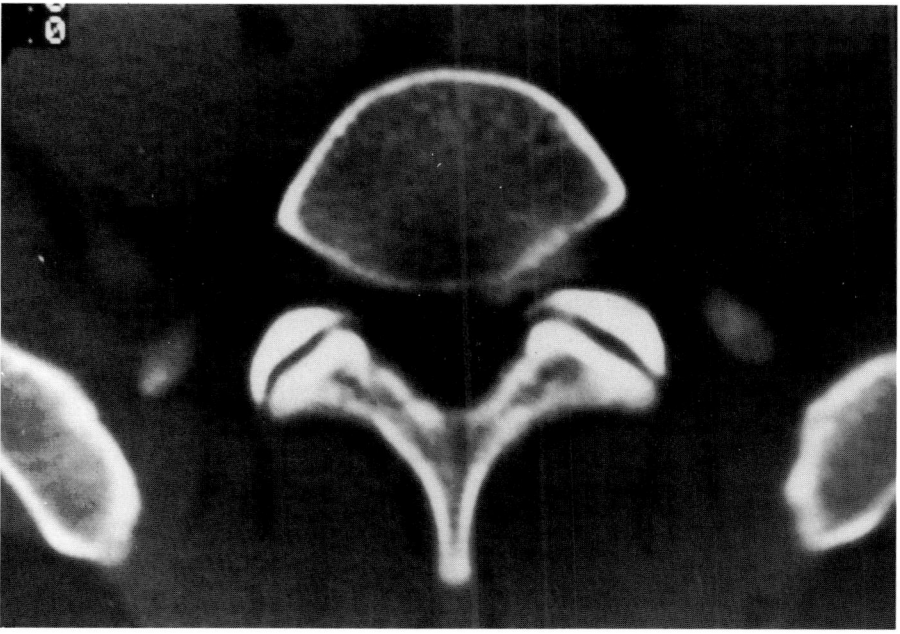

FIGURE 7.
Neural canal stenosis caused by marginal spondylosis. Neurovascular compromise is probable.

course is marked by repeated episodes of low back pain lasting from a few to several days, followed by complete resolution of symptoms. Repeat radiographic examinations reveal progressive narrowing of the involved discal interspace with contiguous marginal vertebral sclerosis. Attending progressive posterior osteophytes and articular joint arthrosis result in narrowing of the spinal canal. This spondylosis and associated upward migration of the superior facet, the result of loss in disk height, results in subarticular and intervertebral canal narrowing. This stenosis is usually bilateral. In the early course of this condition some patients may have unilateral sciatica. It is important to differentiate this condition from herniated nucleus pulposus because treatment by standard laminectomy may provide inadequate nerve decompression.

As important as bony and cartilaginous changes of degenerative spondylosis are, any attempt at complete understanding of this entity would be hollow without full realization of the importance that attending soft tissue changes contribute, particularly in stenosis. Degenerative spondylosis is nearly always associated with hyperplasia, fibrosis, and cartilaginous metaplasia of the annulus, posterior longitudinal ligament, and ligamentum flavum. An increase in the thickness of the ligamentum flavum from its normal of 2 to 5 mm[144] to as much as 5 to 10 mm in patients with spondylosis is not uncommon.[1] Ciricillo and Weinstein[145] report that the hypertrophied ligamentum flavum causes the most notable compression of the neural elements (Fig 8), and it may be the major cause of lumbar stenosis in some patients.[146–149] Surgical specimens reveal at histological examination that the ligamentum flavum demonstrates with fragmentation, degeneration, and disappearance of elastic fibers that do not regenerate after injury. These specimens also show increased vascularity, resulting in excessive collagen deposition and fibrosis. Some evidence of old hemorrhage and residual granulation tissue is occasionally found.[17, 150, 151]

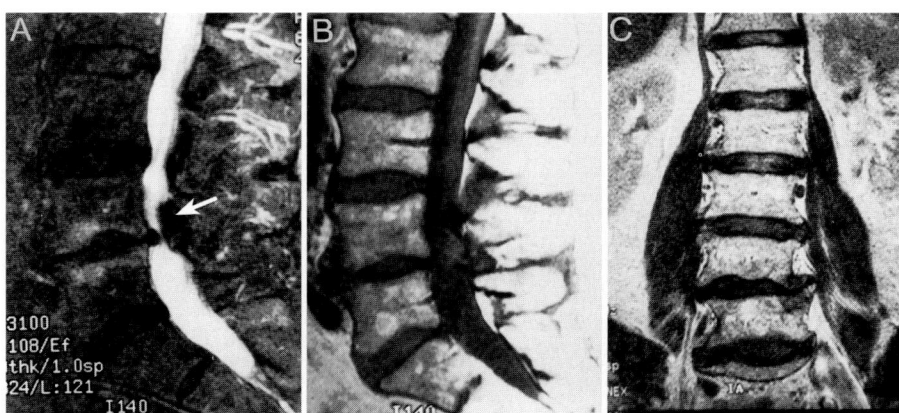

FIGURE 8.
A, L4-5 spinal stenosis due to discal herniation, hypertrophy of the ligamentum flavum *(arrow)* and facet arthrosis. **B,** anterior discal protrusion at L4-5. **C,** the axial views (not presented) also demonstrated far lateral discal herniation at L5-S1 on the right with neural canal stenosis, seen vaguely on this coronal view.

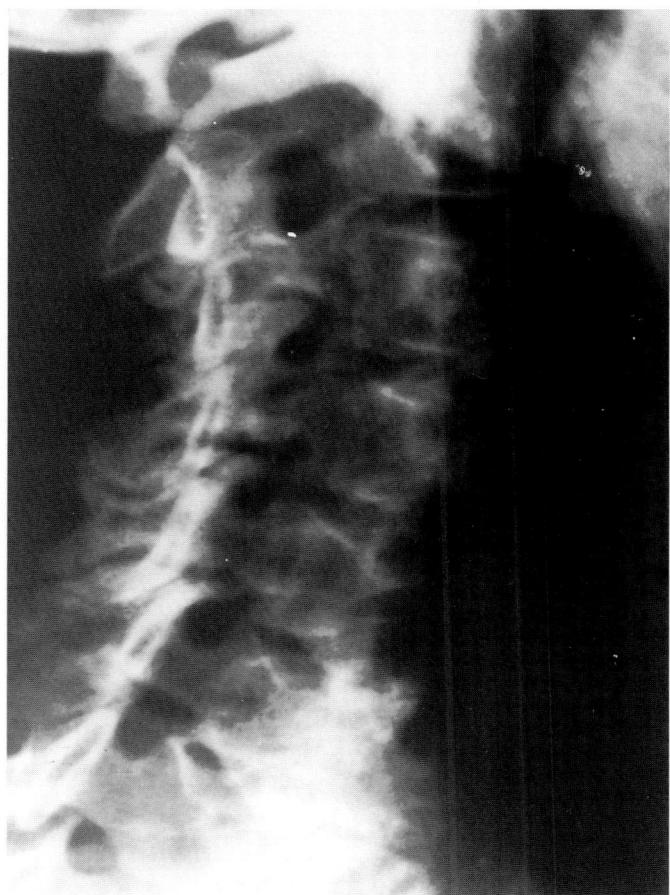

FIGURE 9.
Oblique cervical spine with multilevel posterior vertebral joint arthrosis (PVJA). Facet hypertrophy, suggesting spinal stenosis at C3-4 and C4-5, is suspect.

Narrowing with *stenosis of the lateral recesses* of the spinal canal is common. It may be associated with herniation of the nucleus pulposus or more frequently the result of articular facet hypertrophy (Figs 9 and 10), spondylosis, or other pathophysiological changes of the intervertebral canal.[9, 13, 66, 135, 152–160] Clinically lateral nerve root entrapment manifests during the fifth or sixth decades, as opposed to the earlier age of discal herniation. Often the central and lateral recess stenoses are indistinguishable from a symptom standpoint, and clinical findings frequently overlap. CT or MRI evaluation is frequently helpful in differentiation. From a surgical standpoint this differentiation is necessary because the surgical approach for these two entities is quite different.[152, 159] The fifth lumbar nerve root is the most common spinal nerve root involved in lateral recess stenosis.[161]

Spondylolisthesis
Two distinct forms of spondylolisthesis are reported: spondylolytic, which manifests with an isthmic or pars interarticularis defect, and the

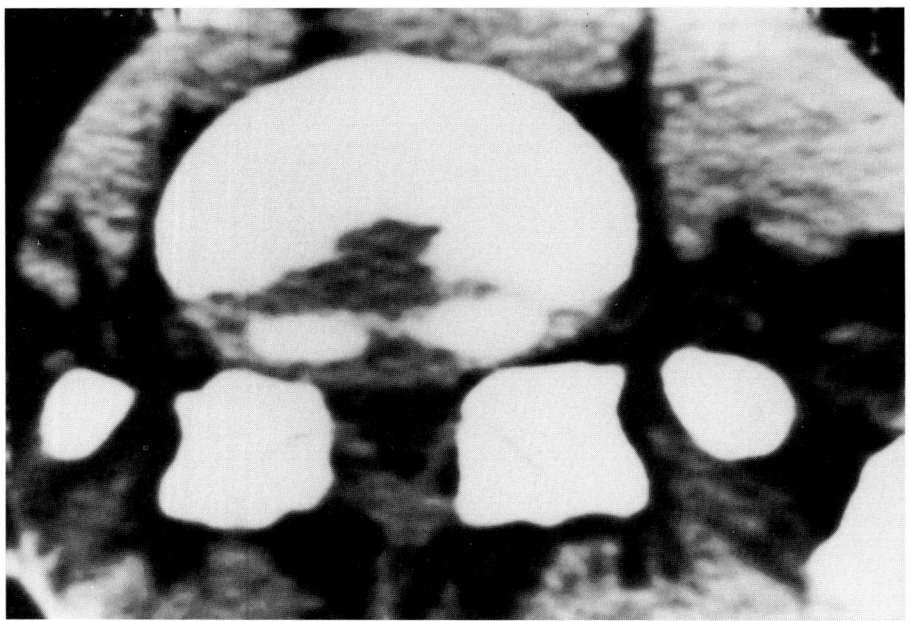

FIGURE 10.
Facet arthrosis and thickening of the ligamentum flavum, resulting in spinal canal and neural canal stenosis.

nonspondylolytic, degenerative, or pseudospondylolisthesis, where no pars defect is demonstrated.

The spondylolytic spondylolisthesis is most common at L-5.[47, 78, 162] It occurs more often in men than women; the articular facets are normal and maintain their correct relationship with one another.

The isthmic or pars interarticularis defect represents a separation in the neural arch typically caused by a stress or fatigue fracture.[163, 164] Traumatic spondylolysis does occur but is less frequent. The resultant forward slippage of one vertebral body on another rarely causes stenosis of the central canal, because as the body slips forward, it does not carry with it the neural arch, and there is little tendency for constriction of the spinal canal. Severe anterior slippage must occur before significant compression of the dural sac will occur.[78, 162, 165, 166] In unilateral spondylolysis, a less common finding, stenosis is not found because of the remaining anchoring effect provided by the intact pars interarticularis.[163, 164] In long-standing cases of typical, bilateral spondylolytic spondylolisthesis, the inferior articular processes of the subluxated vertebra can become densely sclerotic with hypertrophy and cause lateral encroachment of the canal.[162, 165]

In contrast, the nonspondylolytic or degenerative spondylolisthesis, previously referred to as pseudospondylolisthesis, is of frequent concern in clinical stenosis. No neural arch defects are present, and when forward slippage of the vertebra occurs, the unchanged neural arch is carried forward, causing dural sac or nerve root compression. This is frequently found at the L4-5 level, seldom discovered before age 50, and affects women four to six times as frequently as men.[133, 138, 162, 165, 167–176] The pathomechanics include discal and ligamentous degeneration, which precedes facet degeneration, sclerosis, and hypertrophy. This allows forward slippage to occur. The inferior articular facets of the slipping vertebra develop severe degenerative changes (i.e., posterior vertebral joint arthrosis) that grind their way between the superior facet of the vertebra below in a forward direction. The anatomical arrangement of the superior articular facets apparently limits progression of this forward displacement, and the facets have never been observed to move more than one third of the diameter of the vertebral body.[173, 174] As forward displacement of the vertebra occurs, the dural sac is compressed between the posterior margin of the intervertebral disk and the intact neural arch of the anteriorly subluxated vertebra. Degenerative spondylolisthesis causes symptoms of stenosis of the spinal canal or the lateral recesses more frequently than other types of spondylolisthesis.[47, 162] Because of degenerative facet hypertrophy, a concurrent hypertrophy of the ligamentum flavum has been demonstrated[183] that further increases the degree of stenosis to both the dural sac and neural canal.

Scoliosis

Both idiopathic and degenerative scoliosis can cause spinal stenosis.[178–186] Long-standing scoliosis is frequently associated with degenerative changes in elderly patients, most typically within the scoliotic curve. These changes are variable but include posterior or apophyseal joint arthrosis, laminar hypertrophy, spondyloarthrosis, marginal osteophytosis, and hypertrophy of the ligamentum flavum. The resultant stenosis can produce disabling back pain, usually of the low back, with lower extremity pain and neurogenic claudication.[177, 181] Vertebral subluxation, the result of discal and ligamentous degeneration, may also produce spinal or neural canal stenosis with neurocompressive symptoms. The development of clinical signs of stenosis may be superimposed on adolescent idiopathic thoracolumbar scoliosis or may occur as a degenerative process associated with the aging process.[187] Osteoporosis is considered as a significant contributory factor in the development of degenerative scoliosis, often associated with vertebral compression and positional changes that lead to spinal or neural canal stenosis.[179, 181, 186, 188, 189]

Calcification or Ossification of Posterior Longitudinal Ligament

Extensive ossification of the posterior longitudinal ligament (OPLL), initially noted in association with cervical myelopathy, was first recorded in the Japanese population in 1960. Since then numerous other cases have been reported in the literature that suggest the condition to be both common and widely distributed. It has been discovered in other Asian and non-Asian ethnic groups, is well known in whites, but is rare in Indians.[61, 190–199] No evidence of familial tendencies or association with other systemic diseases has been established. Resnick[190] reports that OPLL may be apparent in as many as 50% of cases with DISH; yet, conversely, DISH has been observed in only 20% of OPLL cases. Because both conditions are characterized by ligamentous calcification or ossification, it has been suggested that a common cause and pathogenesis are possible but as yet unproved.[78, 196, 197] Trauma has been suggested as an etiological agent in the development of acquired spinal stenosis secondary to hypertrophic ossification of the ligamentum flavum (OLF) and of the OPLL, but it has never been substantiated.[190, 194, 200] Although it has been reported in all areas of the spine, most cases have been limited to the cervical region. The levels of involvement vary from one to several, and radiographically the unorganized calcification or true ossification of the ligament manifests as linear vertical ossification within the OPLL.[196, 197, 200–206] It is usually asymptomatic and at times overlooked on routine radiographs due to overlay of bone or spondylosis. When sufficient bony outgrowth occurs within the OPLL, it may produce marked flattening with compression of the spinal cord; cervical myelopathy symptoms may be encountered, or a variety of clinical manifestations may be associated with this disorder. Symptoms are initiated by trauma in approximately 20% of cases.[190, 335] OPLL is more frequent in men than women and is typically diagnosed between the fifth and seventh decades of life. In addition to DISH, this condition has also been reported in patients with ankylosing spondylitis and those with fluorosis.[197, 206, 207]

Calcification, Ossification, or Hypertrophy of the Ligamentum Flavum
Considered an unusual cause of spinal stenosis, calcification, ossification, or hypertrophy of the ligamentum flavum has been seen in a few patients with calcium pyrophosphate dihydrate deposition disease (CPPD), hydroxyapatite deposition disease (HADD), and chondrocalcinosis, suggesting that this lesion is part of a calcium crystal deposition disease.[208, 209] It is most often associated with degenerative stenosis, such as spondylosis and arthrosis. Secondary change due to thickened lamina or shortened interpedicular distance has been suggested.[210] The condition occurs primarily in the thoracic and lumbar regions but has occurred less commonly in the cervical spine.[211–217]

Histologically the hypertrophied ligamentum flavum shows a decrease and fragmentation of elastic fibers, marked proliferation of collagen fibers, fibrous tissue substitution, fatty infiltration, and cartilaginous plaques. Hyaline degeneration and spotty calcification are also seen.[177, 201, 228, 229] The specific etiology of ligamentous hypertrophy is unclear, although mechanical injury causing fibrous tissue formation and hypertrophy of the ligamentum flavum has been documented.[220] Mechanical instability secondary to degenerative disk disease or accelerated facet arthrosis associated with asymmetrical facet joint orientation appears likely.[78, 171]

In the absence of degenerative changes, as in the younger patient, the degree of hypertrophy is related primarily to soft tissue compression of the dural tube by the ligamentum flavum or disk,[221] the result of mechanical injury with subsequent fibrocartilage change due to overgrowth of type II collagen.[177] Translational and rotational instability based on discal degenerative changes associated with the aging process may act as the mechanical stress[222] to produce hyperplasia of the extracellular matrix accompanied by cell proliferation, particularly at the enthesis, such as the site at which the ligamentum flavum attaches to the facet joint.[223, 224] This enthesopathy is more marked in the capsular portion than in the interlaminar portion of the ligament and may cause nerve root entrapment in the lateral recess.[177, 210, 222, 225]

Although rare ossification of the ligamentum flavum has been reported in cases associated with ankylosing spinal hyperostosis, the hypertrophy is the result of cartilaginous tissue proliferation. An unusual ossification of the ligament in the thoracic spine has been reported, characterized by endochondral ossification process with phenotypic changes of the collagen matrix.[226, 227] In hypertrophy associated with calcium crystal deposition disease, the degenerative hypertrophy of the ligamentum flavum is characterized with granulomatous tissue, including foreign body giant cells, induced by crystal deposition. The hypertrophy is marked and frequently associated with adhesion formation with the dural tube.[208]

The thickened ligamentum flavum, with or without bulging annulus fibrosus, may be associated with little or no bony hypertrophy seen on CT examination. This combination, however, may result in stenosis of either central or subarticular canals and must be included in any differential diagnosis with clinical findings of neurovascular compression of spinal origin.

Intraspinal Synovial Cysts

An uncommon cause of lumbar nerve root compression, intraspinal synovial cysts are demonstrated by CT and occasionally by myelography. They are most frequently found at the L4-5 spinal level. They develop by herniation of synovium and synovial fluid through the joint capsule, by differentiation of synovial cells derived from the degenerating cartilage of the joint capsule, or both.[228] Sites of origin include the facet joints,[228–230] zygoapophyseal joints,[231] posterior root ganglia,[232] or ligamentum flavum.[215, 233] Extradural compression secondary to synovial cysts has been reported in rheumatoid arthritis.[236, 240]

Most synovial cysts are adequately demonstrated by CT. When located medial to the ligamentum flavum at the L4-5 level, they appear as a nearly round structure that displaces epidural fat and may indent the dural sac. In 75% of cases capsular calcification is present, and in many cases the fluid in the cyst is replaced with gas (i.e., vacuum phenomenon). Intraspinal synovial cysts are nearly always associated with degeneration in the adjacent apophyseal joint.[228]

POSTOPERATIVE SPINAL STENOSIS

Postoperative spinal stenosis may occur after various types of decompressive surgery such as laminectomy and fusion but has also been reported after chemonucleolysis. It is rather common, occurring in as many as 30% to 40% of cases in some studies.[53, 241–248]

Issues of inappropriate patient or procedure selection enter into the explanation of postoperative sequelae, such as stenosis, but these will be discussed later in the section relating to treatment. Most postoperative patient symptoms are nonspecific and varied, often resulting in a delay of diagnosis. Patients may have long-standing motor weakness that has been overlooked or attributed to a poor surgical result from another cause.[152, 241] Clinical recognition of signs and symptoms resulting from postoperative sequelae is typically slow, and these signs and symptoms are often attributed to other nonrelated disorders such as preexisting osteoarthritis.

Stenosis after *postlaminectomy* may occur because of progressive deterioration of the intervertebral disk, which can enhance the development of lateral or foraminal stenosis. Interarticular facet hypertrophy, fibrotic scar tissue formation, and continuation of discal protrusion (Fig 11) may also contribute to the compression of the dural sac.* From a clinical standpoint the patient will have persistent pain and continuation of neurogenic claudication when lateral spinal stenosis is not recognized and treated at surgery. In one 10-year study involving 225 patients treated with surgery for a diagnosis of herniated disk, 56% were found to have concomitant lateral stenosis or lateral spinal stenosis alone.[258] Unsuccessful *chemonucleolysis* most frequently results from sequestration of the intervertebral disk and lateral stenosis.[50, 249, 251] A more insidious and progressive clinical picture may follow chemonucleolysis and certain discectomy procedures, related to decrease or loss of disk volume. This loss of disk volume is frequently associated with relative upward and forward displacement or creep of the superior articular facet and lowering of the pedicle, resulting in narrowing of the foramen and lateral nerve root canal.[133, 245, 250, 253-255]

Other less frequent but reported causes of postoperative stenosis include fibrosis or scar tissue formation at sites of prior hemorrhage or from chemical irritants such as dye, which may result in subarachnoid adhesions or dural fibrosis.[256-258] Even with the use of water-soluble contrast media used during myelograms, one study reports a 6% frequency of fibrous spinal stenosis development.[256] Ossification or hypertrophy of the ligamentum flavum may also develop stenosis after surgery. An acute cauda equina syndrome secondary to local edema, hematoma formation, or coexisting bony spinal stenosis may occur immediately after surgery.[1, 259, 260]

Postfusion surgical procedures are not without reported incidents of postoperative stenosis. Segmental stenosis may occur at the disk levels adjacent to posterolateral or anterior fusion.[241, 245, 261] Entrapment of nerve roots and lateral recesses may occur secondary to postoperative bony overgrowth. Occasionally stenosis may occur beneath the fusion mass itself.†

Patients with osteoarthritis of the hip with unrecognized spinal stenosis and flexion contracture of the hip joint may be at risk of developing postoperative paraplegia during a hip replacement procedure if they are placed in a supine position while they are fully anesthetized. Osteoarthritis of the hip is found with increased frequency in patients with spinal stenosis compared with the general population of the same age (33% vs. 0.15%).[156] Accordingly, if lumbar stenosis is not discovered before surgery, the increased pressure from the stenotic canal on the cauda equina roots during the hip replacement procedure may produce acute

---

*References 152, 160, 241, 242, 244, 249-251.
†References 1, 47, 241, 244, 245, 261, 262.

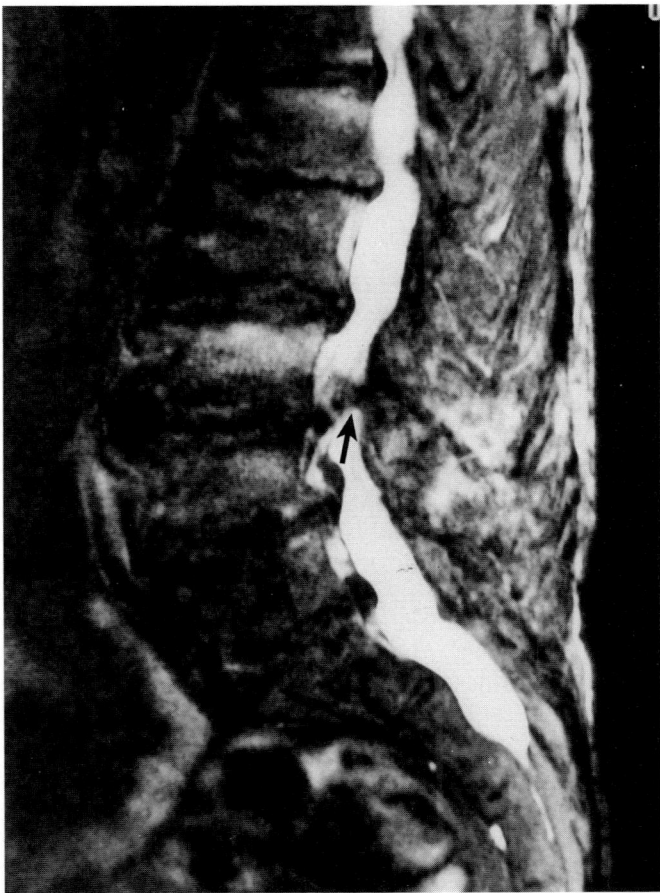

FIGURE 11.
Postlaminectomy L-2 through L-5. At L3-4 is stenosis as a result of remaining discal bulge and posterior epidural fibrosis (arrow). Bulging annulus is seen at L2-3 and L5-S1 with minimal thecal sac compromise.

postoperative paraplegia.[156, 263, 264] Not infrequently, lumbar spinal stenosis has been implicated as a cause of continuing pain and disability after postoperative hip replacement. The concurrent osteoarthritis of the lumbosacral spine may explain intermittent neurogenic claudication and neurological changes seen in some patients before and after hip replacement. Given the increased weight-bearing activity permitted after surgery, with increased stress to the vertebral segments, the degree and severity of lumbar spinal stenosis may increase and explain continuing pain and disability.[265]

POSTTRAUMATIC SPINAL STENOSIS

Both the burst-type fracture of the vertebral bodies and the posterior arch fracture can result in central or lateral canal stenosis. Acute neurocompressive signs and symptoms immediately after trauma may result from direct compression by bone or soft tissue, hematoma formation, or developing edema. Immediate decompression procedures may be necessary to preclude permanent neurological insult. The burst-type fracture can frequently be asymptomatic (relating to stenosis) for several months after injury because ligamentous calcification or hypertrophy, sclerosis, and new bone formation at the site of vertebral fracture will require many months or years to develop to a point of stenosis with symptom development. The lower thoracic and upper lumbar vertebrae (T-12 to L-2) are most frequently involved.[133, 134, 256-261, 262]

METABOLIC AND ENDOCRINE DISORDERS WITH STENOSIS

Although they are rare, a number of endocrine and metabolic disorders have recorded concurrent spinal stenosis. Typically the stenosis is secondary to the patient having received exogenous corticosteroid therapy for treatment and not necessarily from the underlying disorder being treated. Conditions reporting this secondary stenosis formation include Cushing's syndrome, renal and heart transplants, asthma, chronic active hepatitis, polyarteritis nodosa, Graves' ophthalmopathy, systemic juvenile rheumatoid arthritis, and polyarthritis. The thoracic and lumbar sections of the spine are the only reported areas involved. The mechanism of stenosis in these corticosteroid-use conditions is epidural lipomatosis with encroachment of the dural structures. Epidural lipomatosis has been associated with high-dose, prolonged corticosteroid therapy but has also been induced by low-dose corticosteroids used for a long period. Fortunately, spinal stenosis secondary to epidural lipomatosis is uncommon.[272-280]

Secondary spinal stenosis may occur in *osteoporosis*. It occurs with degenerative scoliosis with narrowing of the neural canal, but spinal canal narrowing has also been reported. Less frequent but often more serious is the retropulsed fragments of bone from vertebral compression fractures, which may result in spinal cord impingement.[186, 189, 281]

Spinal stenosis has been reported in *acromegaly* due to vertebral enlargement and osteophytic formations. Radiographic findings in the thoracic and lumbar spine include marked increase of the anteroposterior diameter of the vertebral bodies, the result of both anterior and lateral new bone growth. The lumbar segments frequently have scalloping of their posterior margins. Both neural and spinal canal narrowing may result.[282-286]

Numerous other conditions with concomitant spinal stenosis such as CPPD disease, hypoparathyroidism, renal osteodystrophy, and oxalosis have been reported. In each reported study the frequency and development of spinal stenosis have been unpredictable and without question a secondary finding to the underlying pathological condition.[137, 213, 287-290] Associated findings include crystalline deposition within the ligamentum flavum, cartilage, muscle, and tendon, which may result in calcification; occasionally ossification of ligamentous insertions and muscle; and osteophytosis. Each has the potential of spinal stenosis.

MISCELLANEOUS DISORDERS WITH SPINAL STENOSIS

The etiology of *Paget's disease* is not clear, although a viral cause of the disease has gained support in recent years.[291] The pathophysiological manifestations are varied, as are the neurological complications associated with concurrent spinal stenosis. Radiologically Paget's manifests during its osteoblastic phase with bony overgrowth or expansion of bone, cortical thickening, and coarsened prominent trabeculae, which may occur in any bone or bony compartment but predominates in the axial skeleton. This increase in osteoid with enlargement of bone may cause compression or distortion of nervous tissue. The lumbosacral area is most frequently involved, although all levels of the spine may be affected. The severity of neurological complications varies according to the level of the spine involved. Paresis is most common in patients with thoracic spine involvement. Other neurological deficits such as muscle weakness, paralysis, and rectal or vesical incontinence result from impingement on the spinal cord. As in other conditions, lumbar stenosis of Paget's disease varies from an asymptomatic condition to a markedly severe neurological syndrome. Degenerative arthritis with osteophytosis and spondylosis of the spine and peripheral joints is common.[291-310]

Recently some authors[291] have offered five different mechanisms to explain the pathogenesis of neurological complications: collapse of affected vertebral bodies; increased vascularity of pagetic bone, which steals blood from the spinal cord; mechanical interference with the spinal cord blood supply; narrowing of the spinal canal owing to new bone formation; and stenosis of neural foramina resulting from involvement of the vertebral posterior elements. Previously the vascular steal syndrome (i.e., diverting blood into the hyperemic pagetic bone and producing relative ischemia of neural tissues) had been the favored hypothesis.* The search for an adequate understanding of pathogenesis has occurred because of frequent disappointment in clinical response of patients after some decompressive surgical procedures.[1]

Spinal stenosis is an uncommon development in patients with *ankylosing spondylitis.* Reported are cases due to severe subluxation of the atlantoaxial complex; a stenosing noninfectious inflammatory mass within the posterior epidural space of the midthoracic spine; destructive lesions of the disks and vertebral bodies associated with stress fractures or inflammatory noninfectious processes that have produced dislocation and angular kyphosis; and, finally, the insidious onset of neurological symptoms, the result of a cauda equina syndrome. Due to the slow progressive nature of ankylosing spondylitis, the neurocompressive signs and symptoms of developing stenosis may be ascribed to other clinical causes in the initial stage of manifestation.[311-323]

Other entities such as DISH disease, Forestier's disease, chronic fluoride intoxication, and rarely rheumatoid arthritis have been reported associated with spinal stenosis. The stenosis is generally the result of osteophytosis or ligamentous calcification except for rheumatoid arthritis, which will rarely manifest with the rheumatoid intraspinal nodule or cyst. In each of these conditions, the developing spinal stenosis is secondary, and neurocompressive signs are slow to appear. Anomalous conjoined nerve roots, when found in conjunction with a herniated disk or subarticular canal stenosis causing nerve root entrapment, may them-

---

*References 293, 296, 298, 299, 302, 306.

selves become a part of the stenotic process, which otherwise would not provoke symptoms.[61, 196, 212, 324-334]

CLINICAL CONSIDERATIONS

Spinal stenosis would be of little clinical consequence if pain and biomechanical dysfunction were not major symptoms, because grave neurological changes are rare.[336] Stenosis may be present with no symptoms at all. One study has demonstrated that 21% of asymptomatic patients more than 60 years of age had spinal stenosis.[337] With or without a small trefoil-shaped canal, the onset of hypertrophic degenerative changes or discal protrusion or herniation is typically associated with the onset of symptoms. Clinical manifestations vary according to the location and severity of the stenosis, as well as its cause. Neurogenic claudication is classical, particularly in lumbar spine stenosis.

A narrow spinal canal may be present at birth. This stenosis can later be accentuated by developmental narrowing produced by postnatal growth abnormalities or by acquired narrowing associated with various disease processes. Although signs and symptoms are occasionally encountered in the young, they are far more frequent in middle-aged and elderly persons. Stenosis in the cervical region may lead to impingement of the cord or, less frequently, of the nerve roots. In the lumbar spine, clinical findings associated with stenosis include low back pain, sciatica, and a cauda equina syndrome.[338]

Due to varying neurocompressive mechanisms in the cervical spine compared with the lumbar spine (i.e., cord impingement vs. nerve root compromise), the typical clinical symptoms are somewhat different. Radicular and long tract signs and symptoms are present in almost all cases. Neck pain and headache are frequently encountered. The Lhermitte sign of sudden electric-like shocks extending down the spine on flexion of the head on the neck may be present. Less common findings include impotence and sphincter disturbances.[78, 341, 352-357] Differentiation between the cervical myelopathic symptoms of cervical stenosis and those of cervical radiculopathy, the result of disk herniation or spondylosis, is often necessary. Cervical myelopathic symptoms include arm and hand weakness, a broad-based staggering gait, and interosseous atrophy. Shoulder and arm pain may be present but is variable and uncommon. In cervical radiculopathy the symptoms include upper extremity paresis and paresthesia, neck stiffness and pain, and interscapular pain. In either condition the onset of symptoms may be insidious.[358] Cervical myelopathy has often been misdiagnosed as multiple sclerosis, amyotrophic lateral sclerosis (ALS), syringomyelia, or subacute combined degeneration of the cord.[353-355] Coexisting cervical and lumbar spinal stenosis has also been reported. Initially findings may be referable to only one region, which dominates clinical manifestation. Gradually the typical triad of intermittent neurogenic claudication, progressive gait disturbances, and mixed myelopathy and radiculopathy in both upper and lower extremities develops. This concurrent multilevel spinal stenosis is referred to as tandem spinal stenosis (TSS). Generally the clinical picture of TSS is similar to the classic cervical spondylotic myelopathy, with the addition of neurogenic claudication of the lower extremities. TSS may mimic and be confused clinically with amyotrophic lateral sclerosis (ALS) and other motor neuron diseases. Decompressive surgery is frequently helpful in TSS but rarely in ALS.[178, 359-362]

The symptoms of lumbar stenosis are often vague and bizarre initially. Before manifestation a long history of 2 to 5 years of episodic intermittent low back pain without palpatory tenderness or neurological dysfunction is frequent. Patients usually complain of discomfort deep within the muscles of the low back.[1, 339, 340] The patient typically reports long-standing intermittent neurogenic claudication or pseudoclaudication characterized by leg pain that is poorly localized, sometimes associated with numbness and weakness, exacerbated by walking or standing, and relieved by spinal flexion.* Patients have usually found temporary relief of symptoms related to compression on the nerve roots by adopting a stooped posture involving flexion of the hips and knees, as well as the lower back. This posture is clinically recognized as the so-called simian stance.[344, 345] One third of patients report transient motor deficits,[342, 363-366] and much less frequently encountered is the uncommon symptom of unwanted or "spontaneous erections with walking." This intermittent or spontaneous priapism most likely results from increased parasympathetic tone precipitated by exertion causing stimulation of the spinal nerve roots along their course through the narrowed intervertebral foramina.[253, 367-370] Impotence may also be a presenting symptom.[188, 339, 366]

The age of onset of symptoms is related in part to the type of spinal stenosis.[346-349] Congenital and developmental stenosis often first manifest in the early thirties. In achondroplastic dwarfism, as well as in a patient with normal stature who has a congenitally narrowed canal, symptoms typically coincide with the development of osteoarthritis in a spinal canal with no available reserve space.[340] The more common form of degenerative stenosis occurs in patients in their middle to late fifties to early sixties.[350, 351]

DIFFERENTIAL DIAGNOSIS

Patient history and physical examination are often similar, and it may be difficult to distinguish between lumbar spinal canal stenosis and a herniated nucleus pulposus (HNP), particularly of the less than acute or insidious form. It is not unusual for the two conditions to be present concurrently.[78, 105, 262, 371] The type and character of pain are considered, and differentiation between neurogenic or vascular claudication is paramount.

In the typical scenario of sciatica due to HNP, the pain is usually limited to one extremity, is sharp or deeply aching, and follows a specific dermatomal distribution. Reflex changes or motor weakness may occur. The fifth lumbar nerve root is most commonly involved, producing extensor hallucis longus or tibialis anterior weakness. Weakness occurs when the nerve root is entrapped in the lateral recess or when a disk her-

---

*References 38, 76, 78, 134, 165, 262, 339, 341-343.

niation is associated with an underlying spinal stenosis.[346, 351, 372-374] Antalgic lateral bending of the torso and spine occurs, and paraspinal myospasm with palpatory tenderness at the level of involvement is frequent. Physical positions that may worsen or improve back pain often help to differentiate HNP and spinal stenosis and are listed in Table 2.[78, 262, 341] The discogenic pain of HNP due to mechanical factors may be decreased with walking or standing, but the same activity may increase pain secondary to spinal stenosis. Often the patient with spinal stenosis will report an inability to go shopping for any period without onset of discomfort, particularly neurogenic claudication. Neurogenic claudication is an unusual manifestation of isolated HNP.[78, 371, 375] Sitting frequently exacerbates pain in HNP but often relieves it in spinal stenosis. More telling is the Valsalva maneuver, bending, or lifting, which may stretch the sciatic nerve and cause an increase in pain of discogenic origin yet cause little change in the pain related to spinal stenosis.

Neurogenic claudication (sometimes referred to as pseudoclaudication due to its neurogenic vs. vascular origin) is the most common form of leg pain associated with spinal stenosis. Patients report pain, numbness, tingling, weakness, or cramping in one or, more commonly, both lower extremities. It frequently manifests with central canal neurocompression associated with an hourglass defect on myelographic examination. Typically the pain originates in the low back or buttocks and radiates into one or both legs without following a specific dermatomal distribution. The symptoms may stop at the knee while sedentary, but as activity increases or the condition progresses, it will radiate into the lower leg and foot. The classic patient reports that walking or standing precipitates symptoms, whereas sitting and leaning forward (the simian posture) or lying down alleviates the extremity discomfort. A sudden worsening of symptoms or progression of neurological findings may indicate a concurrent disk herniation associated with the spinal stenosis.[340]

A recent study[445] suggests that a single level central canal stenosis does not produce neurogenic claudication. A bulging, extruded, or sequestrated disk that produces nerve root entrapment will produce the classical syndrome of nerve root pain, worse on coughing, root tension signs, myospasm, and antalgic posture. Even with a massive and perhaps chronic protrusion, neurogenic claudication is not present. A slowly ex-

TABLE 2.
Differential Pain Patterns

Activity	Discogenic Low Back Pain	Spinal Stenosis
Standing/walking	Decrease	Increase
Sitting	Increase	Decrease
Bending	Increase	No change
Lifting	Increase	No change
Valsalva maneuver	Increase	No change
Bed rest	Decrease	Varies

panding spinal cord tumor, which at times may have bizarre symptoms, does not produce claudication. A single level degenerative facet hypertrophy may cause a subtotal occlusion of the canal but without claudication. Single level stenosis of the lateral recess or the neural canal may cause thickening and inflammation of the nerve root with severe nerve root entrapment and pain but without claudication.

Patients with neurogenic claudication generally have two or more levels of stenosis. There may be two levels of central canal stenosis or a single level of stenosis in the central canal and a more distal nerve root canal stenosis. The former tends to produce bilateral neurogenic claudication and the latter claudication in one lower extremity.[445-447]

It is important to exclude vascular disease as a cause of claudication in the differential diagnosis because of similar clinical features.[262, 343, 365, 376, 377] Patients with claudication secondary to vascular disease usually complain of cramping or tightness in the legs, with symptoms that begin distally and progress proximally. Extremity complaints in patients with spinal stenosis begin proximally and progress distally. Some clinical findings that may be helpful in distinguishing vascular from neurogenic claudication are shown in Table 3.[365] Vascular claudication is often relieved by standing, whereas neurogenic claudication is persistent while standing, which is improved by sitting forward.[378] The claudication of vascular disease usually occurs after walking a fixed or constant distance, whereas patients with spinal stenosis walk a variable distance before symptoms occur. Vascular claudication symptoms may be exacerbated by riding a stationary bicycle, whereas patients with neurogenic claudication can ride the bicycle in comfort. Patients with vascular

TABLE 3.
Differential Clinical Findings Between Neurogenic and Vascular Claudication

	Vascular	**Neurogenic**
Walking distance	Fixed	Variable
Exercise	Worse	Variable
Relief of pain	Standing	Sitting-flexed
Standing	Relief	Worse
Lying flat	Relief	Variable
Walk up hill	Pain	No pain
Stationary bicycle	Pain	No pain
Sensory	Stocking deficits	Poorly localized
Type of pain	Cramp, tightness	Numbness, sharp, ache
Pulses	Absent	Present
Bruit	Present	Absent
Skin	Hair loss	Normal
Atrophy	Rarely	Occasional
Weakness	Rarely	Occasional
Back Pain	Uncommon	Common
Spinal movement limitation	Uncommon	Worse with hyperextension
Genitourinary	Impotence	Variable

disease typically have a stocking sensory loss compared with those with neurogenic claudication, who often have poorly localized sensory deficits.[262] In addition, the presence or absence of pulses or bruits is important in differentiation between these two types of claudication.[262, 365]

In some patients confusion may occur in differentiating neurogenic claudication from peripheral neuropathy.[379] Geriatric patients with diabetes or other conditions that can cause neuropathy frequently manifest with suspected concurrent spinal stenosis. Burning or paresthesias that begins in the feet and progresses proximally is a typical neuropathic symptom. The pain is typically worse at night and has no relation to activity. Patients may also complain of an inability to feel their feet, caused by posterior column involvement. In severe cases weakness may occur in one or both lower extremities. The burning stocking distribution of pain below the knees not related to activity is the classic finding of neuropathy. The diagnosis may be confirmed by prolonged nerve conduction velocities during electrodiagnostic testing.[340]

The pathophysiological explanation of many clinical signs and symptoms of spinal stenosis is poorly understood. The narrowing or stenosis may be local, segmental, or generalized but may also be secondary to soft tissue or bony enlargement. Established are the neurocompressive defects on arteries, capillaries, and veins, as well as compression on the nerve roots themselves.* Also believed important in causing symptoms are arterial obstruction, venous hypertension, and pressure or traction on the sinuvertebral nerves and the primary rami.[251, 375, 381–383] Some authors[352, 384] have suggested that pseudoclaudication is a true vascular insufficiency of the nerve roots, but most others consider it to be secondary to mechanical compression of the spinal cord or nerve roots. Considered another likely source of pain in spinal stenosis and degenerative disk disease is the mechanical irritation or inflammation of the sinuvertebral nerve or the posterior ramus[385–388] secondary to vertebral motor unit instability. Because of their size and difficulty of isolation of these nerves, this mechanical source explanation has alluded firm demonstration as a source of pain. Another explanation of pain in spinal stenosis relates to the arterial and nutritional support systems of the cauda equina.[29, 389–394] Studies have shown that the cauda equina nerve roots are supplied with blood by arteries that emerge from the central spinal artery and its radicular and segmental branches. With exercise arterial dilatation occurs with increased oxygen use and stimulation of the nerve.[393–396] With spinal stenosis the constriction or compression of both blood vessels and neural elements can cause diminished oxygen supply, particularly during exercise, and cause ischemia.[392, 394] In neural canal stenosis involving the dorsal nerve root ganglia, a differing mechanism appears likely. The dorsal nerve root ganglia has a rich and extensive microvascular web, and the vessels are more permeable than other intraneural vessels at other levels. This suggests increased metabolic demand, and studies suggest that the dorsal nerve root ganglia is a site where synthesis of several essential pain-mediating substances, such as substance P, occurs.[391, 397] Compro-

---

*References 132, 133, 211, 262, 375, 381–383.

mise in the blood supply secondary to chronic compression, inflammation, fibrosis, or ischemia may alter the diffusion and permeability processes and further contribute to signs and symptoms of stenosis. Ischemia and metabolic nutritional deficiencies appear as a plausible explanation for symptoms of pain and neurological dysfunction.[336]

DIAGNOSIS

The history and clinical examination of a patient with spinal stenosis may be highly suggestive but rarely definitive. A history of long-standing, repetitive episodes of low back pain and neurogenic claudication would be of great help, but these are not always present. The clinician therefore must be alert to the potential of spinal stenosis and use those diagnostic modalities that hold the greatest promise of adequate and prompt demonstration of this entity.

ELECTRODIAGNOSIS

Electromyography (EMG), dermotomal somatosensory-evoked potentials (DSEPs), somatosensory-evoked potentials (SEPs), and cortical somatosensory-evoked potentials (CSEPs) may each contribute to the total assessment of the patient. Save to exclude neurological abnormality, these tests are typically used to confirm the level or levels of nerve root involvement. The EMG is abnormal more often than the neurological examination.[46, 339, 398] It is suggested that a normal EMG in a patient without neurogenic claudication effectively excludes spinal stenosis.[339] In approximately 80% of patients with proven spinal stenosis, the EMG will demonstrate with abnormality and provide additional confirmatory evidence of the level of nerve root involvement.[399–401] The EMG is of particular usefulness in neural canal stenosis in which evidence is typically much less clear than in spinal canal stenosis.[402] Nerve root abnormalities are usually multiple and often bilateral. The finding of a unilateral multiradiculopathy by EMG indicates a more diffuse problem than a herniated disk.[46, 398, 400, 402] In cases with suspected or verified spinal stenosis a bilateral EMG provides valuable information regarding the degree of neurological involvement and excludes polyneuropathy.[403]

Several studies have shown EMG to be less frequently helpful than DSEP in the work-up of spinal stenosis.[404–407] Patients with multiple root involvement by DSEP have EMG studies that are either normal or demonstrate with only single root involvement. This may be partially explained by the anatomy of the cauda equina (i.e., the motor fibers are positioned anteromedial to their respective sensory fibers). Therefore, motor fibers may be more protected in central canal stenosis, resulting in a normal EMG study. Another explanation may be that slow-onset and low-grade chronic nerve compression may result in conduction slowing and not axonal loss or denervation.[408–410] It is not possible for the EMG or DSEP study alone to distinguish between spinal stenosis, arachnoiditis, herniated disks, and other conditions that affect more than one nerve root.

Several studies have shown that DSEPs, SEPs, and CSEPs may be useful preoperatively in identifying the level of cord compression and intraoperatively in assessing the adequacy of neural compression, often resulting in alteration of the planned surgical procedure.[1, 100, 153-155, 411-414]

DIAGNOSTIC IMAGING

Diagnostic imaging plays an integral part in the diagnosis of spinal stenosis and numerous other spinal abnormalities. Included in the spectrum of diagnostic imaging are plain film radiography, myelography, CT, and MRI, with or without contrast enhancement. For many years the anteroposterior and lateral radiographic projections were available for measurement of spinal canal dimensions, but this was at best an estimation of actual spinal canal size. Numerous variations of spinal canal dimension were not well visualized. Estimation of the neural canal measurement depended almost entirely on extrapolation from the appearance of the intervertebral foramina. Little consideration was given to the variation in size or contents of the medial, central, or lateral portions of the neural canal. The fusiform shape of the dorsal nerve root ganglion and its necessary space requirement within the nerve root canal was often overlooked. Although spinal stenosis was known and recognized from myelographic studies and intraoperative observation, it was not until the advent of axial views of CT or MRI studies that stenosis gained status as a common, frequently encountered clinical entity. Before axial projections became available, most cases of spinal stenosis were considered the result of herniation of the intervertebral disk or the various congenital abnormalities, save by the studious clinician, surgeon, or anatomist.

Conventional Radiographs

It is generally accepted that plain film radiographs are not specific for the determination of spinal canal stenosis. The adequate visualization of degenerative processes, particularly when combined with clinical signs and symptoms, will nonetheless contribute to a clinical suspicion of this entity.* Consideration of variations in the spinal canal size due to age, sex, race, and different levels of the spine make specific mensuration of the normal or average canal diameters difficult. In the final analysis the diagnosis of spinal or neural canal stenosis depends less on the size by measurement of the canal than on the configuration and capaciousness of available space for the thecal sac and nerve roots.[256, 399, 416-418] Variations in size and shape of the neurovascular structures, as well as contiguous soft tissues, are all contributory to the final diagnosis.[419-421]

For many years plain film radiographs have been used as one of the first measurements of suspected spinal canal stenosis, particularly in patients with low back pain and neurogenic claudication. The normal sagittal diameter of the lumbar spinal canal is approximately 15 mm or more. Measurements below this are suggestive of abnormality, with a measurement of 12 mm considered as relative stenosis and a measurement of 10 mm considered absolute stenosis.[422-424] This sagittal diameter is measured from the midpoint of the posterior margin of the vertebral body to the point of junction of its spinous process and laminae. Because the pos-

---

*References 47, 138, 188, 342, 402, 415.

terior boundary of the spinal canal (i.e., the junction of the spinous process and laminae) is often obscured by the articular pillars or the pelvis in the lower lumbar spine, it is often necessary to employ a different measurement landmark. Eisenstein[425, 426] proposed drawing a line connecting the apex of the superior articular facet to the apex of the inferior articular facet of the same vertebra and then to a second line connecting the superior and inferior points at the posterior aspect of the vertebral body. The sagittal diameter was then measured by drawing a line perpendicular to line number 2 at the midpoint of the posterior vertebral body and extending it posteriorly to its intersection with line number 1. Buehler[427] advanced another method using a vertical line drawn at a point half way between the anterior and posterior cortical margins of the inferior articular facet at its superior aspect, which lies approximately at the upper one third of the adjacent intervertebral foramen. A second line is drawn connecting the superior and inferior points of the posterior-most aspect of the vertebral body. The sagittal diameter is then measured by drawing a line perpendicular to line number 2 at the inferior aspect of the pedicles and extending it posteriorly to its intersection with line number 1.[428] A comparative study to assess the accuracy of these two methods compared with CT was done by taking all plain film measurements and multiplying by a magnification factor of 0.77 to compensate for magnification. The results indicate the Buehler method as significantly more accurate than the Eisenstein method at the L-3 level but that at L-4 and L-5 no significant difference was found. The standard deviation showed less dispersity of the measurements with the Buehler method at all three levels examined.[428]

The alignment of the facets can be assessed on the anteroposterior view and the interpedicular distance measured. An anteroposterior diameter of 11.5 mm and an interpedicular distance of less than 16 mm are consistent with spinal canal stenosis.[429] Absolute stenosis, defined as a lumbar spinal canal with a midsagittal diameter of 10 mm or less, is more common in males, although the overall number of males and females with spinal stenosis is essentially equal. Relative stenosis with an anteroposterior midsagittal measurement of 10 to 12 mm occurs more frequently among females.[430]

Plain film measurement of the spinal canal and its midsagittal diameter as just described is of particular importance when congenital or developmental stenosis is considered. When degenerative spondylosis or acquired or pathological alterations are present with attending changes that intrude into the spinal canal, the measurement of the anteroposterior diameter is altered. As an example, should a large posterior osteophyte be identified (Fig 12), the anteroposterior measurement would be taken from the most distal or posterior aspect of the osteophyte, not the posterior margin of the vertebral body. When measuring for narrowing or stenosis of the spinal canal one must measure the actual space available or remaining, not what it is supposed to be. This same logic applies in patients with articular facet arthrosis (posterior vertebral joint arthrosis), uncinate arthrosis, or other proliferative or hypertrophic changes that encroach or intrude into the spinal or neural canal. These considerations explain why and how spinal canal stenosis may be suspected on plain film radio-

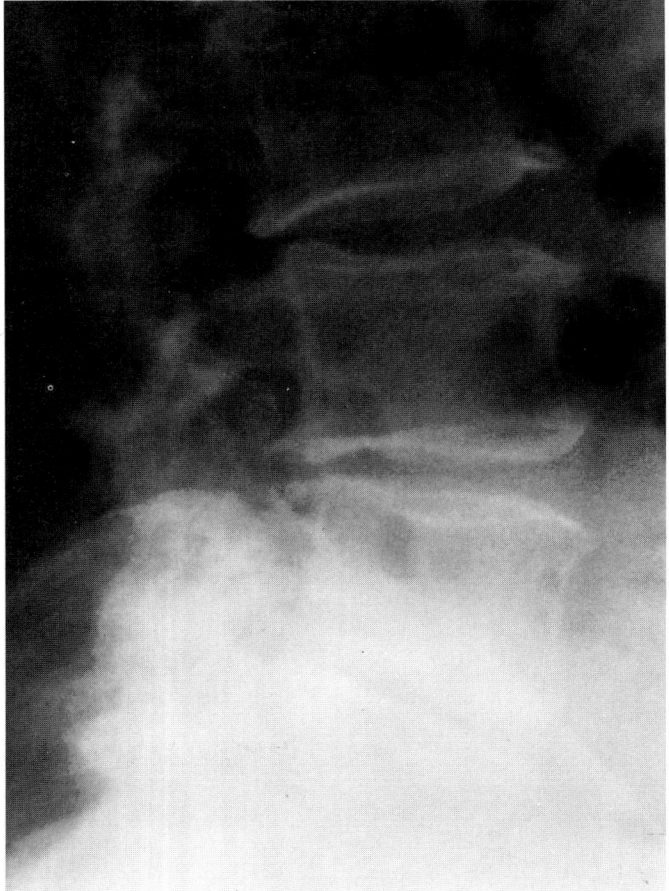

FIGURE 12.
Osteophytic spur from the posterior body plate margin of L-4. Intrusion into the spinal canal with stenosis is likely. By location, nerve root entrapment is doubtful.

graphs, but specific determinations of actual stenosis must rely on other imaging modalities. Plain films are unable to demonstrate the true shape of the canal or the actual relationship of the bone and soft tissue components.

Myelography
Myelography is a safe and effective method for demonstrating the subarachnoid space, spinal cord, and nerve root sheaths. It is more invasive and generally more costly than CT or MRI.[431] Given the current availability of CT and MRI, myelography has found limited usefulness compared with years past. It is now indicated primarily in the investigation of extramedullary-intradural processes for confirming a complete block of the subarachnoid space. It is also helpful in detecting cysts within the spinal cord or subarachnoid space. Occasionally when CT evaluation for cervical radiculopathy is inconclusive, myelography is of value. In spi-

nal stenosis myelographic defects range from complete obstruction to the hourglass appearance of the contrast media.[76, 402, 432] This same defect may also be produced by a central disk protrusion, diffuse bulging of the annulus, and chronic disk degeneration.[433] In the patient with stenotic lumbar spinal canals with complete blockage, myelographic evaluation using the sitting, flexed procedure has been shown to be a quick, simple technique for evaluation.[434, 435] Spinal stenosis of achondroplasia manifests with a distinctive myelographic image of multiple level filling defects but is often technically difficult to perform.[37]

The contrast media used for myelographic examination include gas, water-soluble iodinated media (most often metrizamide), and oily contrast media (most often Pantopaque). Although safe and effective for studying the spinal cord, gas media require multidirectional tomography and special expertise on the part of the examiner and are thus infrequently used. Water-soluble media are at present the standard of choice for most all myelographic studies. They have major advantages in that they provide ideal opacification and are dependable in demonstrating the subarachnoid space and intrathecal structures. Acute side effects from their use may occur but are usually limited to headache, nausea, and other transient symptoms, which typically abate in 48 to 72 hours. Pantopaque does not generally produce acute side effects but may cause a chronic arachnoiditis if it remains in the subarachnoid space after examination.[431]

Myelographic defects result from hypertrophy of the neural arches, spondylotic and arthritic joint changes with bony masses projecting downward into the canal and the lateral recesses, impressions from thickened superior and less often the inferior articular facets, and thickening or hypertrophy of the yellow ligament (ligamentum flavum). Anterior intrusions result from posterior osteophytes and discal herniation (Fig 13). The extent of the myelographic defect may sometimes be increased during hyperextension and relieved in flexion. Occasionally elongated and tortuous nerve roots are seen and frequently confused with venous varicosities.[436] The history of myelography records numerous cases where an inability to identify a specific nerve root entrapment or a far lateral disk protrusion has resulted in poor or inadequate decompressive surgery. This failure of localization is the result of the inherent limitations of the procedure (i.e., the anatomy of the canal) and not the technical aspect of the examination. The advent of CT scanning has probably reduced the frequency of this problem due to better visualization of the nerve canals.[244, 250, 252, 258, 437–440] Where available, myelography is frequently followed by CT scanning and has become a preferred method for identifying any neural encroachment.*

CT and MRI

The recent evolution of both CT and MRI have dramatically changed the imaging approach to spinal stenosis and the appreciation of various spatial characteristics previously underappreciated. Because of certain duplications of imaging detail available with either CT or MRI, these will be discussed simultaneously.

---

*References 47, 76, 135, 138, 344, 402, 437, 441–444.

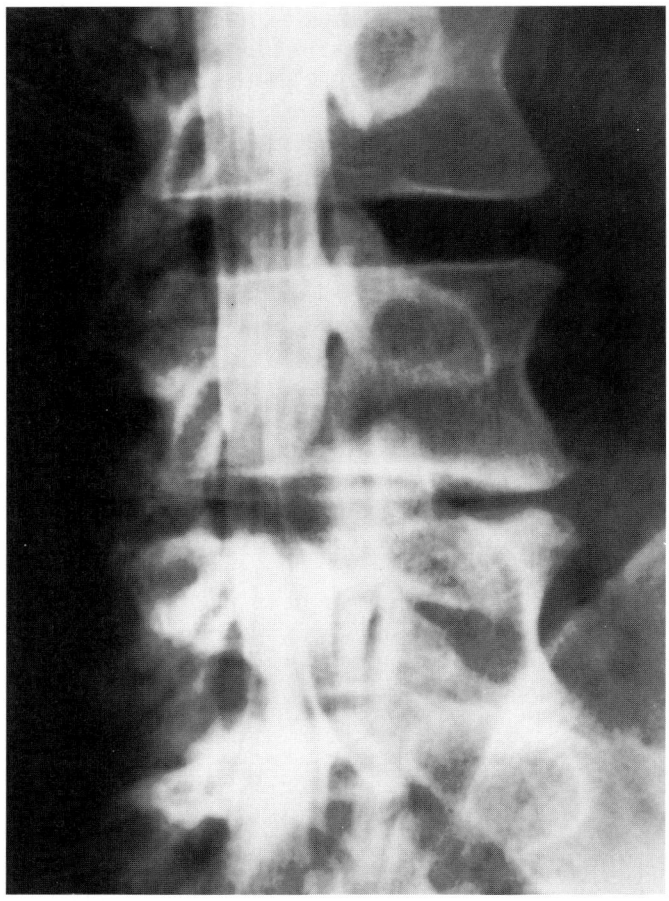

FIGURE 13.
Myelogram demonstrating with large focal defect in the column of dye at L4-5 interspace, the result of discal herniation (thecal sac compression of spinal stenosis).

It is generally acknowledged that CT is less costly than MRI and provides better bony detail than MRI. MRI, however, does not require the use of ionizing radiation, and it provides better soft tissue detail. These factors and those to be discussed will enable the clinician or radiologist to use the procedure best suited for the individual patient.

CT permits the determination of the spinal canal dimensions and configuration, along with any contribution of discal alteration, facet arthrosis, spondylosis, certain soft tissue hypertrophy, neural compression in scoliosis, retropulsed fragments in osteoporotic spines, and occult vertebral fractures.[448–450] Its usefulness in evaluating bony and soft tissue causes of spinal canal narrowing are well established.[244, 412, 437, 442, 451–457] CT is invaluable in visualizing levels below a partial or complete myelographic block[188, 399, 458, 459] and has been shown to direct decompression laminectomy accurately in some cases in which myelography was technically unsatisfactory.[37] CT using a water-soluble intrathecal contrast agent is more sensitive than myelography, which often fails to differentiate posterior from anterior sources of neurocompression and does not demonstrate the configuration of the lateral recesses and foraminae. Contrast-enhanced CT is quite helpful in evaluating persistent postoperative symptoms.[450, 460, 461]

CT features associated with spinal stenosis include broad-based (Fig 14) or central disk bulging (see Fig 4), a congenitally small or developmental trefoil spinal canal, hypertrophic facet changes (Figs 10 and 15), facet or synovial cyst formation, and ligamentous hypertrophy.[462] On axial images taken through the disk space, the absence or marked reduction in the amount of sublaminar epidural fat is a reliable indicator of spinal stenosis. However, on images taken at the level of the pedicles, this may be a normal finding.[463-465]

Although debate continues among various authors regarding myelography vs. CT as it relates to spinal canal stenosis, there is little dispute that in visualizing the lateral recesses and neural canals, CT is far superior. Sagittal reconstruction can provide a clear picture of the neural foramina and the relationships of the existing nerve roots to the pedicles and facets.

MRI is an alternative to CT in the diagnosis of spinal stenosis. Its advantages include the lack of ionizing radiation, the avoidance of invasive intrathecal contrast administration, and the capability of direct multiplanar image construction.[145] This latter option, of viewing both the axial and sagittal planes with equal resolution, is particularly advantageous in

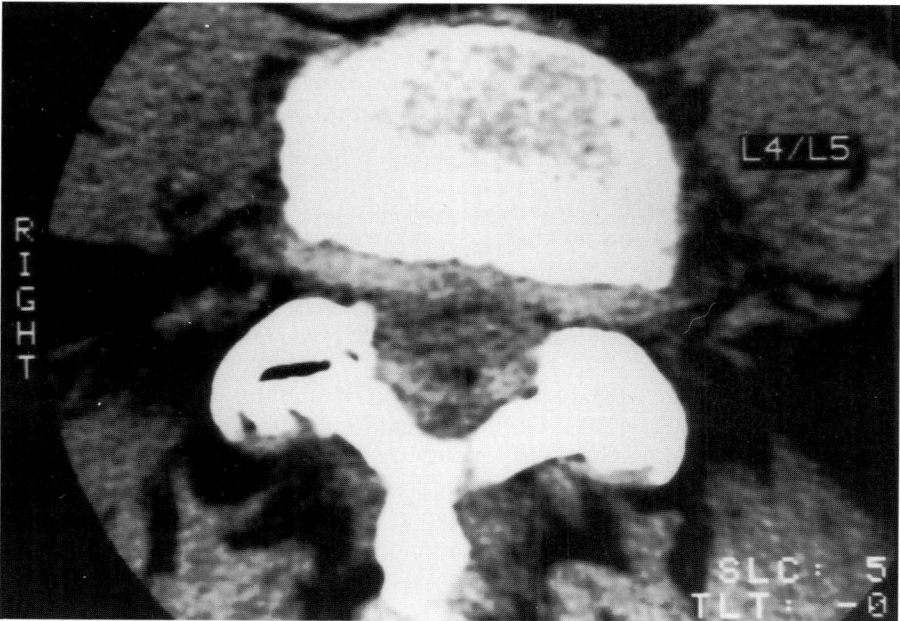

FIGURE 14.
Broad-based annular bulge, bilateral ligamentum flavum and facet hypertrophy. Only minimal thecal sac stenosis is seen, and the neural canals, although narrowed, appear adequate.

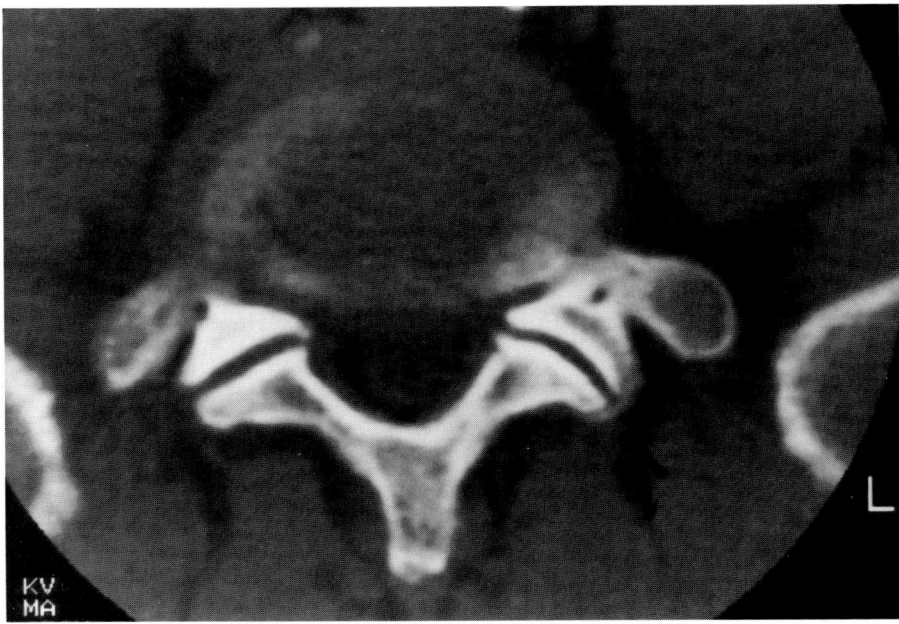

FIGURE 15.
Circumferential discal bulge, particularly of the right, suggesting neural canal stenosis. Clinically, however, symptoms were referred from the osteophytic bridging of the left articular facet, which produces hypomobility.

evaluating the intervertebral canals. MRI has greater sensitivity in detecting disk disease or degeneration (Figs 16 and 17). It can be used to visualize the entire spinal canal, including the conus medullaris and cauda equina.[466] MRI provides better soft tissue detail than CT, particularly within the lateral recesses, but it does not provide the bony detail available with CT.[465–468]

From an evaluation standpoint, MRI appears to combine the best features of CT and myelography. T_1-weighted axial images provide anatomical images similar to CT scans. T_2-weighted images provide a myelographic-like effect of the cerebrospinal fluid (CSF), which demonstrates the extent and degree of stenosis throughout the entire spine examined.[469]

Use of MRI in evaluating cervical foraminal stenosis has been reported with a 90% detection rate.[470, 471] The absence of fat in the cervical epidural space and its paucity in the neural foraminal canal can limit the usefulness of T_1-weighted sequences. Should sufficient MRI spatial resolution be available, however, the T_2-weighted sequences are most helpful because the signal from both the CSF and flow within the intraspinal or canalicular venous plexus may highlight structures such as the spinal cord, nerve roots, and adjacent bone and joint anatomy.[472–474]

Both CT and MRI have the advantage of determining the cross-sectional area of the spinal canal and dural sac dimensions. Spinal stenosis, with or without bony canal pathological conditions, can be identified. The relevance of the diagnosis of spinal stenosis based on measurements alone is problematic. It must be emphasized that pathological findings on CT and MRI indicating spinal stenosis are common and have been reported to occur in up to 28% of asymptomatic patients.[475] This reiterates the absolute need for clinical correlation of patient symptoms with imaging findings before establishment of any treatment regimen, particularly surgical intervention.[476] In a recent study of asymptomatic people, MRI examination of the lumbar spine demonstrated that 64% without back pain had an intervertebral disk abnormality, and 38% had an abnormality at more than one level. Among the abnormalities were disk bulges, protrusions, and extrusions (assumptive stenosis). Seven percent were diagnosed with stenosis of the central canal, and 7% had stenosis of the neural foramen.[477] These findings suggest caution in the early use of MRI in patients with back pain or sciatica. Some would recommend that MRI be reserved for patients who have signs and symptoms of radiculopathy and who have not responded to conservative treatment over 4 to 6 weeks.[478]

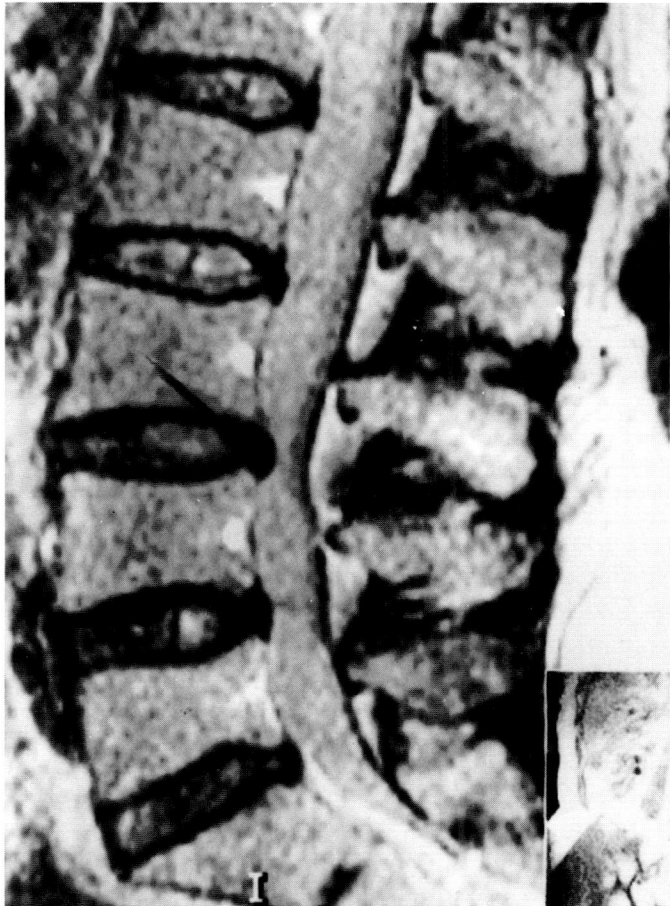

FIGURE 16.
Spinal stenosis with thecal sac compression at L3-4. Minimal posterior bulging at all discal levels without significant loss of vertical disk height.

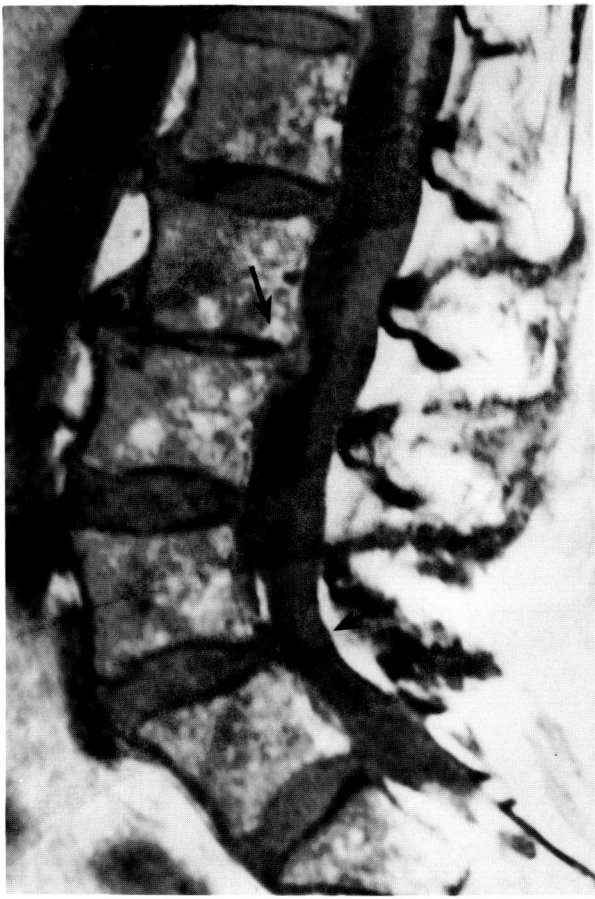

FIGURE 17.
L2-3 disk herniation causing anterior extradural defect and thecal sac stenosis (arrow). Moderate thecal sac stenosis at L4-5 is caused by anterolisthesis of L-4 on L-5, minimal disk herniation and hypertrophy of the ligamentum flavum (arrowhead).

TREATMENT

Regardless of origin or etiology, spinal stenosis of either the central canal or neural canal is often asymptomatic. With the advent of newer imaging technologies, its discovery has increased and all too frequently has resulted in a rush to more invasive tests or treatment based on incidental or irrelevant findings. This activity may result in the development of illness-related behavior and absence from work or other activity by the patient, a pattern previously described in the management of hypertension.[479] Instead of providing reassurance to the patient that the findings are insignificant at the present time, the activity of more testing and active conservative treatment may increase the patients' anxiety and dependence on health care services.[478] It is the physician's responsibility in cases of asymptomatic spinal stenosis to inform and explain to the patient its possible future consequence but to await the onset of clinical symptoms before engaging in active treatment or further testing. Some preventive measures such as posture improvement, ergonomic suggestions, and exercise may be helpful in delaying symptom onset, but these must be done with both the patient and physician fully cognizant that all activity is based on possible, not definite, future clinical events.

In cases of spinal stenosis that are symptomatic such as back pain, neurogenic claudication, and loss of spinal motoricity where no evidence of sphincter disturbances or paralysis is found, nonoperative, conservative management should be the initial management selected.[40, 138, 165, 262, 342] Medical treatment usually consists of nonsteroidal anti-inflammatory medications and exercise programs to strengthen abdominal muscles and reduce the lumbar lordosis.* Bed rest, analgesics, muscle relaxants, local heat, and other physical modalities of pain control are used in the acute stage, with postural exercises, lumbosacral support, and occasionally transcutaneous nerve stimulation used between acute attacks.[132, 262, 481, 482] The use of an exercise bicycle, which allows aerobic activity and strengthens the back and leg muscles while the lumbar spine is flexed forward, may be better tolerated than walking.[145] These treatments have been shown to diminish symptoms in some patients with lateral stenosis[483] and should be used in all patients without significant neurological findings. In patients with Paget's disease, the use of calcitonin, diphosphonates, and mithramycin have been shown to reduce both pain and neurological symptoms.[292-310]

Chiropractic treatment includes many of the same noninvasive, drugless modalities described earlier. In addition, the use of conservative spinal manipulation directed to the level or levels of involvement, soft tissue massage, and physiological therapeutic measures, including short wave diathermy, therapeutic ultrasound, and myoelectric stimulation, are frequently employed. Although no controlled studies are available, the use of spinal manipulation has demonstrated the ability to increase motoricity of the spinal segments involved, lessen the degree of inflammatory response responsible for pain production (presumably by lessening mechanical neurocompressive factors), and permitting increased tolerance of aerobic muscular activity. The use of cryotherapy has been found useful in control of acute pain.

Although the use of these conservative measures may provide control of symptom expression, sometimes for prolonged periods, they do not prevent or permanently inhibit the recurrence of painful radiculopathy with increased patient activity, stress, or fatigue. At times conservative management may be the only alternative in the geriatric patient with concurrent systemic illness in whom surgical intervention is contraindicated.[484]

Surgical treatment for spinal stenosis appears indicated when intolerable pain in activities of daily living, progressively limited walking distances or standing endurance, and major neurological deficits or progressive neurological changes are identified.[1, 48, 138, 363] It should be considered only after adequate conservative treatment fails to provide relief or

---

*References 132, 138, 165, 262, 342, 480.

betterment in the quality of life for the patient, and the natural history of spinal stenosis has been recognized as being characterized by fairly slow progression of symptoms.[485] Surgical decompression of the stenotic area is the typical procedure. Many surgical approaches have been described, but the goal of each is to decompress the thecal sac and exiting nerve roots while minimizing the possibility of subsequent spinal instability.* Wide laminectomy with bilateral foraminotomies is the standard decompressive procedure.[493, 495] When this technique is used, postoperative spinal instability occurs in about 2% of patients older than 35 years of age,[496] although rates as high as 15% have been reported.[497] Fusion of the spine generally is not performed unless degenerative spondylolisthesis is present, because this degenerative process tends to progress, and fusion is needed to prevent or inhibit postoperative instability.[165, 488, 498] Dweyer instrumentation or other internal fixation devices and fusion may by necessary in patients with scoliosis.[179, 180]

Decompression of the lateral recesses requires resection of the medial third of both inferior and superior facets and additional undercutting of hypertrophic facet bone and ligament or joint capsule. Complete facetectomy is rarely required. In elderly patients with spondylosis, complete facetectomy is usually well tolerated if it is unilateral. Unless disks are extruded, they should not be removed because discectomy may increase the possibility of spinal instability after wide decompressive laminectomy and medial facetectomy.[145, 493]

Most patients treated surgically for spinal stenosis obtain good or excellent results, being able to find relief of symptoms and return to most levels of activity. Many, however, are unable to return to work that requires strenuous lifting, prolonged walking or sitting, or riding in an automobile for long distances.[48] Patients with preoperative muscle atrophy or sphincter dysfunction should not anticipate full recovery because of the likelihood of irreversible nerve root damage having already occurred.[145] Mechanical low back pain of interarticular facet origin is the symptom least often relieved by surgical decompression, because although the procedure alleviates nerve root entrapment, it does not alter the underlying degenerative changes that cause synovial or facet insult.[499]

In general the longer the duration of the disease and the more severe the preoperative symptoms, the worse the postoperative results.[48] Preoperative sphincter disturbances, psychosomatic disorders, insurance or medicolegal issues, and poor patient selection all have been associated with poor surgical results.[173, 344]

DISCUSSION

Spinal stenosis is a common condition that, because of its sometimes bizarre and protean symptoms, has frequently been overlooked or underappreciated until irreversible nerve damage has occurred. Patients often have minimal or no abnormal physical findings. When symptoms of adaptation are present, they are often confused with other conditions such

---

*References 36, 37, 77, 78, 146, 165, 363, 486–494.

as osteoarthritis. Typically consideration of stenosis of either the spinal or neural canal is not suspect until the practitioner becomes aware of postural accommodation or neurogenic claudication.

The most commonly encountered cause of stenosis is degenerative disease, but patients with congenital or developmental stenosis may become symptomatic in their second or third decades. Numerous metabolic and systemic diseases and posttraumatic and postsurgical changes are also associated with spinal stenosis.

Many patients with spinal stenosis have a slow, insidious clinical onset before persistent back pain, neurogenic claudication, or radiculopathy are recognized and appreciated as being the result of something other than an acute disk syndrome or some other acute disorder. Most patients respond well to conservative management for long periods and may not require surgical intervention. In some the progressive nature of symptoms and the danger of permanent nerve root injury will indicate the need for operative intervention. Early diagnosis and treatment of spinal stenosis may prevent persistent intractable pain and the permanent neurological sequelae of chronic nerve root entrapment.

The advent of CT and MRI with their ability to visualize the spinal and nerve root canals in both the sagittal and axial plane has dramatically enhanced the identification and measurement of stenosis. Thecal sac or nerve root entrapment can be adequately demonstrated and appropriate clinical or surgical management selected.

ACKNOWLEDGMENT

The assistance of Russell Iwami, reference librarian at the National College of Chiropractic, and staff is greatly appreciated.

REFERENCES

1. Moreland LW, Lopez-Mendez A, Alarcon GS: Spinal stenosis: A comprehensive review of the literature. *Semin Arthritis Rheum* 19:127–149, 1989.
2. Portal A: *Cours d'anatomie medicale on elemens de l'anatomie del'homme.* Paris, Baudovin, 1803, pp 293–319.
3. Bailey P, Casamajor L: Osteoarthritis of the spine as a cause of compression of the spinal cord and its roots: With report of 5 cases. *J Nerv Ment Dis* 38:588–609, 1911.
4. Towne EB, Reichert FL: Compression of the lumbosacral roots of the spinal cord by thickened ligamenta flava. *Ann Surg* 94:327–336, 1931.
5. Verbiest H: A radicular syndrome from developmental narrowing of the lumbar vertebral canal. *J Bone Joint Surg (Br)* 36B:230–237, 1954.
6. Mirkovic S, Garfin S, Rydevik B, et al: Pathophysiology of Spinal Stenosis. *Instruct Course Lect* 41:165–177, 1992.
7. Moreland L, Lopez-Mendez A, Alarcon G: Spinal stenosis as seen by rheumatologists in a University-based practice. *Arthritis Rheum* 32:R38, 1989.
8. Kent DL, Haynor DR, Larson EB, et al: Diagnosis of lumbar spinal stenosis in adults: A metaanalysis of the accuracy of CT, MR, and myelography. *AJR* 158:1135–1144, 1992.
9. Naylor A: Factors in the development of the spinal stenosis syndrome. *J Bone Joint Surg (Br)* 61:306–309, 1979.
10. Blau JN, Logue V: Intermittent claudication of the cauda equina: An unusual

syndrome resulting from central protrusion of a lumbar intervertebral disc. *Lancet* 1:1081–1086, 1961.
11. Arnoldi CC, Brodsky AE, Cauchoix J, et al: Lumbar spinal stenosis and nerve root entrapment syndrome: Definition and classification. *Clin Orthop* 115:4–5, 1976.
12. Postacchini F: Lumbar spinal stenosis and pseudostenosis, definition and classification of pathology. *Ital J Orthop Traumatol* 9:339–350, 1983.
13. Bowen V, Shannon R, Kirkaldy-Willis WH: Lumbar spinal stenosis: A review article. *Childs Brain* 4:257–277, 1978.
14. Epstein BS, Epstein JA, Jones MD: Lumbar spinal stenosis. *Radiol Clin North Am* 15:227–239, 1977.
15. Postacchini F: The diagnosis of lumbar spinal stenosis, analysis of clinical and radiographic findings in 43 cases. *Ital J Orthop Traumatol* 11:5–21, 1985.
16. Verbiest H: Stenosis of the bony lumbar vertebral canal, in Wackenheim A, Babin E (eds): *The Narrow Lumbar Canal: Radiologic Signs and Surgery.* New York, Springer-Verlag 1980, p 115.
17. Weinstein PR: The application of anatomy and pathophysiology in the management of lumbar spine disease. *Clin Neurosurg* 27:517–540, 1980.
18. Epstein BS, Epstein JA, Lavine L: The effect of anatomic variations in the lumbar vertebrae and spinal canal on cauda equina and nerve root syndromes. *AJR* 91:1055–1063, 1964.
19. Angevine JB Jr: Clinically relevant embryology of the vertebral column and spinal cord. *Clin Neurosurg* 20:95–113, 1973.
20. Epstein JA, Malis LI: Compression of spinal cord and cauda equina in achondroplastic dwarfs. *Neurology* 5:875–881, 1955.
21. Sarpyener MA: Congenital stricture of the spinal canal. *J Bone Joint Surg (AM)* 27:70–79, 1945.
22. Verbiest H: A radicular syndrome from developmental narrowing of the lumbar vertebral canal. *J Bone Joint Surg (Br)* 36:230–237, 1954.
23. Morgan DF, Young RF: Spinal neurological complications of achondroplasia. Results of surgical treatment. *J Neurosurg* 52:463–472, 1980.
24. Alexander E Jr: Significance of the small lumbar spinal canal: Cauda equina compression syndrome due to spondylosis: 5. Achondroplasia. *J Neurosurg* 31:513–519, 1969.
25. Pyeritz RE, Sack GLH Jr, Udvarhely GB: Genetics clinics of the John Hopkins Hospital. Surgical intervention in achondroplasia. Cervical and lumbar laminectomy for spinal stenosis in achondroplasia. *Johns Hopkins Med J* 146:203–206, 1980.
26. Bailey JA II: Orthopaedic aspects of achondroplasia. *J Bone Joint Surg (Am)* 52A:1285–1301, 1970.
27. Bergstrrom K, Gaurent U, Lundberg PO: Neurological symptoms in achondroplasia. *Acta Neurol Scand* 47:59–70, 1971.
28. Caffey J: Achondroplasia of pelvis and lumbo-sacral spine. Some roentgenographic features. *AJR* 80:449–457, 1958.
29. Duvoisin RC, Yahr MD: Compressive spinal cord and root syndromes in achondroplastic dwarfs. *Neurology* 12:202–207, 1962.
30. Freund E: Spastic paraplegia in achondroplasia. *Arch Surg* 27:859–867, 1933.
31. Hancock DO, Phillips DG: Spinal compression in achondroplasia. *Paraplegia* 3:23–33, 1965.
32. Lutter LD, Langer LO: Neurological symptoms in achondroplastic dwarfs: Surgical treatment. *J Bone Joint Surg (Am)* 59A:87–92, 1977.

33. Schreiber F, Rosenthal H: Paraplegia from ruptured discs in achondroplastic dwarfs. *J Neurosurg* 9:648–651, 1952.
34. Spillane JD: Three cases of achondroplasia with neurological complications. *J Neurosurg* 15:246–252, 1952.
35. Yamada H, Nakamura D, Tajima M, et al: Neurological manifestations of pediatric achondroplasia. *J Neurosurg* 54:49–57, 1981.
36. Wynne-Davies R, Walsh WK, Gormley J: Achondroplasia and hypochondroplasia. Clinical Variation and spinal stenosis. *J Bone Joint Surg (Br)* 63B:508–515, 1981.
37. Morgan DF, Young RF: Spinal neurological complications of achondroplasia. Results of surgical treatment. *J Neurosurg* 52:463–472, 1980.
38. Joffe R, Appleby A, Arjona V: Intermittent ischaemia of the cauda equina due to stenosis of the lumbar canal. *J Neurol Neurosurg Psychiatry* 29:315–318, 1966.
39. Postacchini F: Lumbar spinal stenosis and pseudostenosis, definition and classification of pathology. *Ital J Orthop Traumatol* 9:339–350, 1983.
40. Bowen V, Shannon R, Kirkaldy-Willis WH: Lumbar spinal stenosis: A review article. *Childs Brain* 4:257–277, 1978.
41. Verbiest H: Fallacies of the present definition, nomenclature, and classification of the stenosis of the lumbar vertebral canal. *Spine* 1:217–225, 1976.
42. Dauser RC, Chandler WF: Symptomatic congenital spinal stenosis in a child. *Neurosurgery* 11:61–63, 1982.
43. Sarpyener MA: Congenital stricture of the spinal canal. *J Bone Joint Surg (AM)* 27:70–79, 1945.
44. Echeverria T, Lockwood RC: Lumbar spinal stenosis: Experience at a community hospital. *NY State J Med* 79:872–873, 1979.
45. Blau JN, Logue V: The natural history of intermittent claudication of the cauda equina: A long-term follow-up study. *Brain* 101:211–222, 1978.
46. Dharker SR, Raman PT, Mathai KV: Congenital stenosis of the lumbar canal, a study of 60 cases. *Neurol India* 26:1–6, 1978.
47. Schatzker J, Pennal GF: Spinal stenosis—a cause of cauda equina compression. *J Bone Joint Surg (Br)* 50B:606–618, 1968.
48. Lee CK, Hansen HT, Weiss AB: Developmental lumbar spinal stenosis: Pathology and surgical treatment. *Spine* 3:246–255, 1978.
49. Verbiest H: Further experiences on the pathological influence of the developmental narrowness of the lumbar vertebral canal. *J Bone Joint Surg (Br)* 37:576–583, 1955.
50. Verbiest H: Results of surgical treatment of idiopathic developmental stenosis of the lumbar vertebral canal, a review of twenty-seven years' experience. *J Bone Joint Surg (Br)* 59:181–188, 1977.
51. Roberson GH, Llewellyn HJ, Taveras JM: The narrow lumbar spinal canal syndrome. *Radiology* 107:89–97, 1973.
52. Verbiest H: Pathomorphologic aspects of developmental lumbar stenosis. *Orthop Clin North Am* 6:177–196, 1975.
53. Tile M, McNeil SR, Zarino RK, et al: Spinal stenosis, results of treatment. *Clin Orthop* 115:104–108, 1976.
54. McIvor GWD, Kirkaldy-Willis WH: Pathologic and myelographic changes in the major types of lumbar spinal stenosis. *Clin Orthop* 115:72–76, 1976.
55. Paine KWE: Results of decompression for lumbar spinal stenosis. *Clin Orthop* 115:96–100, 1976.
56. Jacobson RE, Gargano FP, Rosomoff HL: Transverse axial tomography of the spine: 2. The stenotic spinal canal. *J Neurosurg* 42:412–419, 1975.
57. Sheldon JJ, Russin LA, Gargano FP: Lumbar spinal stenosis, radiographic

diagnosis with special reference to transverse axial tomography. *Clin Orthop* 115:53–67, 1976.
58. Russin LA, Sheldon JJ: Spinal stenosis. Report of series and long term follow-up. *Clin Orthop* 115:101–103, 1976.
59. Birkenfield R, Kasdon DL: Congenital lumbar ridge causing spinal claudication in adolescents: Report of 2 cases. *J Neurosurg* 49:441–444, 1978.
60. Sarpyener MA: Spina bifida aparta and congenital stricture of the spinal canal. *J Bone Joint Surg (AM)* 29:817–821, 1947.
61. Becker DH, Conely FK, Anderson ME: Quadraplegia associated with narrow cervical canal, ligamentous calcification and ankylosing hyperostosis. *Surg Neurol* 11:17–19, 1979.
62. Epstein BS, Epstein JA, Jones MD: Cervical spinal stenosis. *Radiol Clin North Am* 15:215–226, 1977.
63. Hinck VC, Sachdev NS: Developmental stenosis of the cervical spinal canal. *Brain* 89:27–36, 1966.
64. Varughese G, Quartey GR: Familial lumbar spinal stenosis with acute disc herniations: Case report of four brothers. *J Neurosurg* 51:234–236, 1979.
65. Kornbery M, Rechtine GR, Dupuy TE: The treatment of a herniated disc in a young adult with developmental spinal stenosis. *Spine* 9:541–545, 1984.
66. Paine KWE, Huang PWH: Lumbar disc syndrome. *J Neurosurg* 37:75–82, 1972.
67. Nurick S: The pathogenesis of the spinal cord disorder associated with cervical spondylosis. *Brain* 95:87–100, 1972.
68. Clark GA, Panjabi MM, Wetzel FT: Can infant malnutrition cause adult vertebral stenosis? *Spine* 10:165–170, 1985.
69. Verbiest H: The significance and principles of computerized axial tomography in idiopathic developmental stenosis of the bony lumbar vertebral canal. *Spine* 4:369–378, 1979.
70. Edwards WC, LaRocca SH: The developmental segmental sagittal diameter in combined cervical and lumbar spondylosis. *Spine* 10:42–49, 1985.
71. Eisenstein S: Measurements of the lumbar spinal canal in 2 racial groups. *Clin Orthop* 115:42–46, 1976.
72. Porter RW, Wicks M, Ottewell D: Measurement of the spinal canal by diagnostic ultrasound. *J Bone Joint Surg (Br)* 60B:481–484, 1978.
73. Hibbert CS, Porter RW: Relationship between the spinal canal and other skeletal measurements in a Romano-British population. *Ann R Coll Surg Engl* 63:437, 1981.
74. Rich EA: Roentgenology of the spine and pelvis, in *Atlas of Clinical Roentgenology*. Indianapolis, RAE Publishing, 1965, p 162.
75. Postacchini F: Familial lumbar stenosis, case report of three siblings. *J Bone Joint Surg (Am)* 67A:321–323, 1985.
76. Epstein BS, Epstein JA, Jones MD: Lumbar spinal stenosis. *Radiol Clin North Am* 15:227–239, 1977.
77. Bethem D, Winter RB, Luther L, et al: Spinal disorders of dwarfism. *J Bone Joint Surg (Am)* 63A:1412–1425, 1981.
78. Dorwart RH, Vogler JB III, Helms CA: Spinal stenosis. *Radiol Clin North Am* 21:301–325, 1983.
79. Epstein JA, Malis LI: Compression of spinal cord and cauda equina in achondroplastic dwarfs. *Neurology* 5:875–881, 1955.
80. Cartwright DW, Masel JP, Latham SC: The lumbar spinal canal in hypophosphatemic vitamin D–resistant rickets. *Aust NZ J Med* 11:154–157, 1981.
81. Cartwright DW, Latham SC, Masel JP, et al: Spinal cord stenosis in adults with hypophosphatemic vitamin D–resistant rickets. *Aust NZ J Med* 9:705–708, 1979.

82. Yoshikawa S, Shiba M, Suzuki A: Spinal cord compression in untreated adult cases of vitamin D–resistant rickets. *J Bone Joint Surg (Am)* 50A:743–752, 1968.
83. Johnston CC, Kurlander GJ, Smith DM, et al: Familial vitamin D–resistant rickets in untreated adult. *Arch Intern Med* 117:141–147, 1966.
84. Dugger GS, Vandiver RW: Spinal cord compression caused by vitamin D–resistant rickets, case report. *J Neurosurg* 25:300–303, 1966.
85. Newman PH: Stenosis of the lumbar spine in spondylolisthesis. *Clin Orthop* 115:116–121, 1976.
86. Cauchoix J, Benoist M, Chassaing V: Degenerative spondylolisthesis. *Clin Orthop Rel Res* 115:122–129, 1976.
87. Hensinger RN, Lang JR, MacEwen GD: Surgical management of spondylolisthesis in children and adolescents. *Spine* 1:207–216, 1976.
88. Simmons EH, Jackson RP: The management of nerve root entrapment syndromes associated with the collapsing scoliosis of idiopathic lumbar and thoracolumbar curves. *Spine* 4:533–541, 1979.
89. Epstein JA, Epstein BS, Lavine LS: Surgical treatment of nerve root compression caused by scoliosis of the lumbar spine. *J Neurosurg* 41:449–454, 1974.
90. Epstein JA, Epstein BS, Jones MD: Symptomatic lumbar scoliosis with generative changes in the elderly. *Spine* 4:542–547, 1979.
91. Coventry MD, Ghormley RK, Kernohan JW: Discs: Microscopic anatomy and pathology; anatomy, development, and physiology. *J Bone Joint Surg (AM)* 27:105–112, 1945.
92. Kirkaldy-Willis WH: Pathology and pathogenesis of lumbar spondylosis and stenosis. *Spine* 3:319–328, 1978.
93. Weinstein PR: Pathology of lumbar stenosis and spondylosis, in Weinstein PR, Ehni G, Wilson CB (eds): *Lumbar Spondylosis: Diagnosis, Management and Surgical Treatments.* St. Louis, Mosby, 1977, pp 43–91.
94. Epstein JA, Epstein BS, Rosenthal AD, et al: Sciatica caused by nerve root entrapment in the lateral recess: The superior facet syndrome. *J Neurosurg* 36:584–589, 1972.
95. Briggs H, Krause J: The intervertebral foraminotomy for relief of sciatic pain. *J Bone Joint Surg (AM)* 27:475–478, 1945.
96. Epstein JA, Epstein BS: Neurological and radiological manifestations associated with spondylosis of the cervical and lumbar spine. *Bull NY Acad Med* 35:370–386, 1959.
97. Friedmann E: Narrowing of the spinal canal due to thickened lamina: A cause of low back pain and sciatica. *Clin Orthop* 21:190–197, 1961.
98. Schnitker MT, Curtzwiler FC: Hypertrophic osteosclerosis (bony spur) of the lumbar spine. *J Neurosurg* 14:121–128, 1957.
99. Hadley A: Intervertebral joint subluxation, bony impingement and foramen encroachment with nerve root changes. *AJR* 65:377–402, 1951.
100. Herron LD, Trippi AC, Gonyeau M: Intraoperative use of dermatomal somatosensory-evoked potentials in lumbar stenosis surgery. *Spine* 12:379–383, 1987.
101. Epstein JA, Epstein BS, Lavine LS, et al: Obliterative arachnoiditis complicating lumbar spinal stenosis. *J Neurosurg* 48:252–258, 1978.
102. Keim HA: Diagnostic problems in the lumbar spine. *Clin Neurosurg* 25:184–192, 1979.
103. Bohl WR, Steffe AD: Lumbar spinal stenosis. A cause of continued pain and disability in patients after total hip arthroplasty. *Spine* 4:168–173, 1979.
104. Boccanera L, Lelliccioni S, Laus M: Stenosis of the lumbar vertebral canal (a study of 25 cases operated on). *Ital J Orthop Traumatol* 10:227–236, 1984.

105. Macnab I: Negative disc exploration, an analysis of causes of nerve root involvement in sixty-eight patients. *J Bone Joint Surg (Am)* 53A:891–903, 1971.
106. Tsitsopoulos P, Fotiou F, Papakostopoulos D, et al: Comparative study of clinical and surgical findings and cortical somatosensory evoked potentials in patients with lumbar spinal stenosis and disc protrusion. *Acta Neurochir (Wein)* 84:54–63, 1987.
107. Dvonch V, Scarfft, Bunch WH, et al: Dermatomal somatosensory evoked potentials: Their use in lumbar radiculopathy. *Spine* 9:291–293, 1984.
108. Keim HA, Hajdu M, Gonzalez EG, et al: Somatosensory evoked potentials as an aid in the diagnosis and intraoperative management of spinal stenosis. *Spine* 10:338–344, 1985.
109. Surin V, Hedelin E, Smith L: Degenerative lumbar spinal stenosis: Results of operative treatment. *Acta Orthop Scand* 53:79–85, 1982.
110. Natarajan M: Lumbar stenosis. *Int Surg* 60:544–545, 1975.
111. Choudhury AR, Taylor JC: Occult lumbar spinal stenosis. *J Neurol Neurosurg Psychiatry* 40:506–510, 1977.
112. Chahal AS, Mundkur YJ, Sancheti HK, et al: Lumbar canal stenosis. *Paraplegia* 20:288–295, 1982.
113. Weir B, Leo RD: Lumbar stenosis: Analysis of factors affecting outcome in 81 surgical cases. *Can J Neurol Sci* 8:295–298, 1981.
114. Munro D: Lumbar and sacral compression radiculitis (herniated lumbar disc syndrome). *N Engl J Med* 254:243–252, 1956.
115. Schlesinger PT: Low lumbar nerve root compression and adequate operative exposure. *J Bone Joint Surg (Am)* 39A:541–553, 1957.
116. Hasue M, Kida H, Inoue K, et al: Lumbar spinal stenosis, a clinical study of symptoms and therapeutic results. *Int Orthop* 1:133–137, 1977.
117. Frymoyer JW: Backpain and sciatica. *N Engl J Med* 318:291–300, 1988.
118. Uden A, Johnsson KE, Johnsson K, et al: Myelography in the elderly and the diagnosis of spinal stenosis. *Spine* 10:171–174, 1985.
119. Auguier L, Hirsch JF, Paolaggi JB, et al: Stenosis of the lumbar spinal canal and sciatic claudication: A study of 29 cases, thirteen of which were operated upon. *Ann Rheum Dis* 29:691–692, 1970.
120. Gerry CJ: Lumbar spinal stenosis. *J Bone Joint Surg (Br)* 62B:481–485, 1980.
121. Sheldon JJ, Sersland T, Leborgne J: Computed tomography of the lower lumbar vertebral column. *Radiology* 124:113–118, 1977.
122. Ehni G: Significance of the small lumbar spinal canal: Cauda equina syndrome due to spondylosis: IV. Acute compression artificially induced during operation. *J Neurosurg* 31:507–512, 1969.
123. Helms CA: CT of the lumbar spine: Stenosis and arthrosis. *Comput Radiol* 6:359–369, 1982.
124. Schonstrom NS, Bolender NF, Spengler DM: The pathomorphology of spinal stenosis as seen on CT scans of the lumbar spine. *Spine* 10:806–811, 1985.
125. Reynolds AF, Weinstein PW, Wachter RD: Lumbar monoradiculopathy due to unilateral facet hypertrophy. *Neurosurgery* 10:480–486, 1982.
126. Sutro CJ: Lumbar facets—spinal stenosis and intermittent claudication: A mini review. *Bull Hosp Joint Dis* 40:13–37, 1979.
127. Johnsson KE, Willner S, Johnsson K: Postoperative instability after decompression for lumbar spinal stenosis. *Spine* 11:107–110, 1986.
128. Horwitz T: Lesions of the intervertebral disc and ligamentum flavum of the lumbar vertebrae: Anatomic study of 75 human cadavers. *Surgery* 6:410–425, 1939.
129. Grabis SL, Mankin HJ: Pain in the lower back. *Bull Rheum Dis* 30:1040–1045, 1980.

130. Tsuji H: Laminoplasty for patients with compressive myelopathy due to so-called spinal stenosis in cervical and thoracic regions. *Spine* 7:28–34, 1982.
131. Kallina C: Degenerative lumbar stenosis. *Clin Geriatr Med* 1:391–400, 1985.
132. Kirkaldy-Willis WH: The relationship of structural pathology to the nerve root. *Spine* 9:49–52, 1984.
133. Kirkaldy-Willis WH, Wedge JH, Yong-Hing K, et al: Pathology and pathogenesis of lumbar spondylosis and stenosis. *Spine* 3:319–328, 1978.
134. Brodsky AE: Low back pain syndromes due to spinal stenosis and posterior cauda equina compression. *Bull Hosp Joint Dis* 36:66–79, 1975.
135. Keim HA: Diagnostic problems in the lumbar spine. *Clin Neurosurg* 25:184–192, 1979.
136. Reynolds AF, Weinstein PW, Wachter RD: Lumbar monoradiculopathy due to unilateral facet hypertrophy. *Neurosurgery* 10:480–486, 1982.
137. Resnick D, Niwayama G: Entheses and enthesopthy. Anatomical, Pathological and radiological correlation. *Radiology* 146:1–9, 1983.
138. Frymoyer JW: Backpain and sciatica. *N Engl J Med* 318:291–300, 1988.
139. Crock HV: Isolated lumbar disk resorption as a cause of nerve root canal stenosis. *Clin Orthop* 115:109–115, 1976.
140. Venner RM, Crock HV: Clinical studies on isolated disc resorption in the lumbar spine. *J Bone Joint Surg (Br)* 63B:491–494, 1981.
141. Kirkaldy-Willis WH, Hill RJ: A more precise diagnosis for low back pain. *Spine* 4:102–109, 1979.
142. Burton CV, Kenneth BH, Kirkaldy-Willis W, et al: Computed tomographic scanning and the lumbar spine: II. Clinical considerations. *Spine* 4:356–368, 1978.
143. Lancourt JE, Glenn WV, Wiltse LL: Multiplanar computerized tomography in the normal spine and in the diagnosis of spinal stenosis. A gross anatomic-computerized tomographic correlation. *Spine* 4:379–390, 1979.
144. Horwitz T: Lesions of the intervertebral disc and ligamentum flavum of the lumbar vertebrae: Anatomic study of 75 human cadavers. *Surgery* 6:410–425, 1939.
145. Ciricillo SF, Weinstein PR: Lumbar spinal stenosis. *West J Med* 158:171–177, 1993.
146. Ehni G: Surgical treatment of spondylitic caudal radiculopathy, in Weinstein PR, Ehni G, Wilson CB (eds): *Lumbar Spondylosis: Diagnosis, Management and Surgical Treatment*. St. Louis, Mosby, 1977, pp 146–183.
147. Kirkaldy-Willis WH: Pathology and pathogenesis of lumbar spondylosis and stenosis. *Spine* 3:319–329, 1978.
148. McIvor GWD, Kirkaldy-Willis WH: Pathological and myelographic changes in the major types of lumbar spinal stenosis. *Clin Orthop* 115:72–76, 1976.
149. Brown HA: Enlargement of the ligamentum flavum: Cause of low back pain with sciatic radiation. *J Bone Joint Surg (AM)* 20:325–338, 1938.
150. Meredith JM, Lehunan EP: Hypertrophy of the ligamentum flavum. *Surgery* 4:587–596, 1938.
151. Dockerty MB, Love JG: Thickening and fibrosis (so-called hypertrophy) of the ligamentum flavum: A pathological study of fifty cases. *Proc Staff Meet Mayo Clin* 15:161–166, 1940.
152. Macnab I: Negative disc exploration, an analysis of causes of nerve root involvement in sixty-eight patients. *J Bone Joint Surg (Am)* 53A:891–903, 1971.
153. Tsitsopoulos P, Fotiou F, Papakostopoulos D, et al: Comparative study of clinical and surgical findings and cortical somatosensory evoked potentials in patients with lumbar spinal stenosis and disc protrusion. *Acta Neurochir (Wien)* 84:54–63, 1987.

154. Dvonch V, Scarfft, Bunch WH, et al: Dermatomal somatosensory evoked potentials: Their use in lumbar radiculopathy. *Spine* 9:291–293, 1984.
155. Keim HA, Hajdu M, Gonzalez EG, et al: Somatosensory evoked potentials as an aid in the diagnosis and intraoperative management of spinal stenosis. *Spine* 10:338–344, 1985.
156. Surin V, Hedelin E, Smith L: Degenerative lumbar spinal stenosis: Results of operative treatment. *Acta Orthop Scand* 53:79–85, 1982.
157. Natarajan M: Lumbar stenosis. *Int Surg* 60:544–545, 1975.
158. Choudhury AR, Taylor JC: Occult lumbar spinal stenosis. *J Neurol Neurosurg Psychiatry* 40:506–510, 1977.
159. Ciric I, Mikhael MA: Lumbar spinal—lateral recess stenosis. *Neurol Clin* 3:417–423, 1985.
160. Quimjian JD, Matrka PJ: Decompression laminectomy and lateral spine fusion in patients with previously failed lumbar spine surgery. *Orthopedics* 4:563–569, 1988.
161. Herkowitz HN: Spinal stenosis: Clinical evaluation. *Instruct Course Lect* 41:183–185, 1992.
162. Newman PH: Stenosis of the lumbar spine in spondylolisthesis. *Clin Orthop* 115:116–121, 1976.
163. Maurer EL: Spondylolisthesis, in *Practical Applied Roentgenology*. Baltimore, Williams & Wilkins, 1983, p 73.
164. Gehweiler JA Jr, Osborne RL Jr, Becker RF: Spondylolisthesis without spondylolysis, in *The Radiology of Vertebral Trauma*. Philadelphia, WB Saunders, 1980.
165. Wiltse LL, Kirkaldy-Willis WH, McIvor GWD: The treatment of spinal stenosis. *Clin Orthop* 115:83–91, 1976.
166. Epstein BS, Epstein JA, Jones MD: Lumbar spondylolisthesis with isthmic defects. *Radiol Clin North Am* 15:261–274, 1977.
167. Cauchoix J, Benoist M, Chassaing V: Degenerative spondylolisthesis. *Clin Orthop* 115:122–129, 1976.
168. Hensinger RN, Lang JR, MacEwen GD: Surgical management of spondylolisthesis in children and adolescents. *Spine* 1:207–216, 1976.
169. Epstein JA, Epstein BS, Lavine LS, et al: Obliterative arachnoiditis complicating lumbar spinal stenosis. *J Neurosurg* 48:252–258, 1978.
170. Fitzgerald JA, Newman PH: Degenerative spondylolisthesis. *J Bone Joint Surg (Br)* 58B:184–192, 1976.
171. Macnab I: Spondylolisthesis with an intact neural arch, the so-called pseudospondylolisthesis. *J Bone Joint Surg (Br)* 32B:325–333, 1950.
172. Newman PH, Stone KH: The etiology of spondylolisthesis. *J Bone Joint Surg (Br)* 45B:39–59, 1963.
173. Feffer HL, Weisel SW, Cuckler JW, et al: Degenerative spondylosis. To fuse or not to fuse. *Spine* 10:287–289, 1985.
174. Rosenberg NJ: Degenerative spondylolisthesis. *J Bone Joint Surg (Am)* 57A:467–474, 1975.
175. Rosenberg NJ: Degenerative spondylolisthesis: Surgical treatment. *Clin Orthop* 117:112–120, 1976.
176. Epstein BS, Epstein JA, Jones MD: Degenerative spondylolisthesis with an intact neural arch. *Radiol Clin North Am* 15:274–288, 1977.
177. Yoshida M, Shima K, Taniguchi Y, et al: Hypertrophied ligamentum flavum in lumbar spinal canal stenosis. *Spine* 17:1353–1360, 1992.
178. Nelson MA: Lumbar spinal stenosis. *J Bone Joint Surg (Br)* 55B:506–512, 1973.
179. Simmons EH, Jackson RP: The management of nerve root entrapment syn-

dromes associated with the collapsing scoliosis of idiopathic lumbar and thoracolumbar curves. *Spine* 4:533–541, 1979.
180. Epstein JA, Epstein BS, Lavine LS: Surgical treatment of nerve root compression caused by scoliosis of the lumbar spine. *J Neurosurg* 41:449–454, 1974.
181. Epstein JA, Epstein BS, Jones MD: Symptomatic lumbar scoliosis with degenerative changes in the elderly. *Spine* 4:542–547, 1979.
182. San Martino A, D'Andria FM, San Martino C: The surgical treatment of nerve root compression caused by scoliosis of the lumbar spine. *Spine* 8:261–265, 1983.
183. Ruhlin CA, Albert S: Scoliosis complicated by spinal cord involvement. *J Bone Joint Surg (AM)* 23:877–886, 1941.
184. Gortavi P, Fairburn B: Kyphoscoliosis with paraplegia. *J Neurosurg* 33:60–66, 1970.
185. Kleinberg S, Kaplan A: Scoliosis complicated by paraplegia. *J Bone Joint Surg (Am)* 34A:163–167, 1952.
186. Nasca RJ: Surgical management of lumbar spinal stenosis. *Spine* 12:809–816, 1987.
187. Verbiest H: Stenosis of the lumbar vertebral canal and sciatica. *Neurosurg Rev* 3:75–89, 1980.
188. Epstein JA, Epstein BJ, Lavine L: Nerve root compression associated with narrowing of the lumbar spinal canal. *J Neurol Neurosurg Psychiatry* 25:165–176, 1962.
189. Lawrence JS, Sharp J, Ball J, et al: Rheumatoid arthritis of the lumbar spine. *Ann Rheum Dis* 23:205–217, 1964.
190. Resnick D: Calcification and ossification of the posterior spinal ligaments and tissues, in *Bone and Joint Disease*. Philadelphia, WB Saunders, 1989, pp 452–457.
191. Dietemann, JL, Dirheimer Y, Babin E, et al: Ossification of the posterior longitudinal ligament (Japanese disease). A radiological study in 12 cases. *J Neuroradiol* 12:212–222, 1985.
192. Nose T, Egashira T, Enomoto T, et al: Ossification of the posterior longitudinal ligament: A clinico-radiological study of 74 cases. *J Neurol Neurosurg Psychiatry* 50:321–326, 1987.
193. Ono K, Ota H, Tada K, et al: Ossified posterior longitudinal ligament. A clinico-pathologic study. *Spine* 2:126–138, 1977.
194. Resnick D: Ossification of the posterior longitudinal ligament of the spine, in *Diagnosis of Bone and Joint Disorders*. Resnick D, Niwayama G (eds): Philadelphia, WB Saunders, 1981, pp 1453–1461.
195. Yonenobu K, Ebara S, Fujiwara K, et al: Thoracic myelopathy secondary to ossification of the spinal ligament. *J Neurosurg* 66:511–518, 1987.
196. Resnick D, Guerra J, Robinson CA, et al: Association of diffuse idiopathic skeletal hyperostosis (DISH) and Calcification and ossification of the posterior longitudinal ligament. *AJR* 131:1049–1053, 1978.
197. Chin WS, Don CL: Ossification of the posterior longitudinal ligament of the spine. *Br J Radiol* 52:865–869, 1979.
198. Minagi H, Gronner AT: Calcification of the posterior longitudinal ligament: A cause of cervical myelopathy. *AJR* 105:365–369, 1969.
199. Hyman RA, Merten CW, Liebeskind AL, et al: Computed tomography in ossification of the posterior longitudinal ligament. *Neuroradiology* 13:227–228, 1977.
200. Ono K, Ota K, Tada K: Ossified posterior longitudinal ligament: A clinico-pathologic study. *Spine* 2:126–138, 1977.

201. Beamer YB, Garner JT, Sheldon CH: Hypertrophied ligamentum flavum. *Arch Surg* 106:289–292, 1973.
202. Bakay L, Cares HL, Smith RJ: Ossification in the region of the posterior longitudinal ligament as a cause of cervical myelopathy. *J Neurol Neurosurg Psychiatry* 33:263–268, 1970.
203. Beatty RA, Sugar O, Fox TA: Protrusion of the posterior longitudinal ligament simulating herniated lumbar intervertebral disc. *J Neurol Neurosurg Psychiatry* 31:61–66, 1968.
204. Murakami N, Muroga T, Sobue I: Cervical myelopathy due to ossification of the posterior longitudinal ligament. *Arch Neurol* 35:33–36, 1978.
205. Onji Y, Akiyama H, Shimomura Y, et al: Posterior paravertebral ossification causing cervical myelopathy. *J Bone Surg (Am)* 49A:1314–1328, 1967.
206. Yagan R, Khan MA, Bellon EM: Spondylitis and posterior longitudinal ossification in the cervical spine. *Arthritis Rheum* 26:226–230, 1983.
207. Olivieri I, Trippi D, Gemignani G, et al: Ossification of the posterior longitudinal ligament in ankylosing spondylitis. *Arthritis Rheum* 31:452, 1988.
208. Yoshida M, Taniguchi Y, Yamaoto Y, et al: Lumbar canal stenosis associated with calcium crystal deposition in the ligamentum flavum [in Japanese]. *J Japan Med Soc Paraplegia* 5:132–133, 1992.
209. Yoshida M, Funaoka N, Taniguchi Y, et al: Calcification of the ligamentum flavum of the cervical spine [in Japanese]. *Cent Japan J Orthop Surg Traumatol* 34:1333–1334, 1991.
210. Yong-Hing K, Reilly J, Kirkaldy-Willis WH: The ligamentum flavum. *Spine* 1:226–234, 1976.
211. Kubota M, Baba I, Sumida T: Myelopathy due to ossification of the ligamentum flavum of the cervical spine. A report of two cases. *Spine* 6:553–559, 1981.
212. Karpman RR, Weinstein PR, Gall EP: Lumbar spinal stenosis in a patient with diffuse idiopathic skeletal hypertrophy syndrome. *Spine* 7:598–603, 1982.
213. Kawano N, Yoshida S, Ohwada T: Cervical radiculomyelopathy caused by deposition of calcium pyrophosphate dihydrate crystals in the ligamenta flava. *J Neurosurg* 52:279–283, 1980.
214. Omojola MF, Cardoso ER, Fox AJ, et al: Thoracic myelopathy secondary to ossified ligamentum flavum. *J Neurosurg* 56:448–450, 1982.
215. Moiel RH, Ehni G, Anderson MS: Nodule of the ligamentum flavum as a cause of nerve root compression. *J Neurosurg* 27:456–458, 1967.
216. Kamakura K, Namko S, Furukawa T, et al: Cervical Radiculomyelopathy due to calcified ligamenta flava. *Ann Neurol* 5:193–195, 1979.
217. Miyasaka K, Kaneda K, Ito T, et al: Ossification of spinal ligaments causing thoracic radiculomyelopathy. *Radiology* 143:463–468, 1982.
218. Yamamoto R: Operative findings of the lumbar canal stenosis [in Japanese]. *Nippon Seikeigeka Gakkai Zoshi* 51:729–731, 1977.
219. Dockerty MB, Love JG: Thickening and fibrosis (so-called hypertrophy) of the ligamentum flavum: A pathological study of fifty cases. *Proc Staff Meet Mayo Clin* 15:161–166, 1940.
220. Ramsey RH: The anatomy of the ligamenta flava. *Clin Orthop* 44:129–140, 1966.
221. Helms CA: CT of the lumbar spine: Stenosis and arthrosis. *Comput Radiol* 6:359–369, 1982.
222. Naylor A: Factors in the development of the spinal stenosis syndrome. *J Bone Joint Surg (Br)* 61B:306–309, 1979.
223. Sato M: Pathological studies on the lumbar facet joints. *Nippon Seikeigeka Gakkai Zashi* 65:1078–1090, 1991.

224. Niepel GA, Sitaj S: Enthesopathy. *Clin Rheum Dis* 5:857–871, 1979.
225. Rauschning W: Normal and pathologic anatomy of the lumbar root canals. *Spine* 12:1008–1019, 1987.
226. Karpman RR, Weinstein PR, Gall EP, et al: Lumbar spinal stenosis in a patient with diffuse idiopathic skeletal hypertrophy syndrome. *Spine* 7:598–603, 1982.
227. Kurihara A, Tanaka Y, Tsumura N, et al: Hyperostotic lumbar spinal stenosis: A review of 12 surgically treated cases with roentgenographic survey of ossification of the yellow ligament at the lumbar spine. *Spine* 13:1308–1316, 1988.
228. Resnick D: Synovial cysts, Imaging Techniques in Intraspinal Diseases. In Haughton V (ed): *Bone and Joint Imaging*. WB Saunders, Philadelphia, 1989, p 146.
229. Baum JA, Hanley EN Jr: Intraspinal synovial cysts simulating spinal stenosis: A case report. *Spine* 11:487–489, 1986.
230. Sypert GW, Leech RW, Harri AB: Post-traumatic lumbar epidural true synovial cyst: A case report. *J Neurosurg* 39:246–248, 1973.
231. Reust P, Wendling D, Lagier R, et al: Degenerative spondylolisthesis, synovial cyst of the zygoapophyseal joints, and sciatic syndrome: Report of two cases and review of the literature. *Arthritis Rheum* 31:288–294, 1988.
232. Kao CC, Winkler SS, Turner JH: Synovial cyst of spinal facet: A case report. *J Neurosurg* 41:372–376, 1974.
233. Abdullah AF, Chambers RW, Daut DP: Lumbar nerve root compression by synovial cysts of the ligamentum flavum: Report of four cases. *J Neurosurg* 60:617–620, 1984.
234. Haase J: Extradural cyst of ligamentum flavum L-4: A case report. *Acta Orthop Scand* 43:32–38, 1972.
235. Hemminghytt S, Daniels DL, Williams AL, et al: Intraspinal synovial cysts: Natural history and diagnosis by CT. *Radiology* 145:375–376, 1982.
236. Lindquist PR, McDonnell DE: Rheumatoid cyst causing extradural compression. *J Bone Joint Surg (Am)* 52A:1235, 1970.
237. Maresca L, Meland NB, Maresca C, et al: Ganglion cysts of the spinal canal. *J Neurosurg* 57:140–142, 1987.
238. Bland JH, Schymidek HH: Symptomatic intraspinal synovial cyst in a 66 year old marathon runner. *J Rheumatol* 12:1006–1010, 1985.
239. Kurz LT, Garfin SR, Unger AS, et al: Intraspinal synovial cyst causing sciatica. *J Bone Joint Surg (Am)* 67A:865–871, 1985.
240. Jacob JR, Weisman MH, Mink JH, et al: Reversible cause of the back pain and sciatica in rheumatoid arthritis: An apophyseal joint cyst. *Arthritis Rheum* 29:431–435, 1986.
241. Brodsky AE: Post-laminectomy and post-fusion stenosis of the spine. *Clin Orthop* 115:130–139, 1976.
242. Brosky AE: Cauda equina arachnoiditis. A correlative clinical and roentgenologic study. *Spine* 3:51–60, 1978.
243. Phytinen J, Lahde S, Tanska EL, et al: Computed tomography after lumbar myelography in lower back and extremity pain syndrome. *Diagn Imaging* 52:19–22, 1983.
244. Quencer RM, Murtagh FR, Post JD, et al: Postoperative bony stenosis of the lumbar spinal canal: Evaluation of 164 symptomatic patients with axial radiography. *Am J Roentgenol* 131:1059–1064, 1978.
245. Finnegan WJ, Fenlin JM, Marvel JP, et al: Results of surgical intervention in the symptomatic multiple-operated back patient. Analysis of sixty-seven cases followed for three to seven years. *J Bone Joint Surg (Am)* 61A:1077–1082, 1979.

246. Hutter CG: Spinal stenosis and posterior lumbar interbody fusion. *Clin Orthop* 193:103–114, 1985.
247. Jacobs RR, McClain O, Neff J: Control of postlaminectomy scar formation: An experimental and clinical study. *Spine* 5:223–229, 1980.
248. Hirsch C, Nachemson A: The reliability of lumbar disc surgery. *Clin Orthop* 29:189–195, 1963.
249. Benoist M, Deburge A, Heripret G, et al: Treatment of lumbar disc herniation by chymopapain chemonucleolysis. A report of 120 patients. *Spine* 7:613–617, 1982.
250. Deburge A, Rocolle J, Benoist M: Surgical findings and results of surgery after failure of chemonucleolysis. *Spine* 10:812–815, 1985.
251. McCulloch JA: Chemonucleolysis. *J Bone Joint Surg (Br)* 59B:45–52, 1977.
252. Burton CV, Kirkaldy-Willis WH, Young-Hiugk, et al: Causes of failure of surgery on the lumbar spine. *Clin Orthop* 157:191–199, 1981.
253. Hopkins A, Clarke C, Brindley G: Erections on walking as a symptom of spinal canal stenosis. *J Neurol Neurosurg Psychiatry* 50:1371–1374, 1987.
254. Carruthers CC, Kousaie KN: Surgical treatment after chemonucleolysis failure. *Clin Orthop* 165:172–175, 1982.
255. Smith L: Failure with chemonucleolysis. *Orthop Clin North Am* 6:255–259, 1975.
256. DeVilliers PD, Booysen EL: Fibrous spinal stenosis, a report of 850 myelograms with a water-soluble contrast medium. *Clin Orthop* 115:140–144, 1976.
257. Ciappetta P, Delfini R, Cantore GP, et al: CT evaluation of epidural scars following multiple operations for lumbar disc arthrosis. *Eur Neurol* 21:129–135, 1982.
258. Ray CD: New techniques for decompression of lumbar spinal stenosis. *Neurosurgery* 10:587–592, 1982.
259. McLaren AC, Bailey SI: Cauda equina syndrome: A complication of lumbar discectomy. *Clin Orthop* 204:143–149, 1986.
260. Boccanera L, Laus M: Cauda equina syndrome following lumbar spinal stenosis surgery. *Spine* 12:712–715, 1987.
261. Hirabayashi K, Marusjama T, Wakano K, et al: Post-operative lumbar canal stenosis due to anterior spinal fusion. *Keio J Med* 30:133–139, 1981.
262. Kirkaldy-Willis WH, Paine KW, Cauchoix J, et al: Lumbar spinal stenosis. *Clin Orthop* 99:30–50, 1974.
263. Wilkes LL: Paraplegia from operating position and spinal stenosis in non-spinal surgery: A case report. *Clin Orthop* 146:148–149, 1980.
264. Crock HV: Internal disc disruption: A challenge to disc prolapse fifty years on. *Spine* 11:650–653, 1986.
265. Bohl WR, Steffee AD: Lumbar spinal stenosis. A cause of continued pain and disability in patients after total hip arthroplasty. *Spine* 4:168–173, 1979.
266. Weisz GM: Post-traumatic spinal stenosis. *Arch Orthop Trauma Surg* 106:57–60, 1986.
267. Nykamp PW, Levy JM, Christesen F, et al: Computed tomography for a bursting fracture of the lumbar spine. *J Bone Joint Surg (AM)* 60:1108–1109, 1978.
268. Hasue M, Kihuchi S, Inoue K, et al: Posttraumatic spinal stenosis of the lumbar spine: Report of a case caused by hyperextension injury; review of the literature. *Spine* 5:254–263, 1980.
269. Bohlman HH: Late, progressive paralysis and pain following fractures of the thoracolumbar spine. *J Bone Joint Surg (Am)* 58A:728, 1976.
270. Shuman WP, Rogers JV, Sickler ME, et al: Thoracolumbar burst fractures: CT dimensions of the spinal canal relative to postsurgical improvement. *AJR* 145:337–341, 1985.

271. Esses SI: The placement and treatment of thoracolumbar spine fractures, an algorithmic approach. *Orthop Rev* 17:571–584, 1988.
272. Lee M, Lekias J, Gubbay SS, et al: Spinal cord compression by extradural fat after renal transplantation. *Med J Aust* 1:201–203, 1975.
273. Butcher DL, Sahn SA: Epidural lipomatosis: A complication of corticosteroid therapy. *Ann Intern Med* 90:60, 1979.
274. Lipson SJ, Naheedy MH, Kaplan MM, et al: Spinal stenosis caused by epidural lipomatosis in Cushing's syndrome. *N Engl J Med* 302:36, 1980.
275. Chapman PH, Martuza RL, Poletti CE, et al: Symptomatic spinal epidural lipomatosis associated with Cushing's syndrome. *Neurosurgery* 8:724–727, 1981.
276. Archer CR, Smith KR: Extradural lipomatosis simulating an acute herniated nucleus pulposus. *J Neurosurg* 57:559–562, 1982.
277. Russell NA, Belanger G, Benoit BG, et al: Spinal epidural lipomatosis: A complication of glucocorticoid therapy. *Can J Neurol Sci* 11:383–386, 1984.
278. George WE Jr, Wilmot M, Greenhouse A: Medical management of steroid induced epidural lipomatosis. *N Engl J Med* 308:316–319, 1983.
279. Guegan Y, Fardoum R, Launois B, et al: Spinal cord compression after corticosteroid therapy. *J Neurosurg* 56:267–269, 1982.
280. Arroyo IL, Barron KS, Brewer EJ Jr: Spinal cord compression by epidural lipomatosis in juvenile rheumatoid arthritis. *Arthritis Rheum* 31:447–451, 1988.
281. Kaplan PA, Orton DF, Asleson RJ: Osteoporosis with vertebral compression fractures, retropulsed fragments, and neurologic compromise. *Radiology* 165:533–535, 1987.
282. Kaufman HH, Ommaya AK, Dopman JL, et al: Hypertrophy of the ligamentum flavum, secondary cord syndrome in an acromegalic. *Arch Neurol* 25:256–259, 1971.
283. O'Connell JEA: Involvement of the spinal cord by intervertebral disk protrusions. *Br J Surg* 43:225–247, 1955.
284. Epstein H, Whelan M, Benjamin V: Acromegaly and spinal stenosis. *J Neurosurg* 56:145–147, 1982.
285. Hornstein S, Hambrook G, Eyerman E: Spinal cord compression by vertebral acromegaly. *Trans Am Neurol Assoc* 96:254–256, 1971.
286. Efird TA, Genart HK, Wilson CB: Pituitary gigantism with cervical spinal stenosis. *AJR* 134:171–173, 1980.
287. Resnick D, Miwayama G, Goergen TG, et al: Clinical, radiographic and pathological abnormalities in calcium pyrophosphate dihydrate deposition disease (CPPD): Pseudogout. *Radiology* 122:1–15, 1977.
288. Bywaters EGL, Hamilton EBD, Williams R: The spine in idiopathic haemochromatosis. *Ann Rheum Dis* 30:453–465, 1971.
289. Spatola MA, Appelbaum RI: Lumbar spinal stenosis associated with renal osteodystrophy. *Neurosurgery* 20:319–321, 1987.
290. Knight RE, Taddonio RF, Smith FB, et al: Oxalosis: Cause of degenerative spinal stenosis. *Orthopedics* 11:955–958, 1988.
291. Resnick D, Niwayama G: Paget's disease, in Haughton V (ed): *Bone and Joint Imaging*, Philadelphia, WB Saunders, 1989, pp 603–606.
292. Weisz GM: Lumbar canal stenosis in Paget's disease. The staging of the clinical syndrome, its diagnosis and treatment. *Clin Orthop* 206:223–227, 1986.
293. Ravichandran G: Spinal cord function in Paget's disease of the spine. *Paraplegia* 19:7–11, 1981.
294. Walpin LA, Singer FR: Paget's disease, reversal of severe paraparesis with calcitonin. *Spine* 4:213–219, 1979.

295. Cartlidge NET, McCollum JPK, Ayyar RPA: Spinal cord compression in Paget's disease. *J Neurol Neurosurg Psychiatry* 35:825–828, 1972.
296. Herzberg L, Bayliss E: Spinal cord syndrome due to non-compressive Paget's disease of bone: A spinal artery steal phenomenon reversible with calcitonin. *Lancet* 2:13–15, 1980.
297. Schmidek HH: Neurological and neurosurgical sequelae of Paget's disease of bone. *Clin Orthop* 127:70–77, 1977.
298. Chen JR, Rhee RSC, Wallach S, et al: Neurologic disturbances in Paget's disease of bone: Response to calcitonin. *Neurology* 29:448–457, 1979.
299. Hartman JT, Dohn DF: Paget's disease of the spine with cord and nerve root compression. *J Bone Joint Surg (Am)* 48A:1079–1084, 1966.
300. Melick RA, Ebeling P, Hjorth RJ: Improvement in paraplegia in vertebral Paget's disease treated with calcitonin. *BMJ* 1:627–628, 1976.
301. Sadar ES, Walton RJ, Gossman HH: Neurological dysfunction in Paget's disease of the vertebral column. *J Neurosurg* 37:661–665, 1972.
302. Weisz GM: Lumbar spinal canal stenosis in Paget's disease. *Spine* 8:192–198, 1983.
303. Diredze M, Milnes JN: Spinal cord compression in Paget's disease. *Br J Surg* 57:239–240, 1970.
304. Ravichandran G: Neurologic recovery of paraplegia following use of salmon calcitonin in a patient with Paget's disease of the spine. *Spine* 4:37, 1979.
305. Franck WA, Bress NM, Singer FR, et al: Rheumatic manifestations of Paget's disease of bone. *Am J Med* 56:592–603, 1974.
306. Douglas DL, Duckworth T, Kanis JA, et al: Spinal cord dysfunction in Paget's disease of bone. *J Bone Joint Surg (Am)* 63A:495–503, 1981.
307. Schumacher M, Levy A, Beck U, et al: Paget's disease with spinal cord compression: Favourable course after decompression and calcitonin treatment in two cases. *Eur Neurol* 15:116–120, 1977.
308. Shai F, Baker RK, Wallach S: The clinical and metabolic effects of porcine calcitonin on Paget's disease of bone. *J Clin Invest* 50:1927–1940, 1971.
309. Epstein BS, Epstein JA: The association of cerebellar tonsillar herniation with basilar impression incident to Paget's disease. *AJR* 107:535, 1969.
310. Kleverman L: Cauda equina and spinal cord compression in Paget's disease. *J Bone Joint Surg (Br)* 48B:365–370, 1966.
311. Weinstein PR, Karpman RR, Gall EP, et al: Spinal cord injury, spinal fracture, and spinal stenosis in ankylosing spondylitis. *J Neurosurg* 57:609–616, 1982.
312. Good AE, Keller TS, Weatherbee L, et al: Spinal cord block with a destructive lesion of the dorsal spine in ankylosing spondylitis. *Arthritis Rheum* 25:218–222, 1982.
313. Dihlmann W, Delling G: Discovertebral destructive lesions (so-called Anderson lesions) associated with ankylosing spondylitis. *Skeletal Radiol* 3:10–16, 1978.
314. Russell ML, Gordon DA, Ogryzlo MS, et al: The cauda equina syndrome of ankylosing spondylitis. *Ann Intern Med* 78:551–554, 1973.
315. Gordon AL, Yudell A: Cauda equina lesion associated with rheumatoid spondylitis. *Ann Intern Med* 78:555–557, 1973.
316. Bowie EA, Glasgow GL: Cauda equina lesions associated with ankylosing spondylitis. *BMJ* 2:24–27, 1961.
317. Hauge T: Chronic rheumatoid polyarthritis and spondyloarthritis associated with neurological symptoms and signs occasionally simulating an intraspinal expansive process. *Acta Chir Scand* 120:395–401, 1961.
318. Lee MLH, Waters DJ: Neurological complication of ankylosing spondylitis. *BMJ* 1:798, 1962.

319. McGill IG: An unusual neurological syndrome associated with ankylosing spondylitis. *Guys Hosp Rep* 115:33–36, 1966.
320. Matthews WB: The neurological complications of ankylosing spondylitis. *J Neurol Sci* 6:561–573, 1968.
321. Rosenkrang W: Ankylosing spondylitis: Cauda equina syndrome with multiple spinal arachnoid cysts. *J Neurosurg* 34:241–243, 1971.
322. Kramer LD, Krouth GJ: Computerized tomography. An adjunct to early diagnosis in the cauda equina syndrome of ankylosing spondylitis. *Arch Neurol* 35:116–118, 1978.
323. Thomas DJ, Kendall MJ, Whitfield AGW: Nervous system involvement in ankylosing spondylitis. *BMJ* 1:148–150, 1974.
324. Alenghat JP, Hallet M, Kido DK: Spinal cord compression in diffuse idiopathic skeletal hyperostosis. *Radiology* 142:119–120, 1982.
325. Utsinger PD, Resnick D, Shapiro R: Diffuse skeletal abnormalities in Forestier's disease. *Arch Intern Med* 136:763–768, 1976.
326. Resnick D, Shall SR, Robins JM: Diffuse idiopathic skeletal hyperostosis (DISH): Forestier's disease with extraspinal manifestations. *Radiology* 115:513–524, 1975.
327. Forestier J, Rotes-Querol J: Senile ankylosing hyperostosis of the spine. *Ann Rheum Dis* 9:321–330, 1950.
328. Weisz GM: Stenosis of the lumbar spine in Forestier's disease. *Int Orthop* 7:61–64, 1983.
329. Weinstein PR: Forestier's disease and lumbar stenosis. *Spine* 8:919, 1983.
330. Epstein JA, Carras R, Ferras J: Conjoined lumbosacral nerve roots. *J Neurosurg* 55:585–589, 1982.
331. Cannon BW, Hunter SE, Picaza JA: Nerve root anomalies in lumbar-disc surgery. *J Neurosurg* 19:208–214, 1962.
332. Helms CA, Dorwart RH, Gray M: The CT appearance of conjoined nerve roots and differentiation from a herniated nucleus pulposus. *Radiology* 144:803–807, 1982.
333. Rask MR: Anomalous lumbosacral nerve roots associated with spondylolisthesis. *Surg Neurol* 8:139–140, 1977.
334. Bouchard JM, Copty M, Langelier R: Preoperative diagnosis of conjoined root anomaly with herniated lumbar disks. *Surg Neurol* 10:229–231, 1978.
335. Sharma RR, Ramakantan B, Bhama A, et al: Late post-traumatic spinal stenotic progressive myelo-radiculopathy. *J Postgrad Med* 36:33–37, 1990.
336. Mirkovic S, Garfin SR, Bjorn R, et al: Pathophysiology of spinal stenosis. *Instruct Course Lect* 41:165–177, 1992.
337. Boden SD, Davis DO, Dina TS, et al: Abnormal magnetic resonance scans of the lumbar spine in asymptomatic subjects. A positive investigation. *J Bone Joint Surg (Am)* 72A:403–408, 1990.
338. Resnick D, Niwayama G: Degenerative disease of the spine, in Haughton V (ed): *Bone and Joint Imaging*. Philadelphia, WB Saunders, 1989, p 435.
339. Hall S, Bartleson JD, Onofrio BM, et al: Lumbar spinal stenosis, clinical features, diagnostic procedures, and results of surgical treatment in 68 patients. *Ann Intern Med* 103:271–275, 1985.
340. Herkowitz HN: Spinal stenosis: Clinical evaluation. *Instruct Course Lect* 41:183–185, 1992.
341. Paine KWE: Clinical features of lumbar spinal stenosis. *Clin Orthop* 115:77–82, 1976.
342. Spengler DM: Degenerative stenosis of the lumbar spine. *J Bone Joint Surg (Am)* 69A:305–308, 1987.
343. Salibi BS: Neurogenic intermittent claudication and stenosis of the lumbar spinal canal. *Surg Neurol* 5:269–272, 1976.

344. Kallina C: Degenerative lumbar stenosis. *Clin Geriatr Med* 1:391–400, 1985.
345. Simkin PA: Simian stance: A sign of spinal stenosis. *Lancet* 2:652–653, 1982.
346. Spengler DM: Current concepts review: Degenerative stenosis of the lumbar spine. *J Bone Joint Surg (Am)* 69A:305–308, 1987.
347. Blau JN, Logue L: Intermittent claudication of the cauda equina: An unusual syndrome resulting from central protrusion of a lumbar intervertebral disc. *Lancet* 1:1081–1086, 1961.
348. Lipson S: Clinical diagnosis of spinal stenosis. *Semin Spine Surg* 1:143–144, 1989.
349. Nelson MA: Lumbar spinal stenosis. *J Bone Joint Surg (Br)* 55B:506–512, 1973.
350. Jones RAC, Thomson JLG: The narrow lumbar canal: A clinical and radiological review. *J Bone Joint Surg* 50B:595–605, 1968.
351. Kirkaldy-Willis WH, Paine KWE, Cauchoix J, et al: Lumbar spinal stenosis. *Clin Orthop* 99:30–50, 1974.
352. Harris P: Cervical spine stenosis. *Paraplegia* 15:125–132, 1977.
353. Veidinger OF, Colwill JC, Smyth HS, et al: Cervical myelopathy and its relationship to cervical stenosis. *Spine* 6:550–552, 1981.
354. Crandall PM, Gregorius FK: Long-term follow-up of surgical treatment of cervical spondylitic myelopathy. *Spine* 2:139–146, 1977.
355. Brain WR, Northfield DW, Wilkinson M: The neurological manifestations of cervical spondylosis. *Brain* 75:187–225, 1952.
356. Epstein JA, Epstein BA, Lavine LA, et al: Cervical myeloradiculopathy caused by arthritic hypertrophy of the posterior facets and laminae. *J Neurosurg* 49:387–392, 1978.
357. Tammela TLJ, Heiskari MJ, Lukkarinen OA: Voiding dysfunction and urodynamic findings in patients with cervical spondylotic spinal stenosis compared with severity of the disease. *Br J Urol* 70:144–148, 1992.
358. Jahnke RW, Hart BL: Cervical stenosis, spondylosis, and herniated disc disease. *Radiol Clin North Am* 29:777–791, 1991.
359. Dagi TF, Tarkington MA, Leech JJ: Tandem lumbar and cervical spinal stenosis. Natural history, prognostic indices, and results after surgical decompression. *J Neurosurg* 66:842–849, 1982.
360. Teng P, Papatheodorou C: Combined cervical and lumbar spondylosis. *Arch Neurol* 10:298–307, 1964.
361. Epstein NE, Epstein JA, Carras R, et al: Coexisting cervical and lumbar stenosis: Diagnosis and management. *Neurosurgery* 15:489–496, 1984.
362. Edwards WC, LaRocca SH: The developmental segmental sagittal diameter in combined cervical and lumbar spondylosis. *Spine* 10:42–49, 1985.
363. Grabis S: The treatment of spinal stenosis. *J Bone Joint Surg (Am)* 62A:308–313, 1980.
364. McKinley LM, Davis GL: The narrow lumbar spinal canal or lumbar spinal stenosis. *Clin Orthop* 114:319–325, 1976.
365. Wilson CB: Significance of the small lumbar spinal canal: Cauda equina compression syndromes due to spondylosis. *J Neurosurg* 31:499–506, 1969.
366. Sonntag VK: Unusual presentations of lumbar stenosis. *Ariz Med* 41:228–234, 1984.
367. Brish A, Lerner MA, Braham J: Intermittent claudication from compression of cauda equina by a narrowed spinal canal. *J Neurosurg* 21:207–211, 1964.
368. Ravindran M: Cauda equina compression presenting as spontaneous priapism. *J Neurol Neurosurg Psychiatry* 42:280–282, 1979.
369. Laha RK, Dujovny M, Huang PS: Intermittent erection in spinal canal stenosis. *J Urol* 121:123–124, 1979.

370. Ram Z, Findler G, Spiegelman R, et al: Intermittent priapism in spinal canal stenosis. *Spine* 2:377–378, 1987.
371. Wilson CB, Ehni G, Grollmus J: Neurogenic intermittent claudication. *Clin Neurosurg* 18:62–85, 1971.
372. Grabias S: Current concepts review: The treatment of spinal stenosis. *J Bone Joint Surg (Am)* 62A:308–313, 1980.
373. Hall S, Bartleson JD, Onfrio BM, et al: Lumbar spinal stenosis: Clinical features, diagnostic procedures and results in surgical treatment in 68 patients. *Ann Intern Med* 103:271–275, 1985.
374. Schatzker J, Pennal GF: Spinal stenosis: A cause of cauda equina compression. *J Bone Joint Surg (Br)* 50B:606–618, 1968.
375. Blau JN, Logue V: Intermittent claudication of the cauda equina. An unusual syndrome resulting from central protrusion of a lumbar intervertebral disc. *Lancet* 1:1081–1086, 1961.
376. Dodge LD, Bohlman HH, Rhodes RS: Concurrent lumbar spinal stenosis and peripheral vascular disease. *Clin Orthop* 230:141–148, 1988.
377. Hawkes CH, Roberts GM: Neurogenic and vascular claudication. *J Neurosurg Sci* 38:337–345, 1978.
378. Dyke P, Doyle JB: "Bicycle test" of Van Gelderen in diagnosis of intermittent cauda equina compression syndrome. *J Neurosurg* 46:667–670, 1977.
379. Thomas PK: Clinical features and differential diagnosis, in Dyck P, Thomas P, Lambert E, et al (eds): *Peripheral Neuropathy*, ed 2. Philadelphia, WB Saunders, 1984, pp 1169–1190.
380. Kirkaldy-Willis W, Hill RJ: A more precise diagnosis for low back pain. *Spine* 4:102–109, 1979.
381. Hanaig K: Dynamic measurement of interosseous pressures in lumbar spinal vertebrae with reference to spinal canal stenosis. *Spine* 5:568–574, 1980.
382. Edgar MA, Ghadially JA: Innervation of the lumbar spine. *Clin Orthop* 115:34–41, 1976.
383. Mooney V, Robertson J: The facet syndrome. *Clin Orthop* 115:149–156, 1976.
384. Gooding MR: Pathogenesis of myelopathy in cervical spondylosis. *Lancet* 1:1180–1181, 1974.
385. Sinclair DC, Feindel WH, Weddell G, et al: The intervertebral ligament as a source of segmental pain. *J Bone Joint Surg (Br)* 30B:515–521, 1948.
386. Edgar MA, Ghadially JA: Innervation of the lumbar spine. *Clin Orthop* 115:35–41, 1976.
387. Inman VT, Saunders JB: Referred pain from skeletal structures. *J Nerv Ment Dis* 99:660–667, 1944.
388. Stillwell DL: Nerve supply of vertebral column. *Anat Rec* 125:139–142, 1956.
389. Dommisse GF: Morphological aspects of the lumbar spine and lumbosacral region. *Orthop Clin North Am* 6:163–175, 1975.
390. Crock HV, Yoshizawa H: *The Blood Supply of the Vertebral Column and Spinal Cord in Man*. New York, Springer-Verlag, 1977.
391. Arvidson B: Distribution of intravenously injected protein tracers in peripheral ganglia of adult mice. *Exp Neurol* 63:388–410, 1979.
392. Watanabe R, Parke WW: Vascular and neural pathology of lumbosacral spinal stenosis. *J Neurosurg* 64:64–70, 1986.
393. Parke WW, Gammell K, Rothman RH: Arterial vascularization of the cauda equina. *J Bone Joint Surg (Am)* 63A:53–62, 1981.
394. Parke WW, Watanabe R: The intrinsic vasculature of the lumbosacral spinal nerve roots. *Spine* 10:508–515, 1985.
395. Blau JN, Logue V: Intermittent claudication of the cauda equina: An unusual

syndrome resulting from central protrusion of a lumbar intervertebral disc. *Lancet* 1:1081–1086, 1961.
396. Blau JN, Rushworth G: Observations on the blood vessels of the spinal cord and their responses to motor activity. *Brain* 81:354–363, 1958.
397. Olsson Y: The involvement of vasa nervorum in the diseases of peripheral nerves, in Vinken PJ, Bruyn GW (eds): *Handbook of Clinical Neurology. Vascular Diseases Of The Nervous System, Part II*. New York, American Elsevier, 1972, vol 12, pp 644–664.
398. Clark K: Significance of the small lumbar spinal canal: Cauda equina compression syndrome due to spondylosis: 2. Clinical and surgical significance. *J Neurosurg* 31:495–498, 1969.
399. Schonstrom NS, Bolender NF, Spengler DM: The pathomorphology of spinal stenosis as seen on CT scans of the lumbar spine. *Spine* 10:806–811, 1985.
400. Jacobson RE: Lumbar stenosis, an electromyographic evaluation. *Clin Orthop* 115:68–71, 1976.
401. Eisen A, Hoirch M: The electrodiagnostic evaluation of spinal root lesions. *Spine* 8:98–106, 1983.
402. Postacchini F: The diagnosis of lumbar spinal stenosis, analysis of clinical and radiographic findings in 43 cases. *Ital J Orthop Traumatol* 11:5–21, 1985.
403. Johnsson K, Rosen I, Uden A: Neurophysiological investigation of patients with spinal stenosis. *Spine* 12:483–487, 1985.
404. Dvonch V, Scarff T, Bunch W, et al: Dermatomal somatosensory evoked potentials: Their use in lumbar radiculopathy. *Spine* 9:291–293, 1984.
405. Scarff TB, Dallmann DE, Toleikis JR, et al: Dermatomal somatosensory evoked potentials in the diagnosis of lumbar root entrapment. *Surg Forum* 32:489–491, 1981.
406. Slimp JC, Rubner DE, Snowden ML, et al: Dermatomal somatosensory evoked potentials: Cervical, thoracic and lumbosacral. *Electroencephalogr Clin Neurophysiol* 84:55–70, 1992.
407. Stolov WC, Slimp JC: Dermatomal somatosensory evoked potentials in lumbar spinal stenosis. American Association of Electromyography and Electrodiagnosis, American Electroencephalography Society Joint Symposium, San Diego, 1988, pp 17–22.
408. Wall EJ, Cohen MS, Massie JB, et al: Cauda equina anatomy: I. Intrathecal nerve root organization. *Spine* 15:1244–1247, 1990.
409. Wall EJ, Cohen MS, Massie JB, et al: Cauda equina anatomy: II. Extrathecal nerve roots and dorsal root ganglia. *Spine* 15:1248–1251, 1990.
410. Snowden ML, Haselkorn JK, Kraft GH, et al: Dermatomal somatosensory evoked potentials in the diagnosis of lumbosacral spinal stenosis: Comparison with imaging studies. *Muscle Nerve* 15:1036–1044, 1992.
411. Scarff TB, Dallmann DE, Toleikis JR: Dermatomal somatosensory evoked potentials in the diagnosis of lumbar root entrapments. *Surg Forum* 32:489–491, 1981.
412. Gonzalez EG, Hajdu M, Bruno R, et al: Lumbar spinal stenosis: Analysis of pre- and postoperative somatosensory evoked potentials. *Arch Phys Med Rehabil* 66:11–15, 1985.
413. Larsen SJ: Somatosensory evoked potentials in lumbar stenosis. *Surg Gynecol Obstet* 157:191–196, 1983.
414. Machida M, Weinstein SL, Yamada T, et al: Spinal cord monitoring, electrophysiological measures of sensory and motor function during spinal surgery. *Spine* 10:407–413, 1985.
415. Johnsson KE, Willner S, Pettersson H: Analysis of operated cases with lumbar recess stenosis. *Acta Orthop Scand* 52:427–433, 1981.

416. Larsen JL: The lumbar spinal canal in children: II. The interpedicular distance and its relation to the sagittal diameter and transverse pedicular width. *Eur J Radiol* 1:312–321, 1981.
417. Eisenstein S: Lumbar vertebral canal morphometry for computerized tomography in spinal stenosis. *Spine* 8:187–191, 1983.
418. Eisenstein S: Measurement of the lumbar spinal canal in 2 racial groups. *Clin Orthop* 115:42–46, 1976.
419. Schonstrom NSR, Bolender NF, Spengler DM, et al: Pressure changes within the cauda equina following construction of the dural sac. *Spine* 9:604–607, 1984.
420. Schonstrom NSR, Bolender NF, Spengler DM: The pathomorphology of spinal stenosis as seen on CT scans of the lumbar spine. *Spine* 10:806–812, 1985.
421. McCall IW: Radiology of spinal stenosis. *Acta Orthop Scand* 64(suppl 251):59–60, 1993.
422. Verbiest H: Further experiences on the pathological influence of a developmental narrowness of the bony lumbar vertebral canal. *J Bone Joint Surg (Br)* 37B:576, 1955.
423. Verbiest H: Neurogenic intermittent claudication with absolute and relative stenosis of the lumbar vertebral canal (ASLC and RSLC), in cases with narrow lumbar intervertebral foramina, and in cases with both entities. *Clin Neurosurg* 20:204, 1972.
424. Verbiest H: Results of surgical treatment of idiopathic developmental stenosis of the lumbar vertebral canal: A review of twenty-seven years experience. *J Bone Joint Surg (Br)* 59B:181–188, 1977.
425. Eisenstein SM: The morphometry and pathological anatomy of the lumbar spine in South African Negroes and Caucasoids with specific reference to spinal stenosis. *J Bone Joint Surg (Br)* 54:173–180, 1977.
426. Eisenstein S: Measurements of the lumbar spinal canal in two racial groups. *Clin Orthop* 115:42–46, 1976.
427. Buehler MT: Spinal stenosis. *J Manipulative Physiol Ther* 1:103–112, 1978.
428. Dailey EJ, Buehler MT: Plain film assessment of spinal stenosis: Method comparison with lumbar CT. *J Manipulative Physiol Ther* 3:192–199, 1989.
429. Ullrich CG, Binet EF, Sanecki MG, et al: Quantitative assessment of the lumbar spinal canal by computed tomography. *Radiology* 134:137–143, 1980.
430. Epstein NE, Epstein JA: Individual and coexistent lumbar and cervical spinal stenosis: Diagnosis and management. *Spine* 1:401–420, 1987.
431. Resnick D: Imaging techniques in intraspinal diseases, in Haughton V (ed): *Bone And Joint Imaging*. Philadelphia, WB Saunders, 1989, pp 142–153.
432. Uden A, Johnsson KE, Jonsson K, et al: Myelography in the elderly and the diagnosis of spinal stenosis. *Spine* 10:171–174, 1985.
433. Rothman RH, Campbell RE, Mankowitz E: Myelographic patterns in lumbar disk degeneration. *Clin Orthop* 99:18–29, 1974.
434. Crane R, Margolis MT: Use of sitting position to relieve myelographic obstruction. *AJNR* 7:502–503, 1986.
435. Kapila A, Chakeres DW: Flexed sitting maneuver for complete lumbar myelography in patients with severe spinal stenosis and apparent block. *Radiology* 160:265–267, 1986.
436. Epstein BS, Epstein JA, Jones MD: Lumbar spinal stenosis. *Radiol Clin North Am* 15:227–239, 1977.
437. McAfee PC, Ullrich CG, Yuan HA, et al: Computed tomography in degenerative spinal stenosis. *Acta Orthop Scand* 52:427–433, 1981.
438. Galanski M, Weidner A, Vogelsang H: Der Enge Lumbale Spinalkanal. *Roentgenblatter* 31:450, 1982.
439. Lackner K, Schroeder S, Koester O: Quantitative Auswertung, Indikationen

und Wertigkeit der Computer Tomographic der Lendenwirbelsaeule. *ROFO* 137:309, 1982.
440. Nagase J: Experimental and clinical studies on the diagnostic value of CT-myelography using a water-soluble contrast medium, metrizamide. *Nippon Seikeigeka Gakkai Zasshi* 56:1569, 1982.
441. Bolender NF, Schonstrom NSR, Spengler DM: Role of computerized tomography and myelography in the diagnosis of central spinal stenosis. *J Bone Joint Surg (Am)* 67A:240–245, 1985.
442. Dublin AB, McGahan JP, Reid MH: The value of computed tomographic metrizamide myelography in the neuroradiological evaluation of the spine. *Radiology* 146:79–86, 1983.
443. Natelson SE: The injudicious laminectomy. *Spine* 11:966–969, 1986.
444. Bell GR, Rothman RH, Booth RE, et al: A study of computer assisted tomography. *Spine* 9:552–556, 1984.
445. Porter RW, Ward D: Cauda equina dysfunction. The significance of two-level pathology. *Spine* 17:9–15, 1992.
446. Olmarker K, Rydevik B: Single versus double level nerve root compression. An experimental study on the porcine cauda equina with analysis of nerve impulse conduction properties. *Clin Orthop* 279:35–39, 1992.
447. Ooi Y, Mita F, Satoh Y: Myeloscopic study on lumbar spinal canal stenosis with special reference to intermittent claudication. *Spine* 15:544–549, 1990.
448. Bolender NF, Schonstrom NSR, Spengler DM: Role of computerized tomography and myelography in the diagnosis of central spinal stenosis. *J Bone Joint Surg (AM)* 67:240–245, 1985.
449. Weisz GM: Post-traumatic spinal stenosis. *Arch Orthop Trauma Surg* 106:57–60, 1986.
450. Simeone FA, Rothman RH: Clinical usefulness of CT scanning in the diagnosis and treatment of lumbar spine disease. *Radiol Clin North Am* 21:197–200, 1983.
451. Williams DM, Gabrielson TO, Latack JT, et al: Ossification in the cephalic attachment of the ligamentum flavum: An anatomical and CT study. *Radiology* 150:423–426, 1984.
452. Arroyo IL, Barron KS, Brewer EJ: Spinal cord compression by epidural lipomatosis in juvenile rheumatoid arthritis. *Arthritis Rheum* 31:447–451, 1988.
453. Urso S, Postacchini F: The value of transverse axial tomography in the diagnosis of lumbar stenosis. *Ital J Orthop Traumatol* 4:213–221, 1978.
454. Simeone FA, Rothman RH: Clinical usefulness of CT scanning in the diagnosis and treatment of lumbar spine disease. *Radiol Clin North Am* 21:197–200, 1983.
455. Postacchini F, Petteri G: CT scanning versus myelography in the diagnosis of lumbar stenosis, a preliminary report. *Int Orthop* 5:209–215, 1981.
456. Lee BCP, Kazam E, Neuman AD: Computed tomography of the spine and spinal cord. *Radiology* 128:95–102, 1978.
457. Hammerschlag SB, Wolpert SM, Carter BL: Computed tomography of the spinal canal. *Radiology* 121:361–367, 1976.
458. Weinstein PR: Diagnosis and management of lumbar spinal stenosis. *Clin Neurosurg* 30:677–697, 1983.
459. Herkowitz HN, Garlin SR, Bell GR, et al: The use of computerized tomography in evaluating non-visualized vertebral levels caudad to a complete block on a lumbar myelogram, a review of thirty-two cases. *J Bone Joint Surg (Am)* 69A:218–224, 1987.
460. Pyhtinen J, Lahde S, Tanska EL, et al: Computed tomography after lumbar myelography in lower back and extremity pain syndromes. *Diagn Imaging* 52:19–22, 1983.

461. Quencer RM, Murtagh FR, Post JD, et al: Postoperative bony stenosis of the lumbar spinal canal: Evaluation of 164 symptomatic patients with axial radiography. *AJR* 131:1059–1064, 1978.
462. Pleatment CW, Lukin RR: Lumbar spinal stenosis. *Semin Roentgenol* 23:106–110, 1988.
463. Kaiser MC, Capesius P, Roilgen A, et al: Epidural venous stasis in spinal stenosis—CT appearance. *Neuroradiology* 26:435–438, 1985.
464. Helms CA: CT of the lumbar spine—stenosis and arthrosis. *Comput Radiol* 6:359–369, 1982.
465. Gaskill MF, Lukin R, Wiot JG: Lumbar disc disease and stenosis. *Radiol Clin North Am* 29:753–764, 1991.
466. Schnebel B, Kingston S, Watkins R, et al: Comparison of MRI to CT in the diagnosis of spinal stenosis. *Spine* 14:332–337, 1989.
467. Crawshaw C, Kean DM, Mulholland RC, et al: The use of nuclear magnetic resonance in the diagnosis of lateral canal entrapment. *J Bone Joint Surg (AM)* 66:711–715, 1984.
468. Modic MT, Masaryk T, Boumphrey M, et al: Lumbar herniated disk disease and canal stenosis: Prospective evaluation by surface coil MR, CT, and myelography. *AJR* 147:757–765, 1986.
469. Gaskill M, Lukin R, Wiot G: Lumbar disc disease and stenosis. *Radiol Clin North Am* 29:753–764, 1991.
470. Modic MT, Masaryk TJ, Mulopulos GP, et al: Cervical radiculopathy: Prospective evaluation with surface coil MR imaging, CT with metrizamide, and metrizamide myelography. *Radiology* 161:753–759, 1986.
471. Modic MT, Masaryk TJ, Ross JS, et al: Cervical radiculopathy: value of oblique MR imaging. *Radiology* 163:227–231, 1987.
472. Hedberg MC, Drayer BP, Flom RA, et al: Gradient echo (GRASS) MR imaging in cervical radiculopathy. *AJR* 150:683–689, 1988.
473. Van Dyke C, Ross JS, Tkach J, et al: Gradient-echo MR imaging of the cervical spine: Evaluation of extradural disease. *Am J Neuroradiol* 10:627–632, 1989.
474. Yousem DM, Atlas SW, Goldberg HI, et al: Degenerative narrowing of the cervical spine neural foramina: Evaluation with high-resolution 3DFT gradient-echo MR imaging. *Am J Neuroradiol* 12:229–236, 1991.
475. Kent DL, Haynor DR, Larson EB, et al: Diagnosis of lumbar spinal stenosis in adults: A metaanalysis of the accuracy of CT, MR, and myelography. *Am J Radiol* 158:1135–1144, 1992.
476. Rydevik B: Spinal stenosis—conclusions. *Acta Orthop Scand* 64:81–82, 1993.
477. Jensen MC, Brant-Zawadzki MN, Obuchowski N, et al: Magnetic resonance imaging of the lumbar spine in people without back pain. *N Engl J Med* 331:69–73, 1994.
478. Deyo RA: Magnetic resonance imaging of the lumbar spine. [editorial]. *N Engl J Med* 331:115–116, 1994.
479. Haynes RB, Sackett DL, Taylor DW, et al: Increased absenteeism from work after detection and labeling of hypertensive patients. *N Engl J Med* 299:741–744, 1978.
480. Lee CK, Hansen HT, Weiss AB: Development lumbar spinal stenosis: Pathology and surgical treatment. *Spine* 3:246–255, 1978.
481. Guegan Y, Fardoum R, Launois B, et al: Spinal cord compression after corticosteroid therapy. *J Neurosurg* 56:267–269, 1982.
482. Moreland LW, Lopez-Mendez A, Alarcon GS: Spinal stenosis: A comprehensive review of the literature. *Semin Arthritis Rheum* 19:127–149, 1989.
483. Ciric I, Mikhael MA: Lumbar spine—lateral recess stenosis. *Neurol Clin* 3:417–423, 1985.

484. Johnsson KE, Uden A, Rosen I: The effect of decompression on the natural course of spinal stenosis—a comparison of surgically treated and untreated patients. *Spine* 16:615–619, 1991.
485. Johnsson KE, Uden A, Rosen I: The effect of decompression on the natural course of spinal stenosis—a comparison of surgically treated and untreated patients. *Spine* 16:615–619, 1991.
486. Jonsson B, Akesson M, Johnsson K, et al: Low risk of vertebral slipping after decompression with facet-joint preserving technique for lumbar stenosis. *Eur Spine J* 1:100–104, 1992.
487. Fast A, Robin GC, Floman Y: Surgical treatment of lumbar spinal stenosis in the elderly. *Arch Phys Med Rehabil* 66:149–151, 1985.
488. Grabis S: The treatment of spinal stenosis. *J Bone Joint Surg (AM)* 62:308–313, 1980.
489. Hutter CG: Spinal stenosis and posterior lumbar interbody fusion. *Clin Orthop* 193:103–114, 1985.
490. Ray CD: New techniques for decompression of lumbar spinal stenosis. *Neurosurgery* 10:587–592, 1982.
491. Kawai S, Hattori S, Oda H, et al: Enlargement of the lumbar vertebral canal in lumbar canal stenosis. *Spine* 6:381–387, 1981.
492. Rosomoff HL: Neural arch resection for lumbar spinal stenosis. *Clin Orthop* 154:83–89, 1981.
493. Lin PM: Internal decompression for multiple levels of lumbar spinal stenosis: A technical note. *Neurosurgery* 11:546–549, 1982.
494. Shenkin HA, Hash CJ: A new approach to the surgical treatment of lumbar spondylosis. *J Neurosurg* 44:148–155, 1976.
495. Weinstein PR: Lumbar stenosis, in Hardy RW (ed): *Lumbar Disc Disease*. New York, Raven Press, 1982, pp 257–276.
496. White AH, Wiltse LL: Postoperative spondylolisthesis, in Weinstein PR, Ehni G, Wilson CB (eds): *Lumbar Spondylosis: Diagnosis, Management and Surgical Treatment*. St. Louis, Mosby, 1977, pp 184–194.
497. Shenkin HA, Hash CJ: Spondylolisthesis after multiple bilateral laminectomies and facetectomies for lumbar spondylosis. *J Neurosurg* 50:45–47, 1979.
498. Nachemson A: Lumbar spine instability: A critical update and symposium summary. *Spine* 10:290–292, 1985.
499. Grabias S: The treatment of spinal stenosis. *J Bone Joint Surg (AM)* 62:308–313, 1980.

Low Back Pain and Pregnancy

Paula J. Stern, B.Sc., D.C., F.C.C.S.C.
Private Practice, Saskatoon, Saskatchewan, Canada

Low back pain during pregnancy is common and often results in significant morbidity. In Sweden, it was estimated that 70% of pregnant women took an average of 9 weeks of sick leave for different health problems.[1] Back pain was by far the most common condition for work absenteeism. Unfortunately, few studies have identified the risk factors enabling clinicians to determine who may be prone to developing low back pain during pregnancy.

It is a well-known fact that pregnancy places additional biomechanical stresses on the musculoskeletal system. This is believed to originate from postural alterations and ligamentous laxity. These and other physiological changes make the musculoskeletal system susceptible to injury during pregnancy. The ability of a woman's body to adapt to the unique physical, hormonal, and emotional changes experienced during pregnancy is truly remarkable. For many women, pregnancy is smooth sailing. Unfortunately for many others, pregnancy is plagued with numerous aches and pains. As chiropractors, our expertise lies in the ability to diagnose and treat neuromusculoskeletal conditions.

The intent of this chapter is to provide the clinician with a better understanding of back pain and related disorders in pregnancy. The treatment of neuromusculoskeletal conditions in pregnant women may elicit apprehension in some patients and clinicians. However, armed with the proper knowledge, the treatment of these patients can be just as simple and rewarding as in the nonpregnant woman.

PHYSIOLOGY

During pregnancy the physiology of the musculoskeletal system is temporarily modified by hormonal and biomechanical changes. These changes specifically target the lumbar spine and pelvis and may predispose pregnant women to develop low back pain.

The effects of hormonal changes during pregnancy are vast. Of these, the ones produced by relaxin are known to specifically affect the musculoskeletal system. Relaxin is a hormone present throughout the normal menstrual cycle. It peaks during pregnancy and reaches its highest level during the first trimester.[2] During the first 3 months, it is released from the corpus luteum and targets the cervix, uterus, and pelvic ligamentous structures.[2,3] It produces alterations in the biomechanical properties of connective tissue, resulting in ligamentous laxity.[2,4] Relaxin promotes widening and an increased flexibility of the symphysis pubis and sacroiliac joints to facilitate delivery.[2]

Chiropractors have a special interest in the biomechanical alterations on the spine and pelvis. These changes are dynamic and evolve with the continuously growing fetus and uterus. It is estimated that by term, the size of the uterus will increase by 150 times and its weight by 20 times.[4]

As the fetus grows, a forward shift in the mother's center of gravity is observed. This is further amplified by the enlarging breasts. To compensate, the lumbar lordosis increases, which results in anterior rotation of the pelvis. The center of gravity subsequently shifts back over the pelvis. As a consequence of the increased lumbar lordosis, the thoracic and cervical curves develop compensatory sagittal curves.

EPIDEMIOLOGY

Low back pain is often regarded as an integral component of the physical symptoms of pregnancy. Although it is a well-recognized clinical problem, few scientific studies address this issue. It is estimated that more than 50% of pregnant women experience low back pain.[5-8] In a large prospective study, Ostgaard et al.[8] determined an incidence rate of 27% and a point prevalence of 25% for low back pain during pregnancy. Low back pain usually develops in the second trimester between the fifth and seventh month.[5,7]

Several epidemiological studies investigating the problem of low back pain in society have established risk factors for its development. However, the specific risk factors for developing low back pain during pregnancy have not yet been firmly demonstrated.

Attempts at identifying the risk factors associated with low back pain during pregnancy have led to conflicting results. According to Mantle et al.,[5] the prevalence of back pain increases with age at a rate of 5% for every 5 years of age and with parity. This is in partial contradiction with Berg et al.,[6] who found that parity was not responsible for an increase in incidence. Ostgaard et al.,[8] studying a cohort of 855 pregnant women from their third month until delivery, found that back pain occurred twice as often in women with prepregnancy back pain and that it lasted longer in this group. The younger women were more at risk of developing low back pain.[8,9]

Strenuous physical work and a previous history of low back pain are also believed to increase the risk of suffering from low back pain during pregnancy.[6] However, no association has been found between low back pain and maternal weight and height, maternal weight gain, fetal weight at birth, or parity.[5-7,9,10]

Typically low back pain in pregnancy is reported to be located over the sacroiliac joints.[1,6,11,12] However, involvement of the sacroiliac joints in the cause of low back pain remains empirical. Further support comes from several authors[1,6] who reported that the sacroiliac provocation test results (Patrick-Fabere, Gaenslen's, Yeoman's) are often positive in pregnant women suffering from low back pain. Berg et al.,[6] in a study of 862 pregnant women, concluded that the most common cause of severe low back pain was sacroiliac dysfunction. In a prospective study of the prevalence of back pain in pregnant women, Ostgaard et al.[8] categorized the location of pain into three areas: pain above the lumbar region, pain in the lumbar region with or without leg radiation, and pain over the sacroiliac joint with or without thigh radiation. As pregnancy progressed, there was an increase in the total number of patients in the sacroiliac group. This corresponded to a decrease in the low back group.

In a questionnaire distributed to 180 women within 24 hours postpartum, Mantle et al.[5] found that the most common aggravating factors for low back pain were standing, ironing, making beds, and fatigue, and almost half the patients obtained relief by placing a cushion behind the back.

ETIOLOGY

There is much speculation regarding the cause of low back pain in pregnancy. Most researchers believe that the cause is multifactorial. Of all the proposed theories, it is well accepted that it likely results from hormonal and mechanical changes.

It is postulated that the effects of relaxin on the spinal and pelvic ligamentous structures are responsible for the majority of low back pain in pregnancy. It is reported that the sacroiliac joint is the most common affected articulation in a pregnant woman.[6,12] This is likely to be secondary to an elevated relaxin level, which causes ligamentous laxity and encourages motion at otherwise minimally moving joints. Consequently, inflammation and pain result.[3] Further, sacroiliac symptoms commonly occur in the first trimester, which is before any significant weight gain or postural alteration.[3] Machennan et al.[13] studied the relationship between relaxin and pelvic pain during late pregnancy by comparing the serum relaxin levels of 35 women with severe pelvic pain and instability to 368 controls. A highly significant positive correlation was found between relaxin levels and pelvic pain. It is therefore plausible that high levels of relaxin predispose women to develop low back pain during pregnancy.

Postural factors are believed to promote the development of back pain during pregnancy. Subtle changes in posture are seen in the early stages of pregnancy, and as the pregnancy progresses, the increasing weight applies a significant amount of added stress to the weight-bearing joints. As mentioned earlier, the growing uterus causes the body's center of gravity to shift anteriorly, thereby altering the lumbar lordosis. When the alignment of the spine begins to change, the muscles, ligaments, and disks are placed at a biomechanical disadvantage.[3,14] With the increase in lumbar lordosis, the paraspinal muscles are shortened and are unable to be aided by the overstretched abdominal muscles. Because the optimal function of these muscles is affected, excess stress is applied to the posterior elements of the lumbar spine and intervertebral disks. The paravertebral muscles therefore fatigue more quickly, and the ligaments and disks absorb more of the mechanical stress. The nociceptive innervation of the lumbar posterior elements is well documented.[15] Stimulation of these nociceptors may produce pain and radiation into the buttock or thigh.[16]

One school of thought believes that the hyperlordosis seen in pregnancy is responsible for the development of low back pain. However, several authors[10, 17] have questioned its validity. Bullock et al.[17] examined the changes in lumbar lordosis, pelvic tilt, and thoracic kyphosis in an attempt to determine if these changes correlated with the complaint of back pain. Thirty-four women without back pain before pregnancy were examined three times throughout their pregnancy. A significant increase was seen in magnitude of both the thoracic and lumbar curves. Although 88% of the women reported back pain before the fifth month of pregnancy, no statistically significant relationship was found between back pain and postural changes.

To further support the argument that biomechanical change may not be a primary cause of low back pain in this group, Ostgaard et al.[8] observed that the point prevalence of back pain remained constant throughout pregnancy. In another study they found that back pain significantly correlated with the increasing transverse and sagittal diameter of the abdomen and the lumbar lordosis at 12 weeks' gestation.[10] No correlations were found with regard to weight gain and ulnar deviation as a measure of joint laxity.

Although biomechanical factors may contribute to the development of low back pain, it is unlikely that they are the only responsible factors, or a continuous increase in prevalence would be observed with advancing pregnancy. In addition, many women state that their back pain began before the twelfth week of pregnancy.[8] Therefore, biomechanical changes are considered a secondary but not primary cause of low back pain.

Other risk factors involved in the cause of low back pain during pregnancy include poor physical fitness before pregnancy,[1] previous history of back trouble,[6, 8] and physically demanding employment.[6]

HISTORY AND PHYSICAL EXAMINATION

The information gathered by conducting a history is the single most important aspect of diagnosing. This process will allow the clinician to establish a differential diagnosis and to exclude a multitude of disorders that can mimic spinal pain. The purpose of the history is to determine if the back pain is mechanical or not. Table 1 presents a list of nonmechanical causes of low back pain during pregnancy. The clinician should also ensure that the pregnancy is uncomplicated and that the patient is followed by an obstetrician or family physician.

Often early warning signs will alert the clinician to the possible presence of complications. Specific questions should address previous miscarriages, history of spotting, menstrual-like cramps, pelvic pressure, increased vaginal discharge, and uterine contractions. Suspicion or evidence of a nonmechanical cause for low back pain warrants an immediate referral to a physician.

No office visit is complete without a proper physical examination. The history has generated a list of differential diagnoses, and the examination helps rule in a specific diagnosis.

The examination can usually be performed in the same manner as with any other patient. However, by midpregnancy, the protuberant abdomen makes it uncomfortable for the woman to lie on her stomach, and

TABLE 1.
Nonorthopedic Conditions with Low Back Pain That Should Alert the Clinician*

Preterm labor
Bladder problems
Fibroid enlargement
Intra-abdominal pathological conditions (e.g., biliary, pancreatic, gastric, duodenal)
Bone tumors
Spinal infection

*Adapted from Pruzansky ME, Siffert RS, Levy RN: Orthopaedic complications, in Cherry SH, Merkatz IR (eds): *Complications of Pregnancy: Medical, Surgical, Gynecologic, Psychosocial and Perinatal*, ed 4. Baltimore, Williams & Wilkins, 1991, pp 996–1005.

the examination has to be modified. Using a doughnut pillow will allow more comfort for the prone examination (Fig 1). Gaenslen's and Yeoman's sacroiliac tests can be performed in the lateral recumbent position (Fig 2).

When a diagnosis of mechanical low back pain has been made, a list of potentially involved structures should be ascertained. The sacroiliac joint, apophyseal joints, intervertebral disks, and musculotendinous tissues may be involved in the pain syndromes.

Sacroiliac syndrome is suspected when pain is located directly over the posterior superior iliac spine. It can refer to the buttock, greater trochanter, or down the posterior or lateral side of the thigh to the knee. Common complaints include difficulty getting up from a chair and rolling in bed. On examination lumbar range of motion is restricted and painful in extension. Sacroiliac stress tests, although not specific are often

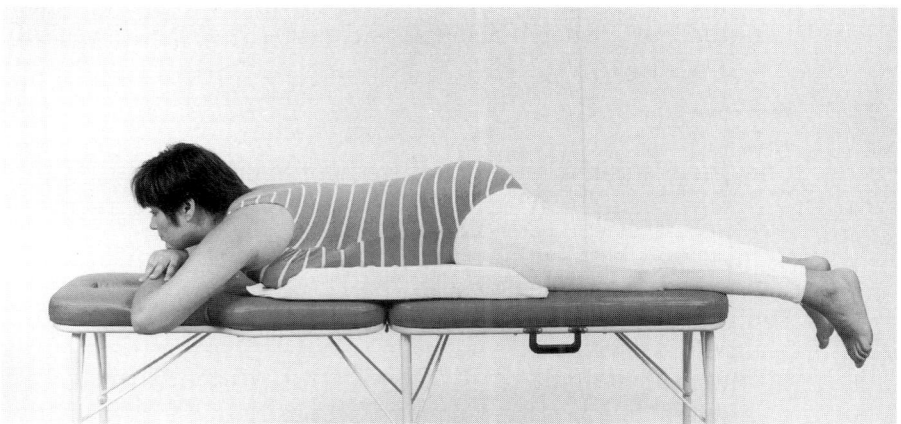

FIGURE 1.
A doughnut pillow placed under the abdomen can help alleviate pressure on the stomach.

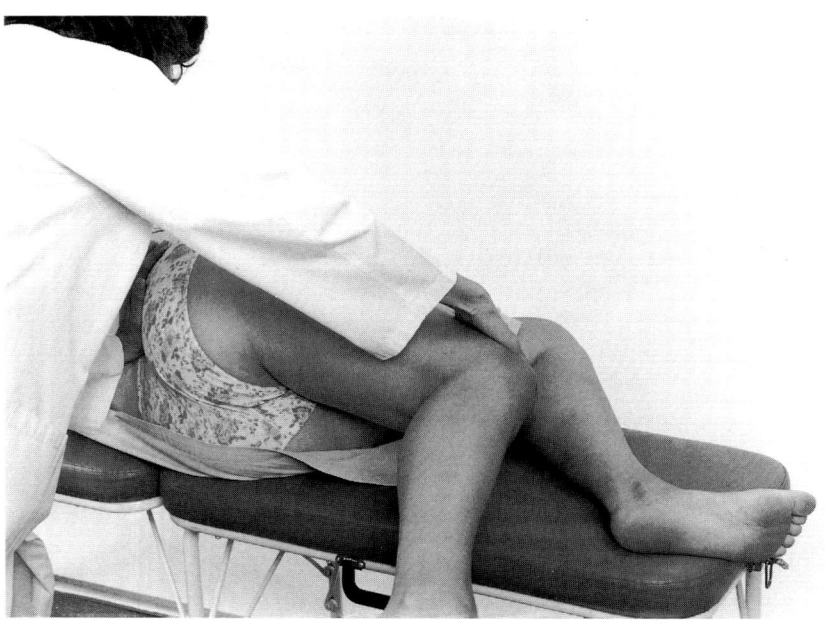

FIGURE 2.
Technique for performing a lateral recumbent sacroiliac stress test. The woman should be lying on her side with the bottom leg straight. With the top leg bent at the knee, place one hand over the sacroiliac joint to be stressed (the joint facing up) and the other hand on the anterior knee. Gently pull the knee backward while applying pressure to the sacroiliac joint. If pain is elicited in the joint, the test result is positive.

positive (Faber-Patrick, Yeoman's, Gaenslen's, direct compression).[18] Sacroiliac pain can be mimicked by many conditions (Table 2).

Strain injuries of the posterior joints, which usually occur after a minor trauma, result in synovitis and contraction of the segmental muscles.[19] Low back pain is the predominant complaint, and pain referred to the greater trochanter and posterior thigh may be present. It

TABLE 2.
Conditions Mimicking a Sacroiliac Joint Syndrome*

Posterior facet joint syndrome
Lumbar disk herniation
Lateral recess spinal stenosis
Hip joint disease
Maigne's syndrome
Myofascial syndromes

*Adapted from Bernard TN, Cassidy JD: The sacroiliac joint syndrome—pathophysiology, diagnosis and management, in Frymoyer JW (ed): *The Adult Spine: Principles and Practice.* New York, Raven Press, 1991, vol 2, pp 2107–2130.

rarely travels past the knee. Rest relieves the pain, and motion aggravates the condition. Lumbar range of motion is affected, with extension being the most limited.

The erector spinae, quadratus lumborum, and gluteal muscles are common causes of myofascial pain during pregnancy. Both the gluteus maximus and quadratus lumborum can refer to the sacroiliac joint and mimic sacroiliac pain.[18] Palpation of trigger points that reproduces the pain pattern in the area of complaint suggests the involvement of these muscles.

DIFFERENTIAL DIAGNOSIS

Mechanical low back pain with or without leg pain should be differentiated from other orthopedic conditions that it may mimic.

DISK HERNIATION

Disk herniation in the nongravid woman is a well-recognized disorder.[20, 21] During pregnancy, it is estimated that it will be present in 1:10,000 deliveries.[22] Controversy exists regarding pregnancy as a predisposing factor of lumbar spine disk herniation. In a series of 347 women with surgically proven disk herniation, O'Connell[23] found that 70 complained of back pain and sciatica during pregnancy. Seventy-six percent of these women had never suffered from symptoms of disk herniation before pregnancy. This elevated rate may be explained by the highly selected population that was investigated. Based on his findings, he claimed that pregnancy was a predisposing factor for lumbar disk herniation.

It is proposed that the added stress of the fetus, combined with the ligamentous laxity, makes the intervertebral disk (IVD) more susceptible to herniation.[23, 24] However, LaBan et al.[22] challenged this theory. They argued that if mechanical and postural factors put women at a greater risk, disk herniation would be more prevalent in women.

The point prevalence of lumbar disk herniation is higher in the third trimester. Signs and symptoms of disk herniation are no different in the pregnant patient than in the nonpregnant women. The presence of severe back pain, sciatica, a positive straight leg raise test result, and objective neurological findings should increase the suspicion of a disk herniation.

When a disk herniation occurs during pregnancy, conservative therapy is the treatment of choice.[25] However, evidence of cauda equina lesions (manifesting with bowel and bladder problems) or rapidly progressive neurological deficit that does not improve after bed rest warrants immediate neurosurgical referral.[25]

There are many options and much debate regarding the most effective nonoperative treatment of disk herniation in the nonpregnant patient. A few studies have suggested that manipulation may be an effective treatment for disk herniation in the nonpregnant population.[20, 26–28] However, there are no reports or trials addressing the issue of manipulation for disk herniations in pregnant individuals. In fact, in most studies pregnancy is an exclusion criteria.

Most authors believe that the majority of disk herniation cases in pregnancy are best treated with up to 6 weeks of bed rest.[25, 29] Once symptomatic relief is obtained, use of a corset, application of heat, or transcutaneous neurostimulation may help.[22, 25] As the acute pain diminishes, the patient can gradually return to daily activities. Avoidance of all aggravating activities is important. As well, beginning an exercise program may aid in decreasing the likelihood of a relapse.[29] However, as reported by LaBan et al.,[22] nonremitting back pain and sciatica that fail to respond to a course of nonoperative treatment during and after pregnancy may have to be treated surgically.

PUBIC PAIN

Symphysis Pubis Diastasis

This condition refers to the rupture of the soft tissue structures surrounding the symphysis pubis. It usually occurs at the time of delivery, but it can be seen during the pregnancy.[30] It is a rare condition, with an incidence between 1:600 and 1:20,000 deliveries.[31, 32] It causes joint widening and increased motion. Clinically, pain may be present in the symphyseal region or in the low back, with the sacroiliac most commonly affected. Radiations into the groin, thigh, and leg may be associated with it.[33, 34] According to some, walking, standing, climbing stairs and turning in bed typically aggravate the complaint.[30, 33, 34]

On examination there is tenderness over the symphysis pubis, and pain with hip flexion or abduction. A palpable gap is often observed at the symphysis pubis. Gentle joint play reveals increased motion in the vertical or horizontal plane.

Treatment is conservative and generally includes bed rest and a pelvic support.

Osteitis Pubis

The softening of the pelvic ligaments is thought to be responsible for this painful condition.[35] Clinically there is gradual onset of pain in the symphysis pubis, which progresses to severe pain over a few days. The pain is located in the symphysis pubis and pubic rami area with radiations into the medial thigh.[35] The pain is aggravated by activity, especially hip adduction. Local tenderness is present over the adductor insertion in the pubic rami.[36] Treatment is bed rest with the legs flexed and adducted over a pillow.[35] Ice may be beneficial.

LEG CRAMPS

Leg cramps are common during pregnancy. Between 15% and 30% of pregnant woman suffer from cramps, which usually beginning during the second trimester.[37]

Although the exact cause is unknown, it has been suggested that a calcium or magnesium deficiency is the culprit. Studies have shown that pregnant women are deficient in calcium, most likely as a result of the poor oral intake and the fetal demand.[14, 37]

The cramps often begin while the woman is sleeping, and they are severe enough to awaken her from her slumber. They usually occur in the calf muscles, but thigh and buttock involvement has been reported.[37] These painful contractions last anywhere from seconds to minutes. Hammar et al.,[37] in a randomized control trial of 42 pregnant women suffering from leg cramps, reported improvement in the cramps in those women treated with orally ingested calcium.

Thus, there appears to be support for calcium supplementation. Other suggestions include massaging, stretching, or attempting to walk when the cramps begin.

OSTEOPOROSIS

Although a rare condition, idiopathic osteoporosis of pregnancy is important to recognize. Patients complaining of back pain and loss of height, usually in the last trimester of pregnancy or soon after delivery, should be suspected of suffering from a compression fracture.[38] Transient osteoporosis has been documented in other parts of the body.[14] Heckman[14] states that because of the vague symptoms of pelvic, hip, thigh or groin pain, this condition is difficult to diagnose. The pain gradually increases in severity and results in an inability to bear weight. If undetected, a stress fracture of the femoral neck can result.

The majority of these patients will be asymptomatic within 4 to 6 months after delivery. Osteoporosis of pregnancy does not tend to recur with future delivery.

OTHER CAUSES

It is important to remember that although they are rare, more serious causes of low back pain exist, including tumors and infections.

NEUROLOGICAL CONDITIONS

Few neurological diseases are directly caused by pregnancy. Usually preexisting conditions are exacerbated and will manifest themselves clinically. The differential diagnosis of back pain and sciatica should include the common neurological disorders seen during pregnancy. In this section their clinical diagnosis and management are discussed.

MERALGIA PARESTHETICA

Compression of the lateral femoral cutaneous nerve can occur either under the inguinal ligament or retroperitoneally over the sacroiliac joint. Compression is caused by the weight gain and the increased lumbar lordosis. Patients complain of severe pain and paresthesia in the anterolateral side of the thigh. It is aggravated by standing and relieved by sitting or lying down. The condition is benign and resolves spontaneously after delivery.[39] Treatment can be aimed at decreasing the sacral tilt by wearing a lumbosacral corset and postural exercises that strengthen the abdomen.[35]

MULTIPLE SCLEROSIS

The incidence of multiple sclerosis is highest in the childbearing years.[39] Although the cause is still unknown, pregnancy has been implicated as a precipitating factor for an attack. As well, it is believed that pregnancy can adversely alter the course of multiple sclerosis.[39] It has been shown that 50% of all exacerbations occur during the first 3 months postpartum.[39] The most common presenting symptoms include combinations of limb weakness or numbness, diplopia, monocular visual loss, vertigo, facial weakness or numbness, ataxia, and nystagmus.[40]

TARSAL TUNNEL SYNDROME

Important in the differential diagnosis of leg and foot pain is tarsal tunnel syndrome. It results from compression of the posterior tibial nerve underneath the ankle flexor retinaculum. Complaints include numbness, tingling, burning and pain in the sole or medial side of the foot that can extend up the leg.[25] Aggravating factors include standing and walking. Because it often occurs at night, it must be differentiated from leg cramps. A positive Tinel sign is present over the posterior tibial nerve. Treatment is aimed at decreasing ankle motion and applying ice packs.[35] If pain is severe, injections may be beneficial.

COMPLICATIONS OF PREGNANCY

Numerous complications can arise from a pregnancy. This section includes the most frequent ones and their associated signs and symptoms. It is the role of the chiropractor to recognize the signs and symptoms of complications when treating a pregnant woman. It is imperative that the woman be sent directly to her obstetrician or family physician if one of the following conditions is suspected.

SPONTANEOUS ABORTION (MISCARRIAGE)

Approximately 10% to 20% of pregnancies result in spontaneous abortions.[41] The most common alerting sign is uterine bleeding. As well, symmetrical or bilateral lower abdominal cramping pain may be present.[41, 42]

ECTOPIC PREGNANCY

With an incidence of 1/200 pregnancies, ectopic pregnancy occurs when the fertilized ovum implants in an abnormal location.[42] In the majority of cases, this site is tubal.[42, 43] Because the tubal musculature is unable to maintain a gestation of any size, rupture is inevitable. More than 50% of ectopic pregnancies occur between the ages of 23 and 34 years.[44]

Unilateral or generalized abdominal pain is present in 99% of ectopic pregnancies.[43] Irregular bleeding is the initial sign in 40% of women.[43] Because there is intraperitoneal bleeding, the pain is usually accompanied by pallor, fainting, diaphragmatic or shoulder pain, abdominal distention, and tenderness on palpation.[42]

Patients at risk include those with tubal abnormalities (congenital or due to pelvic inflammatory disease), a history of previous ectopic pregnancy, or a history of intra-abdominal surgeries.[44]

PRETERM LABOR

The concern regarding preterm labor is significant because of its large contribution to infant morbidity and mortality. Infants born prematurely are at a higher risk for developing cerebral palsy and other chronic childhood disabilities.[45] Although the cause of preterm labor is known in some instances, the cause remains unknown in the majority of cases.[45, 46] The signs and symptoms of preterm labor are similar to the experiences of a normal pregnancy, thus making the recognition of this condition at times very difficult. However, preterm labor patients experience both painful and painless contractions at a greater frequency than normal pregnant patients. As well the complaints of menstrual cramps, back pain, and increased vaginal discharge are also seen more frequently in preterm labor patients.

To aid in determining whether a woman is experiencing preterm labor, Iams et al.[47] suggest that the presence and persistence of several symptoms mentioned earlier warrant prompt investigation and referral to her obstetrician.

PREECLAMPSIA-ECLAMPSIA

The term preeclampsia-eclampsia is also known as pregnancy-induced hypertension. Its cause remains unknown. In general, hypertension results from an increase in either cardiac output or peripheral vascular resistance. Because the cardiac output remains within normal limits during most pregnancies, preeclampsia-eclampsia is believed to result from increased peripheral vascular resistance.

A diagnosis of preeclampsia-eclampsia is confirmed when hypertension is combined with proteinuria or edema after the twentieth week of pregnancy. It is more commonly seen during the first pregnancy, usually in the teenager or women more than 35 years of age.[48] Therefore, it is recommended that the blood pressure be checked at regular intervals during pregnancy.

The term eclampsia refers to the development of convulsions and coma. There are several obvious warning signs to alert the clinician, including acceleration of hypertension, epigastric or right upper quadrant pain, blurred vision, scotomas, headaches, and tremulousness.[49]

PLACENTA PREVIA

Placenta previa refers to the placenta covering the entire or a part of the cervix. Studies report an incidence of 1/100 to 1/250, and it is more commonly seen in multiparous women.[50] The most common sign is significant, painless vaginal bleeding during the third trimester.

ABRUPTIO PLACENTAE

Abruptio placentae is defined as premature separation of the normally implanted placenta. Although the cause is unknown, approximately 47% of patients with this condition suffer from pregnancy-induced or chronic hypertension.[51] Recurrence of abruptio placentae is 10 to 15 times more common in a woman with a previous history of this condition. Women with a history of spontaneous abortion are also at risk. Clinically patients complain of abdominal pain, vaginal bleeding, contractions, and uterine tenderness.

DEEP VENOUS THROMBOSIS AND PULMONARY EMBOLISM

Although a rare condition in pregnancy, deep venous thrombosis is a serious complication because of its potentially fatal results. An incidence of 0.5 to 1 in 1,000 pregnancies is observed during pregnancy, and the incidence increases five times postpartum.[52] During pregnancy the potential for coagulation and thrombosis is increased because of the combination of increased plasma coagulation factors and venous stasis that accompanies pregnancy.[52] The risk is greatest at term and immediately after delivery. Risk factors are women older than 35 years, obesity, multiparity, and prolonged immobilization.[52, 53] Clinical signs and symptoms include muscle pain, tenderness, edema, change in limb color, a palpable cord, and Homan's sign (pain when the foot is passively dorsiflexed).

It is important to recognize that on occasion, the first sign of deep venous disease is the occurrence of pulmonary embolus. The main signs and symptoms include dyspnea, chest pain, cough, tachypnea, and tachycardia.

MANAGEMENT

The treatment of mechanical low back pain in pregnant women requires few modifications from the treatment of nonpregnant patients. Clinicians should avoid using interferential current, ultrasound, or any electrical modality due to the unknown effects on the fetus. However, one suspected complication is that these modalities may cause uterine contractions, leading to spontaneous abortion.[54]

At our center in Saskatoon, the plan of management usually consists of manipulation, education, and exercises.

SPINAL MANIPULATION

Substantial evidence supports the use of spinal manipulation as a safe and effective treatment for low back pain in the general population.[55-58] In the majority of studies pregnancy was an exclusion criteria. Unfortunately, no randomized controlled trials have yet been performed to test the effectiveness of manipulation for the treatment of low back pain during pregnancy. At our clinic, we found a short course of gentle side posture manipulation is beneficial in relieving pain and stiffness. According to Sands,[12] manipulation is an effective form of treatment for mechanical lumbosacral back pain. Further, Berg et al.[6] reported complete relief in 7 out of 10 women treated with mobilization for severe sacroiliac joint dysfunction.

Although it may be technically difficult to position and manipulate the pregnant patient, there is no contraindication to manipulation in a woman suffering from mechanical low back pain.[59]

Diakow et al.,[60] in a review of 400 pregnancies involving 170 women, found that of 25 women who had manipulation for low back pain, 84% reported relief.

These studies, although weak methodologically, do support the notion that manual therapy may be a beneficial form of treatment for back pain during pregnancy. The need for well-designed randomized control trials is required.

EDUCATION

Home Advice

One of the most important aspect of treatment includes patient education. In many cases, the treatment may provide only temporary relief.

Therefore, lifestyle adjustments may be necessary to avoid aggravation of the complaint. Simple suggestions may be rewarding for the patient:

1. Use of pillows when lying down. Many women experience difficulty getting comfortable in bed. Incorporating pillows in body positioning can often help (Fig 3).
2. Stretching and strengthening program. As soon as the woman discovers she is pregnant, she should begin a daily stretching and strengthening routine. As the abdomen enlarges, it presses on the inferior vena cava, and it is recommended that supine stretches be replaced by standing or side lying exercises. Exercises should include knee-to-chest pull, straight leg raise, curl-ups, and pelvic tilt, all of which will likely aid in relieving backaches and increasing flexibility (Fig 4). All stretches should be held for 5 to 8 seconds and repeated 10 times. The pelvic tilt exercise can be done supine or standing. When supine, assume the starting position described in Figure 4, A, with the feet apart and the knees touching. Tighten the buttock and press the lower back to the floor. Hold for 5 to 8 seconds and relax. The standing pelvic tilt is described in Figure 5.
3. Sitting and standing. Adaptation of the sitting posture can aid in decreasing stress on the lumbar curve and lumbar pain. Placing a small pillow in the small of the back can help. Feet should be flat on the floor or up on a stool. When standing for long periods (e.g., in the

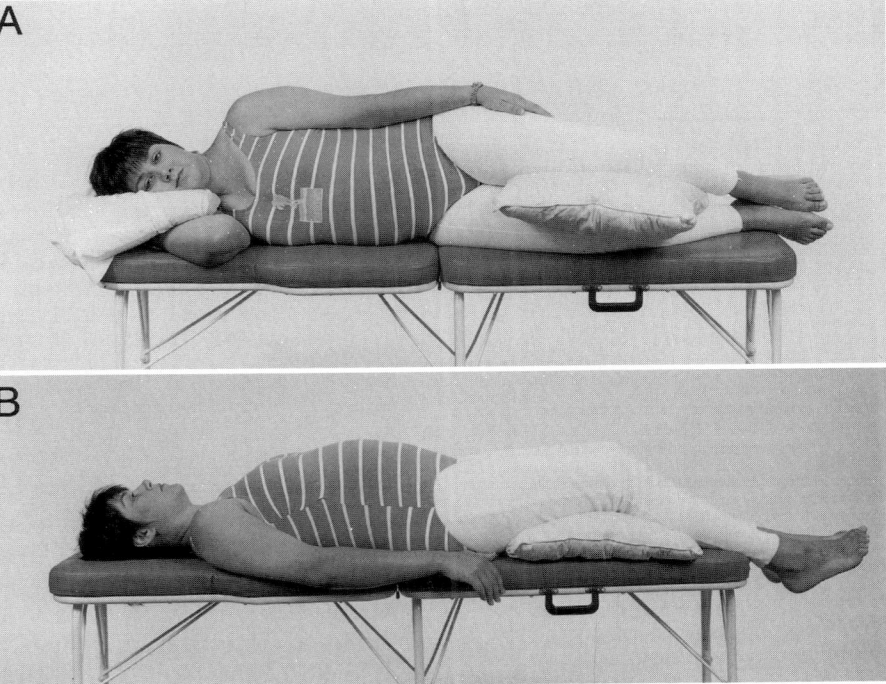

FIGURE 3.
Pillow position while lying in bed. **A,** if sleeping on the side, place a pillow between the flexed legs. **B,** if lying on the back, place pillows under the knees to aid in flattening the lower back.

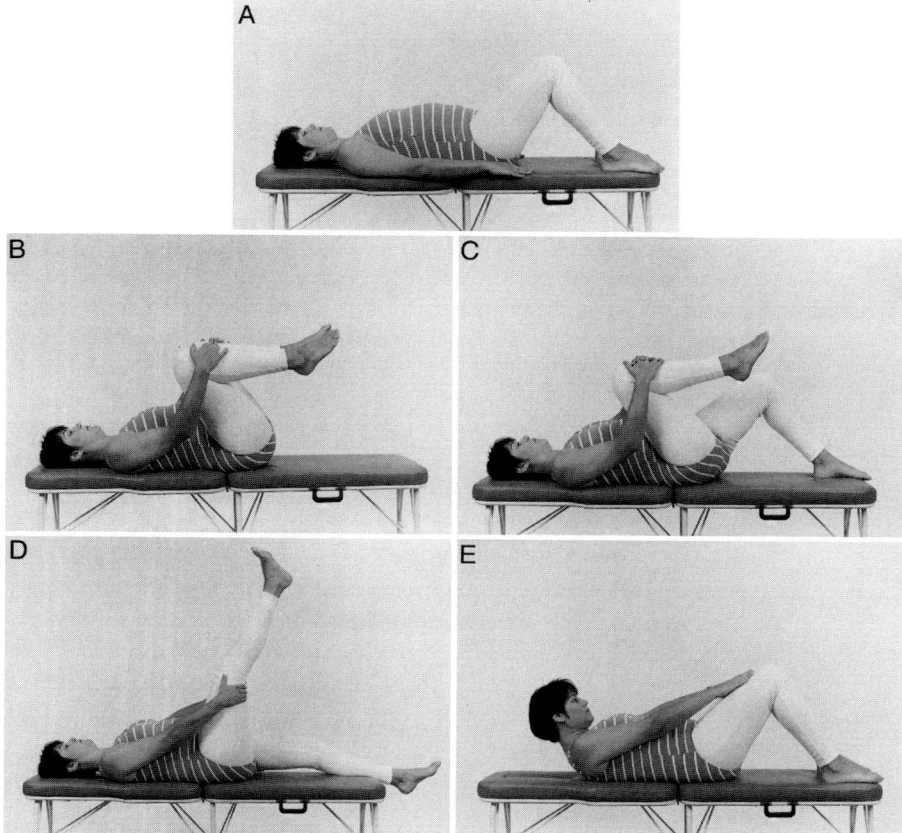

FIGURE 4.
A, for all of the following stretches, instruct the woman to lie on her back with both knees bent and feet flat on the floor. This is the starting position. Depending on the size of the abdomen, either both legs **(B)** or a single knee **(C)** can be gently pulled up toward the chest. When feeling a gentle pull in the low back, stop and hold the stretch for 5 to 8 seconds. **D,** with one leg bent or straight, using both hands behind the thigh, raise the other leg until a gentle stretch is felt in the back of the thigh. **E,** tuck the chin toward the chest and tighten the stomach. Slowly slide the hands toward the knees while lifting the head and shoulders off the floor. Slowly lower back to the floor. Relax.

kitchen or ironing), place one foot on a stool or telephone book to alleviate stress in the low back (Fig 6).

4. Lifting and carrying. A pregnant women should avoid bending from the waist only. She should use the hips and knees. Squatting is recommended because her balance will be better, and there will be less strain on the lower back. The object to be lifted should be as close to her as possible. This also applies to carrying (see Fig 6).

5. Ice and heat. It is believed that application of ice or heat to the low back can give symptomatic relief.

6. Family support. I often advise pregnant women to decrease the amount of housework, especially vacuuming, ironing, and washing

dishes. Support from the family to perform these activities should be encouraged.

7. High heel shoes. These shoes increase the lumbar lordosis and place strain on the back ligaments and muscles. Therefore, their use should be discouraged.

Back Education Classes

There has been an increased amount of interest in the role of a structured back program for the relief of low back pain in pregnancy. It is assumed that if a patient is properly educated about back care, future back pain will either be prevented or reduced in severity.[61] Back care education can be provided in the prenatal class or in a formal back school. Mantle et al.[5] reported that women attending prenatal classes during their third trimester had slightly less severe back pain. In a later study designed to as-

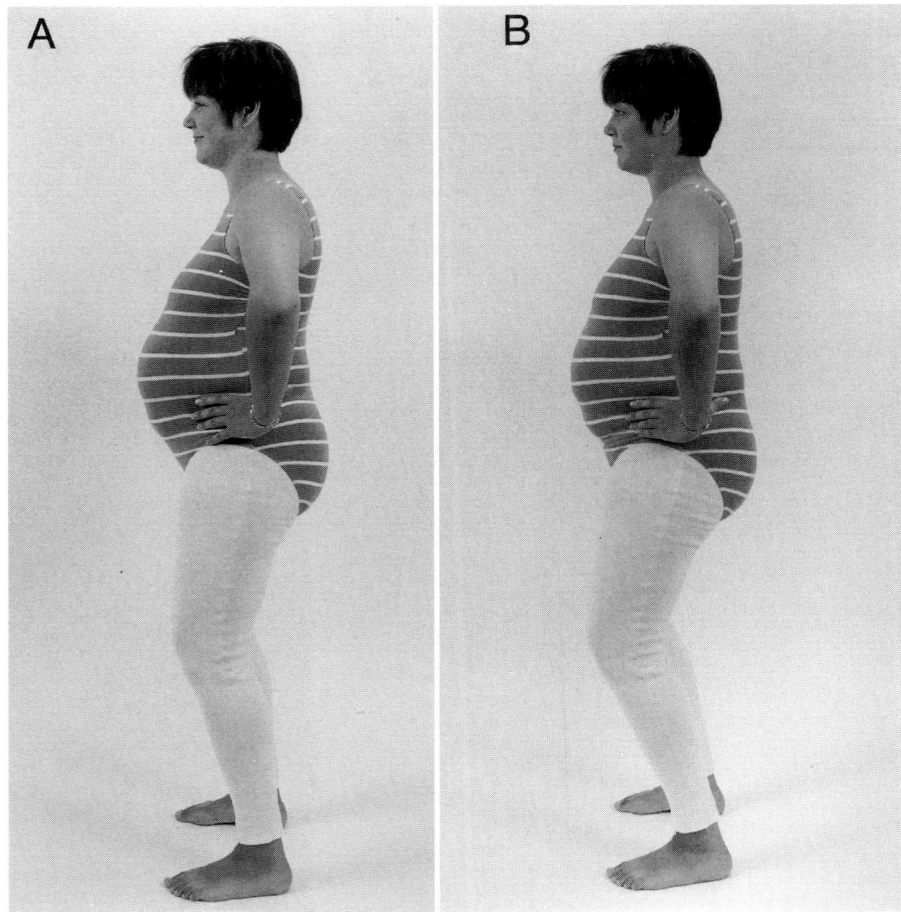

FIGURE 5.
Standing pelvic tilt. **A,** when one is standing, the feet should be shoulder width apart with the knees slightly bent and hands on the hips. **B,** contract the buttock and abdominal muscles and gently thrust the pelvis forward. Hold for 5 to 8 seconds.

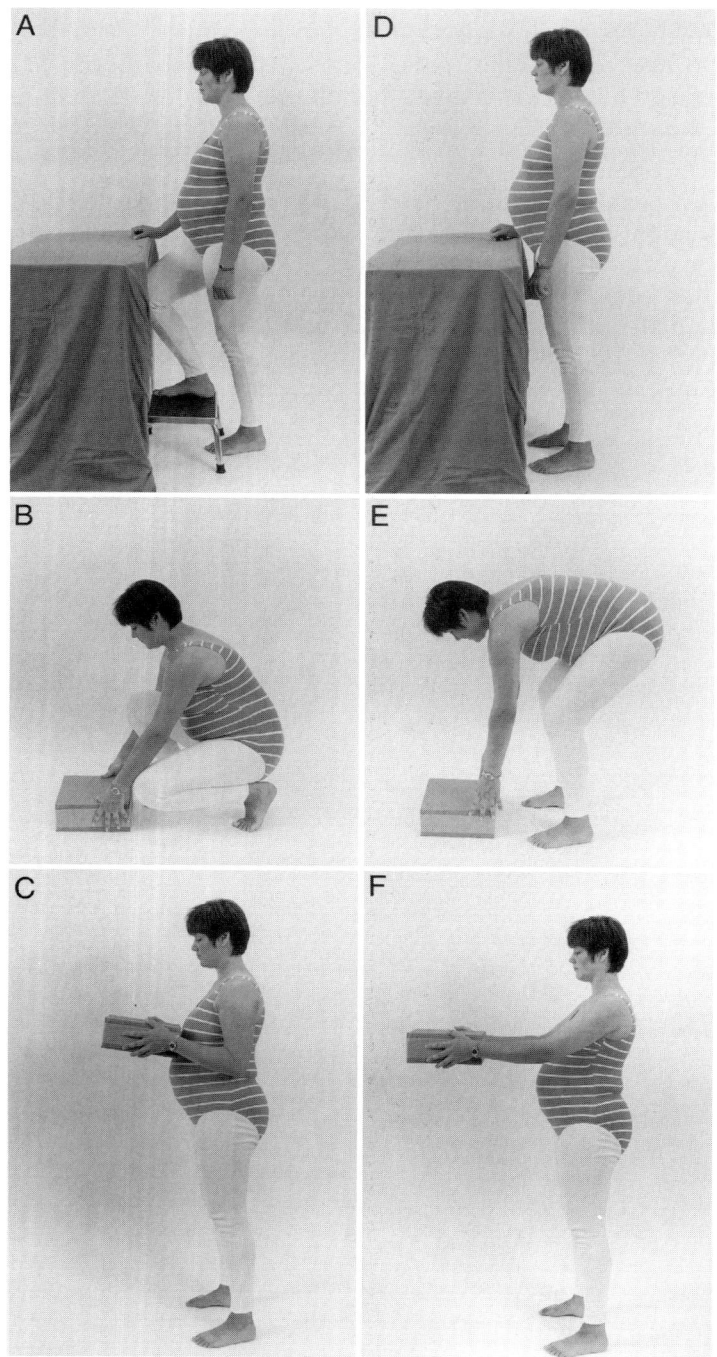

FIGURE 6.
Advice for standing, lifting, and carrying. **A, B,** and **C,** Dos—use a footstool or telephone book; bend at hip and knee; hold object close to you. **D, E,** and **F,** Don'ts—do not bend only at the waist.

sess the role of back care in pregnancy, women were offered two sessions of back school within the first 4 months of pregnancy.[62] Although benefit was reported in those attending class, no statistical significance was reached.

Ostgaard et al.[1] conducted a recent randomized control trial to determine the effectiveness of an education and training program in reducing back and pelvic pain during pregnancy. Of the 407 women included in the study, those receiving information either in a group or individually fared better than those serving as controls. The classes given individually were more effective in reducing back pain than those receiving information as a group. As well, although the pain intensity during pregnancy was the same in all three groups, the women receiving individual instruction reported less sick leave and less pain 8 weeks postpartum. More important, it was found that the women who were physically active for 45 minutes or more per week before pregnancy reported less sick leave.

Although there is some evidence supporting the effectiveness of back education classes in reducing the severity and frequency of back pain, its effectiveness in decreasing the incidence of low back pain in pregnancy remains to be demonstrated.

Sacroiliac and Trochanteric Belts and Lumbar Corsets

The primary purpose of belt and corset wear is to provide stability and support to the low back. In general, studies have reported good results with belts and corsets when the pain appears to be originating from the sacroiliac joints.[1, 6, 14]

Berg et al.[6] reported that 72% of women wearing a trochanteric belt for severe sacroiliac dysfunction or symphysiolysis experienced improvement of their complaint when wearing the belt. In another study, Ostgaard et al.[1] prescribed nonelastic sacroiliac belts to 59 women attending back education classes. Eighty-three percent of women were able to walk greater distances when wearing the belt. However, no pain relief was provided at work or while resting when the sacroiliac belt was worn. Heckman[14] described results of a small group of patients in whom either a trochanteric belt or lumbar corset was prescribed for low back pain. Significant pain relief was obtained in at least 75% of the sample.

Thus, there appears to be support for the prescription of a sacroiliac and trochanteric belt or lumbar corset.

EXERCISE

Exercise has become increasingly popular over recent years. Women have shown more interest in becoming active and when pregnant many wish to continue with some form of exercise. Studies have shown that fit individuals report less back pain than those not physically fit.[63, 64] To date, exercise standards have not been set for pregnant women. Although the scientific literature is limited, it is generally believed that during pregnancy, exercise is beneficial for most women.

Before recommending an exercise routine, all clinicians should be aware of the potential effects of exercise on the mother and fetus. All pregnant women should have a medical examination to ensure that there are no contraindications to exercise (Table 3).

Exercising during pregnancy may have beneficial and harmful effects. The beneficial effects of exercise include maintenance of muscle tone, strengthening, and endurance. Strengthening the lumbar and abdominal muscles is believed to protect against the development of low back pain. There are also obvious psychological benefits that enhance well-being and self-image.[65] It has also been proposed that regular exercise before and during pregnancy may be associated with shorter labor, fewer complications during pregnancy, and faster recovery from labor and delivery.[65, 66] More research is needed, however, to substantiate these claims.

The potential harmful effects of exercises affect primarily the fetus. During an uncomplicated pregnancy, fetal injury is unlikely.[67] However, because exercising is associated with an increase in body temperature and decreased blood flow to the uterus, caution is warranted. When a pregnant woman exercises strenuously or for prolonged periods, the body temperature elevates, and the fetus may be in danger. In addition, blood being diverted from the uterus to the exercising muscles may alter the fetal

TABLE 3.
Contraindications to Exercising in Pregnancy*

Absolute contraindications
  Cardiac disease
  Thrombophlebitis
  At risk or diagnosed with premature labor, multiple gestations,
    incompetent cervix, placenta previa, ruptured membranes
  Severe hypertension
  Uterine bleeding
  History of intrauterine growth retardation
  No prenatal care
  Suspected fetal distress
  Acute infectious disease
  Recent pulmonary embolism
  Severe isoimmunization
Relative contraindications
  Essential hypertension
  Diabetes
  Thyroid disease
  Anemia or other blood disease
  Excessive obesity or extreme underweight
  Breech presentation in last trimester
  History of sedentary lifestyle

*Adapted from Mittelmark RA, Wiswell RA, Drinkwater BL, et al: Exercise guidelines in pregnancy, in Mittelmark RA, Wiswell RA, Drinkwater BL (eds): *Exercise in Pregnancy*, ed 2. Baltimore, Williams & Wilkins, 1991, pp 299–312; Artal R: Exercise in pregnancy, in Cherry SH, Merkatz JR (eds): *Complications of Pregnancy: Medical, Surgical, Gynecologic, Psychosocial and Perinatal*, ed 4. Baltimore, Williams & Wilkins, 1991, pp 68–77.

cardiac function and result in a 20% decrease in fetal heart rate.[65, 67] It is still unknown whether these events lead to lasting effects on the fetus because no prospective studies have addressed these issues.[67] It has also been suggested by various epidemiological studies that there is a potential association between strenuous physical activity and intrauterine growth retardation of the fetus. However, these reports are preliminary, and more investigations are required.

Other risks associated with exercise include a predisposition for musculoskeletal injuries resulting from increased joint and ligamentous laxity.[67] Pregnant women enrolled in an exercise program should be instructed of the warning signs of complication (Table 4).

Each woman should be assessed individually, and the exercise program should reflect her needs. The level of physical fitness before pregnancy will help to determine the level of exercise to be recommended during the following months. A woman may often decide to become physically active shortly after the confirmation of pregnancy. It should be explained to her that if she has never exercised before, this is not the time to start a vigorous routine. According to the American College of Sports Medicine, it is not necessary to exercise strenuously to obtain the benefits of working out.[66] The program should start with a gentle stretching, combined with daily walking. Many local community centers offer fitness or aquafit classes geared to pregnant women.

The competitive athlete with an uncomplicated pregnancy who is anxious to train may continue her activities throughout the first and second trimester. As she enters her third trimester, exercising becomes difficult as her weight increases and her endurance decreases. It is recom-

TABLE 4.
Some Warning Signs and Symptoms of Exercising*

Pain
Vaginal bleeding
Shortness of breath
Dizziness or faintness
Palpitations or tachycardia
Persistent nausea or vomiting
Back, pubic, or hip pain
Generalized edema
Visual disturbances
Difficulty walking
Decreased fetal activity

*Adapted from Mittelmark RA, Wiswell RA, Drinkwater BL, et al: Exercise guidelines in pregnancy, in Mittelmark RA, Wiswell RA, Drinkwater BL (eds): *Exercise in Pregnancy*, ed 2. Baltimore, Williams & Wilkins, 1991, pp 299–312; ACOG guidelines: Exercise during pregnancy and the postnatal period, in Mittelmark RA, Wiswell RA, Drinkwater BL (eds): *Exercise in Pregnancy*, ed 2. Baltimore, Williams & Wilkins, 1991, pp 313–319.

mended that the competitive athlete remain under strict medical supervision throughout her training. She should be reminded not to become overheated or to exercise to the point of exhaustion.

The following are general guidelines summarized from the American College of Obstetricians and Gynecologists on exercises during pregnancy[68]:

1. To avoid injury, warm-up and cool-down stretches are advised. Because joint and ligamentous laxity predisposes women to injury, excessive stretching should be avoided.
2. The strenuous portion of exercising should be less than 15 minutes to avoid hyperthermia and musculoskeletal injury.
3. Maintaining proper caloric and fluid intake is important to avoid hyperthermia. Drinking before and after exercise is advised.
4. When one exercises in an unsupervised environment, the heart rate should not exceed 140 beats per minute. This recommendation is based on the fact that cardiovascular complications occur more commonly during strenuous exercise.
5. If no complications are present, a woman may continue to exercise as she did before pregnancy. However, to eliminate potential risks, one should avoid the following:
   a. Exercises in the supine position after the fourth month
   b. Exercises involving the Valsalva maneuver
   c. Hyperthermia; body core temperature should not exceed 38°C.
   d. Ballistic movements and deep flexion and extension of the joints
   e. Exercises performed in hot, humid weather

POSTPARTUM

Back pain immediately after delivery has been reported in 67% of women.[69] Although it tends to disappear within 1 to 6 months after delivery, a high percentage of patients continue to have pain for up to 1 year.[3, 6, 69, 70] Ostgaard et al.,[70] in a prospective study of 817 women followed for 18 months postpartum, found that 42% had back pain at 6 months and 37% had back pain at 18 months. In another study they found several factors that correlated to persistent postpartum back pain. These included back pain both before and during pregnancy, physically heavy work, and multiparity.[69]

Chiropractic care has an important role in the treatment of postpartum low back pain. A proper history and physical examination are of importance to rule out any complicating conditions.

Injuries to the pelvic nerves or lumbosacral plexus can result from delivery. The fourth and fifth lumbar and high sacral roots, which supply the sciatic nerve and superior gluteal nerve, are most at risk.[25] Clinically there is pain or sensory loss in the corresponding dermatome. Foot drop or calf muscle weakness may be evident. If foot drop is present, one must differentiate between compression of the lumbosacral root or peroneal nerve as it wraps around the fibular head. The hip muscles are weak if the gluteal, femoral, or obturator nerve is damaged. These conditions are usually self-limiting and reversible over time. Thus, the main role is reassurance. In the presence of foot drop, an orthosis may help.[25] As well, exercises should be performed to strengthen and prevent contracture or disuse atrophy.

In the absence of complications, patients with postpartum low back pain can be treated like any other patient. However, care must be given when manipulating women the first 3 months after delivery. Although relaxin appears to return to nonpregnant levels within 3 to 7 days postpartum, it is believed that the anatomic changes take approximately 6 to 12 weeks to resolve.[13, 66]

All women should begin gentle stretching as soon as possible after delivery. This includes the knee-to-chest pulls, straight leg raising, and pelvic tilts. Because many women still experience back pain postpartum, a strengthening program for the back, abdomen and legs should commence after 12 weeks. Extreme stretching, heavy weight lifting, and ballistic movements should be avoided the first 12 weeks postpartum.

ACKNOWLEDGMENTS

I would like to thank Dr. N. Podilsky M.D., F.R.C.S.C., for reviewing my manuscript. As well I would like to thank the Chiropractor's Association of Saskatchewan and the Chiropractic Foundation for Spinal Research for financial assistance in preparing this manuscript and the Department of Medical Photography at the Royal University Hospital for assistance with photography.

REFERENCES

1. Ostgaard HC, Zetherstrom G, Roos-Hansson E, et al: Reduction of back and posterior pelvic pain in pregnancy. *Spine* 19:894–900, 1994.
2. Sherwood OD: Relaxin, in Knobil E, Neill JD, et al (eds): *The Physiology of Reproduction*. New York, Raven Press, 1988, vol 1, pp 585–674.
3. Rungee JL: Low back pain during pregnancy. *Orthopedics* 16:1339–1344, 1993.
4. Romem Y, Masaki DI, Mittelmark RA: Physiological and endocrine adjustments to pregnancy, in Mittelmark RA, Wiswell RA, Drinkwater BL (eds): *Exercise in Pregnancy*, ed 2. Baltimore, Williams & Wilkins, 1991, pp 9–28.
5. Mantle MJ, Greenwood RM, Currey HLF: Backache in pregnancy. *Rheum Rehabil* 16:95–101, 1977.
6. Berg G, Hammar M, Moller-Nielsen J, et al: Low back pain during pregnancy. *Obstet Gynecol* 71:71–75, 1989.
7. Fast A, Shapiro D, Ducommun EJ, et al: Low back pain in pregnancy. *Spine* 12:368–371, 1987.
8. Ostgaard HC, Andersson GBJ, Karlsson K: Prevalence of back pain in pregnancy. *Spine* 16:549–552, 1991.
9. Ostgaard HC, Andersson GBJ: Previous back pain and risk of developing back pain in a future pregnancy. *Spine* 16:432–436, 1991.
10. Ostgaard HC, Andersson GBJ, Schultz AB: Influence of some biomechanical factors on low-back pain in pregnancy. *Spine* 18:61–65, 1993.
11. Andersson GBJ: Low back pain in pregnancy, in Weinstein JN, Weisel SW (eds): *The Lumbar Spine*. Philadelphia, WB Saunders, 1990, pp 841–845.
12. Sands RX: Backache of pregnancy: A method of treatment. *Obstet Gynecol* 12:670–676, 1958.

13. Machennan AH, Nicolson R, Green RC, et al: Serum relaxin and pelvic pain of pregnancy. *Lancet* 2:243–245, 1986.
14. Heckman JD: Managing musculoskeletal problems in pregnant patients. *J Musculoskeletal Med* 1(7):14–24, 1984.
15. Bogduck N, Twomey LP: Nerves of the lumbar spine, in *Clinical Anatomy of the Lumbar Spine*. New York, Churchill Livingstone, 1987, pp 92–102.
16. McCall IW, Park WM, O'Brien JP: Induced pain referral from posterior lumbar elements in normal subjects. *Spine* 4:441–446, 1979.
17. Bullock JE, Jull GA, Bullock MI: The relationship of low back pain to postural changes during pregnancy. *Aust J Physiother* 33:10–17, 1987.
18. Bernard TN, Cassidy JD: The sacroiliac joint syndrome—pathophysiology, diagnosis and management, in Frymoyer JW (ed): *The Adult Spine: Principles and Practice*. New York, Raven Press, 1991, vol 2, pp 2107–2130.
19. Kirkaldy-Willis WH: The three phases of the spectrum of degenerative disease, in Kirkaldy-Willis WH (ed): *Managing Low Back Pain*, ed 2. New York, Churchill Livingstone, 1988, pp 117–131.
20. Nwuga VCB: Relative therapeutic efficacy of vertebral manipulation and conventional treatment in back pain management. *Am J Phys Med* 61:273–278, 1982.
21. Saal JA, Saal JS: Nonoperative treatment of herniated lumbar intervertebral disc with radiculopathy. An outcome study. *Spine* 14:431–437, 1989.
22. LaBan MM, Perrin JCS, Latimer FR: Pregnancy and the herniated lumbar disc. *Arch Phys Med Rehabil* 64:319–321, 1983.
23. O'Connell JEA: Lumbar disc protrusions in pregnancy. *J Neurol Neurosurg Psychiatry* 23:138–141, 1960.
24. DePalma AF, Rothman RH: *The Intervertebral Disc*. Philadelphia, WB Saunders, 1970, p 285.
25. Felsenthal G: Peripheral nervous system disorders and pregnancy, in Goldstein PJ, Stern BJ (eds): *Neurological Disorders of Pregnancy*, ed 2. New York, Futura, 1992, pp 223–267.
26. Stern PJ, Cote P, Cassidy JD: A descriptive study of low back pain with sciatica treated by chiropractors, *J Manipulative Physiol Ther*, in press.
27. Cassidy JD, Thiel HW, Kirkaldy-Willis WH: Side posture manipulation for lumbar intervertebral disc herniation. *J Manipulative Physiol Ther* 16:96–103, 1993.
28. Kuo PP, Loh ZC: Treatment of lumbar intervertebral disc protrusions by manipulation. *Clin Orthop* 215:47–55, 1987.
29. Pruzansky ME, Siffert RS, Levy RN: Orthopaedic complications, in Cherry SH, Merkatz IR (eds): *Complications of Pregnancy: Medical, Surgical, Gynecologic, Psychosocial and Perinatal*, ed 4. Baltimore, Williams & Wilkins, 1991, pp 996–1005.
30. Stern PJ, Cote P, O'Connor S, Mior SA: Symphysis pubis diastasis—a complication of pregnancy. *J Neuromusculoskeletal System* 1:74–78, 1993.
31. Taylor RN, Sonson RD: Separation of the pubic symphysis: An underrecognized peripartum complication. *J Reprod Med* 31:203–206, 1986.
32. Eastman NJ, Hellman LM: *Williams Obstetrics*, ed 13. New York, Appleton-Century-Crofts, 1966, pp 820–821.
33. Lindsey RW, Leggon RE, Wright DG, et al: Separation of the symphysis pubis in association with childbearing: A case report. *J Bone Joint Surg* 70A:289–292, 1988.
34. Sequeira W: Diseases of the pubic symphysis. *Semin Arthritis Rheum* 16:11–21, 1986.
35. Karzel RP, Friedman MJ: Orthopedic injuries in pregnancy, in Mittelmark RA,

Wiswell RA, Drinkwater BL (eds): *Exercise in Pregnancy*, ed 2. Baltimore, Williams & Wilkins, 1991, pp 123–132.
36. DeFinney J, Clemenys D, Staines M, et al: Osteitis pubis: A clinical challenge. *J Can Chiropr Assoc* 34:206–211, 1990.
37. Hammar M, Larsson L, Tegler L: Calcium treatment of leg cramps in pregnancy. *Acta Obstet Gynecol Scand* 60:345–347, 1981.
38. Smith R, Stevenson JC, Winearls CG, et al: Osteoporosis of pregnancy. *Lancet* 1:1178–1180, 1985.
39. Yahr MD, Ellis SJ, Gudesblatt M, et al: Neurological complications of pregnancy, in Cherry SH, Merkatz IR (eds): *Complications of Pregnancy: Medical, Surgical, Gynecologic, Psychosocial and Perinatal*, ed 4. Baltimore, Williams & Wilkins, 1991, pp 1008–1022.
40. Adams RD, Victor M: *Principles of Neurology*, ed 4. New York, McGraw-Hill, 1991, pp 304–307.
41. Strasberg ER: Abortion, in Rivlin ME, Morrison JC, Bates GW (eds): *Manual of Clinical Problems in Obstetrics and Gynecology with Annotated Key References*. Boston, Little, Brown, 1982, pp 5–8.
42. Renaer M: Gynaecological pain, in Wall PD, Melzack R (eds): *Textbook of Pain*. New York, Churchill Livingstone, 1984, pp 359–376.
43. Rivlin ME: (Think) ectopic pregnancy, in Rivlin ME, Morrison JC, Bates GW (eds): *Manual of Clinical Problems in Obstetrics and Gynecology with Annotated Key References*. Boston, Little, Brown, 1982, pp 8–12.
44. Leipzig S: Ectopic pregnancy, in Cherry SH, Merkatz IR (eds): *Complications of Pregnancy: Medical, Surgical, Gynecologic, Psychosocial and Perinatal*, ed 4. Baltimore, Williams & Wilkins, 1991, pp 1029–1035.
45. Andersen HF, Merkatz IR: Preterm labor, in Cherry SH, Merkatz IR (eds): *Complications of Pregnancy: Medical, Surgical, Gynecologic, Psychosocial and Perinatal*, ed 4. Baltimore, Williams & Wilkins, 1991, pp 1104–1125.
46. Lipshitz J: Preterm labor, in Rivlin ME, Morrison JC, Bates GW (eds): *Manual of Clinical Problems in Obstetrics and Gynecology with Annotated Key References*. Boston, Little, Brown, 1982, pp 107–111.
47. Iams JD, Stilson R, Johnson FF, et al: Symptoms that precede preterm labor and preterm premature rupture of the membranes. *Am J Obstet Gynecol* 162:486–490, 1990.
48. Anderson GD: Pregnancy-induced hypertension, in Rivlin ME, Morrison JC, Bates GW (eds): *Manual of Clinical Problems in Obstetrics and Gynecology with Annotated Key References*. Boston, Little, Brown, 1982, pp 31–36.
49. Anderson GD: Eclampsia, in Rivlin ME, Morrison JC, Bates GW (eds): *Manual of Clinical Problems in Obstetrics and Gynecology with Annotated Key References*. Boston, Little, Brown, 1982, pp 36–39.
50. Rhaman FR: Placenta previa, in Rivlin ME, Morrison JC, Bates GW (eds): *Manual of Clinical Problems in Obstetrics and Gynecology with Annotated Key References*. Boston, Little, Brown, 1982, pp 16–21.
51. Rhaman FR: Abruptio placentae, in Rivlin ME, Morrison JC, Bates GW (eds): *Manual of Clinical Problems in Obstetrics and Gynecology with Annotated Key References*. Boston, Little, Brown, 1982, pp 21–24.
52. Sibai BM: Deep vein thrombosis and pulmonary embolism, in Rivlin ME, Morrison JC, Bates GW (eds): *Manual of Clinical Problems in Obstetrics and Gynecology with Annotated Key References*. Boston, Little, Brown, 1982, pp 198–202.
53. Jacobsen JH, Haimov M: Treatment of venous disease in pregnancy, in Cherry SH, Merkatz IR (eds): *Complications of Pregnancy: Medical, Surgical, Gynecologic, Psychosocial and Perinatal*, ed 4. Baltimore, Williams & Wilkins, 1991, pp 495–500.

54. Penna M: Pregnancy and chiropractic care. *Am Can Assoc J Chiropr* Nov:31–33, 1989.
55. Meade TW, Dyer S, Browne W, et al: Low back pain of mechanical origin: Randomised comparison of chiropractic and hospital outpatient treatment. *BMJ* 300:1431–1437, 1990.
56. Postacchini F, Facchini M, Palieri P: Efficacy of various forms of conservative treatment in low back pain: A comparative study. *Neuroorthopedics* 6:28–35, 1988.
57. Hoehler FK, Tobis JS, Buerger AA: Spinal manipulation for low back pain. *JAMA* 245:1835–1838, 1981.
58. Hadler N, Curtis P: A benefit of spinal manipulation as adjunctive therapy for acute low back pain: A stratified controlled trial. *Spine* 12:703–706, 1987.
59. Maitland GD: *Vertebral Manipulation*, ed. 4. New York, Butterworths, 1977, p 2.
60. Diakow PRP, Gadsby TA, Gadsby JB, et al: Back pain during pregnancy and labor. *J Manipulative Physiol Ther* 14:116–118, 1991.
61. Nordin M, Weiser S, Halpern N: The prevention and treatment of low back disorders, in Frymoyer JW (ed): *The Adult Spine: Principles and Practice*. New York, Raven Press, 1991, vol 2, pp 1641–1651.
62. Mantle MJ, Holmes J, Currey HLF: Backache in pregnancy: II. Prophylactic influence of back care classes. *Rheumatol Rehabil* 20:227–232, 1981.
63. Cady LD, Bischoff PC, O'Connell ER, et al: Strength and fitness and subsequent back injuries in fire fighters. *J Occup Med* 21:269–272, 1979.
64. Lindstrom I, Ohlund C, Eek C, et al: Mobility, strength and fitness after a graded activity program for patients with subacute low back pain. *Spine* 17:641–649, 1992.
65. Heckman JD: Managing musculoskeletal problems in pregnant patients. *J Musculoskeletal Med* 1(8):35–40, 1984.
66. Mittelmark RA, Wiswell RA, Drinkwater BL, et al: Exercise guidelines in pregnancy, in Mittelmark RA, Wiswell RA, Drinkwater BL (eds): *Exercise in Pregnancy*, ed 2. Baltimore, Williams & Wilkins, 1991, pp 299–312.
67. Artal R: Exercise in pregnancy, in Cherry SH, Merkatz IR (eds): *Complications of Pregnancy: Medical, Surgical, Gynecologic, Psychosocial and Perinatal*, ed 4. Baltimore, Williams & Wilkins, 1991, pp 68–77.
68. ACOG guidelines: Exercise during pregnancy and the postnatal period, in Mittelmark RA, Wiswell RA, Drinkwater BL (eds): *Exercise in Pregnancy*, ed 2. Baltimore, Williams & Wilkins, 1991, pp 313–319.
69. Ostgaard HC, Andersson GBJ: Postpartum low-back pain. *Spine* 17:53–55, 1992.
70. Ostgaard HC, Andersson GBJ, Wennergren M. The impact of low back and pelvic pain in pregnancy outcome. *Acta Obstet Gynecol Scand* 70:21–24, 1991.

Running Injuries: A Fresh Perspective

William C. Toth, D.C., D.A.C.B.S.P.
Instructor, Post Graduate Division, National College of Chiropractic, Lombard, Illinois

The popularity of running as a form of exercise and recreation has grown rapidly during the past 20 years. Running has become a sport in its own right due in part to the fitness revolution in America and to the economics of the sport. To participate in running, an athlete needs only a good pair of running shoes and some loose fitting clothing. Running can be done anytime, anywhere, and with anyone. Reasons for running range from improving health and fitness through personal performance or competition.

Each year more people are taking part in running events worldwide. The number of runners participating in major events, such as the Hawaiian Ironman and the Boston, New York, and Chicago marathons, has risen steadily and astronomically since their respective inceptions. Further, according to Walter,[1] the number of Canadians running doubled from 15% in 1976 to 31% in 1983. Here in the United States there are an estimated 30 million runners of all levels.[2]

Actual numbers of runners are difficult to obtain, because most runners are not members of any sports group, club, or organization. Then too, one must consider those runners who participate in running as a portion of another sport such as baseball and basketball.

Because the number of runners is so difficult to ascertain, we then have considerable challenges in relation to determining the *incidence* of running injuries. This task is complicated further by the way some authors report their data. Some will report data based on the number of injured runners per 100 runners (person incidence) or as the number of injuries per 100 runners (injury incidence). More recently data have been reported as the number of injuries per 1,000 hours of running (injury per exposure). Additional variables to consider include the definition of injury, runner characteristics, research design, and length of study.

For purposes of this discussion, running injury is defined as a musculoskeletal-biomechanical event that causes a runner to cease, decrease, or alter his or her running for a time. This definition and discussion will focus on those individuals for whom running is their primary sport as opposed to those who run as part of another sport. The reader may extrapolate to the latter group as appropriate.

It is estimated that of the millions of people who run, more than 70% of them will at some time experience a running-related injury.[3] Although the majority of these are minor strains and sprains, some injuries are major or life threatening. All running injuries have the potential to become chronic if left untreated by the patient or physician.

Several studies have shown that running injuries are independent of gender, age, weight, height, running surface, and mileage.[4] In fact, the single largest predictor regarding running injuries is a prior injury.[4] Therefore, the role of the sports physician is not just to diagnose and treat the runner's injury but to educate the runner as to the prevention of future injuries.

BIOMECHANICS OF RUNNING

The purpose of this section is to provide the reader with some fundamental biomechanics as related to running. This is done so injuries, examinations, and preventive measures can be evaluated with respect to proper biomechanical function.

GAIT CYCLE

The gait cycle consists of what occurs from the initial heel strike of one lower extremity through the point at which the same heel strikes the ground again. During this cycle each extremity passes through a stance phase and a swing phase. This means that each cycle consists of two stance phases and two swing phases.

The stance phase begins at heel strike and ends when only the great toe of the same lower extremity is just touching the ground. This point is often referred to as "toe off." While walking, the stance phase comprises approximately 60% of the gait cycle. This figure becomes less as the individual begins to run and seems to be inversely proportional to the runner's speed. This percentage is smallest in the group of runners known as "forefoot runners" (see the discussion of heel strike). Altogether 80% of runners are heel-toe runners, and only 20% are forefoot runners.

The swing phase begins as the toe of one lower extremity leaves the ground and ends just before that extremity begins heel strike. This phase is the shortest in a walker and longest in forefoot runners.

Each of these phases consist of a variety of significant biomechanical events. A fault in any of these events, whether it be biomechanical or anatomical, can lead to a running injury.

HEEL STRIKE

Heel strike dynamics vary with the level of running expertise. The most elite runners use a technique known as "forefoot running." This is where the runner lands on the ball of the foot with the heel barely or never touching the ground. This group has a unique set of injuries, which are discussed later. The majority of runners contact the ground with the middle to lateral aspect of their heel. During this phase their forefoot is in a position of inversion. The amount of inversion is more pronounced in forefoot runners. During this time the tibia is externally rotated, the subtalar joint is supinated, and the patellar tendon is angulated laterally, thereby increasing the Q angle.

STANCE PHASE

After the heel contacts the ground and as the body moves forward, several events occur nearly simultaneously. The lateral aspect of the foot rapidly contacts the ground, which causes the forefoot to evert. Also, the tibia internally rotates, which causes the subtalar joint and medial aspect of the foot to pronate. This pronation and internal tibial rotation serve as a mechanism to reduce the Q angle, thereby decreasing lateral knee forces. Concurrently during this time the knee flexes 30 to 40 degrees.

As the stance phase progresses, the ground reaction forces (which began at the heel) are transferred along the lateral aspect of the foot. Once they have reached the head of the fifth metatarsal, the foot pronates and everts. This serves to transfer the forces across the metatarsal heads to the first metatarsal-phalangeal joint in preparation for toe off. Just before toe off, the tibia externally rotates, the foot inverts, and the subtalar joint again supinates.

SWING PHASE

The swing phase begins just after toe off and ends just before that same extremity reaches heel strike. During this phase the tibia remains externally rotated. The subtalar joint maximally supinates and the forefoot maximally inverts again.

During running these cycles occur approximately 800 to 2,000 times per mile, or 50 to 70 times per minute per foot.[3] Ground force reaction has been measured to be approximately two to four times the runner's body weight.[6] When you consider total mileage times total force, you are faced with tons of force per mile being imparted to the body. This is why small abnormalities in function or anatomy, which are asymptomatic with walking, become symptomatic with running.

MUSCULAR CONTROL OF THE ANKLE WHILE RUNNING

Taunton[7] has shown that the majority of running injuries below the knee are a result of muscle dysfunction, fatigue, or both. The physician should be aware of the action of these muscles during the phases of the gait cycle for proper diagnosis, treatment, and prevention of injuries.

The recent work of Reber[8] has changed some popular misconceptions regarding muscle action below the knee during running. Their study used a fine-wire needle electromyelogram, and high-speed photography to document muscle action of a selected group of runners.

During the stance phase the posterior muscles of the leg (gastrocnemius, soleus, tibialis posterior) showed peak activity at midstance. This can be interpreted to mean that these muscles are eccentrically loading to control ankle dorsiflexion as the center of gravity passes over the ankle point. This is contrary to what was previously believed, namely, that the posterior muscles were most active during toe off.

The tibialis posterior muscle was determined to be most active during the early stance phase. This supports the common belief that this muscle serves to control pronation of the foot. Hyperpronation problems for runners are extremely common, and therefore this knowledge would appear to confirm that preventive measures should focus on rehabilitation of this muscle.

The posterior group of muscles significantly decreased their activity after midstance. They remained essentially "dormant" until the next heel strike.

During the swing phase the anterior lower leg muscles become more active. This is particularly true of the tibialis anterior muscle. This is considered to be necessary to maintain the inverted/supinated position of the forefoot as previously discussed. This muscle was shown to have a higher sustained level of activity than any of the other muscles tested by Reber.[8] This translates into a higher potential for injury.

All of the lower leg muscles were shown by Reber to increase their activity as the pace of running increased. This was especially true of the peroneus brevis muscle. This makes sense if one considers that as pace increases, the ground contact point tends to move forward on the plantar surface of the foot.[9] This, in turn, causes more force to be supported, during midstance, at the midfoot and forefoot region. This occurs at a time when the subtalar joint is relatively "loose packed" or, in other words, less stable than at other times of the gait cycle. To compensate for the relative lack of stability, the peroneus brevis muscle contracts more forcibly.

Knowledge of proper biomechanics during the phases of the gait cycle allows the physician to more accurately diagnose the runner's injury. After that, proper rehabilitation may be prescribed for recovery, and then a training program can be written that corrects the underlying weakness or dysfunction.

CATEGORIES OF RUNNERS

Injuries that runners experience can be classified into two categories: training errors and anatomical faults. Of these two categories, training errors are the most significant. Many anatomical faults or biochemical aberrations remain symptomatically silent during activities of daily living. However, these situations often become symptomatic when an individual begins a running program. In addition, most injuries seem to occur when runners change their program through intensity, distance, or both. Therefore, *how* a runner is running often becomes more significant to the physician.

To assist in the assessment of the runner, the physician should categorize the type of running the patient does because of the fact that certain injuries occur within certain running groups or levels. Table 1 is a somewhat arbitrary classification scheme that some physicians may find useful. It does not account for those running injuries or runners who are injured while playing a certain sport such as football or racquetball.

CATEGORIES OF RUNNING INJURIES

TRAINING ERRORS

Training errors are the most frequent cause of running injuries. These range from improper technique to premature return to running after an

TABLE 1.
Categories of Runners

Level	Miles/Week	Time/Mile
Jogger	1–10	10–12
Recreational	11–30	7–9
Competitive	31–60	6–8
Marathoner	≥60	5–7

injury. This is the area where the sports physician can have the most beneficial impact. It is also the area where athletes are likely to "forget" details when reporting to the physician.

Probably the most common training error is "too much too soon." This applies to both beginners and elite runners. All training programs must start slow in terms of speed and distance and gradually progress over weeks or months. Beginners typically have no idea what their physiological limits are and frequently run too far or too fast early in their program. Many quit after such an experience. Those who do not quit and then try to maintain the same pace or distance usually end up in the physician's office.

Many elite runners foolishly start the new season at the same pace and distance at which they finished the prior season. Fortunately, this group of runners tends to have less serious injuries than the beginners and consequently are able to return to running shortly after some rehabilitation and coaching.

The next most common training error is the athlete's choice of running surface. Recreational runners are the group most at risk in this case because they typically run on "pitched" or "crowned" road surfaces. This, combined with the habit of running the same route, can lead to injuries. Biomechanically the downside leg has more external rotation of the tibia and supination of the foot. This places a greater than normal amount of stress on the lateral side of the knee. The upside leg is subjected to greater internal tibial rotation and pronation. This leads to greater stress on the medial side of the knee. Two other injuries common to runners who run on banked surfaces are iliotibial band syndrome and bursitis over the greater trochanter.

The next area of concern is stretching too much, too little, or improperly. The research on this topic is not clear. There seems to be a negative rather than positive correlation between stretching and running injuries.[14] The discrepancies in the research probably result from nonstandardization of stretching techniques and reporting thereof.

It may well be that some types of stretching may be effective, whereas others are not. Conversely, "when" an athlete stretches may be more important than "how." This issue needs further investigation. Stretching before and after running are common practices that have not been significantly successful in preventing injuries. Stretching before running is probably more common.

The sports physician can be fairly comfortable with the following widely accepted stretching axioms. First, no runners should stretch "cold" muscles. All muscle groups should be warmed up *before* being stretched. A reasonable warm-up consists of 3 to 5 minutes of calisthenics or running in place. Second, no stretches should be done in a ballistic manner, which means no bouncing while stretching. A slow stretch and hold seems to work the best. I have found it helpful to instruct athletes to exhale as they actively stretch the muscle. This serves to decrease the pain and seems to allow them to stretch the muscle further.

Probably the most important muscles that need to be stretched in runners are the hamstring and the calf muscles, especially the hamstrings. This is because running causes the hamstrings to strengthen to a greater degree and at a greater rate than the quadriceps or gluteal muscles. Along with this strengthening comes some shortening of the hamstring muscles. The subsequent imbalance in the normal quad to hamstring ratio (3:2) often leads to knee pain, injury, or both.

One strengthening technique that seems to work well for many runners for their hamstrings is the "standing hurdler's stretch." This technique seems to be more effective if the athlete keeps the lower back straight and bends the upper torso from the waist toward the knee as opposed to most runners who try to touch their forehead to their knee.

For the gastrocnemius and soleus muscles, the perennial favorite stretch is to hang the rearfoot off the edge of a stair by supporting the bodyweight on the ball of the foot. After an injury to the lower leg, these muscles are stretched while sitting by using a towel or strap to pull the forefoot into a position of dorsiflexion.

One final common training error is the athlete's choice of shoes. With the proliferation of media hype regarding athletic shoes that promise to make you run faster, longer, jump higher, and so forth, it is easy to understand why many athletes buy the wrong shoes. Athletes make one of two mistakes when buying an athletic shoe: They either buy the wrong shoe for their sport or buy the wrong shoe for their foot or body type.

There are hundreds of shoe types on the market for athletes and physicians to choose from. Because I have agreed to limit the discussion to people for whom running is their primary sport, this category may be narrowed down to three types of shoes: cross trainers, running shoes, and running cleats.

Cross trainers are shoes that are designed to be used for several different sports. Very commonly, the cross trainer is a combination running shoe, court shoe, and strength-training shoe. As a general rule, this type of shoe is heavier and stiffer and has more lateral support than a typical running shoe. This type of shoe is ideally suited for someone who is indulging in a general fitness program that would involve some running in a sport such as racquetball or volleyball and some limited track or road running. Cross trainers should not be used for running if the running portion of the athlete's program is more than 10 miles per week at 10 to 12 minutes per mile (jogger).

Literally hundreds of models of running shoes are available from dozens of manufacturers. Because excessive pronation has found wide acceptance as an indicator for running injuries, most of these shoes are designed to limit pronation. Manufacturers know that the least amount of pronation takes place while running barefoot,[16] so they make their shoes torsionally stiff to limit pronation. This torsional stiffness occurs in the longitudinal plane and causes a smaller torsion angle but has an end result of greater torsional force at the ankle joints. These effects are taking place primarily at heel strike and are the principal reasons that manufacturers are so concerned with shock absorption at heel strike.

Manufacturers use primarily two materials in the midsole for shock absorption, either ethylene vinyl acetate (EVA) or polyurethane. Polyurethane is more expensive and softer than EVA, so it is used less and wears out more quickly. Then too, softer is not necessarily better, because what you gain in shock absorption, you lose in foot control. In general, midsoles cause loss of foot control, and with softer midsoles that loss is greater.

To counter the loss of control, manufacturers build running shoes with a midsole and sole that is wider than the upper portion of the shoe. This increases both foot and ankle control and also leads directly to greater angular velocities of foot and ankle joints, which some believe cause greater injury. The companies also add a thermoplastic heel counter to the heel of the shoe upper. Within 1 or 2 hours of walking or running, the athlete's body heat softens the thermoplastic and therefore allows it to deform to the shape of the athlete's ankle. This cups the ankle, thereby leading to greater stability in the shoe. This is important because there is growing concern in the literature relative to the interaction that *might* occur between the athlete's foot *inside* the shoe *while running*.

The third type of shoe available to runners is the running cleat or spikes. These shoes have a very thin soft sole except for the forefoot where there is a stiff plate used to mount the spikes. The shoe upper is also very soft, including the heel region. This type of shoe is definitely not torsionally stiff; therefore, the torsional angle and force that occur are very close to those that occur while running barefoot. Unfortunately, the lack of support in the heel allows hyperpronation to take place.

The next logical question is which shoe is used when? Each athlete is different and will develop different preferences. However, most runners will generally follow the trend (i.e., what are other runners doing, especially ones that are faster than they are). I have seen the majority of runners use their spikes on running tracks, especially for interval training and running races. For the rest of their training and for road races, these runners use running shoes. The groups of runners I am referring to are the recreational runners, competitive runners, and marathoners.

SHOE FIT

Determining the type of shoe needed is only half the battle. The right shoe and the best shoe will not work properly unless the shoe fits properly. The most important message you can give to your runners is to get the best fit possible.

First, have runners visit the shoe store at the end of a run or at the end of a day when their feet are the largest. They should wear the same socks they wear when they run, and they should fit the shoe to their largest foot. They should make sure there is one thumb's width from the end of the longest toe to the end of the toe box. This will prevent hammer toes and damage to the nail beds. The toe box should be wide enough so that the foot does not force the shoe upper to protrude past the midsole.

Second, the shoes should be checked carefully. Even within the same manufacturer's shoe line, shoe size can vary from style to style or within the same style. It is not uncommon to find that the same brand, make, and model number of shoe will look and feel different because it was made in another country.

Next, the shoes are placed sole to sole and heel to heel. Observing the shoes from a lateral aspect, they should make sure the length of the soles are equal. If not, the salesperson should get another pair, because a few millimeters' difference in length translates to larger differences in torsion and force at the ankle and eventually the knee.

The shoes should then be flexed through the toe box perpendicular to the long axis of the shoe. The point of flexion may differ because of different midsole thickness or even different amounts of glue between midsole and outer sole. If a difference is present, the process should be started over again until the runner finds a pair in which left and right match.

Also, the runner should consider other design features such as plastic tabs that allow double lacing, stitching in the uppers, logos, high-tech heel counters, and "pumping" mechanisms. In some instances, these features have been known to cause injury. Those special features may or may not be useful to the runner and the runner's style of running.

The physician may want to keep up with technological changes in shoes so as to be the best possible resource for his or her patients. This can be accomplished by contacting either the shoe company directly or the company's technical sales representatives. Most shoe companies have a toll-free number for information regarding their products. This is often a good place to start. By means of the telephone, you may be able to work your way through to the research and development or technical analysis department. They will usually be happy to send you volumes of data regarding every single shoe design and why each particular design is so good. Some of this information will be sales hype, and some will be reliable data. The most important item for the physician to remember is that for an athlete, the shoe is not just another addition to his or her wardrobe. Running shoes are considered to be a piece of equipment that has a specific design for a specific purpose. It is the sports physician's responsibility to educate patients as to the specifics regarding running style, individual biomechanical needs, and appropriate footwear that matches the former.

EVALUATION OF RUNNING INJURIES

DIAGNOSIS

The three groups of runners who do the most running (recreational, competitive, and marathoners) all share a common unique mind-set. Any physician who has worked with runners is aware of this and those who are just beginning will quickly learn of it.

For these groups of runners, running is a very significant part of their social and emotional life. These folks do not run just to increase their fitness. Many of these folks have integrated running into their identity: It is not only something they do; it becomes part of *who they are*. The physician must take this into consideration when treating runners.

The physician must also allow sufficient time for patients to fully express complaints, explain their training methods, and describe previous injuries and treatments. Failure to acquire this information will frequently lead to therapeutic failure.

HISTORY

A thorough patient history is essential for the proper diagnosis of running injuries. The physician should be especially concerned with the patient's cardiorespiratory history and prior injuries to the musculoskeletal system, especially from the umbilicus region to the toes. This is very important because subtle compensatory patterns develop after improperly or untreated injuries. These patterns frequently are asymptomatic in nonrunners or with low-mileage runners and later become symptomatic as mileage increases.

The physician should ask the following questions concerning the patient's running habits:

1. How long have you been running?
2. What mileage do you normally run?
3. How long does that usually take?
4. What type of stretching do you do before or after running (or both)?
5. What type of shoes do you wear?
6. Have there been any changes in your running routine?
7. Have there been any recent injuries?

It is during this line of questioning where the physician usually gets a sense of how important running is to these individuals. The physician will often hear how runners attempted to "train around" an injury because they "have to" run. This is definitely not a time for the doctor to be judgmental. It is best to acknowledge the patient's intent and then offer an alternative that is mutually compatible with both the patient's goals and the physician's therapeutic objectives.

PHYSICAL EXAMINATION

The usual orthopedic and neurological assessments should be performed on each runner. Careful attention should be given to anatomical and functional faults. The patient should be in shorts and barefoot for this portion of the examination.

The patient should be observed in a standing position first (Table 2). The physician should look for gross anatomical abnormality of the lower back, hips, pelvis, legs, and feet. The physician is looking for conditions such as wide pelvis, genu varum, genu valgus, patellar malalignment, pes planus, pes cavus, and femoral neck anteversion or retroversion.

Next, the patient's thoracolumbar range of motion should be evaluated. The flexibility of the lower spine, hamstring, and calf muscles

TABLE 2.
Key Physical Examination Items of Runners

Standing
    Pelvic width
    Genu varus, valgus
    Patellar position
    Pes planus, cavus
    Femoral neck anteversion, retroversion
    Tibial torsion
    Thoracolumbar range of motion
Supine
    Direction and degree of hip rotation
    Q angle
    Hamstring length
Prone
    Leg length
    Leg-heel alignment
    Heel-forefoot alignment
Active running/walking
    Biomechanics of foot/ankle
    Biomechanics of knee/hip

should be assessed and compared bilaterally. Next, the physician should examine the patient in a supine position. The two most significant observations at this point should be to determine the degree and direction of hip rotation and the Q angle. Excessive external hip rotation will cause the runner to run with the feet turned out, whereas internal rotation will cause the reverse. The Q angle is a strong discriminator between injured and noninjured runners.[10] In males Q angles are generally considered normal if they are between 8 and 10 degrees. In females Q angles are generally considered normal if they are between 10 and 15 degrees. Some authors[10] believe that 15 degrees should be considered the upper limit of normal because of the fact that Q angles of injured runners tended to fall in the 15- to 20-degree range. An increased Q angle may result from lateral displacement of the tibial tuberosity, genu valgum, femoral anteversion, or excessive tibial torsion. The increased Q angle causes the patella to deviate laterally as the quadriceps contract. This forces the lateral aspect of the undersurface of the patella to contact the lateral femoral condyle. Too much contact can lead to pain and injury. The presence or absence of patella alta needs to be noted for its contribution to the Q angle.

    Leg length equality or inequality is a must with regard to assessment. Leg length inequality is a relatively common musculoskeletal malalignment related to structural, postural, and environmental factors. If inequality exists, it is considered to be a plausible factor in the development of overuse injuries.[11] This is because it alters the function of the lower limbs, pelvis, and lower back and causes uneven load distribution amongst those structures.

Leg length is measured three ways. Two are easily accomplished in the office with a tape measure. First, the physician can measure from the anterior superior iliac spine to the tip of the medial malleolus. This measurement is commonly referred to as "absolute leg length" and is often interpreted as being the true anatomical leg length. The second method is to measure from the umbilicus to the tip of the medial malleolus. This is commonly referred to as the "relative leg length" and is often interpreted as being the functional leg length. This is because pelvic distortion patterns will easily alter this measurement.

The third and most accurate method for measuring actual leg length is called a "scanogram" and requires an x-ray unit with a table. This technique requires the patient to lie on the table. On an 11 by 17 in. film (divided into thirds lengthwise), anteroposterior radiographs are taken of the hip joints, knees, and ankles (all bilaterally). Measurements are made on the film and compared bilaterally. This is the most accurate measurement procedure for determining anatomical vs. functional leg length. Also, the technique is less susceptible to physician error.

Recently, Hoyle[12] described a noninvasive measurement of leg length inequality using a Metrecom. They reported low intraexaminer and interexaminer variability compared with that using tape measurements. This technique will require further research and review.

The ankle and foot are examined carefully. Callus, blister, and bunion formation warn the physician of either improper footwear or improper biomechanical function. Three types of foot conditions predispose the athlete to injuries. First is the obvious pes planus, or "flat foot." Next is the also obvious pes cavus, or "high arch foot." Both of these situations cause the foot to *transmit* rather than absorb the force of running. Finally, there is "Morton's foot," where the second metatarsal is larger than the first. This too seems to allow the forces of running to be transmitted up the lower extremity. There is some question as to whether this really occurs as a result of this particular anatomical variant (Morton's foot).

With the foot in a neutral position and the patient prone, the physician should check the leg-heel alignment. The calcaneus and leg should be aligned or parallel. Medial or lateral deviation of the calcaneus usually indicates a biomechanical fault of the foot ankle complex.

The heel-forefoot alignment should also be checked with the foot and athlete in this position. Ideally the calcaneus should be perpendicular to the forefoot. Again, medial or lateral deviation usually indicates altered function.

The physician may also choose to use an in-house measurement to determine the degree of pronation. This technique measures "navicular drop" and was first described by Schuster.[13] It is done with the patient standing barefoot on a firm surface.

Ideally the midline of the heel, lower calf, and navicular bone all are marked at their respective midlines. The foot is placed in a neutral position, and an index card is placed on the medial aspect of the foot with its bottom edge on the floor. The level of the navicular is marked, and the foot is then relaxed with weight bearing. The resulting lower position of the navicular bone is marked as well. The distance between the two marks is referred to as the "navicular drop." Normally this distance is approximately 8 to 10 mm, and a distance greater that 15 mm is considered to indicate hyperpronation. Navicular drop of more than 15 to 20 mm would indicate the need for orthotics.

RADIOGRAPHIC EXAMINATION

Plain films are generally considered to be a good starting point for the evaluation of running injuries. In addition to the already mentioned "scanogram," the physician should consider a knee series that includes a tangenital ("sunrise") view because many preexisting conditions, especially malalignments, will be uncovered at this stage.

Appropriate sectional x-ray series should be ordered based on clinical suspicion. For example, if there is a suspected hip problem, a hip series should be ordered. A series of plain films should be ordered only if the clinical examination warrants them. Routine use of plain film is not encouraged.

Occasionally a bone scan is necessary to reveal the presence of stress fractures or early Osgood-Schlatter disease. Stress fractures are relatively common for runners, particularly those who are just beginning or those who run long distance. Common sites for stress fractures in runners include the tibia, metatarsals, and pelvis, with the tibia being the most common site of stress fractures in runners.

BIOMECHANICAL EVALUATION

Today's athletes are increasingly sophisticated in relation to training techniques, supplementation, and their knowledge of evaluation procedures. It is not uncommon for an athlete to request a videotape analysis of his or her biomechanical function. In the past, they were used by research facilities only. Today many sports physicians have treadmills and videotape equipment in their offices. There are many good systems on the market within the reach (economically) of a wider range of sports physicians.

These procedures and setups allow both the athlete and the physician to evaluate the runner's biomechanical mechanism. Very often both the runner and the coach are amazed by the results obtained with this equipment. However, for the physician carefully trained in observation, sometimes all that is necessary is to observe the runner at the track or even in the parking lot of the office. In this case, what is missing is the ability to use slow-motion video technology for review.

SHOE EVALUATION

Just as the eyes are the mirror to the soul, the shoes of a runner are a mirror of the runner's biomechanics. Wear patterns on the soles and the condition of the midsole and uppers all provide information regarding the runner's technique. It is an essential part of the examination to evaluate the runner's shoes.

The doctor should not be fooled by shoes that "look good." A shoe may look okay to the eye and still be functionally impaired. Shoe manufacturers design the midsole to last approximately 300 to 500 miles. For most runners, that is the amount of miles run in one season, or 3 to 6 months. When this part of the shoe wears out, it will feel hard and dry, or it may show signs of compression (i.e., "wrinkling").

Frequently runners are fooled into thinking their shoes have good cushioning because of their bodies' ability to adapt to the shoe. They still think the shoe is comfortable. There are two ways to show runners that their shoes are worn out in addition to the previously mentioned methods. First, place the the shoes on a flat surface and observe them from the heel while at the level of the flat surface. Worn-out midsoles allow the upper part of the shoe to appear turned in or out. Try rolling the shoes side to side; if they roll, roll them right into the garbage. A normal shoe will stay flat on the table. Next, observe the shoe from the heel and pay attention to a line perpendicular to the flat surface that passes through the center of the sole. A runner who pronates will force the heel of the shoe to deviate laterally, whereas a runner who supinates will force it to deviate medially. Second, have the athlete go to the shoe store and try on some new running shoes. The athlete will immediately be able to tell the difference between the old shoes and the new ones.

The sole of the shoe also gives critical information relative to the biomechanics of the runner. Please recall that after heel strike, the foot rolls forward along the lateral edge until the head of the fifth metatarsal contacts the ground. Then the foot pronates across the metatarsal heads, thus transferring the force to the ball of the foot. From there the force goes out through the great toe during toe off. This creates a telltale wear pattern that begins on the lateral aspect of the heel, follows along the lateral aspect of the sole, then crosses over to the ball of the foot and finally out through the great toe region. A foot that is pronating will show a more than normal *lateral* heel strike, very little wear along the lateral sole, and much more wear at the second and third metatarsal heads. This is because the foot that pronates contacts the ground at heel strike and then, instead of rolling, slaps down to the ground at the second and third metatarsal heads. A foot that is supinating excessively will very likely not have a heel strike and instead will show greater wear at the lateral forefoot region. This is also what you will see with forefoot runners.

One final condition that shows prominently on the soles of the shoes is leg length inequality. As a general rule, the shoe on the longer limb will show greater wear patterns of scuffing or smoothing of the sole. This will tend to be generalized. The shorter limb will generally show a more pronounced or deeper normal wear pattern (if foot and ankle are functioning normally).

One note of caution: Wear patterns are also related to running surfaces. This means that if an athlete habitually runs on a banked track or a pitched road, a variety of additional wear patterns may present themselves. This underscores the necessity for the history questions related to running.

The next area to observe is the upper part of the shoe. Observe the area around the toe box (i.e., from the ball of the foot forward). A runner who supinates excessively will "break out" or roll the upper part of the shoe over the sole in a lateral direction. Conversely, a runner who pronates will collapse the medial aspect of the shoe.

ANATOMICAL FAULTS AND CONDITIONS

Running injuries account for a large percentage of sports-related practices. This is because there are a large number of runners in the United States and because approximately 70% of runners experience running-related injuries, aches, and pain.[3,17] These injuries fall into two categories: overuse (training errors) and functional anatomical faults.

The majority of running injuries involve the lower extremities. Those that do not are usually a result of trauma and are not covered in this chapter. In particular, the knee is the most often involved structure, with the ankle-foot complex running a close second and the hip running a not-to-distant third. This section reviews the common anatomical faults and conditions that are common to injured runners. Please bear in mind that some uninjured runners may have these same situations present.

The knee is the largest joint in the body and the most susceptible to injury.[18] Anatomists call it a ginglymus joint, which essentially means its primary sources of support are the ligaments and muscles that control its movement.

PATELLOFEMORAL ARTHRALGIA

The single greatest knee-related problem is patellofemoral pain. This is sometimes referred to as patellofemoral arthralgia, patellalgia, patellofemoral compression syndrome, and of course the great garbage pail diagnosis, chondromalacia patella.

The literature on the condition is quite abundant and confusing. Most research points to changes in the anatomical structure of the anterior knee as being the source of the pain.[19] Examples of said changes are chondromalacia patella, lateral retinacular contracture, and synovial plica. What is confusing to some is that many runners who have said changes have no patellofemoral pain, whereas those who have the pain often do not have the changes. This would suggest that the source of the pain is a result of *functional* changes rather than anatomical changes.

This is to say that patellofemoral pain is the result of malalignment of the patella as it travels within the trochlear groove. This malalignment may have one or more of several possible causes.

The most common cause is likely to be a relative or frank weakness of the vastus medialis oblique muscle. In runners this is particularly common because running puts more demand on the vastus lateralis muscle. This creates a laterally directed vector of force that pulls the patella into contact with the lateral femoral condyle. Other factors that have the same effect include a tight iliotibial band, a tight lateral retinaculum, and an increased Q angle.

Athletes who suffer from the condition will report long-term insidious onset of "burning" retropatellar pain. This burning, achy pain will become sharp with going up or down stairs or with jumping. In general this condition is worse after activity. However, the pain may also become noticeable while sitting for long periods of time; therefore, this condition is one that produces "cinema sign."

The physician will likely be able to elicit palpatory tenderness of the undersurface of the lateral aspect of the patella. Extension of the knee from a flexed position, especially while under load, will often produce significant pain. Manual lateral deviation of the patella will usually reproduce the patient's chief complaint.

This condition will usually resolve with early conservative care such as RICE (rest, ice, compression, and elevation). Correction also is within the purview of conservative care. These patients benefit significantly from isometric quadriceps exercise, followed with graduated resistance exercises that focus on the vastus medialis muscle. Cycling also focuses on the vastus medialis muscle. Most patients will recover enough to resume sports activities. Always a prophylactic program of knee extension, squats, and leg presses is instituted to prevent future recurrence.

ILIOTIBIAL BAND SYNDROME

The next most common cause of knee pain is considered to be iliotibial tract syndrome. This is also probably the single largest cause of lateral knee pain. The cause of the condition is an inflammatory reaction that occurs between the lateral femoral epicondyle and the iliotibial tract in response to friction that occurs with repetitive knee flexion and extension.

Athletes suffering from this condition will report sharp, burning, boring pain over the lateral knee, specifically over the lateral femoral epicondyle. They often report this problem begins with running on pitched or crowned roads and continues afterward. This condition will affect the downside leg first. Also, downhill running causes the problem because the knee stays flexed for longer periods. Other causes include excessive stride lengths, genu varus, crossover gait, hyperpronation, and rapid increases in mileage.

Treatment for this condition focuses on reducing the inflammation presumably with RICE. Patient active care is instituted via a stretching program for this region. A general lower extremity strengthening program would follow.

POSTERIOR TIBIAL SYNDROME

It is not known just how far this diagnosis reaches in terms of impact on the total number of injuries because this term was once widely used to describe any pain between the knee and ankle. Currently this term refers only to pain along the medial distal two thirds of the tibial shaft. This condition is commonly called "shin splints."

Some authors consider this condition to actually be three separate clinical entities that are actually a progression of the same problem. It is thought that shin splints are caused by some altered mechanics that result in traction of the posterior tibialis tendon at its attachments to the interosseous membrane and tibia.

Stage 1 is posterior tibialis tendinitis, which, if left untreated, progresses to periostitis (stage 2). This condition, if let untreated, results in stress fractures of the tibia (stage 3).

Athletes who suffer from this condition will call the physician's office with the complaint of "I can't run anymore." They will report long-term insidious onset of anterior lower leg pain that worsens with activity and gets only partial relief with rest. Pain may be described as burning, throbbing, bloating, heaviness, or sharp and stabbing, especially if the tibia is touched.

Conservative care is appropriate in these cases. Initially RICE is sufficient. After symptoms abate, the return to running should be gradual and on softer surfaces. Some studies have shown that gastrocnemius stretching offers some relief.

POPLITEAL TENDINITIS

Popliteal tendinitis is most often a direct result of downhill running or hyperpronation. This muscle originates on the lateral femoral condyle and inserts on the posterior surface of the tibia.

This tendon acts to prevent the forward displacement of the femur on the tibia and therefore is very active with downhill running and running on a banked surface. (The upside leg is affected first.)

Because this tendon runs intra-articularly, patients report this condition or pain as deep and boring. They report, "I can't put my finger on it." The smart physician will be able to find point tenderness over the posterior lateral joint line.

RICE is the treatment of choice coinciding with a reduction in running. Interval training, hills, and pitched roads should be avoided until symptoms have abated.

ACHILLES TENDINITIS

Achilles tendinitis is the second most common cause of heel pain in a runner. This condition involves an inflammatory process surrounding the Achilles tendon just above its attachment to the calcaneus. This may be caused by downhill running, toe off during up-hill running, improper padding in the heel of the shoe, and shoe soles that are too hard or soft. In addition, pes cavus, tight gastrocnemius, and tight hamstrings have been associated with this condition.

Typically runners will report a burning pain when they first bear weight, which then subsides during the day. If they are still running, the pain is severe in the beginning, lessens during the run, and then worsens after the run.

Aggressive, conservative care is called for because of the potential seriousness of no care. Left untreated, Achilles tendinitis usually progresses to Achilles tendon rupture. The patient must stop running and aggressively pursue anti-inflammatory measures. Ice massage on a hourly basis is not unreasonable for the first 3 days, gradually decreasing frequency to three to four times daily for several days. An ankle rehabilitation program is discussed later.

PLANTAR FASCIITIS

The most common cause of heel pain in runners is plantar fasciitis.[20] This is the result of chronic traction on the plantar fascia, which results in the inflammation of the fascial fibers near the medial tubercle of the calcaneus. A bone spur sometimes forms as a *result* of the inflammatory process and not the reverse, as was previously thought.

Primarily the traction on the tendon results from hyperpronation.

This may be the result of poor shoe construction, pes planus, pes cavus, and running on pitched surfaces. All of these situations allow the navicular bone to descend to such a degree as to cause traction of the aponeurosis near its midpoint. This stress is transferred to the tendon attachment near the medial tubercle of the calcaneus.

Athletes who suffer from this condition frequently report intense pain when they get out of bed in the morning. They report they are "crippled" for the first few steps. This pain gradually abates and settles to a "burning ache" that will usually worsen after more activity. On palpation of the medial tubercle of the calcaneus, the patient will usually respond with sharp outcries.

The first line of defense in this situation is a good offense. The best place to start is to replace the runner's shoes with a pair that has additional medial arch support. Next, add some shock absorption to the shoe such as Sorbothane inner soles. This helps reduce the stress put into the plantar aponeurosis. Educate the athlete on the benefits of self foot massage relative to relaxing the tendon. Numerous home massage units are in abundance in the market place.

For this situation, the following foot-ankle rehabilitation program is also appropriate after RICE.

GENERAL FOOT ANKLE REHABILITATION

RICE

R = Rest from running until symptom subsides.
I = Ice packs, 20 minutes per use, with a warm wet towel between ice and skin; or direct ice massage for 5 minutes.
C = Compression of affected part.
E = Elevation of lower extremity for duration of ice use.

PROPRIOCEPTIVE REHABILITATION

Proprioceptive rehabilitation is often the key to a successful rehabilitation program. All too often runners are sent out to the track or street pain free, with complete range of motion, with normal strength, and with little or no proprioceptive sense.

Proprioceptive rehabilitation can be accomplished at home while the athlete is recovering from the injury. The sports physician can have the patient roll the feet in a clockwise and counterclockwise range of motion while seated and with the feet elevated. Next, the patient, in a seated position, should roll the feet in a clockwise and counterclockwise motion while resting on two golf balls, one under each foot. This is done in stocking feet or barefoot.

These two exercises serve to reinforce proprioception pathways in the remaining proprioceptive fibers of the uninjured tissues. There is an additional benefit of massage with the golf ball technique. These two exercises are begun immediately after injury but then only in a pain-free range. Their purpose is to reinforce the body's sense of position in space and time.

The next stage of proprioceptive rehabilitation is done while weight bearing. This can be done on a BAPS board (a device designed specifically for proprioceptive rehabilitation), or it can be done at home on the floor.

Have the athlete stand on both feet (barefoot) approximately 12 to 18 in. apart. Next, have the athlete flex the knees approximately 30 to 40 degrees and then swivel the hips and trunk in such a way that the knees are traveling in a clockwise and counterclockwise circle.

The proprioceptive exercises should be done daily, as frequently as practical, for 3- to 5-minute intervals. The athlete should perform these exercises first with the eyes open and then with the eyes closed for even greater proprioceptive awareness.

STRENGTHENING

The next phase of foot-ankle rehabilitation consists of strengthening the muscles that support the foot and ankle complex. These exercises help promote a stable ankle complex and thereby decrease the chance of injury.

The fundamental exercise for this region is called the heel raise or calf raise. This involves athletes standing on a ledge or stair such that the weight is supported on the ball of the foot and the heel is free. Then they simply raise the heel as far as they can and hold for a count of 3. They lower the heel until it is below the level of the ledge or stair, again holding for a count of 3. This is primarily for the posterior tibialis and gastrocnemius muscles and their role in controlling pronation.

Weight may be added when the athlete can do three sets of 10 repetitions without pain or subsequent soreness. Weight can be added by placing a barbell across the shoulders, holding a dumbbell in one hand, or supporting his or her weight on one foot with the other foot held behind the heel.

Distance runners should consider seated heel raises because this exercise concentrates on the soleus muscle, which we know to be primarily slow twitch or endurance fibers. To do this, athletes can sit on a chair in front of a stair or ledge with a barbell held across the top of their knees.

All runners should add some peroneal exercises to their program because of the aforementioned importance of these muscles. The peroneal exercises can be performed using some elastic tubing. The emphasis should be maintained on eversion first and dorsiflexion second.

The next phase of rehabilitation involves the progressive return to sport. During the first week or 2 the athletes should focus their attention on running figure eights. These should be run on flat open ground. The figure eights should initially be very large and slow. As the athlete improves, the figure eights become smaller and faster. They should be run in alternating clockwise and counterclockwise patterns.

Because most lower extremity injuries involve the knee, we must direct some attention to rehabilitation of this joint as well. Much of what was done for proprioceptive rehabilitation of the ankle indirectly benefits the proprioceptive sense of the knee. Therefore, our attention is focused on the strengthening of the knee complex.

Before strengthening the knee, one must not overlook the hamstring.

Short hamstrings artificially decrease the knee range of motion, particularly extension. Therefore, the hamstring must first be stretched. This is initially done by the sports physician with any number of proprioceptive neuromuscular facilitation techniques. Once the physician has restored the range of motion to the hamstrings, it becomes the patient's responsibility to retain that increased range of motion.

Most commonly, the hamstrings are stretched by the athlete with a standing hurdler's stretch. I prefer a variant of that stretch as follows. The athlete is instructed to stand with one foot up on a chair with the two feet 90 degrees opposed such that the foot on the chair is pointing straight up while the weight-bearing foot points 90 degrees to the lateral direction as if the two heels were on the floor touching one another. Next the athlete will turn and square off or face the foot on the chair. Then, keeping an eye on the horizon and the lower back straight, he or she will bend at the hips toward the foot and chair. This is to be done slowly, without bouncing. The athlete should exhale as he or she does the stretch, stop when "pain" appears, and continue after the next breath. This should be repeated several times until the athlete feels he or she can go no further. It is important to emphasize that the athlete is not to touch the head to the knees as has been taught in the past. This "old way" actually caused athletes to stretch their middle and upper spines without enough stretch of the hamstrings.

The quadriceps also need to be stretched before strengthening, as do the gastrocnemius muscles. This is because they too affect knee range of motion. The gastrocnemius muscles can be stretched as previously described, and the quadriceps can be stretched by extending at the hip with the knee fully flexed.

The quadriceps strengthening begins with isometrics during the acute phase of injury. Next, a stationary cycling program can be used before the athlete progresses to a resistance program.

It is probably best to begin with three to six sets of 10-repetition knee extensions. They should be done with the toes turned in, out, and straight up. This is because the literature is divided as to where the vastus medialis is actually most active. Thus, we cover our bases by using all three methods. Repetition should be slow, deliberate, and only in a pain-free range. Excessive speed can easily overcome a weak tracking mechanism and actually cause more difficulty. This program should be done every other day initially and should progress such that the athlete does not add weight until he or she can easily do three sets of 12 to 15 repetitions.

The quadriceps need to be balanced by strong hamstrings. It is commonly accepted there should be a strength ratio of 3:2 in favor of the quadriceps group. Usually runners have a reverse ratio, so strengthening the hamstrings is not necessary. However, should an injury or other training error make it necessary, the physician can have the athlete do prone or standing hamstring curls. Some athletes prefer one over the other, and some trainers, coaches, and physicians believe the prone hamstring curls focus more on the upper hamstrings, whereas the standing curls focus more on the lower hamstrings.

Overall strengthening of the legs can be accomplished with squats. There are numerous forms of the exercise, each having a slightly different emphasis. The particular form one chooses depends largely on the individual.

Some general concepts are important to mention with regard to the squat and knee strengthening. First and foremost, the athlete must use strict form and perform repetitions slowly. Because the greatest strength gains come from eccentric loading, one common timing technique is up for a count of 2 and down for a count of 4. This also helps prevent the injuries that occur with increased speed. The athlete should exhale with exertion; in this case, exhale on the way down.

This exercise is started with the feet shoulder width apart, head looking up, and the lower back locked in position. When coming down, the athlete should think of "sitting on the toilet." This will keep the knees in such a position that they do not pass in front of the ball of the foot or center of gravity. This prevents undo shearing stress on knee ligaments. It also prevents the athlete from coming up on the balls of the feet, thereby shortening the gastric muscles.

Again, as with the calf muscles, the athlete should perform three sets of 10 repetitions. He or she should progress up to three sets of 12 to 15 repetitions, keeping the weights "easy." Then more weight may be added to the point where he or she can do just three sets of 10 repetitions.

RETURN TO RUNNING

After an injury, the therapeutic intervention, and subsequent rehabilitation, there comes the inevitable return to running. This is the point of time looked forward to by the athlete and sometimes dreaded by the sports physician.

Returning to running too early leads to recurrent injury and ultimately more time lost from training. This is a situation not desired by either party. The runner wants to do what he or she considers to be a part of his or her life or identity and the physician wants the patient to be happy and satisfied with the care.

Some common threads course through the plethora of running programs. These common threads are the foundation to a safe return to running. They begin with "graduation."

Graduation means starting slow, short, and easy and *gradually* increasing the running parameters. Running speed should be such that the runner can speak without developing shortness of breath. Running distance to start depends on the category of runners and the type of injury. Refer to Table 1 and use 25% of the training distance as a starting point. This increases 10% to 25% per week until the distance is normal for that patient.

"How much is too much" is largely a function of trial and error. Daily telephone monitoring is entirely appropriate during the first week to 10 days. Occasionally frequent rechecks at the office may be necessary.

Patients know their bodies best. It is essential that they be able to be honest with their physician. They should not feel that their doctor is going to be overly cautious and stop their running for a minor injury or setback in training. Yet, they must know when the doctor is certain that they must stop. When this relationship is firmly established, both the runner and physician will enjoy their respective identities.

CONCLUSION

The evidence continues to mount on the importance of staying active for life. Regular exercise is one key to healthy living, and running is but one means of exercise.

This form of exercise is accessible to almost anyone, anywhere, and anytime. To run, all you really "need" is a good pair of shoes and some loose clothing. In excess of 30 million Americans make use of this practical, relaxing form of exercise for a variety of reasons.

About 70% of those runners will suffer an injury severe enough to require time off from running and possibly even other activities of daily living. An unknown number of these will seek the care of a sports physician.

The sports physician must not only be able to diagnose and treat physical injuries but must also be able to deal with runners' lost sense of identity that comes with not being able to run. At times, the runners' mind-set can be a detriment to therapy in that they return to running too soon. This we know leads to further injuries.

Flexibility is the key to understanding and caring for these athletes. Flexibility on the part of the athlete is adopting an alternative to running such as cycling or swimming for the purpose of rehabilitation. Flexibility on the part of the physician is keeping up with shoe technology and running trends. Each physician and each athlete have different needs and goals. *Together* they must make new goals so that both will be satisfied. In the words of the late George Sheehan, M.D., "Everyone is an experiment of one."

REFERENCES

1. Walter SD: The Ontario cohort study of running related injuries. *Arch Intern Med* 149:2561–2564, 1989.
2. Jacobs SJ: Injuries to runners. *Am J Sports Med* 14:151–155, 1986.
3. Brody D: Running injuries. *Clin Symp* 39:1–36, 1980.
4. Macera C: Lower extremity injuries in runners. *Sports Med* 13:50–57, 1992.
5. Powell KE: An epidemiological perspective on the causes of running injuries. *Physician Sports Med* 14:100–114, 1986.
6. Cavanaugh PR: Ground reaction forces in distance running. *Biomechanics* 13:397–406, 1980.
7. Taunton JE: The role of biomechanics in the epidemiology of injury. *Sports Med* 6:107–120, 1988.
8. Reber L: Muscular control of the ankle in running. *Am J Sports Med* 21:805–810, 1993.
9. Williams KR: Biomechanical studies of elite female distance runners. *Int J Sports Med* 8:107–118, 1987.
10. Messier SP: Etiologic factors associated with patellofemoral pain in runners. *Med Sci Sports Exerc* 23:1008–1015, 1991.
11. McCaw ST: Leg length inequality. *Sports Med* 14:422–429, 1992.
12. Hoyle DA: Intraexaminer, interexaminer and interdevice comparability of leg length measurements obtained with measuring tape and metrecom. *J Orthop Sports Phys Ther* 14:263–268, 1991.
13. Schuster R: Children's foot survey. *J Podiatr Soc* 17:13–14, 1956.
14. Mechelen Van W: Running injuries, a review of the epidemiological literature. *Sports Med* 14:320–335, 1992.

15. Wichmann S: Athletic shoes; finding the right fit. *Physician Sports Med* 21:204–211, 1993.
16. Stacoff A: The effects of shoes on the torsion and rearfoot motion in running. *Med Sci Sports Exer* 23:482–490, 1991.
17. Dugas R: Causes and treatment of common overuse injuries in runners. *J Musculoskeletal Med* 8:107–116, March 1991.
18. Newell SG: Overuse injuries to the knee in runners. *Physician Sports Med* 12:81–92, 1984.
19. Galea M: Patellofemoral pain. *Physician Sports Med* 22:48–56, 1994.
20. Ellis J: The match game; finding the right shoe for you. Biomechanics and running gait. *Runners World* Oct:66–71, 1985.

The Temporomandibular Joint

Darryl D. Curl, D.D.S., D.C.
Director, Pacific Coast Faculty Resource Group, Whittier, California; Associate Professor, Department of Diagnosis, Los Angeles College of Chiropractic, Whittier, California

This chapter is organized for the reader who is not readily familiar with the terminology, definitions, diagnosis, and treatment of the temporomandibular (TM) joint (TMJ) and associated structures. However, it is assumed the reader is familiar with the anatomy and biomechanics of the TMJ. The reader may want to consult the chiropractic literature on this subject if a review is needed.[1]

The following outlines my train of thought while I composed this chapter to enable the nonspecialist reader to quickly become caught up with the advances in TM disorders:

- The role of the chiropractor in TM disorders
- Screening procedures for TM disorders
- Examination of the TM apparatus
- Common TM disorders and how to recognize them
- Treatment: Should the TMJ be adjusted?
- Injuries resulting from delayed diagnosis
- Common questions

These seven principal headings will advance the reader's skills on a fascinating subject and hopefully answer some common questions on how to approach these sometimes elusive conditions—TM disorders.

The often disclosed intercausal relation between cervical whiplash and TM disorders has resulted in an increased involvement by chiropractors in an area heretofore managed almost exclusively by dentists. This is fortunate because, in many ways, chiropractors provide care for patients having or suspected of having a TM disorder that a dentist simply cannot offer.

Beyond providing initial care, the chiropractor also plays an important role in communicating the presence of these disorders to dental specialists or involved third parties. This means, more than ever, chiropractors are being asked to be effective communicators not only to their patients' other health care providers but to a larger degree to third-party interests, be they indemnity, managed care, personal injury, or a legal representative of the patient.

Now more than at any other time communication is the key to a successful practice regardless of professional affiliation. No other business requires the comprehensive and detailed documentation of the services (evaluation and management) provided to the client (patient) than that of the business of health care. Like it or not, as part of the legal duty owed to patients, every chiropractor is ethically and legally required to record clinically relevant historical, diagnostic, and treatment-related information about his or her patients and to maintain that information in the form of a legible patient file.

The chiropractic-patient relationship gives rise to a host of duties for the chiropractor that go beyond providing health care. Completing forms and reports for patients in a manner that is not misleading, deceptive, untrue, or fraudulent is one of these obligations. The courts have repeatedly ruled the chiropractor's duty to complete forms and reports in a timely and proper way is an extension of the legal obligation to bear witness on behalf of his or her patient.[2]

It should come as no surprise, then, that the purposes of this chapter are to establish a groundwork for interprofessional relations between the chiropractor and dentist, for effective communications to interested third parties, and for effective care of patients suspected as having a TM disorder. It is hoped these goals can be achieved by defining and explaining current advances in the areas of diagnosis and treatment of various common jaw complaints, as well as a brief discussion on the practical documentation of such efforts.

It has been my experience that what needs to be emphasized is the perspective of the nonspecialist—the one who is the first contact in most cases. Specifically, attention must be placed on good screening skills, as well as diagnostic and treatment skills. These abilities are essential to successful therapy.

TM disorder is in vogue. Its rise in popularity coincides with the development of advanced imaging techniques, enhanced physiotherapy devices, and the advancement of microsurgical techniques, and this technology is within easy grasp of most clinicians. It is now possible to detect very subtle changes from the "ideal" TMJ. However, this improved ability to "find" TM disorders is not without its problems; the overdiagnosis of TM dysfunction is an acknowledged problem.[3] Studies consistently show only 3% to 5% of the population having signs or symptoms of TM dysfunction need treatment.[4] Overdiagnosis creates many problems for the patient, who may be treated for a condition prematurely. Worse yet, they may be subjected to treatment for some condition that will not benefit from the therapy provided. Imagine, by analogy, a surgeon ordering a 28-year-old woman to undergo hip replacement surgery on finding mild osteoarthritis on x-ray film and doing so on the basis that the degenerative changes might lead to an increased probability of hip fracture when the patient is 75 years old! With regard to TM disorders, beware of therapy based on the belief that something must be done now because it will prevent some "terrible" pathological condition that "may" happen in the distant future.

Easy access to technology also creates problems for the clinician. The fact that abnormalities of the TMJ can be detected well before they produce any clinical signs or symptoms creates confusion in two critical areas of clinical decision making: establishing how much disease there is and defining how well the treatment works. For instance, electronic jaw-tracking devices are able to detect very minute changes in jaw movements, whereas careful observation with the naked eye detects less than one tenth the changes seen via electronic enhancement. When does the TM disorder begin—with electronically enhanced variations (if so, which of the minute changes actually mark the beginning) or with traditional methods? Then, presuming an answer can be found, the next logical question arises: What is appropriate treatment? Is aggressive intervention indicated at the first detection of an abnormality (e.g., an "irregular" electromyogram of the jaw muscles), or should intervention wait until more traditional signs and symptoms develop? Current knowledge forewarns the clinician that the increasing use of sophisticated diagnostic methods promotes a cycle of increasing intervention that often confers little or no benefit to the patient.[5] Current wisdom tell us it is safer and more effective to initiate treatment of TM disorders when functional impairment is demonstrated via traditional signs and symptoms.

Many chiropractors become involved in litigation of TMJ injuries, and they do so because they are caregivers for patients who are plaintiffs. In these cases the chiropractor will play a crucial role in determining the nature and extent of injury to the TMJ. As such, a proper diagnosis is crucial. TMJ disorder is not an appropriate diagnosis, nor is lateral condyle, restricted condyle, or subluxation. TMJ refers to a body part, as does the word knee. A record stating the doctor is treating TMJ casts doubt on the credibility of the doctor.[6,7] Likewise, imagine the disbelief on seeing a physician report that he or she is treating for, say, elbow.

It is essential the diagnosis appropriately relates the findings in the case to the treatment rendered. Diagnosis is and always will be the cornerstone for appropriate therapy. If the diagnosis is not logically connected to the historical findings and consistent with the physical examination findings, failure is inevitable and may result in malpractice action, denial of payment for services, or an investigation for suspected insurance fraud.[8]

In addition to diagnosis and treatment, a chiropractor may be called on to assess the degree of impairment and disability relative to the patient's condition. Impairment is a medical condition involving loss of function, and its degree of severity is determined by the treating chiropractor only after a maximum response to therapy has been achieved. Rarely do TMJ injuries result in permanent disability; the resulting impairment typically does not prohibit the person's ability to engage in gainful employment.

In cases where impairment is claimed, the combined data from the history and the physical examination serve as a powerful lever should disability be judged necessary. When viewed as a whole, the accumulated data (i.e., history, physical examination, and additional studies) speak powerfully toward the stated diagnosis and resulting impairment. In other words, the reader of the doctor's medical report will have a high degree of confidence that the doctor is in a good position to treat the patient's impairment in such a way as to assure maximum response to treatment and is in the best position to make the most intelligent and effective decision regarding disability.

SCREENING PROCEDURES FOR TM DISORDERS

The decision to treat or not to treat patients with a TM disorder is one that every chiropractor must make with each patient. However, with regard to head and neck pain, every chiropractor has the responsibility to screen and identify patients with a TM disorder. This responsibility (to properly screen and identify) holds true no matter what the reason for the patient's head or neck pain.

Whenever a patient has a complaint implicating the TM apparatus after any form of trauma, it is prudent to screen for evidence of a preexisting condition or telltale signs of predisposing factors. Failure to do so ignores the great body of knowledge that tells us that very few TM disorders are solely caused by a single traumatic event. Further, such failure practically assures poor treatment outcome.

DISTANT SOURCES OF PAIN

The head, jaw, and facial areas are virtual megaphones through which pain arising from distant sites may sound off. Therefore, any screening for a TM disorder begins with a quest to remove clinical suspicion for non-TM apparatus etiologies.

Problems arising from inside the cranial vault, specialized organs of the head and face, cervical spine and muscles, cranial nerves, autonomic system, vascular elements, and the psyche may be confused with a TM disorder (Table 1). This confusion may exist in the patient, clinician, or both. Failure to recognize problems in one of these areas or treating an erroneous diagnosis can have serious consequences for the patient and the chiropractor.

Chiropractors are often the portal-of-entry providers for their patients, and in this light the patient is depending on the chiropractor to oversee his or her general health. Although no chiropractor can provide for every need of his or her patients, all chiropractors are capable of recognizing conditions that may be harmful to the patient and those that are benign or innocent. If doubt exists in ruling out problems in the areas mentioned in Table 1, the chiropractor can proceed more confidently after obtaining an appropriate consultation (Table 2).

HEAD POSTURE

The head literally teeters on top of the cervical spine with a center of gravity anterior to the spine, and it is tethered to the body by the muscles of the anterior and posterior neck (Fig 1). Functional and resting head posture is dependent on tension in these muscles. A standardized method of determining neutral head posture has yet to be established, and there are many methods to choose from.[9-12] One method I have carefully studied measures the plane of the rim of the orbit against the plane of the sternal notch. This method appears to be superior due to the fact that the

TABLE 1.
Differential Diagnoses

Diagnostic Group	Possible Origin of the Complaint
Cranial vault	Brain, circle of Willis and associated vessels, cranial sinuses
Specialized organs of the head and face	Eyes, ears, nose, throat, salivary glands, sinuses
Cervical spine and muscles	Vertebrae, ligaments, intervertebral discs, facet joints, muscles, vertebrobasilar system, esophagus, trachea, thyroid gland, lymph tissue
Cranial nerves	Any of the 12 cranial nerves
Autonomic system	Sympathetic plexus
Vascular elements	Beyond those already mentioned, carotid artery, jugular vein, temporal artery, facial artery
Psyche	Depression, anxiety, somatoform disorder

head carriage is measured from relatively fixed points with the lower reference point as close to the head as possible. Most all other measurement procedures fall prey to optical illusion, migrating inferior landmarks or inconsistent positioning against the inferior landmark. Measures taken from the plane of the rim of the orbit and the plane of the sternal notch have been shown to be reliable. An additional advantage to this method is that it is simple, does not require expensive equipment, and is quickly performed (Fig 2).

TABLE 2.
Potential Referrals for TM Disorder Patients

Dental specialist (orthodontist, periodontist, oral surgeon, etc.)
Endocrinologist
General dentist
Gynecologist
Internist
Neurologist
Neurosurgeon
Ophthalmologist
Orthopedic surgeon
Otolaryngologist
Physical medicine
Psychiatrist
Psychologist
Rheumatologist
Vascular surgeon

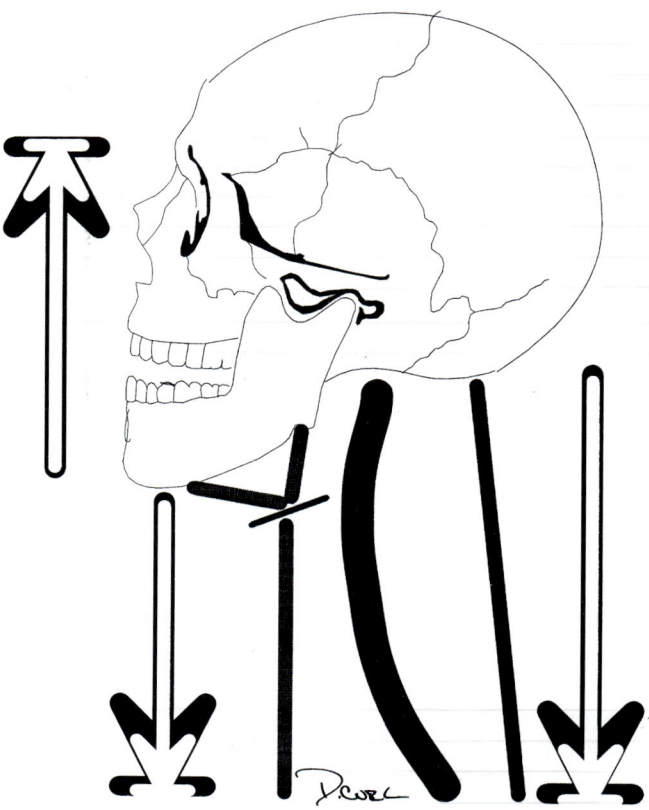

FIGURE 1.
Reciprocal relationship between the posterior neck muscles, anterior neck muscles, and the muscles of the jaw. Any change in tension in one group is experienced in the other two groups due to the many postural reflexes that control head and jaw position. For instance, shortening of the posterior neck muscles causes a compensatory contracture of the anterior neck muscles and the jaw muscles.

Head posture and the resting position of the mandible are intimately related, and a change in one necessarily affects the others. This becomes clinically obvious when the body is examined as it attempts to (1) preserve the relationship of the horizontal planes of the skull to the vertical axis of the spine while (2) maintaining a patent airway and (3) performing the complex functions of the TM apparatus (e.g., swallowing, speech, and chewing).

As the head migrates forward, the distance between the origins and insertions of the suprahyoid and infrahyoid muscles increases. This forward migration tends to concurrently induce a posterior cranial rotation, contributing further to inframandibular muscle tension. This tension, referred to as light passive or light elastic force, will induce depression and retrusion of the mandible.[13]

Posterior cranial rotation is thought to produce increased jaw muscle activity in the temporalis, masseter, and anterior digastric muscles.[14] The increased mandibular elevator activity produces opposing forces on the inframandibular tissues, and synergistic forces of mandibular retrusion.

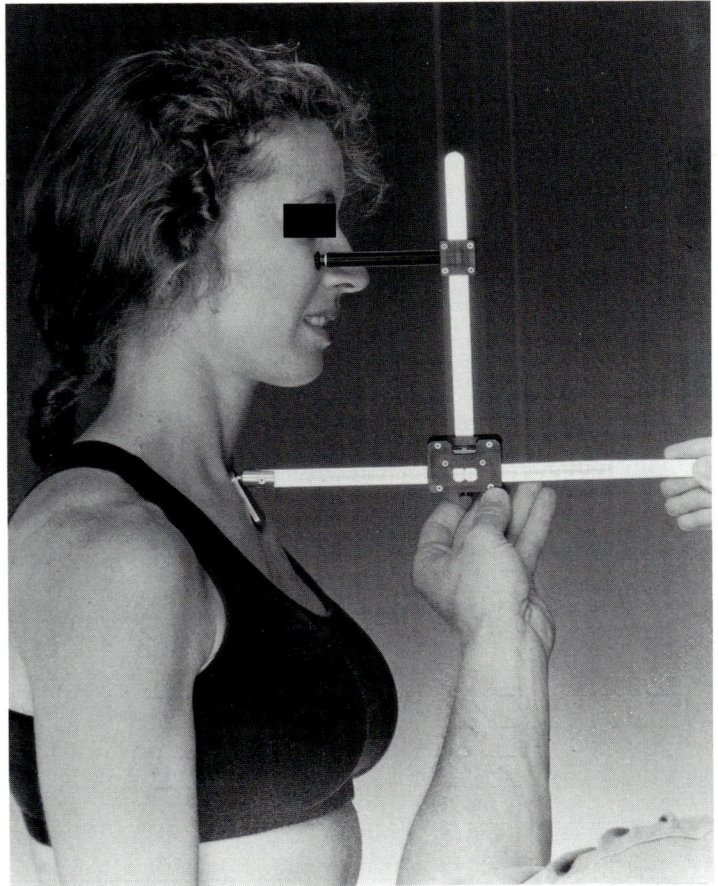

FIGURE 2.
Forward head carriage can be measured by comparing the difference between the planes of the sternal notch and the inferior rim of the right orbit. Here the Chek device is used to demonstrate this method.

This mandibular retrusion created by the forward head is nonphysiological and may induce microtrauma to the TMJ.[15]

Mandibular retrusion and altered closing trajectory are also associated with the forward positioned head. In other words, forward head position not only influences the mandibular postural rest position but also can change the habitual pattern of jaw closure to the intercuspal position.[16] Neuromuscular alterations in the arc of closure are generated to compensate for the new closing arc and do so at the expense of additional muscle activity.[16] The magnitude of this additional muscle activity can be appreciated when one realizes that the TMJ opens and closes 1,500 to 2,000 times daily during the motions of chewing, talking, kissing, yawning, and snoring and another 1,000 to 2,000 times during swallowing.[17] The results of this phenomenon are commonly seen as persistent muscle soreness and hypertonicity secondary to mild ischemia and conducive to trigger point development.

The increased tonicity of the masseter muscle secondary to changes in the trajectory of the closing arc may lead to entrapment of the maxillary vein where it emerges between the masseter and the mandible,[18] the result of which is retardation of venous flow from the infraorbital subcutaneous tissues. This may be clinically evident as puffiness beneath the ipsilateral eye and narrowing of the palpebral fissure.

As the musculoskeletal system fatigues with the burden of compensation for the forward head, trigger point activity and ischemia become increasingly potent sources of pain. When the muscles involved in correction of the occlusal engram can no longer handle the burden, parafunctional recruiting of the suboccipital muscles can occur.[19] This may be identified by a bobbing action of the head during speech, talking, and mastication.

MANDIBULAR POSTURAL REST POSITION

Normal mandibular postural rest position (MPRP) is an equilibrium between the downward pull of gravity and myotactic reflex contraction of the mandibular elevators. This equilibrium depends on the inherent elasticity of the elevator musculature and proprioceptive input from the TMJs and airway receptors. MPRP is the result of a very sensitive neuromuscular system and is heavily influenced by head posture, body posture, occlusion, muscle activity, and psychogenic factors.

Neutral MPRP is easily determined in the clinical setting. When the mandible is at rest, a freeway space of about 3 to 5 mm exists between the relaxed position and full closure (Fig 3). Head posture is probably the single most important physical factor governing MPRP. This is easily demonstrated by placing the head in an extended position and taking note of the increased freeway space created by this movement. Conversely, the freeway space decreases with head flexion. Bear in mind that any dys-

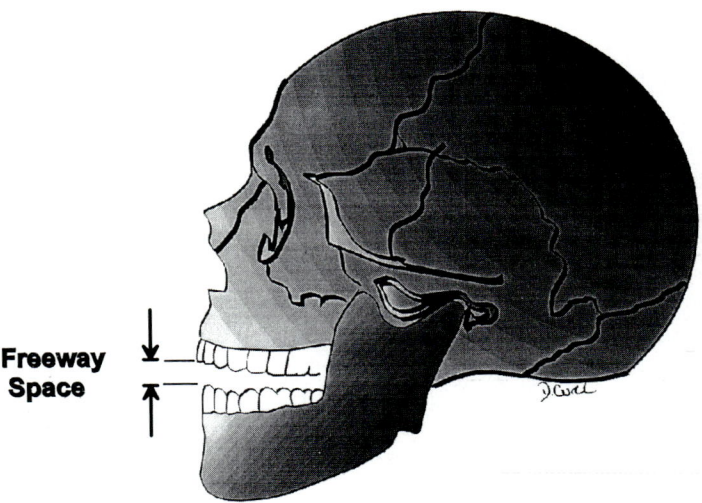

FIGURE 3.

Freeway space is simply that space that exists between the closed position of the jaw and when the jaw is at rest. Freeway space is also known as interocclusal clearance.

function in the cervical spine has the potential to alter head posture and therefore MPRP.

Determination of MPRP is best done when the patient is unaware he or she is being observed, and MPRP should be evaluated over the course of the entire doctor-patient interaction. Does the patient carry the jaw in MPRP 100%, 90%, 80%, and so forth of the period of observation? When

•	Please answer each question by marking the appropriate response.	Never	None at present	Mild	Mod	Severe
1.	Do your jaw joints make clicking or popping noises?					
2.	Does it hurt when you open wide or yawn?					
3.	Does your jaw ever lock so you cannot close it?					
4.	Does your jaw get stuck momentarily or longer so that you cannot open fully?					
5.	Does it hurt when you chew, or use your jaws?					
6.	Does your pain continue when you are not using your jaw?					
7.	Is your pain worse upon awakening in the morning?					
8.	Do you have pain in front of your ears or in your ears?					
9.	Do you have pain in your temples?					
10.	Do you have jaw muscle (cheek) pain?					
11.	Do you have frequent headaches (more than once a week)?					
12.	Are you aware of any teeth clenching or grinding during the day?					
13.	Has anyone heard you grind your teeth at night?					
14.	Has your bite felt uncomfortable or unusual?					

FIGURE 4.
There are many types of useful screening questionnaires for TM disorders depending on the needs of the clinician. This questionnaire is appropriate to the chiropractic setting.

the jaw is not in MPRP, is there evidence of masseter contraction? If so, this suggests a clenching habit. Give the patient instructions to relax the jaw. Following these instructions, can the patient sustain the relaxed position comfortably, or does he or she have to move, close, or clench the jaw? Such behavior suggests the TM apparatus may be reacting to abnormalities in head posture, general body posture, occlusion, underlying abnormal muscle activity (clenching habit), or psychogenic factors.

SCREENING QUESTIONNAIRE

Literally dozens of TM disorder screening questionnaires have been developed over the last 50 years, with many of them falling by the way side. Clark et al.[20] reviewed the literature with respect to the utility and validity of the different questionnaires that have been used to assess TM disorder patients. They determined that many of these questionnaires have not been validated and that there is a lack of standardization in the use of them. In other words, questionnaires are not the proper method of classifying patients suspected of having a TM disorder into better-defined diagnostic subgroups. To reach a diagnosis the chiropractor still must rely on the traditional, and powerful, history and physical examination.

This is not to say that questionnaires cannot serve a good purpose for the chiropractor. In fact, the chiropractor is encouraged to use them. Questionnaires serve as an excellent tool to elicit information from the patient that enables the chiropractor to target key issues for further exploration. However, a word of caution is in order when questionnaires are used, be it the one supplied in this chapter or one developed by the doctor (Fig 4). Briefly stated, it is virtually impossible to create the "perfect questionnaire." No matter how well designed the questionnaire is, patients tend to overrespond or underrespond to the items in it. This point is easily demonstrated by examining the typical responses to questions about clicking (Fig 5).

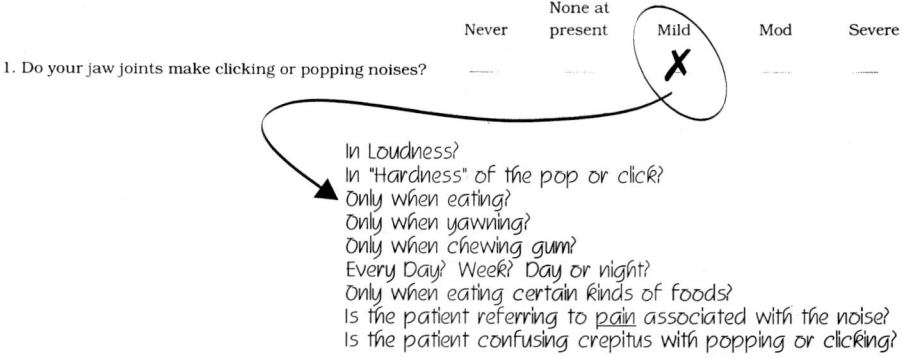

FIGURE 5.
Questionnaires are exceedingly difficult to design if the goal is to elicit complete and accurate responses. Even well-designed questionnaires are able to elicit responses that are either complete or accurate but not both. This analysis of a response to clicking demonstrates this point.

EXAMINATION OF THE TM APPARATUS

PATIENT HISTORY

Sir William Osler once so suitably noted, "Listen to the patient, he is giving you the diagnosis."

The examination of the patient begins, obviously, with a thorough history. Less obvious, though, is the fact that the history is the single most important source of information when one is dealing with a suspected TM disorder patient. Why? At this time, the technology available to the clinician is not sufficient to delve accurately (or cost effectively) into the innermost workings of the vastly complex head and upper neck area. Hence, as Dr. Osler observed, we must depend on the patients to supply the vital details of their condition.

The patient history is the *single most important* adjunct to the physical examination. The *oral* and *written* history will furnish information regarding the mental status of the patient (mental health is a significant factor here), the patient's reaction to the disorder, history of previous treatment, and so forth.

A careful history complements a diligently performed examination of the patient, particularly in TM disorders, because TM disorder patients are usually aware of up to only 50% of those findings that can be found on a careful examination.[21] Without a carefully developed history, the examining doctor may be tempted to label all the examination findings as evidence of some disorder when, in fact, they may represent normal variations or other benign changes.

INSPECTION

General Appearance

FACE.—The examiner notes any facial abnormalities such as asymmetry or a short upper lip. Signs of soft tissue stress such as hypertrophy of the masseter (bruxism), or hypotonicity, as is common in the orbicularis oris (loose, full lipped), should be noted (mouth breather).

HEAD.—Watch the patient as he or she speaks; does the head move excessively or too little? Or is it canted to one side only during speech? Observe the patient as he or she listens. Is the head maintained in a neutral posture, or does the patient turn the head slightly, favoring one ear as you speak?

HANDS.—Rheumatoid arthritis is an example of a common systemic disorder that can also affect the TMJ.[22] Therefore, examination of the hands and wrists may be an important clue. Of course, many other clues to a systemic disorder may be revealed to the clinician in the course of the normal examination.

Certainly it is wise not to ignore the hands as part of the examination of the head pain patient. Many other clues pointing to the nature of the jaw complaint may come to light by careful observation of the hands. Are the nails being bitten? In children, look for a clean digit as a sign of thumb or finger sucking. This likely is the one the child favors. Adults are also known to suck a finger or thumb. Look at the pen in the adult's pocket to see if the ends are being chewed and look at the fingernails. All of these are signs of *parafunctional* uses of the TMJ and may in and of themselves be the cause for TM dysfunction complaints.

NECK AND POSTURE.—Examination of the neck will have already been done in the normal course of a chiropractic evaluation. What needs to be emphasized is the effect the TMJ apparatus has on the neck and vice versa.

The approach to any patient suspected of having a TM disorder, be it by a chiropractor or a dentist, must take into consideration the reciprocal relationship between head carriage, neck posture, and posturing of the mandible. One side of this relationship is nicely described in a study by Winnberg et al.[23] In their 1988 study, synchronized electromyography and videofluorography were used to investigate the influence of altered head posture on various components of TM apparatus function (i.e., hyomandibular movements, suprahyoid muscle length, suprahyoid working angle, and timing of suprahyoid and masseter muscle activity). In their study, several statistically significant observations were made during forward flexion and backward extension of the head. The authors[23] concluded that head posture is a significant factor regulating mandibular and hyoid bone movements and masseter and suprahyoid muscle function.

The second side of this relationship is seen in the changes in cervical spine posture caused by alterations in the way the maxillary and mandibular teeth meet one another (occlusion). Moya et al.[24] conducted a study to determine the effect of occlusal changes on cervical posture in subjects having muscle spasms in the sternocleidomastoid and trapezius muscles. Cephalometric analysis showed that significant changes in occlusion caused a measurable amount of extension of the head on the cervical spine. They also claim to have found a significant decrease in cervical spine lordosis in the first, second, and third cervical segment. They suggest that these cervical changes could be a compensation mechanism caused by the extension of the cranium on the upper cervical spine. From this they conclude that due to the compensatory changes in the cervical curvature it is necessary to periodically evaluate the cervical spine whenever the patient's occlusal status is significantly changed or, better yet, when such changes are in the planning stage of the patient's care.

The muscles of the neck figure prominently in some types of TM disorders. For instance, the sternocleidomastoid muscle is implicated in autonomically induced vascular headaches, as well as in changing the "tone" of the muscles of mastication. Remember too that trigger points in the trapezius can set up secondary trigger point sites in the temporalis muscle. Here, in both instances an ounce of prevention is worth a pound of cure.

The muscles of mastication appear to be reflexly related to the functioning of the smaller muscles surrounding C-1, C-2, and C-3. Accordingly, some argue TM disorders are capable of altering the biomechanics of the upper cervical mechanism. This may explain the presence of suboccipital pain common to so many TM disorder patients.

Here, of course, comes the debate of which comes first—the TM dysfunction and then neck problems or neck problems, followed by TM dysfunction? It is likely that both paths do occur and both problems can and do occur independently of one another. Curiously, some clinicians insist TM disorders have nothing to do with cervical dysfunction and vice versa. Unless one can redefine the principles of kinematic and biomechanical relationships between joint systems, there seems to be little merit to the belief that these two joint systems operate exclusive of one another.

Here is something you may find rather interesting. Evaluate the next patient with joint clicking or deviated mandibular opening for unequal hip levels. Then have the patient stand on some item to level the hips. Recheck the clicking or opening gait. Reverse the stance to make the hip level even more uneven and recheck the clicking or gait. Often you will see a change!

Does this mean that TM dysfunction can be treated only this way? Of course not. The problem is more complicated than that. However, there is merit in addressing any dysfunction occurring in associated joint systems. Certainly this is part of the therapy that may be included in the overall treatment of TM disorders.

Patients with TM dysfunction often have other spinal or postural disorders. Commonly found are scoliosis, increased or decreased lordosis, increased or decreased kyphosis, abnormal head carriage, uneven shoulder height, hip height discrepancy, and so on. Interestingly, there was a study that conveyed that the short leg would be found on the affected TMJ side 70% of the time.[25] Check for it and see what you find.

PALPATION

TMJ Palpation

One reason for palpating the TMJ is to assist in the stethoscopic examination of the TMJ for joint sounds (see the discussion of auscultation). It is not uncommon for the clicking noise to be heard in both joints. However, in the majority of cases only one joint is producing the clicking sound, but because bone is an excellent conductor of sound, the click of one side is readily heard on the unaffected side. Palpation is often used to confirm the true source of the joint sound. Differentiating joint sounds notwithstanding, there are other reasons for performing TMJ palpation.

TMJ palpation (Fig 6) begins with a visual inspection of the area. Signs of external trauma such as small cuts, insect bites, furunculosis, abrasion, or evidence of impact trauma should be noted and may explain the presence of pain. The skin surface overlying the TMJ should be inspected for signs of inflammation or infection (e.g., redness, warmth, swelling, or exudate). Significant swelling is usually seen with acute infection or systemic inflammatory disease.[26] During the time of the visual inspection, muscle activity should be observed. Often evidence of contributing factors such as signs of abusive oral habits (e.g., habitual jaw-jutting or bruxing) may be observed.

Wänman and Agerberg[27] report on the use of a three-point grading scale when the TMJ and surrounding area are palpated (Table 3).[27] In my experience, this scale provides an excellent guide to the palpatory findings. Palpation of the lateral aspect of the TMJ is performed by placing the pad of the index finger immediately in front of the tragus of the ear and lightly palpating an area about 1 cm in diameter. In almost all in-

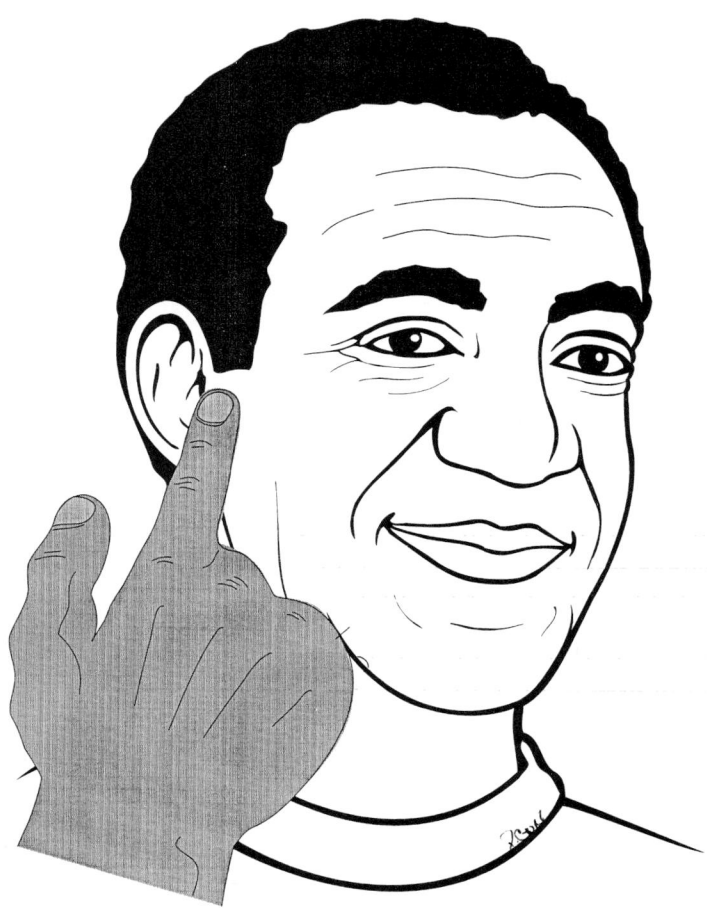

FIGURE 6.
Digital palpation of the TMJ is very informative. Care must be taken to palpate lightly. Heavy palpation tends to injure the joint capsule because it lies so close to the surface and is relatively unprotected on its lateral surface. The TMJ is located immediately in front of the tragus of the ear.

stances the pain elicited within this circle on palpation is suggestive of capsulitis or synovitis. When either condition is present, palpation generally evokes a grade II or III response and is restricted to the area immediately surrounding the TMJ.

Palpation of the posterior aspect of the TMJ is usually performed by placing the distal pad of the smallest finger in the external auditory meatus (EAM). Palpation via the EAM may detect inflammation of the posterior attachment.[28] In addition to detecting inflammation, the EAM palpation has been empirically used to detect a posteriorly positioned condyle, reciprocal clicking, or crepitus.

Muscle Palpation

When muscle palpation is used to corroborate other clinical findings, the information gained is meaningful (Fig 7). However, some muscles that a clinician may want to examine directly by palpation are sometimes im-

TABLE 3.
Palpation Scale*

Grade	Palpation Criteria
I	Patient feels slight tenderness; no obvious pain reaction is involved
II	Pain gives rise to a palpebral reflex
III	Pain gives rise to a protective reflex

*From Wänman A, Agerberg G: J Craniomandib Disord 5:35–44, 1991. Used by permission.

possible to reach.[29] One such muscle is the lateral pterygoid. The best one can achieve during palpation of this muscle is to compress the overlying tissue against the edge of the lateral pterygoid plate or, perhaps, on the very beginning of the lateral pterygoid muscle itself. In fact, the clinician is not really palpating the muscle. Instead, the digital pressure is actually exerted against the rich vascular pterygoid plexus. The information gained from this is quite useful because this plexus happens to be a very reliable indicator of local joint problems (e.g., edema or inflammation).

The medial pterygoid and the posterior digastric are also difficult (some say very unlikely) to be palpated.[30] It is not the intention of this monograph to settle this debate but merely to express and make aware of the arguments some may bring up when certain muscle "palpation" findings are discussed.

Putting debate aside, palpation is a very powerful clinical tool. Clinicians carefully trained in palpatory skills will uncover handy clues when the muscles or their nearby structures lying within the head and neck, small or large, are palpated. For example, take a patient who complains of temporalis pain. Typically palpation of the temporalis will confirm its soreness, but it is only when careful palpation is continued into the neck that it is discovered the trapezius is the primary pain site and the temporalis is the referral zone.

In summary, palpation of the muscles is useful in determining the following:

1. Location of muscle pathological conditions
2. Muscle tone
3. Trigger points
4. Thermal changes
5. Location of swelling
6. Verification of anatomical landmarks.

Muscle palpation can be misleading because

1. Muscle pathological conditions may be mistaken for referred pain
2. Tissue can be compressed against underlying sensitive tissues
3. Inflammation of the salivary, lymph, or thyroid glands can be mistaken for muscle pathological conditions
4. Vascular inflammation can be mistaken for muscle pathological conditions

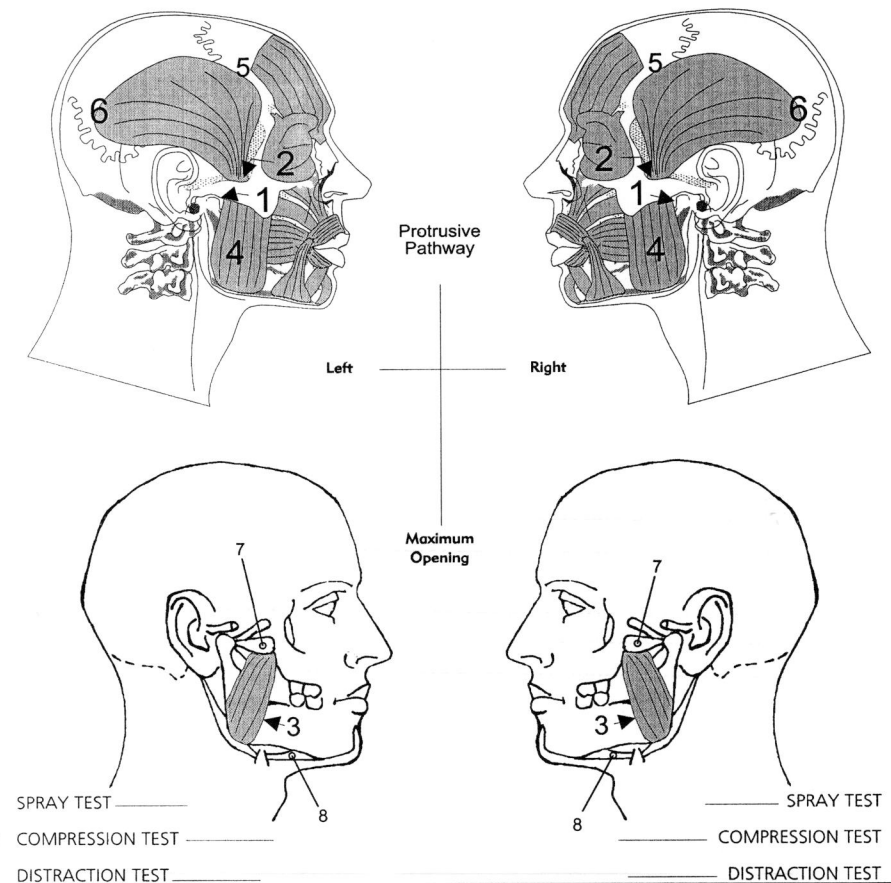

1. External TM joint Capsule
2. Coronoid Process and Tendon of Temporalis
3. Deep Masseter
4. Body of Masseter
5. Anterior Temporalis
6. Posterior Temporalis
7. Internal Pterygoid Area
8. Anterior Belly of Digastric

EXAMINATION CODES

Ⓟ Pain to Palpation   Ⓗ Hard or Nodular Mass   Ⓕ Fibrous or Ropey
Ⓢ Swelling or Edema   Ⓡ Referred   Ⓝ Other - See Notes

FIGURE 7.
Palpatory examination data sheet. Digital palpation of the muscles of the head is a vital part of the examination.

PERCUSSION

Dental pain is one of the most common causes of acute pain in the head. Therefore, a rapid screening procedure would be quite useful to rule out or rule in this type of pain. Two such procedures are available to the chiropractor: general dental percussion and tooth-specific percussion.

To perform a *general percussion*, simply ask the patient to sharply close the teeth together while listening and observing the patient. A single or faint "strike" sound or pain raises the level of clinical suspicion that there is a dental source of pain (acute malocclusion, tooth abscess, periodontal disease, etc.). Generally speaking, a positive finding here should be followed by tooth specific percussion.

To perform *tooth-specific* percussion, simply carefully strike the individual tooth one at a time at approximately 30 degrees from the horizontal against the buccal (cheek-side) surface with a firm, blunt object (Fig 8). Remember, this item used for percussion must be sterilized or discarded after use. The wearing of gloves and eye protection is advised. A tooth that responds painfully raises the level of clinical suspicion for dental pain, and a referral to a dentist is advised.

AUSCULTATION

Joint noises have traditionally been taken to be one of the surest signs of TM dysfunction. However, current studies are altering this concept a bit. There are circumstances where joint noises occur in an otherwise healthy joint. In other words, some joint sounds are nothing more than a normal variant.[31]

Characteristics of joint sounds are best determined by using a stethoscope (preferably one with a deep bell) and listening over the joint while the patient moves the mandible. For those who possess a Doppler-type device, by all means use it because it is considered (by some) to be the state-of-the-art listening and recording device for TMJ noises. For those

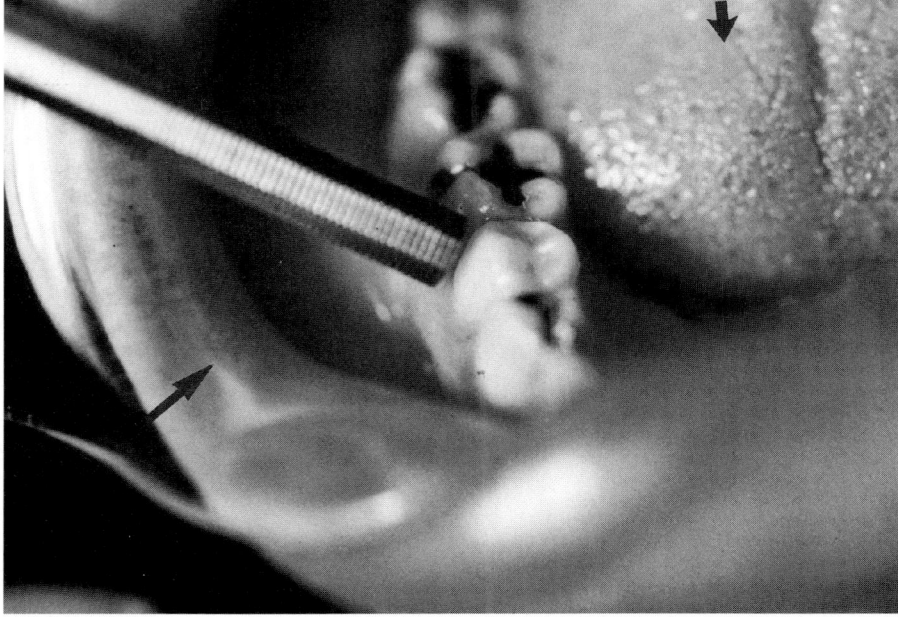

FIGURE 8.
Tooth-specific percussion. Notice a blunt-ended instrument is used to generate a light tapping force on the buccal side of the tooth from an angle of approximately 30 degrees. Arrows indicate tongue and cheek retractor.

skilled in its use there is a plethora of purportedly meaningful sounds to be heard. From another point of view, records of joint sounds may be important when it comes to documentation and data tracking. However, no one is sure just yet what, if any, clinical significance these recorded sounds have.

Auscultating (stethoscopic) joint sounds is one procedure where there is the greatest likelihood to incorporate error. The most frequent error is made when popping occurs in just one joint, but the records show that both joints were making popping sounds. What really happens here is the skull (an excellent conductor of sound) carries the sound readily from one side to the other. It is easy to be fooled.

The best way to keep from being fooled by false-positive stethoscopic findings is with the use of chiropractor's keen sense of digital touch. Palpate the joint via the lateral aspect of the joint and "feel" for sound (digital auscultation).

Finally, once sounds such as crepitus, popping, and clicking are located, note when they occur during the mandible's gait cycle and the duration of the sound, such as right opening crepitus beginning at 17 mm and releasing at 25 mm, with brief reciprocal (closing) click at 28 mm.

INSTRUMENTATION

Amount of Opening

The normal maximal opening is considered to be 40 to 55 mm, incisal edge to incisal edge. Older references use a guide of two and one-half to three knuckles (proximal interphalangeals of the patient's nondominant hand). Although this guide is gross in measure, it is handy for screening purposes.

Limited opening (<40 mm) can be a warning sign for discoid derangements (internal derangement) and should not be taken lightly. However, limitation in mandibular opening can result from pain (protective muscle splinting), muscular, capsular, or hard tissue pathological conditions. Soft tissue pathological conditions are more likely muscular (external derangements) than capsular and can be differentiated by a soft end-feel vs. a springy end-feel due to capsular limitations. A firm end-feel with a very limited opening (≤20 mm) suggests disk derangement, whereas a bony end-feel can occur when the limitation in opening results from coronoid process elongation.

Be aware of hypermobility of the TMJ (generally opening in excess of 55 mm). When hypermobility is present, the joint is likely to be unstable and may dislocate if excessive force is exerted or applied, damaging even further the already lax joint capsule.

Direction of Opening

The normal opening path of a joint is straight down, with the midline staying true. If an opening deviation is seen, note when the deviation occurs and the path it takes (Fig 9). Strong deviations point toward disk derangements, whereas mild deviations point to muscle imbalances.

Protrusive Deviation

Again, the path should be straight, with the midline staying true. Strong deviations in protrusion are usually indicators of internal derangements.

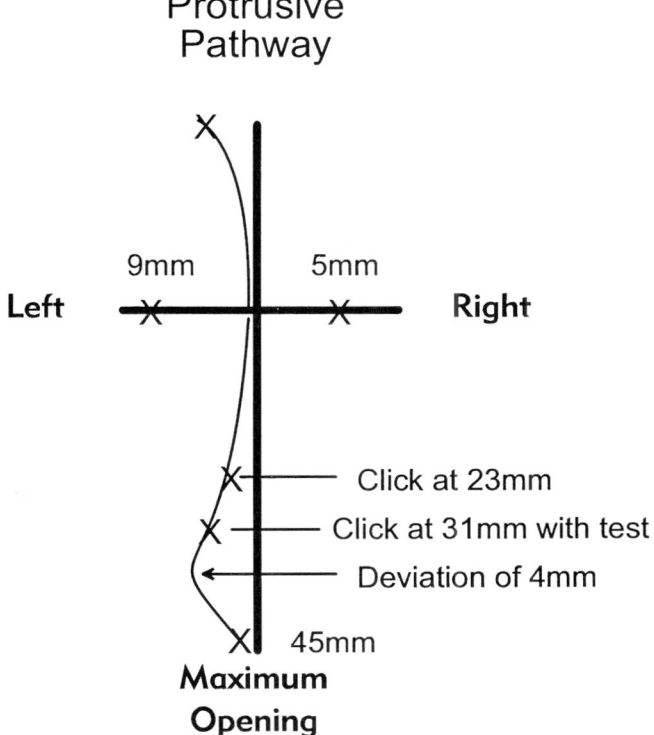

FIGURE 9.
The visual range of motion scale is an appropriate method of documenting the activities of jaw movement.[53] An example of a patient with clicking at 23 mm and a deviation of the mandible to the left of 4 mm on opening is noted. Lateral excursion to the left is restricted when compared with the right, which suggests a hypomobility disorder in the left TMJ. This is also reflected in the deviation to the left on protrusion. When the DCDT is performed, the clicking sound on opening is delayed 8 mm, which suggests the anteriorly displaced disk is not adhered to the articulating surface.

Lateral Excursions
The patient is asked to move the jaw slowly from side to side (to the limit) while the examiner notes the presence of pain or restriction. Objective measures are obtained by using the midline of the maxillary and mandibular teeth as a guide (Fig 10). Pain or limitation to lateral excursion can indicate joint inflammation, muscular dysfunction, coronoid process impingement, or internal derangement (e.g., an anteriorly positioned disk or discoid adhesions).

RANGE OF MOTION

To complete the range of motion (ROM) assessment of the mandible (the active ROM was performed under instrumentation), perform the *passive* assessment. Passive ROM studies of the mandible essentially evaluate the integrity of the ligamentous structures of the TMJ. This study can be done by checking for *medial glide, open end-feel,* and *distractive joint play.*

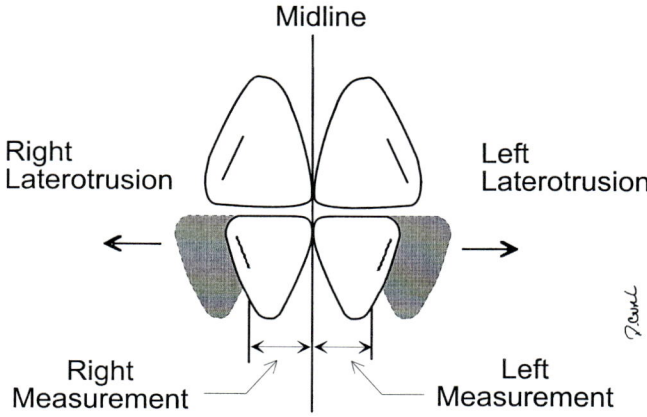

FIGURE 10.
Detailed view of the technique to measure lateral excursion. If the patient's dental midlines do not match up as shown, simply draw a midline on the surface of the mandibular tooth with a sharp pencil.

✓ Medial glide is evaluated by contacting the lateral poles of the TMJ and alternatively pressing medially. This is quite similar to palpating the lateral glide of the atlas (C-1). Significant limitations in medial glide suggest the presence of intracapsular adhesions.

Open end-feel is determined by taking a protected (gloved and padded) contact on the incisal edge of the mandibular incisors and applying a downward and slightly posterior pressure at the end range of mandibular opening. A capsular or ligamentous end-feel is normal.

Distractive joint play is performed by taking a protected (gloved) intraoral contact on the mandibular molars and pressing downward and slightly lateral at about 15 to 20 degrees. A capsular end-feel with little gapping is optimal or normal.

PROVOCATIVE TESTS

Muscle Testing
Masticatory muscle testing is probably the most overlooked part of the examination. By far, most pain associated with TM dysfunction is myogenous pain.

LATERAL PTERYGOIDS.—The lateral pterygoids are primary opening muscles and can be tested by putting one hand under the chin and the other just above the external occipital protuberance. The patient opens slightly, and the clinician applies a strong closing force to the chin. Be careful, because like the hamstrings, these muscles can cramp easily. The examiner is not looking for weakness so much as provocation of pain.

CLOSING MUSCLES.—The masseter, temporalis, and medial pterygoid muscles are tested by placing a folded gauze pad between the molars on each side and instructing the patient to bite very firmly for 5 to 8 seconds. Watch out for loose teeth, caps, dentures, and so on. Note the definition of the musculature during contracture, especially the masseter. The greater the definition, the more likely the person either bruxes or clenches. As usual, observe for provocation of pain and its specific location.

MEDIAL AND LATERAL PTERYGOIDS.—When the medial and lateral pterygoids act unilaterally, they deflect the mandible to the side (lateral excursion) and can be tested by placing one hand on the side of the mandible and the stabilizing hand on the opposite temporal area. The patient is told to resist a lateral pull to the mandible. Because the lateral pterygoid is often involved with TM dysfunction, this test is especially useful and impressive to the patient.

The lateral pterygoids can be tested bilaterally by performing a *protrusive-retrusive test*. Here the patient protrudes the jaw and resists a force that pushes it posteriorly.

DIGASTRIC AND POSTERIOR TEMPORALIS.—Place two protected fingers lingual (on the tongue side) of the mandibular teeth and attempt to pull the mandible forward as the patient resists the pull. Follow the same cautions and advice as for closing muscles.

EXAMPLE.—A patient has positive results to protrusive, right lateral excursive and closing tests and negative results to opening. The clinician is able to define the left medial pterygoid as being the dysfunctional muscle. How? A positive protrusive indicates all four pterygoids may be involved. The negative opening eliminates the lateral pterygoids, leaving the two medial pterygoids. The lateral excursive indicates the side of dysfunction.

A patient tests positive on opening and right lateral excursion but negative to closing. What muscle was isolated? The left lateral pterygoid.

Counterirritant Test

When mandibular motion is limited, the clinician must determine if the limitation is caused by an internal or external derangement. The counterirritant test (CIT) is useful in discovering limitations due to external derangements. The counterirritant (ice or fluoromethane spray) is applied to the muscles that cross the TMJ while a passive distractive pressure is applied to the mandibular front teeth when the mandible is at maximum opening (Fig 11). If a gradual increase in mandibular opening is observed, one can safely rule in an external derangement.

Swallowing Test

Tongue thrust or other abnormal swallowing activity is a considerable stressor of the musculoskeletal system of the head and neck. (We swallow 1,000 to 2,000 times daily!) Fortunately, a quick screening examination for deviated swallowing patterns is available to the clinician. The patient is instructed to take a sip of water while the clinician observes the swallowing mechanism. To fully evaluate the swallowing event, instruct the patient to keep the lips slightly apart at all times. With a little practice, all patients can comply with this instruction.

An indicator of swallowing dysfunction (tongue thrust) is seen when

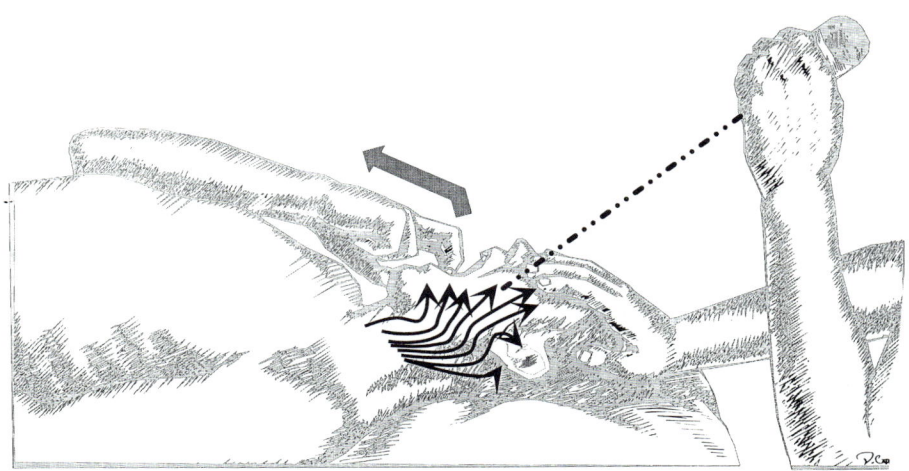

FIGURE 11.
The counterirritant test is an excellent method to distinguish between muscle-based disorders and joint-based disorders. Fluoromethane spray is used to provide the counterirritant of extreme cold. The mandible opens via passive stretch as applied through the patient's fingers. The patient applies the stretch only while the spray is being applied. I suggest substituting a bag of very cold crushed ice for the spray.

the tongue darts forward between the front teeth midway in the swallowing cycle. When tongue thrust is discovered, a consultation with a dental specialist or a speech therapist is advised.

Joint Compression/Distraction Test
The joint compression/distraction test (JCDT) helps the clinician determine the source of pain when internal derangements are suspected.

If palpation reveals pain in the TMJ, the examiner performs the JCDT. If there is pain when the mandible is passively pressed posteriorly and slightly superiorward (compression) but not during distraction, retrodiscoid tissue involvement is suspected (Fig 12,A). This is because the mandible was moved in such a way as to compress the condyle against the retrodiscoid tissue.

If, however, pain is increased when the joint is gapped but not during passive posterior pressure, the capsular or ligamentous tissues are likely the cause (Fig 12,B). Here the distractive pressure placed the load on the capsule and ligaments and removed the load from the intraarticular structures.

Disk Compression/Distraction Test
The disk compression/distraction test (DCDT) is used to help differentiate between disk malposition without adhesions and disk malposition with adhesions. If joint popping is uncovered during active ROM, the examiner performs the DCDT. First measure the exact location of the sound during the opening gait of the mandible. From a closed jaw position, compress the condyle against the articular eminence using a superior and slightly anteriorward pressure exerted from the angle of the mandible (Fig

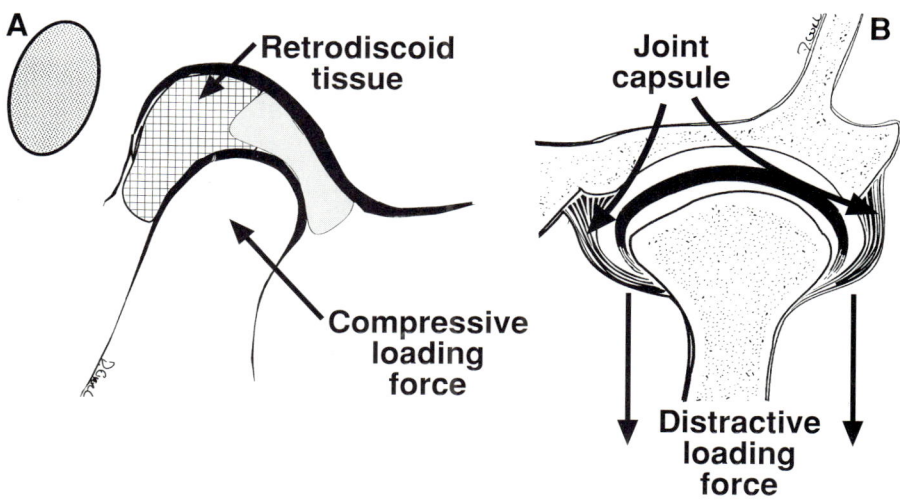

FIGURE 12.
The compression of the condyle against the retrodiscoid tissue evokes a pain response when synovitis is present. Distraction of the joint capsule (A) evokes a pains response when capsulitis is present (B).

13). Repeat the opening gait measurement of the sound. If the sound moved in its location during opening gait, it is likely the disk is freely moving. If the sound does not move in location during opening gait, it is very likely that the disk is immobile (disk malposition with adhesions).

NEUROLOGICAL TESTS

A cranial nerve examination is mandatory! The protocol outlined in the "4-minute neurological examination," which includes evaluations of the vestibular and cerebellar systems, is suitable.[32]

Occlusal Evaluation

There are a myriad of items to look for once the chiropractor decides to look inside the mouth, and a detailed discussion of this area is beyond the scope of this chapter. However, there are some key points a chiropractor can look for once inside the oral cavity.

✓ First, look inside the mouth and determine if any teeth are missing. (There should be 32 unless the wisdom teeth are missing, in which case there will be 28.) Then have the patient bite down. Does the bite look Class II (bucktooth)? Or Class III (prognathic mandible)? (Class I is called a "normal bite.") The teeth should appear clean, and the gingival tissue around them should not be edematous or bleed easily. Using gloved hands, palpate the teeth. Are any mobile? At the same time determine if any part or parts of the teeth appear to be missing. Is the patient wearing dentures, does he or she have a lot of restorations? Do the teeth look flat and worn?

If at this point you see anything suspicious, there is a reasonable likelihood of a dental contribution to the patient's pain or suspected TM dysfunction.

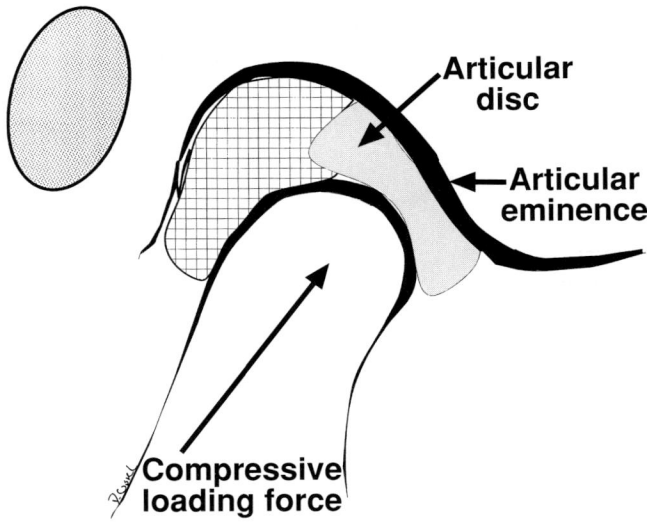

FIGURE 13.
The compression of the condyle against the articular disk (loading) assists in differentiating between disk malpositions with or without adhesions. When adhesions are present, the loading of the joint will not cause the popping sound to change in its location during mandibular gait. However, if no adhesions are present, loading causes the disk to travel further along the gait cycle, thus delaying the appearance of the popping sound.

Be advised that even healthy looking mouths and teeth are not necessarily conducive to proper TMJ function. When in doubt, arrange for a dental consultation.

If other findings are positive in the examination, it is wise to have the dentist do an examination that includes:

- Full-mouth x-ray films
- Periodontal health evaluation
- Study models of the teeth
- TMJ scout films (corrected tomographs) if a TM dysfunction is still suspected

COMMON TM DISORDERS AND HOW TO RECOGNIZE THEM

There are many dozens of types of TM disorders. Some of them are readily uncovered by a routine history and examination, whereas others are elusive, even with sophisticated diagnostic efforts. Fortunately, all of the common TM disorders, the ones we routinely see in our practice, are quickly identified by usual history and examination efforts.

The immediate hint that a TM disorder may exist arises when one or more of the symptoms mentioned in Table 4 are present. The clinician must keep in mind at all times that although some patients may exhibit all of these common symptoms, most experience a unique pattern. Because of these varied symptoms, it is easier to understand and subse-

TABLE 4.
Signs or Symptoms

Painful or painless noises arising from the TMJ
Pain initiated or provoked by jaw activity
Deviations or limitations in jaw movement
Locking of the jaw
Pain arising from the TMJ
Sudden changes in the bite
Swelling arising from the TMJ
Pain of the chief complaint worsened by palpation
Pain of the chief complaint worsened by provocative tests
Abnormal changes as seen in imaging studies
Early fatigue of the jaw muscles with normal activity

---

quently treat the patient's TM disorder by placing the condition into one or more of the following classifications:

1. Disorders involving the TMJ
2. Disorders involving the muscles of mastication
3. Disorders of mandibular mobility

Should the patient's condition not appear to readily fall into one of these classifications, it is very likely it will fall into one of the following three:

1. Disorders relating to the teeth
2. Disorders of growth
3. Disorders that are not musculoskeletal in nature but appear as though they are

When the condition does fall into one of the preceding three categories, a referral to an appropriate specialist is indicated.

DISORDERS INVOLVING TMJ

Capsulitis and Synovitis

Management goals for patients with capsulitis or synovitis are similar to those for patients with other joint related disorders, namely, decrease pain and tenderness, decrease adverse loading, restore normal function and the resumption of activities of daily living.[33] Factors found to be etiologically important must be managed during treatment because those etiologies that initiate capsulitis or synovitis may also perpetuate them. The reader may want to refer to Parker's dynamic model of etiology in TM disorders[34] for a complete review of the major factors that are important considerations in effective TM disorder management.

The initial management of noninfectious capsulitis or synovitis is similar to that prescribed for most any inflamed joint. If the condition is severe, aspirin, nonsteroidal anti-inflammatory medication, mild heat or cold, a soft diet, or instructions to limit mandibular movement should be quickly applied. In the case of synovitis, a stabilization appliance[35] may prove useful because it tends to disengage the condyle from the inflamed posterior attachment. A stabilization appliance such as an Aqualizer[36] may also be used for either capsulitis or synovitis if it has been determined that relaxation of the elevator muscles is needed.[37]

Generally treatment of capsulitis or synovitis includes mild cryotherapy to the area for 10- to 20-minute periods, followed by ultrasound or other physiotherapy. As the acute stage resolves, 20-minute applications of moist heat can be used to further reduce inflammation and associated muscle complaints. Instructions to the patient routinely include resting of the jaw, soft diet, and the taking of a mild analgesic (e.g., aspirin). In the final stages of healing, mobilization and manipulation of the joint have been reported to be useful in accelerating tissue repair.[38]

DISORDERS INVOLVING THE MUSCLES OF MASTICATION

There are dozens of masticatory muscle disorders. Generally the recognition and treatment of their acute manifestations are very similar. When the muscle disorder is refractory to treatment or when the condition recurs, further investigation into a specific diagnostic subgroup is indicated.

Most muscle pain is the result of macrotrauma (e.g., blunt injury), microtrauma (e.g., bruxing), or myofascial dysfunction. Generally the history is sufficient to distinguish between these causes. The physical examination reveals the pain is localized to the involved muscle or muscles and worsens with function. Mandibular opening may be limited because of muscle soreness. Protracted periods of rest improve the complaints, whereas prolonged chewing or speaking leaves notable residual soreness.

Most muscle pain conditions respond well to a soft diet, soft tissue therapy, and avoidance of the initiating cause. When the pain fails to promptly respond to therapy, infectious causes must be considered.

DISORDERS OF MANDIBULAR MOBILITY

Mandibular hypomobility is defined for the purposes of this chapter as the result of the condyle failing to undergo full translation. This means that the articular disk is not traveling with the condyle due to disk displacement, joint surface disk adhesion, or disk deformation. The two most common causes, disk dislocation and adhesion, will be discussed.

Acute Closed Lock

When the disk is in such a position as to prevent normal condylar translation, the condition is known as *anterior disk dislocation* (Fig 14). *Acute* anterior disk dislocation is often spontaneous and usually results from laxity of the TMJ or from trauma. The history may include a specific trauma or multiple previous episodes of joint locking of which the patient was capable of reducing.

Acute closed lock of the TMJ is classically characterized by

1. Pain and tenderness in the TMJ region
2. Restriction of mandibular movement without joint sounds during condylar movement
3. Pain or apprehensive disposition

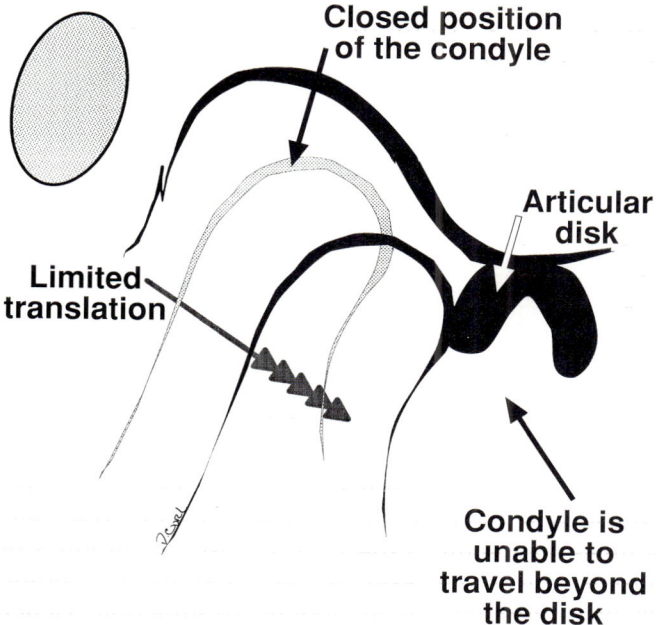

FIGURE 14.
Notice the dislocated disc prevents the condyle's ability to fully translate. Thus, the patient complains of limited opening. Notice also that because the condyle is not able to get under the disk, no popping sounds are made.

4. Acute malocclusion
5. Other minor symptoms (suboccipital pain, dysphagia, tinnitus, etc.)[39, 40]

When this condition is present in its early phase, no joint noises will be heard. Instead, there will be a series of reproducible restrictions during mandibular movement, which are a result of the disk's blocking translatory glide of the condyle. In addition, the patient will have an acute inability to open the mouth normally. Opening distances for these patients are usually only 5 to 20 mm, hence the term closed lock.

Mandibular manipulation is frequently reported to be a successful form of conservative therapy in dislocation disorders when the manipulation is performed properly. The treatment goal for acute closed lock is to increase articular mobility, decrease pain emanating from the TMJ, and reposition or recapture the disk to an anatomically normal position. The key to the therapy is prompt reduction of the disk dislocation. Reduction by manipulation is well reported.[41]

Disk Adhesion

As with all other synovial joints, the TMJ is highly vulnerable to biochemical changes. When the changes are severe enough adhesions form. These adhesions impair normal biomechanics and disk nutrition, thus accelerating the degenerative process. Adhesions may occur in either compartment of the TMJ, but it is far more common to see them form in the superior compartment.[42] Adhesions in the superior joint space impair condylar translation, which typically results in painful and limited mandibular opening (Fig 15).

Generally, disk adhesion is a sequela to traumatic hemarthrosis, disk derangements, inflammatory conditions, or persistent static loading of the TMJ. Almost all anterior disk dislocations that have not been successfully reduced in a timely manner result in the formation of intracapsular adhesions.

Habitual bruxism can also result in the formation of temporary adhesions (i.e., sticky joint) due to prolonged periods of static loading and concurrent microtrauma. Typically this occurs during periods of nocturnal bruxism and, on awakening, the limited jaw motion will be restored with a "click" as the mandible is moved, hence disrupting the adhesions.[43] This click, unlike those from other causes, is not reproducible unless another prolonged period of bruxism occurs.

Permanent adhesions occur any time the temporary adhesions are allowed to remain. The clinical characteristics of chronic anterior disk displacement with reduction complicated by fibrous ankylosis is as follows. Pain, if present, is mild to minimal. There is a very significant history of joint noise, limitation of mandibular opening, or both. Examination reveals moderate to severe limitation of mandibular opening. Opening of the mandible is noted by a slight to moderate deviation on opening to the affected side. Slight to moderate persistent joint popping or clicking is evident on each opening. There may also be slight to moderate limited

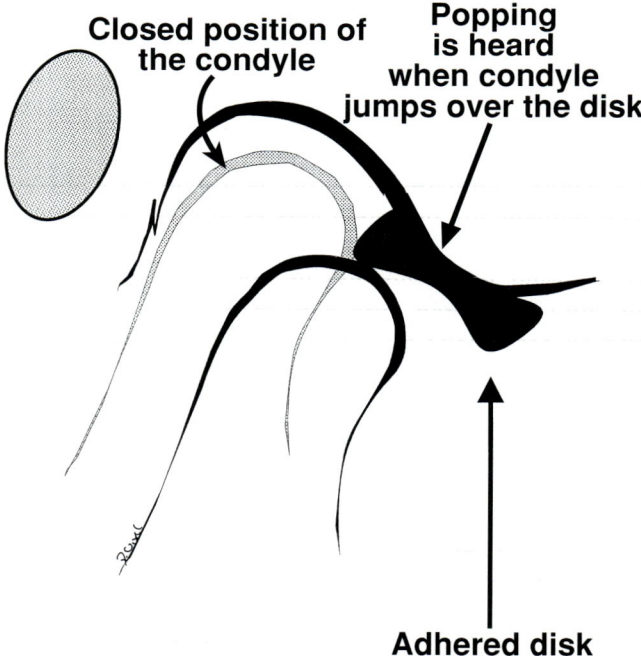

FIGURE 15.
Adhesions located between the articular disk and the articular eminence. Notice that the adhesions prevent the disk from traveling with the condyle. As the condyle passes by the disk, popping sounds are generated.

laterotrusion to the contralateral side. Soft tissue imaging by magnetic resonance imaging (MRI) reveals the displaced disk is stationary during condylar translation.

TREATMENT: SHOULD THE TMJ BE ADJUSTED?

Certain adjustive procedures for the TMJ are appropriate and effective. There are clinical conditions where conservative adjustive attempts should be applied before any decision is made to escalate the patient's care towards more invasive procedures. However, clinical studies specifically addressing the effectiveness of adjustive procedures for the TMJ are severely lacking. Those that do exist tend to be, unfortunately, empirical and are often performed in the context of other forms of treatment. Therefore, it is very difficult to ascribe specific therapeutic benefits of the adjustive procedures. However, some interesting extrapolations can be derived from what we know of the available studies.

INDICATIONS

One such extrapolation, and perhaps the weakest, has to do with one of the mechanisms thought to disrupt jaw movement, namely, muscle hyperactivity or dysynchronicity (nonrhythmic jaw movements). Adjustive approaches are known to influence sensory feedback/reflexes from joints. Although rhythmic jaw movements are elicitable by the stimulation of various cortical and hypothalamic sites, it is now clearly established that a central pattern generator (CPG) for chewing exists. Although chewing movements can be readily evoked on intraoral stimulation, it is suggested that the CPG is sensitive to, and in fact dependent on, sensory feedback for genesis and continual modification of the complex movement pattern. Recent research and clinical therapy, therefore, has focused on the importance of reflexes and their control during jaw movement. Hence, some argue that a general adjustment of the jaw enables a normalization of rhythmic jaw movements via some sort of proprioceptive bombardment to the TMJ.

Second, internal derangements of the TMJ (dislocation, adhesion, subluxation, etc.) associated with disturbed jaw movement are perhaps the best studied conditions for which manipulation has been shown to be valuable. Manipulative approaches have been shown to enhance intraarticular nourishment, reduce dislocations, and possibly break up articular adhesions.[44]

One of the most disturbing influences to normal joint function is "stickiness" of the articular disk. Here, the poor quality or quantity of synovial fluid production is the cause, hence, discoid lubrication and nourishment are impaired. The impairment of normal synovial fluid production predisposes the disk to develop perforations as a consequence of the diminished capability of the synovial fluid to nourish the disk. When joint stickiness occurs, gentle manipulations parallel to the slope of the eminence are indicated to release immature adhesion formation. Gentle gapping manipulations applied in a pumping fashion cause a "washing" of the synovial fluid across the joint surfaces and assist in nourishing the disk.

Adhesion formation is a common problem in the TMJ. Fibrous ankylosis (disk adhesion) can occur in the TMJ after prolonged static loading of the joint, due to trauma induced hemarthrosis, or as a result of disk derangements. The mechanism of adhesion formation is a consequence of a well-known inflammatory cascade.[45] When fully formed, the adhesions cement the disk to the articular eminence and cause considerable, yet sometimes painless, alterations in joint movement. Recently a new method of releasing the adhesions by using manual manipulation has been reported.[46]

Mandibular manipulation is frequently reported to be a successful form of acceptable conservative therapy in dislocation disorders affecting the TMJ. These procedures are technique sensitive but, when performed properly, are quite often effective in treating dislocations of the disk. A study by Segami et al.[47] reports a success rate of nearly 72% using manual manipulation. The selection of the specific variety of the gapping manipulation is dependent on many factors such as the level of skill of the clinician, the nature of the dislocation, and the status of the mandible and dentition. A review and a complete discussion of the many points relating to the use of gapping manipulation to achieve reduction of an acute anterior disk dislocation or a condylar dislocation are readily available in the chiropractic literature.

CONTRAINDICATIONS

When one concludes there are indications for TM manipulation, one implies there are certain instances where it would not be helpful, or, worse yet, injurious. More commonly these circumstances are called contraindications.

Contraindications to TMJ manipulation are greater in number than their companion indications but can be easily identified. Essentially any patient with one or more of the following conditions should not be subjected to manipulation until further clinical investigation or preliminary therapy is performed: pain in the TMJ, muscle splinting, thin cortises of the articular fossa, thin "disk space," infection, recent surgery, or contrary findings on plain films, computed tomography, or MRI. Crepitus and bone weakening conditions are absolute contraindications to manipulation.

INJURIES RESULTING FROM DELAYED DIAGNOSES

FIBROUS ANKYLOSIS OF THE DISK

Fibrous ankylosis (disk adhesion) can occur in the TMJ whenever there has been a delay in controlling joint inflammation. This delay may be as short as 48 to 72 hours. The mechanism of adhesion formation is a consequence of a well-known inflammatory cascade (Fig 16). When fully formed, the adhesions cement the disk to the articular eminence and may cause considerable, yet usually painless, alterations in joint movement. One notable sign of disk adhesion is a characteristic reproducible and sometimes loud pop heard whenever the jaw opens to a predetermined distance. Prompt institution of a series of manipulations to the joint early

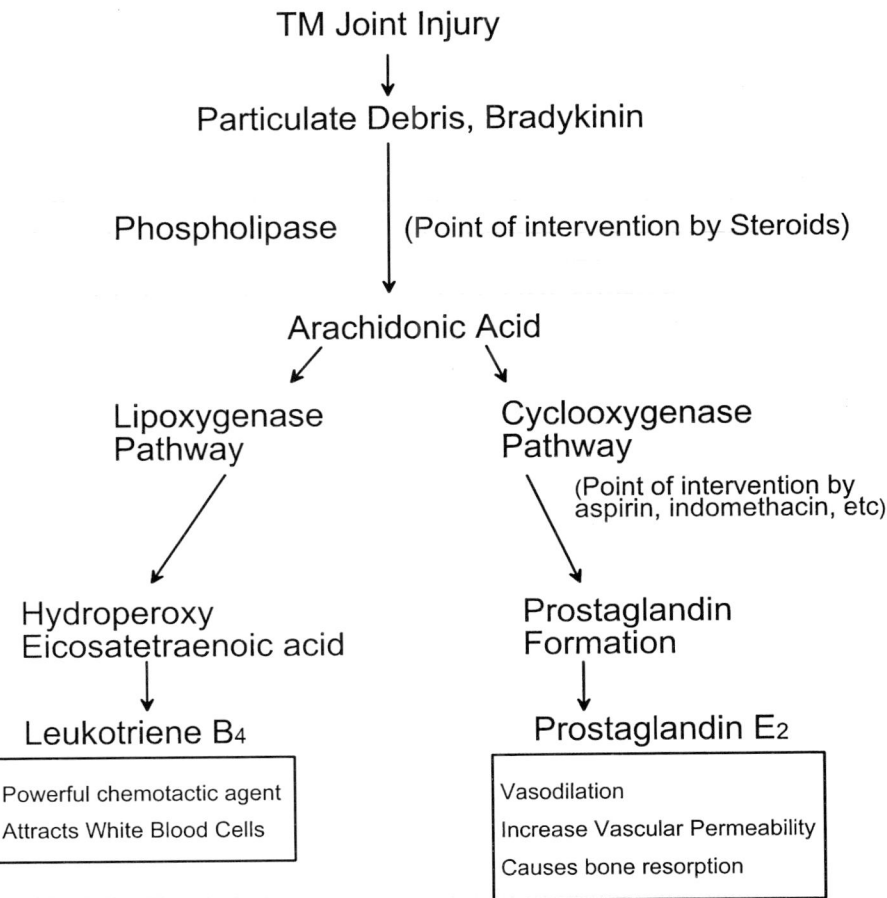

FIGURE 16.
Adhesion formation is made possible by the effects of the well-known inflammatory cascade. The chemical environment conducive to adhesion formation begins as early as 24 to 48 hours after the cascade begins. Therefore, early intervention to control the cascade and then to turn it off is critical to the prevention of adhesion formation.

in the adhesion forming process disrupts the adhesions and prevents permanent sequela.

CAPSULAR CONTRACTURE

Capsular contracture is a painless and persistent resistance of the TMJ to passive stretch. It usually occurs as a result of chronic capsulitis or synovitis but can occur as a complication of surgery to the TMJ.

When capsular contracture is fully developed, the patient complains of limited jaw opening and strong deviation to the involved side. Usually the patient ends up with complaints involving the opposite joint because it decompensates from the chronic stresses placed on it. On examination, a taut and hypomobile end-feel is detected on passive stretch of the involved joint, whereas the opposite joint is usually hypermobile with laxity in the capsular feel. Often a history of chronic joint inflammation or surgery is elicited. Carefully applied gapping manipulations are recommended to release the capsular contractures.

MYOFIBROTIC CONTRACTURE

<u>Muscle contracture (muscle fibrosis) is a painless and persistent resistance of a muscle to passive stretch. It occurs as a result of fibrotic deposition in either the supporting tendons, ligaments, or muscle fibers. Muscle contracture is usually caused by trauma but can result from infection.</u>

When muscle fibrosis is fully developed, the patient complains of limited jaw movement involving the affected muscle, which is usually one of the closing muscles, hence limiting the opening. On examination a leathery end-feel is detected on passive stretch, and the texture of the muscle is dense and ropy. Usually a history of trauma or infection is elicited. When myofibrotic contracture is evident, a consultation with an oral surgeon is advised.

COMMON QUESTIONS

QUESTION

As a new chiropractor, I have worked with many chiropractors and dentists who treat the TMJ and have seen them use techniques ranging from manipulation of the jaw and neck, acupuncture, electronic instrumentation (transcutaneous electrical nerve stimulation), kinesiographs, dental splints, foot orthotics, and physiotherapy. Although I have seen these patients improve with these various methodologies, some doctors seem to get better results. Is it because of the techniques and instruments they use?

ANSWER

Is the success of TMJ treatment dependent on a technique or a particular instrument? There was a time when it was believed certain techniques or a certain type of instrumentation was essential to the successful treatment of a TM disorder. However, time and experience have changed our way of thinking. Knowledgeable clinicians consistently report that any success in treatment depends wholly on an accurate diagnosis of the patient's problem. Therefore, successful practitioners do not fall prey to depending on one adjustive technique or some expensive device for their patients. Instead they base their treatment on knowing what the patient needs, and this is based solely on their diagnosis. More than likely these doctors show a higher success rate because they are better diagnosticians.

QUESTION

The impact of the TM apparatus on the locomotor system is a reality, yet we do not fully understand the dynamics behind the interaction of these two systems. In light of this relationship, should dentists learn to understand the dynamics of the entire locomotor apparatus, and, in turn, should chiropractors learn more about malocclusion, especially the effects of a reduced vertical dimension, incisal edge overload, and so forth and their impacts onto the skull and spine?

ANSWER

Ideally, yes. However, on a practical side, this is very difficult to accomplish. Can dentists be taught to understand the dynamics of the entire locomotor system? No. Simply said, there is too much to learn, and the dental profession does not have the wherewithal to achieve such a lofty goal for all of its members. I believe, however, the chiropractic profession can learn more about malocclusion, reduced vertical dimension, and incisal edge overload, (i.e., dysfunctions of the dental apparatus) and integrate that knowledge into their already existing understanding of the skull and spine. This is a more realistic expectation. Chapters such as this one, scientific articles, and texts on the subject of TM disorders appearing in the chiropractic literature are evidence of the reasonableness of this goal.

QUESTION

Can hyperflexion—hyperextension injury to the muscles of the neck—initiate dysfunction of an otherwise healthy TM apparatus?

ANSWER

Whiplash injury to the TM apparatus can occur by one or more of four mechanisms of injury (Table 5).[48] In the classic sense, Weinberg and LaPointe's[49] description of mandibular whiplash represents the most popular interpretation of injury to the TMJ in a cervical acceleration-deceleration (CAD) accident. However popular this notion of TMJ injury may be, it is by no means the most common unless, of course, the patient was in a major CAD accident. Even then, the incidence is extremely low.[50]

TABLE 5.
Mechanisms of Injury to the TM Apparatus

Category	Description	Comments
Classic mandibular whiplash		Seen almost exclusively in major CAD accidents
Increased vulnerability to injury	Position, preexisting conditions, disease, illness	Seen more common in the minor CAD accidents
Direct trauma to jaw	Contusions, abrasions, lacerations or any form of impact trauma	Seen in both major and minor CAD accidents
Iatrogenic injury	There are many common iatrogenic injuries to the TM apparatus	Iatrogenic injury should not be ignored in whiplash patients

According to this classical description of injury, the (1) motion of the head during neck hyperextension/hyperflexion directly injures the jaw; (2) jaw structures are damaged by the suddenness and velocity of the acceleration/deceleration motion; (3) when the head is forced backward during hyperextension of the neck, the jaw is forcibly opened beyond the physiological limit; and (4) when the vehicle strikes an object or rapidly decelerates, the head rebounds very rapidly forward, causing the jaw to be jammed shut. Accordingly, the hyperextension phase causes stretched or torn posterior attachment tissue and collateral discal ligaments, whereas the hyperflexion phase causes crushing of the retrodiscal tissue. Subsequent masticatory myospasm, particularly of the lateral pterygoid, accentuates the victim's plight. Although considerable debate exists regarding the legitimacy of Weinberg and LaPointe's[49] unproven whiplash theory, most agree that if the injury were to occur as described (i.e., extreme and rapid changes in mandibular position), the forces of the collision would have to be major and the head must be whipped about to its extremes of forward and backward motion.[51, 52]

QUESTION

What is a "splint"? Is there more than one kind? Why do dentists seem to use some form of splint therapy in the majority, if not all, of their TM disorder patients? Is splint therapy really effective in treating TM disorders? Why not?

ANSWER

In a general sense, the dental splint is similar to the foot orthotic in that it occupies a predetermined amount of space. Unlike that of the foot orthotic, the design, composition, principle of use, duration of use, and function of the dental splint are highly varied. This wide array of design potential has made splint therapy difficult for the clinician, sometimes to the point of appearing impossible to understand.

The specific type of dental orthotic to be used is strictly dependent on clinical findings, diagnosis, and treatment goals. Treatment goals, in this case, refer to the intended or final state of the dentition (teeth) as they relate to the maxilla, mandible, and the TMJ.

Splints are either soft or hard. If they are hard, they are either stabilization splints, vertical repositioning splints, horizontal repositioning splints, or both horizontal and vertical repositioning splints (Figs 17–20).

Soft splints are very similar to the mouthguards athletes use. Like the athletic mouthguard, they are made out of a latex-type material. Again, similar to the mouthguard, one of the uses of soft dental splints is to protect the teeth. For instance, a patient who grinds his or her teeth will benefit from a soft splint because of the protection it affords the teeth.

A soft splint is used primarily at night, during sleep, especially with a bruxing (grinding) patient. This is because bruxing activity is often highest during sleep periods, a time in which the patient is least able to control mandibular muscle activity. Soft splints can be used for daytime wear, but the bulkiness of the splint and the fact that the person is more capable of conscious control over mandibular muscle activity limit its daytime utility.

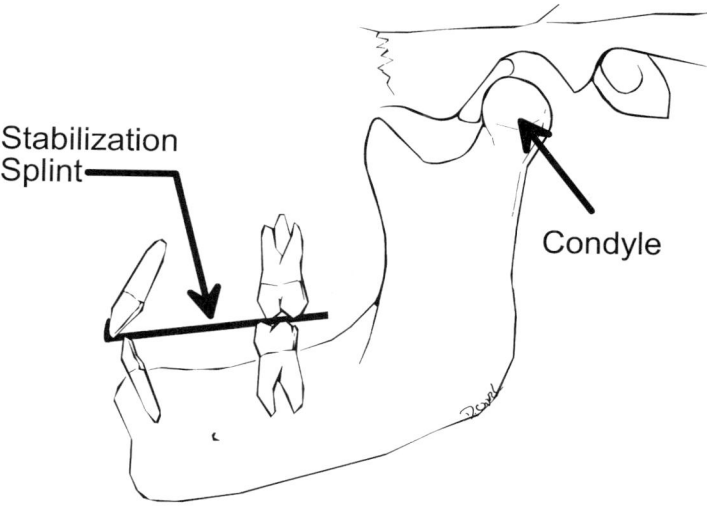

FIGURE 17.
The stabilization splint is the type of splint used most often by dentists. It is a good general purpose device for short-term therapy.

Fortunately smaller soft splints are available for daytime wear. The Aqualizer is the smallest and most comfortable soft splint for daytime use. It requires very little expense, and its design makes it easy for the chiropractor to deliver to the patient.

Hard splints vary in design in about every way imaginable. In the last

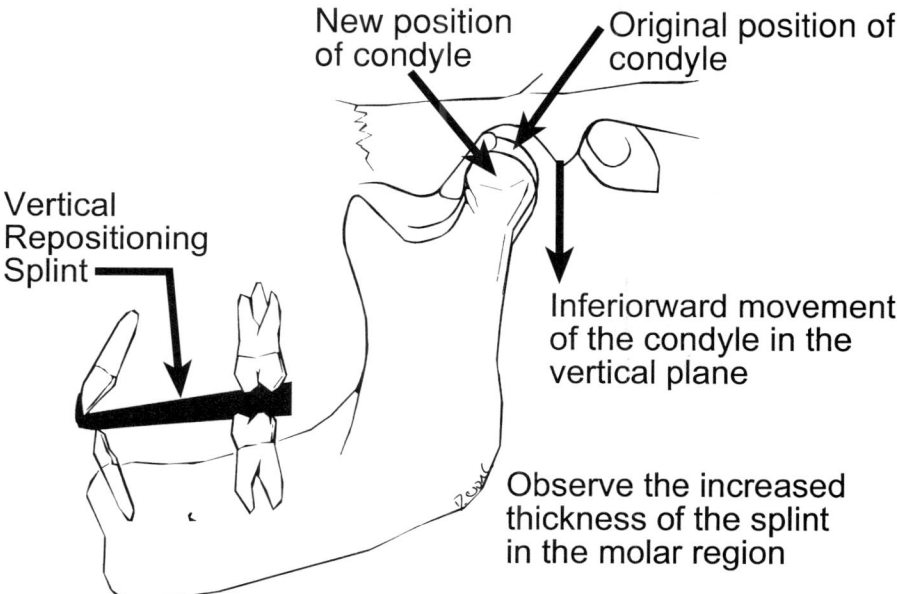

FIGURE 18.
The vertical repositioning split is used when the patient has lost vertical height to the teeth. Extreme wear from bruxing or excessively worn restorations are common causes of lost vertical height.

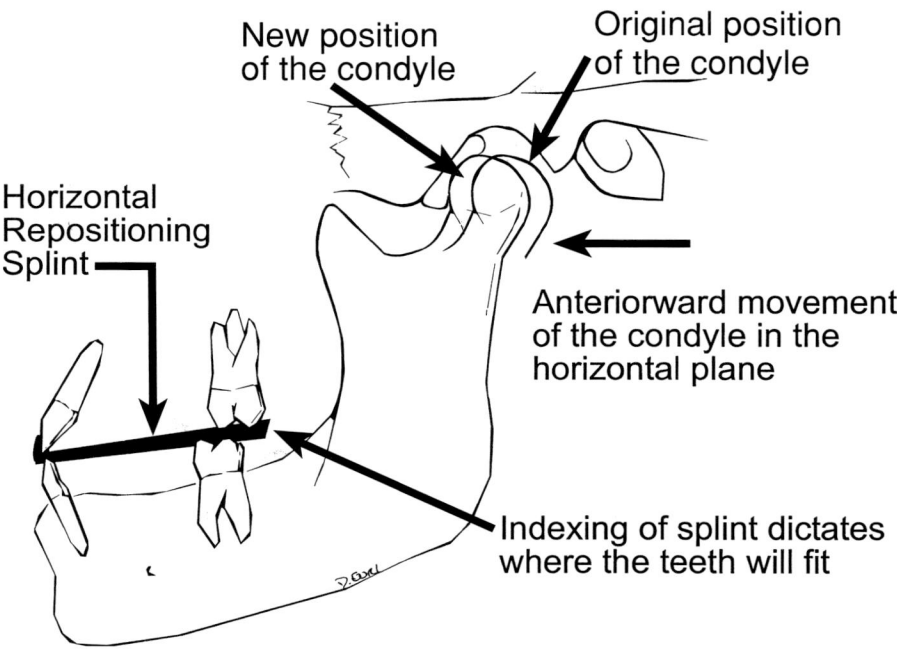

FIGURE 19.
The horizontal repositioning splint is used whenever one attempts to move the condyle away from the fragile retrodiscoid tissue without wanting to alter the patient's vertical dimension. Usually the patient needs orthodontic treatment once the condyle is satisfactorily positioned to position the teeth to the new bite. Horizontal repositioning therapy is of dubious long-term benefit because of the tendency toward relapse.

10 to 15 years dozens upon dozens of splint designs had been developed and experimented with. Some fell by the wayside, whereas others survived and are still being used. It is worth mentioning that among the survivors, some have lingered well past their time of legitimate use.

Of the splint-types currently available, the clinician can choose among two major splint classifications based on design: pivotal or full coverage. Pivotal splints, although once very popular, have lost a lot of their clinical utility. This decrease in utility came about because of some serious untoward effects discovered during clinical trials.

Full occlusion–type splints can be subdivided into two main groups: stabilization and repositioning. Stabilization splints are used when the dentist does not want to alter dental alignment or that of the mandibular condyle. Repositioning splints, on the other hand, attempt to alter condylar position while keeping the dental component as stable as possible.

Like the pivotal splint, full-occlusion splints have failed to show clinical effectiveness. Current studies are beginning to show that dental splints, no matter how popular among dentists, are no better at providing relief than a placebo because the nature of any TM disorder requires much more care than that provided by a splint. Simply said, splints are not effective when it comes to dealing with many of the problems asso-

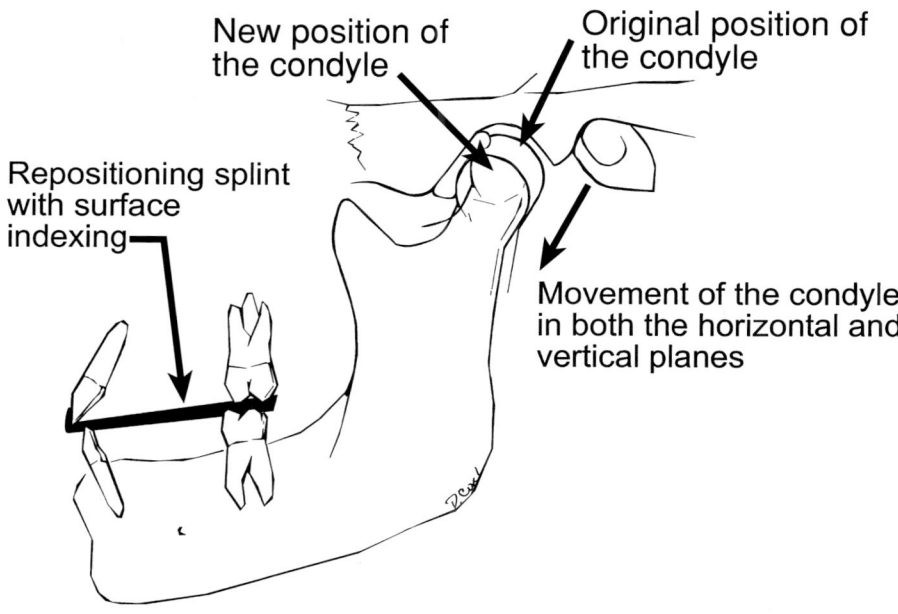

FIGURE 20.
Generally repositioning splints incorporate both changes in the vertical and horizontal dimension. This makes sense given the sloped nature of the articular eminence. This type of splint was most popular when it was believed that the slightly displaced articular disk could be recaptured by this method. However, clinical experience revealed this disc-recapturing therapy was of dubious value because of poor long-term results.

ciated with TM disorders such as reducing disk dislocations or discoid adhesions. For these conditions adjustive procedures are needed. Such therapy should come only from the hands of a skilled chiropractor.

REFERENCES

1. Curl DD: The chiropractic approach to temporomandibular disorders. *Semin Chiropr* 1:34–39, 1990.
2. Sax BM: Fiscal integrity and the civil monetary penalties law. *Health Law Vigil* 8:18–20, 1985.
3. Clark GT, Delcanho RE, Goulet JP: The utility and validity of current diagnostic procedures for defining temporomandibular disorder patients. *Adv Dent Res* 7:97–112, 1993.
4. Solberg WK: Epidemiological findings of importance to management of temporomandibular disorders, in Clark GT, Solberg WK (eds): *Perspectives in Temporomandibular Disorders*. Chicago, Quintessence, 1987, pp 27–41.
5. Black WC, Welch HG: Advances in diagnostic imaging and overestimation of disease prevalence and the benefits of therapy. *N Engl J Med* 326:1237–1243, 1993.
6. McNeill C: *Craniomandibular Disorders: Guidelines for Evaluation. Diagnosis and Management.* Chicago, Quintessence, 1990.
7. Bell W: *Temporomandibular Disorders*, ed 2. St. Louis, Mosby, 1986.
8. Burda D: Court upholds tough definition of false claim. *Mod Health* 21(37):32–33, 1991.

9. Hackney J, Bade D, Clawson A: Relationship between forward head posture and diagnosed internal derangement of the temporomandibular joint. *J Orofac Pain* 7:386–390, 1993.
10. Koncek V, Pollak VA, Yu AM: Analysis of stability of human upright posture based upon the measurement of the head sway. *Med Prog Technol* 19:55–60, 1993.
11. Salonen MA, Raustia AM, Huggare J: Head and cervical spine postures in complete denture wearers. *Cranio* 11:30–35, 1993.
12. Garrett TR, Youdas JW, Madson TJ: Reliability of measuring forward head posture in a clinical setting. *J Orthop Sports Phys Ther* 17:155–160, 1993.
13. Mohl N: Role of head posture in mandibular function, in Solberg WK, Clark GT (eds): *Abnormal Jaw Mechanics, Diagnosis and Treatment*. Chicago, Quintessence, 1981, pp 97–116.
14. Makofsky H: The effect of head posture on muscle contact position: The sliding cranium theory. *Cranio* 7:286–292, 1989.
15. Junghanns H: *Clinical Implications of Normal Biomechanical Stresses on Spinal Function*. Rockville, Md, Aspen, 1990, pp 195–197, 200–203.
16. Korr IM: *The Collected Papers of Irvin M. Korr*. Colorado Springs, Colo, American Academy of Osteotomy, 1979, pp 54–65.
17. Barral JP: *Visceral Manipulation II*. Seattle, Eastland Press, 1989, p 100.
18. Laplace LB, Nicholson JT: Physiologic effects of the correction of faulty posture. *JAMA* 107:1009–1012, 1936.
19. Skillern PG: Clinical observations on (I) cutaneovisceral (somatosympathetic) reflex arcs; (II) the role of hypermyotonia in bodily aches and pains. *J Nerve Ment Dis* 105:449–464, 1947.
20. Clark GT, Delcanho RE, Goulet JP: The utility and validity of current diagnostic procedures for defining temporomandibular disorder patients. *Adv Dent Res* 7:97–112, 1993.
21. Griffiths RH: Report on the president's conference on the examination, diagnosis, and management of temporomandibular disorders. *J Am Dent Assoc* 106:75–77, 1983.
22. Tegelberg A, Kopp S: Short-term effect of physical training on temporomandibular joint disorder in individuals with rheumatoid arthritis and ankylosing spondylitis. *Acta Odontol Scand* 46:49–56, 1988.
23. Winnberg A, Pancherz H, Westesson PL: Head posture and hyo-mandibular function in man. A synchronized electromyographic and videofluorographic study of the open-close-clench cycle. *Am J Orthod Dentofacial Orthop* 94:393–404, 1988.
24. Moya H, Miralles R, Zuniga C, et al: Influence of stabilization occlusal splint on craniocervical relationships: I. Cephalometric analysis. *Cranio* 12:47–51, 1994.
25. Gelb H, Bernstein I: Clinical evaluation of two hundred patients with temporomandibular joint syndrome. *J Prosthet Dent* 49:234–243, 1983.
26. Friedman MH, Weisberg J, Agus B: Diagnosis and treatment of inflammation of the temporomandibular joint. *Arthritis Rheum* 12:44–51, 1982.
27. Wänman A, Agerberg G: Etiology of craniomandibular disorders: Evaluation of some occlusal and psychological factors in 19-year-olds. *J Craniomandib Disord* 5:35–44, 1991.
28. Arlen H: The otomandibular syndrome: diagnosis. *Ear Nose Throat J* 57:553–556, 1983.
29. Johnstone DR, Templeton M: The feasibility of palpating the lateral pterygoid muscle. *J Prosthet Dent* 44:318–323, 1980.
30. Friedman MH, Weisberg J: Pitfalls of muscle palpation in TMJ diagnosis. *J Prosthet Dent* 48:331, 1982.

31. Vincent SD, Lilly GE: Incidence and characterization of temporomandibular joint sounds in adults. *J Am Dent Assoc* 116:203–206, 1988.
32. Goldberg S: *The Four Minute Neurologic Exam*. Miami, Medmaster, 1987.
33. Curl DD, Stanwood G: Chiropractic management of capsulitis and synovitis of the temporomandibular joint. *J Orofacial Pain* 7:283–293, 1993.
34. Parker MW: A dynamic model of etiology in temporomandibular disorders. *J Am Dent Assoc* 20:283–290, 1990.
35. Okeson JP, Kemper JT, Moody PM, et al: A survey of the use of occlusion splints in the treatment of acute and chronic patients with craniomandibular disorders. *J Prosthet Dent* 48:708–712, 1982.
36. Aqualizer. Jumar Corporation, Carefree, Ariz.
37. Okeson JP, Moody PM, Kemper JT, et al: Evaluation of occlusal splint therapy and relaxation procedures in patients with TMJ disorders. *J Am Dent Assoc* 107:420, 1983.
38. Mennell JM: *Joint Pain: Diagnosis and Treatment Using Manipulative Techniques*. Boston, Little, Brown. 1964.
39. Kleinrok M: Anterior shifting of the articular disc in the temporomandibular joint: I. Etiology, diagnosis and treatment principles. *Protet Stomatol* 36:224–230, 1986.
40. Solberg WK: Neuromuscular problems in the orofacial region: Diagnosis—classification, signs and symptoms. *Int Dent J* 31:206–215, 1981.
41. Curl DD: Acute closed lock of the temporomandibular joint: Manipulation paradigm and protocol. *J Chiropr Tech* 3:13–18, 1991.
42. Sanders B: Arthroscopic surgery of the TMJ: Treatment of internal derangement with persistent closed lock. *Oral Surg Oral Med Oral Pathol* 62:361–372, 1986.
43. Okeson J: Nonsurgical management of disc-interference disorders. *Dent Clin North Am* 1:29–51, 1991.
44. Sagahfi D, Curl DD: Chiropractic manipulation of anteriorly displaced disc with adhesion. *J Manipulative Physiol Ther*, 18:98–104, 1995.
45. Appelgren A, Appelgren B, Kopp S, et al: Relation between the intra-articular temperature of the temporomandibular joint and the presence of neuropeptide Y–like immunoreactivity in the joint fluid. A clinical study. *Acta Odontol Scand* 51:1–8, 1993.
46. Curl DD, Sagahfi D: Manual reduction of adhesion in the temporomandibular joint. *J Chiropr Tech* 7:22–29, 1995.
47. Segami N, Murakami K, Matsuki M, et al: Clinical assessment for treatment of patients with TMJ closed-lock by means of manipulation and pumping manipulation technique. *Jpn J Oral Maxillofac Surg* 34:1123–1131, 1988.
48. Curl DD: Whiplash and temporomandibular joint injury: Principles of detection and management, in Foreman S, Croft A: *Whiplash Injuries*, ed 2. Baltimore, Williams & Wilkins, 1994.
49. Weinberg S, LaPointe H: Cervical extension-flexion injury (whiplash) and internal derangement of the temporomandibular joint. *J Oral Maxillofac Surg* 45:653–656, 1987.
50. Heise AP, Laskin DM, Gervin AS: Incidence of temporomandibular joint symptoms following whiplash injury. *J Oral Maxillofac Surg* 50:825–828, 1992.
51. Burgess J: Symptom characteristics in TMD patients reporting blunt trauma and or whiplash injury. *J Orofacial Pain* 5:251–257, 1991.
52. Schneider K, Zernicke RF, Clark G: Modeling of jaw-head-neck dynamics during whiplash. *J Dent Res* 69:1360–1365, 1989.
53. Curl DD: The VROM scale: Analysis of mandibular gait in a chiropractic setting. *J Manipulative Physiol Ther* 15:178–185, 1992.

Reflex Sympathetic Dystrophy and Chiropractic

Howard T. Vernon, D.C., F.C.C.S.(C)
Associate Dean of Research, Canadian Memorial Chiropractic College, Toronto, Ontario

Pain arising from or associated with abnormal activity of the sympathetic nervous system (SNS) is one of the most puzzling and challenging conditions in musculoskeletal medicine. Ever since Weir Mitchell et al.[1] described the agonizing, burning pains of gun shot wounds suffered by Civil War casualties as "causalgia," clinicians have struggled to meet the challenges presented by such painful conditions.

Although terms such as causalgia,[2,3] "reflex sympathetic dystrophy," (RSD)[4-7] and others[8,9] have arisen over the years, it is accepted today that there is a spectrum of conditions that have as their basis altered activity of the SNS and conform to the overall category known as "sympathetically maintained pain" (SMP) syndromes.[10]

DEFINITIONS

The International Association for the Study of Pain[11] defines RSD as "continuous pain in a portion of an extremity after trauma which may include fracture but does not involve a major nerve, associated with sympathetic hyperactivity." A recent consensus definition from experts[12,13] in the field expands the clinical definition somewhat better:

> RSD is a descriptive term meaning a complex disorder or group of disorders that may develop as a consequence of trauma affecting the limbs, with or without obvious nerve lesion. RSD may also develop after visceral diseases, and central nervous system lesions or, rarely, without an obvious antecedent event. It consists of pain and related sensory abnormalities, abnormal blood flow and sweating, abnormalities in the motor system and changes in structure of both superficial and deep tissues ("trophic changes"). It is not necessary that all components are present. It is agreed that the name "reflex sympathetic dystrophy" is used in a descriptive sense and does not imply any specific underlying mechanisms.

According to McMahon,[14] several reasons support the notion that the sympathetic nervous system is involved in these pain syndromes. First, it is quite apparent in these syndromes that there are signs of abnormal sympathetic activity, particularly changes in skin temperature in the affected extremity or extremities, changes in sweating patterns, and dystrophic changes that are likely caused by prolonged alterations in blood

TABLE 1.
Spectrum of Pain Syndromes Associated with the SNS

Causalgia	Reflex Sympathetic Dystrophy	Sympathetically Maintained Pain	Reflex Sympathetic Dysfunction	
High		**Nerve damage**		Low
Low		**Intervertebral dysfunction?**		High?

flow to both superficial (skin) and deep structures (even to bone). The second reason involves the effect of altering sympathetic activity on the clinical course of sympathetic-involved pain syndromes. This applies to activities that either increase or decrease sympathetic activity. It is well known that patients with these syndromes have aggravation of their pain when they are exposed to cold, when they are under extra emotional stress, when the arm is elevated (implicating mechanisms related to hydrostatic pressure in the circulation), and when they are exposed to stressful stimuli. On the other hand, it is the collective clinical wisdom that procedures designed to reduce sympathetic activity are often effective in relieving RSD[15-17] and similar conditions. These procedures will be discussed but consist of attempts to block sympathetic activity by injection of pharmacological agents, by prescribing medication, or even by performing neurolytic surgical procedures. Behavioral therapies designed to increase relaxation may also help.

The spectrum of painful conditions that may involve the SNS is depicted in Table 1 and is based on an axis that has, at one pole, frank damage or injury to nerves, resulting in classic causalgia. Intermediately, the largest category is the well-defined RSD, caused by a variety of noxious or traumatic events. Near the other end of the spectrum is a less well-established category of "sympathetically maintained pains," which are contrasted with "sympathetically independent pains." Finally, at the other pole, a category named by Hooshang[18] as "reflex sympathetic dysfunction," which he describes as a widely present syndrome and, in his opinion, is the basis for the majority of chronic soft tissue pains.

Interestingly, Hooshang's notion of sympathetic dysfunction is highly convergent with Korr's[19] concepts of the "facilitated segment" and "sympathicotonia." This primary clinical model, adopted by chiropractors and osteopaths,[20-22] places great emphasis on the potential for segmental or regional sympathicotonia to be related to spinal mechanical dysfunction, thus predisposing any spinal level (but probably the more common regions of the lower cervical and lumbar) as capable of initiating sympathetic dysfunction. This theory proposes that a crucial link exists between spinal or vertebral sources of prolonged noxious input (i.e., the chiropractic spinal subluxation) and prolonged alterations in sympathetic activity.

EPIDEMIOLOGICAL AND CLINICAL FEATURES OF RSD AND SMP

RSD appears to be more common in the age group 35 to 60 years, but there are reports of cases in pediatric and adolescent age groups.[10,15] There is a slight predilection favoring women over men.[10]

The upper limb is affected more frequently than the lower. Blumberg and Janig[10] cite a rough estimation of annual prevalence as 1:5,000 persons per population; however, the proportion of pain clinic patients with RSD is probably much higher.

The precipitating event for RSD and other sympathetic pain syndromes is characteristically some form of trauma or significant noxious event. As described earlier, nerve injuries from crush, laceration, or gunshot wounds tend to precipitate the more severe form of causalgic symptoms, whereas less severe trauma, such as sprains, fractures, and burns, may precipitate RSD. Other agents of onset may be surgery, occupational macrotrauma or microtrauma, or even a variety of medical conditions such as myocardial infarction, stroke, vascular disease, or infection.[23]

RSD is characterized as a syndrome with symptoms and signs in three distinct categories: autonomic (sympathetic efferent), motor, and sensory. As Blumberg and Janig[10] state: "[The symptoms] are not confined to the innervation zone of an individual nerve, and show a distally generalized (quasi-polyneuropathic) distribution."

Autonomic symptoms are the most characteristic and prevalent and consist of symptoms reflecting both hyperfunction and hypofunction of the SNS. These include generalized swelling (the most prevalent of all findings in Blumberg and Janig's[10] report), warm- and cold-affected extremity, and disturbances in sweating patterns. These autonomic disturbances show high variability between patients and even moderate levels of variability within patients. This is particularly so over time, with early changes reflecting increased heat in the extremity and later changes involving the development of a colder extremity.

One important sign of autonomic dysfunction is the dystrophic changes involving both superficial tissues (i.e., shiny, swollen skin, and subcutaneous tissues) and deep tissues, including the extremity bones, where radionuclide scanning often reveals increased uptake, reflecting circulatory stasis.

The motor symptoms include greatly reduced active motion (often because movement aggravates pain), reduced strength (from disuse and dystrophic changes), myofascial contractures, and tremor, which may be present in 30% to 50% of cases.[10, 15, 23]

The sensory symptoms are among the most puzzling of all. They include the following:

1. *Deep spontaneous pain.*
2. *Hyperalgesia*, defined as an increased pain response to normally noxious stimuli. This is clinically detected as greatly increased tenderness and response to pin-prick testing.
3. *Hyperpathia*, defined as an abnormal and strong persistence of pain well after the noxious stimulus.
4. *Movement-related pain*, defined as pain arising on movement of a joint or joints normally well within the nonnoxious range.
5. *Allodynia*, the most puzzling sensory anomaly, defined as pain evoked by normally nonnoxious sensation. Mechanical allodynia is pain evoked by light touch or brushing and is the basis for the clinical observation of RSD patients protecting the affected limb from any stimulus, no matter how light.

Thermal allodynia is pain evoked by normally nonnoxious thermal stimuli, which is the basis for the common observation that RSD patients complain of aggravation of pain, especially in cold conditions that would not normally be experienced as painful per se.

6. *Hyperasthesia,* defined as abnormal tactile sensitivity to nonnoxious mechanical stimuli. Less frequently, hypoasthesia and hypoalgesia may be present, but RSD is generally characterized by hyperexcitable sensory disturbances.

A final category of symptoms to consider in RSD is those reflecting psychological disturbance. It is generally accepted that these reflect the effects of chronic debilitating pain as opposed to being causative factors in the development of RSD. These symptoms run the gamut from anxiety to depression, irritability, withdrawal behaviour, disturbance of sleep, and, finally, as Charlton[23] states, hopelessness.

CLINICAL COURSE OF RSD

Charlton[23] summarizes three stages through which RSD evolves. Stage one is the early stage, which begins within days or weeks of the precipitating event. This stage is described as "mild," although the degree of pain and dysfunction may be well above that normally seen with peripheral injury. Local pain is typically burning and sharp. According to Blumberg and Janig,[10] allodynia is absent at this stage. The signs of autonomic (edema) and motor (spasm) dysfunction are well established. The patient holds the limb immobile, and there may be considerable sensitivity to external stimuli.

In stage two ("moderate"), chronicity sets in. Changes distal to the site of injury become more prominent and signs of excessive sympathetic activity become increasingly severe. The limb is cold, moist, with mottling of the skin and edema. Extreme pain, tenderness, and sensitivity are present. The joints become progressively stiffer, with myofascial contractures existing. This stage may last for many months and may be refractory to treatment.

The third, or "severe," stage involves a full-blown, intractable syndrome in which even psychological effects are present. Constant aching and throbbing pain are present in a virtually immobilized limb. Extreme sensitivity and tenderness and severe myofascial contractures are present. Dystrophic changes in skin, nails, and subcutaneous tissues are highly visible, along with muscular atrophy. Osteoporosis (i.e., Sudeck's atrophy) is quite advanced as imaged on plain bone films[19, 15] and technetium scintigraphy.[23] This stage is more or less permanent and fully resistant to treatment.

Blumberg and Janig[10] take a different approach to the issue of staging of RSD. They are more skeptical of the idea of discrete stages evolving over predicted time intervals. Rather, they state: "what is probably more important is that patients with RSD should be graded according to the intensity of the sensory, autonomic motor and trophic changes as being mild, moderate or severe."[10]

Although treatment approaches will be discussed, it should be quite clear to the reader that it is paramount to arrive at as early a diagnosis as possible. Initiating treatment as early as possible is the single most important element in the prognosis. The longer RSD persists, the more resistant it becomes to treatment and the more morbidity develops.

DIAGNOSTIC METHODS

CLINICAL METHODS[23]

Autonomic Signs
Palpation may reveal bilateral temperature differences in the extremities. Skin coloration, subcutaneous thickening, and edema may be observed. Temperature readings can be performed with thermistors or thermography.[24-26]

Sensory Signs
Light touch, pin prick, and temperature sensitivity are assessed in standard fashion. Deep palpation for tenderness in muscle bellies and over bony prominence establishes the presence of hyperalgesia. A pressure pain threshold meter[27] may be used to quantify hyperalgesia.

Motor Signs
Motor signs consist of observation of muscular atrophy; range of motion testing for joint stiffness, myofascial contractures, and abnormal pain on movement (mechanical allodynia); and manual muscle testing for weakness.

Radiological Signs
Demineralization of the distal end of long bones can be seen in advanced RSD (Sudeck's atrophy[23]). Three-phase bone scan or scintigraphy has become the gold standard in this area and is characterized by increased uptake on the affected side, indicating "increased flow, pooling, and delay."[23]

NEURAL BLOCKADE TESTING

The most common diagnostic test used in RSD is the diagnostic sympathetic ganglion block. A local anesthetic is carefully (under fluoroscopic guidance, and with double blind protocol) injected into either the stellate ganglion (C-7 to T-1 for the arm) or lumbar paravertebral ganglia. A positive test result is confirmed if there is documented increase in skin temperature. Blumberg and Janig[10] point out that if temporary pain relief is obtained, this indicates that the sympathetic *efferents* are involved in the pain mechanism (see later discussion).

Charlton[23] cautions that a false-positive response, chiefly due to the placebo effect, can occur in up to 40% of patients. This, he notes, diminishes with repeated procedures. As well, the therapeutic effects of the diagnostic block may outlast the known time course for the blocking agent. This phenomenon may be caused by the central neural changes, which may underly RSD, and whose interruption by peripheral neural blockade may have important therapeutic implications (see later discussion).

As an alternative to diagnostic blocks, a systemic agent known as guanethidine may be given intravenously.[17] This agent depletes presynaptic noradrenaline stores and thus produces an initial, short-lived exacerbation of symptoms, followed by a relief of symptoms.

The phentolamine test[23] is another possible test involving the α-adrenoreceptor-blocking agent phentolamine. Relief of pain and improvement of symptoms indicate increased peripheral sympathetic activity, the reduction of which may prove beneficial therapeutically.

MECHANISMS

A variety of theories and models have been proposed over the 125 years since Weir Mitchell's report. Perl[28] cites Leriche as the first to implicate the sympathetic nervous system as the underlying basis for causalgic symptoms. Table 2 lists several of the recent and current theories that have been proposed to explain RSD, and a brief discussion of these follow. The reader is referred to Blumberg and Janig,[10] McMahon,[14] and Hendler[15] for much more comprehensive reviews of the basic science evidence supporting these theories.

It should be said that all of these theories have their strengths and weaknesses. The strengths often relate to the degree to which they are innovative in bringing coherence to the variety of basic science and clinical evidence available at the time they are proposed. The weaknesses often relate to those very same findings that are often not accounted for by one theory or another. As such, the search has continued for a unified, comprehensive theory, with strong clinical utility.

PERIPHERAL MECHANISMS

McMahon[14] has summarized the proposed peripheral mechanisms related to nerve injury. Basically, peripheral nerve injury results in reorganization of reflex activity and signal transmission within the axon, at the peripheral receptors and, as we will see, within the spinal cord as well.

Earlier theories focused on structural reorganization within the axon at or near the site of injury. During nerve repair and regeneration, abnormal structural developments were proposed consisting of ephaptic connections between sympathetic efferents and primary sensory afferents. It was thought that by "cross talk" between these fibers at these ectopic synapses, normal sensory transmission would result in efferent sympathetic activation. This theory lacked sufficient experiment support and was replaced by the notion of axonal sprouting resulting in abnormal transmission within fibers.

Further studies of the sites of nerve injury resulted in the proposal that damaged nerves became abnormally sensitive to circulating norepinephrine. This might lead to ectopic discharges from the healing neuroma, leading to abnormal sensory bursts, particularly of C fibers (leading to persistent pain) and sympathetic efferents, leading to vascular changes in the periphery.

Finally, this theory of chemosensitivity and changes in receptor mechanisms was applied to the peripheral tissues themselves. Perl,[28] McMahon,[14] and Devor[29] have implicated the peripheral β-adrenergic receptor on the primary nociceptor, as well as within vascular tissues, as the site of primary activity. According to this theory, when a nerve is damaged, there is a *reduction* of adrenergic outflow in the sympathetic efferents (not the originally proposed increase!). This leads to a denervation

TABLE 2.
Theories of RSD

Theory	Pathophysiological Mechanism	Clinical Implications
Historic		
Increased sympathetic outflow	Activation of adrenergic receptors	Vasoconstriction Ischemia Possible pain symptoms.
Peripheral		
Ephaptic connections between sympathetic and sensory neurons due to nerve damage	"Cross talk" and abnormal activation	Allodynia Vasoconstriction
Nerve sprouts from peripheral injury	Abnormal neural firing	Allodynia Vasoconstriction
Direct injury-induced activation of nociceptive afferents	C fiber activation	Burning pain
Abnormal activation of receptors in		Vasoconstriction Allodynia
Primary afferents	Hypersensitivity leading to abnormal firing patterns	
	Neurogenic inflammatory mechanisms (related to substance P)	Vasoconstriction leading to vasodilation.
Sympathetic efferents	Denervation supersensitivity due to eventual depletion of released norepinephrine but up-regulation of β-adrenergic receptors	Abnormal sensation and pain
Central		
Sensitization of wide dynamic range (convergent neurons in dorsal horn)	Alterations in sensory-motor processing.	Allodynia Vasoconstriction (?)

hypersensitivity of the peripheral β-adrenergic receptors, which undergo a process known as "up-regulation."[28] This may consist of an activation of latent receptors, leading to a quantitative increase in synaptic connections and a qualitative increase in receptor strength. Both mechanisms lead to an increase in synaptic efficacy and exaggerated responses to normal or even lowered neurotransmitter loads. This theory is currently much in favor, because it explains two important clinical observations:

the not-uncommon lack of response to sympathectomy and the favorable response to peripheral adrenergic blocking agents (e.g., phentolamine or clonidine).

CENTRAL MECHANISMS

This theory is generally attributed to Roberts[30] and implicates changes in convergent dorsal horn neurones (wide dynamic range cells). Persistent pain from injury to nerves or soft tissue alters (lowers) the excitability of these cells, a process termed by Woolf[31] as "central sensitization." Once sensitized, the nonnoxious inputs from large α-afferent fibers (touch, proprioceptive sense) are able to trigger firing of these convergent neurones leading to the central signalling of pain, hence, the term touch-evoked allodynia. This process may be initiated by discharges from the periphery, that is, the nociceptors may become supersensitive to norepinephrine (as described earlier). This creates a coupling between normal sympathetic outflow and abnormal afferent inflow from both nociceptors and nonnociceptive afferents. This leads to persistent pain (with a burning quality if C fiber receptors are activated), along with touch-evoked allodynia.

This leads to a final point in the area of mechanisms of RSD, which is the notion of multifaceted models in which several of these mechanisms might interact together. McMahon[14] and Blumberg and Janig[10] describe this as a "vicious cycle" of positive feedback in which noxious stimuli create altered central nervous system processing of sensory stimuli, which leads to pain, dysasthesias, and allodynia, and of sympa-

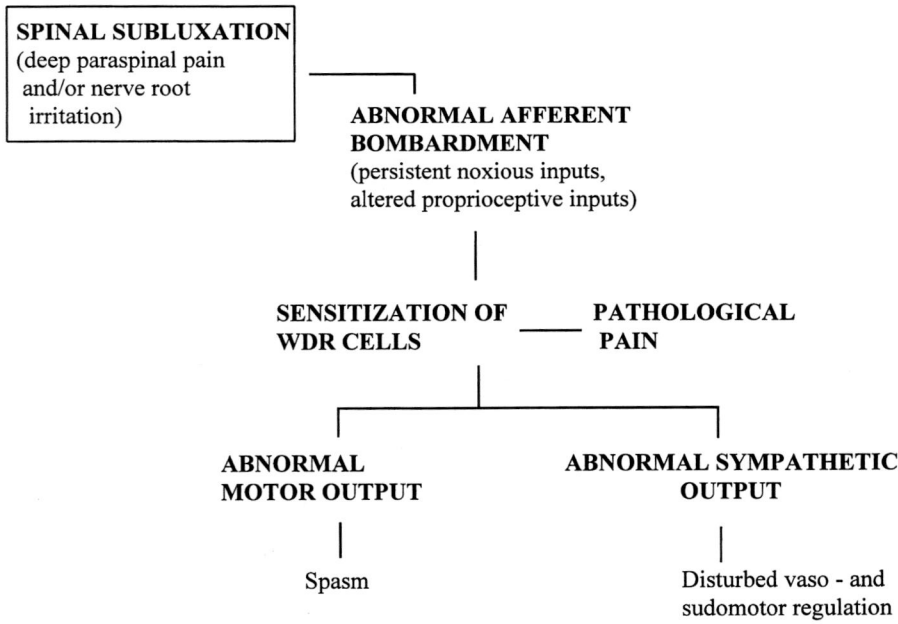

FIGURE 1.
Chiropractic theory of RSD. WDR = wide dynamic range.

thetic and motor efferent activity, which leads to spasm and alteration of vasomotor and sudomotor control in the periphery, all of which make up the panoply of symptoms seen in RSD.

This, of course, is highly reminiscent of Korr's model of "central facilitation" and "sustained sympathicotonia" models, which have been linked, at least conceptually and empirically, if not experimentally, to the chiropractic spinal subluxation. As such, a "chiropractic" version of these vicious cycles would look something like Figure 1.

TABLE 3.
Therapeutic Approaches in RSD

Sympathetic nerve blocks
  Local
    Stellate ganglion block
    Lumbar sympathetic block
  Regional
    Guanethidine block
  Somatic nerve blocks
Medications
  α- and β-adrenergic blockers
    Phentolamine
    Clonidine
    Reserpine
  Calcium channel blockers
  Corticosteroids
Neurosurgery
  Sympathectomy
    Radiofrequency
    Phenol block
  Implanted neurostimulators
Physical therapy
  Heat
  Exercise
  Stretching
  Mobilization
  Manipulation
  Transcutaneous electrical nerve stimulation
  Electroacupuncture
Behavioral therapy
  For
    Depression
    Anxiety
    Phobias
    Pain-avoidance behaviors
  By
    Counseling/cognitive therapy
    Biofeedback
    Relaxation therapy

TREATMENT

The treatment of RSD is based primarily on reduction of excess sympathetic activity, supported by physical and psychological modalities. Table 3 lists the current common therapies for RSD. The reader is referred to Charlton's[23] excellent review for greater detail.

CHIROPRACTIC IMPLICATIONS

No chiropractic report or study has yet been published on RSD and manipulation. However, several studies have appeared dealing with manipulation, pain in one of the limbs, and altered vasomotor reflexes. Figar et al.[32] and Stary et al.[33] published several reports employing plethysmography and documenting relief of pain and improvement of vasomotor regulation after manipulation.

I[34] published a case report documenting relief of arm pain and numbness and improvement in vascular regulation as measured by photoplethysmography (Fig 2). Several reports employing thermography have shown changes in the limb, putatively due to improved vasoregulation after manipulation. These reports, however, have focused on radicular type of pains[35] or local pains originating from myofascial trigger points.[36] These mechanisms are probably similar to those involved in RSD, with the exception of the magnitude and intractability of the RSD condition.

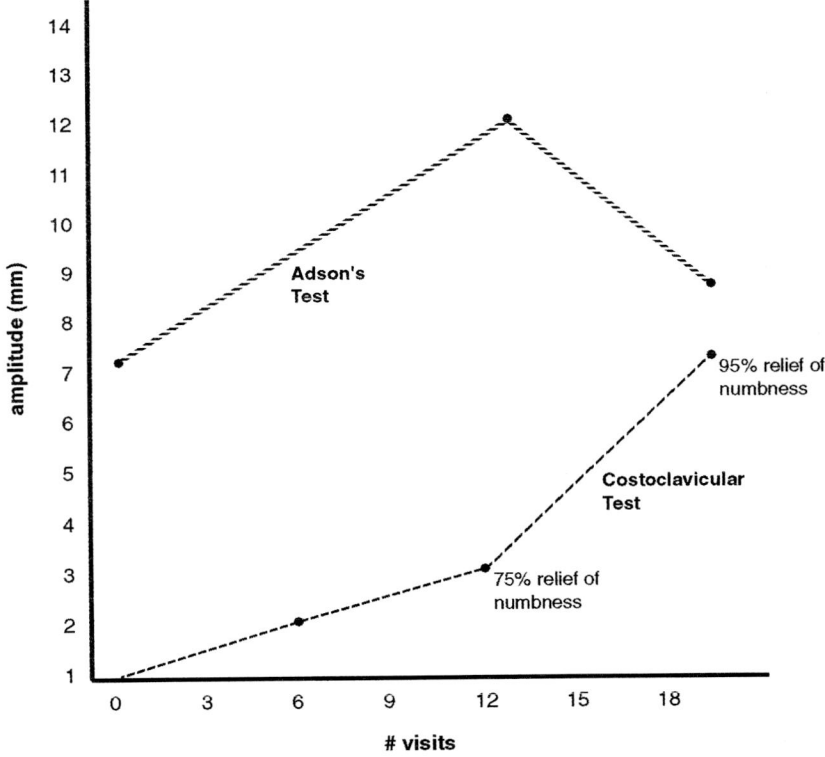

FIGURE 2.
Results of a case study of peripheral vascular response to manipulation.

As such, it behooves chiropractors to put their clinical and neurophysiological theories to the test with RSD. RSD offers an ideal combination of elements as a test of these theories, even as it offers one of the most difficult and challenging conditions those of us involved in treating pain will ever encounter.

REFERENCES

1. Mitchell SW, Morehouse GR, Keen WW: *Injuries of Nerves and Their Consequences.* Philadelphia, JB Lippincott, 1864.
2. Livingston WK: *Pain Mechanisms, a Physiologic Interpretation of Causalgia and its Related States.* New York, MacMillan, 1943.
3. Richards RL: Causalgia. A centennial review. *Arch Neurol* 16:339–350, 1967.
4. Park TJ, Martin GM, Magness JL: Reflex sympathetic dystrophy. *Minn Med* 53:507–512, 1970.
5. Payne R: Neuropathic pain syndromes with special reference to causalgia and reflex sympathetic dystrophy. *Clin J Pain* 2:59–73, 1986.
6. Bonica JJ: Causalgia and other reflex sympathetic dystrophies, in Bonica JJ (ed): *Advances in Pain Research and Therapy.* New York, Raven Press, 1970.
7. Loh L, Nathan PW: Painful peripheral states and sympathetic blocks. *J Neural Neurosurg Psychiatry* 41:664–671, 1978.
8. Glick EN: Reflex dystrophy [algoneuro-dystrophy]. Results of treatments by corticosteroids. *Rheumatol Rehabil* 12:84–88, 1973.
9. Kozin F, McCarty DJ, Sims J, et al: The reflex sympathetic dystrophy syndrome: 1. Clinical and histologic studies: Evidence for bilaterality, response to corticosteroids and articular involvement. *Am J Med* 60:321–331, 1976.
10. Blumberg H, Janig W: Clinical manifestations of reflex sympathetic dystrophy and sympathetically maintained pain, in Wall PD, Melzack R (eds): *Textbook on Pain.* New York, Churchill-Livingstone, 1993.
11. International Association for the Study of Pain: Classification of chronic pain: Descriptions of chronic pain syndromes and definitions of pain terms. *Pain* 3(suppl):S29, 1986.
12. Abram SE, Blumberg H, Boas RA: Proposed definition of reflex sympathetic dystrophy, in Stanton-Kicks M, Janig W, Boas RA (eds): *Reflex Sympathetic Dystrophy.* Boston, Kluwer, 1990, pp 209–210.
13. Janig W, Blumberg H, Boas RA, et al: The reflex sympathetic dystrophy syndrome: Consensus statement and general recommendations for diagnosis and clinical research, in Bond MR, Charlton JE, Woolf CJ (eds): *Pain Research and Clinical Management (Proceedings of the Sixth World Congress on Pain).* New York, Elsevier, 1991.
14. McMahon SB: Mechanisms of sympathetic pain. *Br Med Bull* 41:584–600, 1991.
15. Hendler N: Reflex sympathetic dystrophy and causalgia, in Tollison DC (ed): *Handbook of Chronic Pain Management.* Baltimore, Md, Williams and Wilkins, 1989, pp 444–454.
16. Boas RA: Sympathetic nerve blocks: Their role in sympathetic pain, in Stanton-Hicks M, Janig W, Boas RA (eds): *Reflex Sympathetic Dystrophy.* Boston, Kluwer, 1990.
17. Hannington-Kiff JG: Relief of causalgia in the limbs by regional intravenous guanethidine. *BMJ* 2:367–368, 1979.
18. Hooshang H: *Chronic Pain: Reflex Sympathetic Dystrophy Prevention and Management.* Boca Raton, Fla, CRC Press, 1993.

19. Korr IM: The neural basis of the osteopathic lesion. *J Am Osteopath Assoc* 47:191–198, 1947.
20. Denslow JS: An analysis of the irritability of spinal reflex arcs. *J Am Osteopath Assoc* 44:357–362, 1945.
21. Denslow JS, Korr IM, Krebs AD: Quantitative studies of chronic facilitation in human motoneurone pools. *Am J Physiol* 105:229–238, 1947.
22. Patterson MM: A model mechanism for spinal segmental facilitation. *J Am Osteopath Assoc* 76:62–72, 1976.
23. Charlton JE: Management of sympathetic pain. *Br Med Bull* 47:601–618, 1991.
24. Sherman PA, Karstetter KW, Damiano M, et al: Stability of temperature asymmetries in reflex sympathetic dystrophy over time and changes in pain. *Clin J Pain* 10:71–77, 1994.
25. Uematsu S: Thermographic imaging of cutaneous sensory segment in patients with peripheral nerve injury: Skin temperature stability between sides of the body. *J Neurosurg* 62:716–720, 1985.
26. Perelman RB, Alder D, Humphreys M: Reflex sympathetic dystrophy: Electronic thermography as an aid to diagnosis. *Orthop Rev* 16:561–566, 1987.
27. Fischer AA: Pressure threshold measurement for the diagnosis of myofascial pain and evaluation of treatment results. *Clin J Pain* 2:207–214, 1987.
28. Perl E: Causalgia: Sympathetically-aggravated chronic pain from damaged nerves. *Pain (Clin Update)* 7:371–384, 1993.
29. Devor M: Nerve pathophysiology and mechanisms of painful causalgia. *J Auton Nerv Sys* 7:371–384, 1983.
30. Roberts WJ: A hypothesis on the physiological basis for causalgia and related pain. *Pain* 24:297–311, 1986.
31. Woolf CJ: Evidence for a central component of post-injury pain hypersensitivity. *Nature* 306:686–688, 1983.
32. Figar S, Stary O, Hladka V: Changes in vasomotor reflexes in painful vertebrogenic syndromes. *Rev Czech Med* 10:238–246, 1964.
33. Stary O, Figar S, Andelova E, et al: The analysis of disorders of vasomotor reactions in lumbosacral syndromes. *Acta Univ Carol (Med) (Praha)* 21:70–72, 1965.
34. Vernon H: The role of plethysmography in the chiropractic management of costo-clavicular syndromes: Review of principles and case report. *J Manipulative Physiol Therap* 5:17–20, 1982.
35. Ben Eliyahu DJ, Duke SG: Pathoneurophysiology assessed by infra-red thermography in patients with lumbar facet syndrome. *Chiropractic* 8:3–9, 1992.
36. Diakow PR: Differentiation of active and latent trigger points by thermography. *J Manipulative Physiol Therap* 7:439–441, 1992.

Pronation and Associated Disorders

Neil Fried, D.C., D.P.M.
Instructor and Senior Staff Clinician, National College of Chiropractic, Lombard, Illinois; Attending, Department of Surgery, Doctor's Hospital of Hyde Park, Chicago, Illinois

WHAT IS PRONATION?

Pronation is a motion of the subtalar joint and the midtarsal joints (talonavicular joint and calcaneal-cuboid joint) that occurs in all three cardinal planes simultaneously. The motions include dorsiflexion, eversion, and abduction.

The joints involved in pronation go through several motions to achieve pronation. These motions are dependent on the axes of motion about these joints. The subtalar joint, which affects rearfoot motion and position, has a single axis of motion. The greater the axis is from a cardinal plane, the greater the motion that will occur within that plane. The subtalar joint axis deviates 48 degrees from the frontal plane, 16 degrees from the sagittal plane, and 42 degrees from the transverse plane; therefore, its primary function is to invert and evert the foot. Dorsiflexion and plantarflexion occur primarily at the ankle joint, whose axis deviates 75 degrees from the sagittal plane and only 15 degrees from the frontal plane and has little ability to invert and evert the foot. The midtarsal joint, which affects forefoot position and motion, has two axes of motion, oblique and transverse. The oblique axis deviates 38 degrees from the frontal plane, 57 degrees from the sagittal plane, and 52 degrees from the transverse plane; therefore, its primary motion is dorsiflexion and plantarflexion of the forefoot, as well as abduction and adduction of the forefoot. It has little ability to invert and evert the forefoot. The transverse axis deviates 75 degrees from the frontal plane and therefore primarily inverts and everts the forefoot; it has negligible ability to function in the sagittal and transverse axes of motion.

When the subtalar joint is in its neutral position (i.e., the joint surfaces are congruous and neither supinated or pronated), and when the midtarsal joint is in its neutral position, which is maximal pronation, the rearfoot will be parallel to the forefoot in a subtalar joint that has a neutral position of 0 degrees (neither inverted or everted).

The main function of the foot is threefold: mobile adapter, shock absorber, and rigid lever. These functions are intimately related to subtalar joint function and position, along with its relationship to the function and position of the midtarsal joint.

In gait there are four phases, two of which are swing phase and stance phase. The latter is separated into three phases: heel strike, midstance, and propulsion. This discussion will concentrate primarily on the stance phase. Knee flexion is essential in the shock absorption at heel strike. Subtalar joint pronation is necessary for faster internal rotation of the tibia than the femur to allow for smooth knee flexion.

At heel contact the subtalar joint should be supinated approximately 2 degrees; the midtarsal joint will also be supinated or inverted. The position of the foot will be with the heel and forefoot inverted to the ground. For the forefoot to contact the ground, the subtalar joint must pronate from its inverted or supinated position to approximately 4 degrees of pronation. At this point the forefoot should be flat on the ground. In this heel strike phase the foot is a shock absorber and a mobile adapter. In midstance the subtalar joint will begin to resupinate from 4 degrees of pronation to 2 degrees of supination to allow for maximal pronation of the midtarsal joint, which, in turn, creates a stable forefoot for propulsion or toe off (Fig 1). If full resupination does not occur, the subtalar joint will still be pronated at toe off, which allows for greater ability for the midtarsal joint to pronate; thus, it will not be locked at toe off, and the forefoot will be unstable and therefore the foot loses its ability to be a rigid lever. This can lead to many clinical conditions, which are discussed later in the chapter.

It would be beneficial at this time to discuss the function of the extrinsic foot muscles on pronation and supination. The function of these muscles can be easily divided. Those muscles, whose tendons pass medial to the subtalar joint axis, are supinators of the foot, and those that pass lateral to the subtalar joint axis are pronators. The supinators include the extensor hallucis longus, extensor digitorum longus, tibialis anterior, flexor hallucis longus, flexor digitorum longus, and tibialis posterior. The

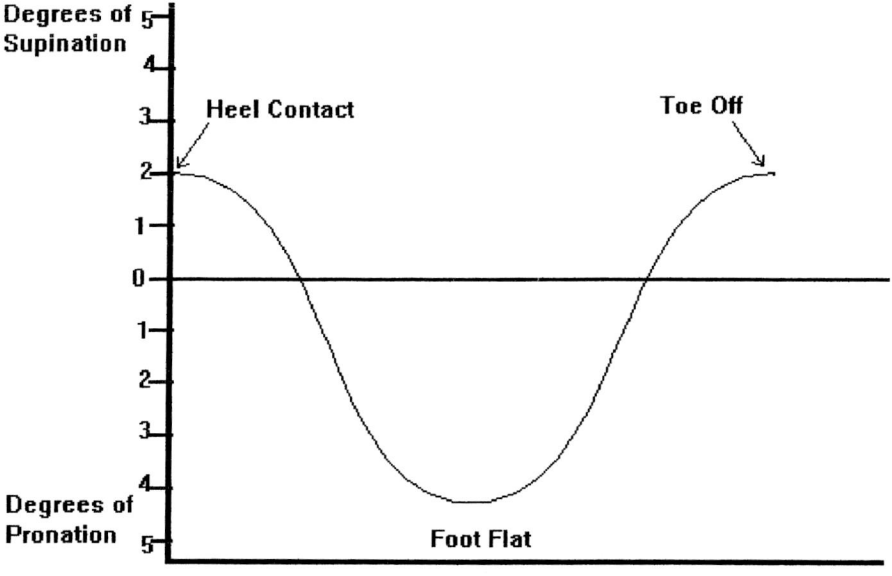

FIGURE 1.
The subtalar joint in the stance phase of gait.

pronators include the peroneus tertius, peroneus longus, and peroneus brevis. The peroneus longus is unique, however, because of its dual ability to pronate and supinate the foot. When the subtalar joint resupinates, it puts the peronus longus in a mechanically advantageous position to plantarflex the first ray. (It takes its attachment at the plantar aspect of the first cuneiform and the plantar aspect of the base of the first metatarsal.) This creates the rigid lever function of the foot. Pronation results from intrinsic causes, extrinsic causes and disease processes.

The most common causes are intrinsic, including rearfoot varus, forefoot valgus, and rearfoot valgus. Extrinsic causes include internal tibial torsion, femoral antetorsion and retroversion, metadductus, equinus, tibia varum, genu valgus, and limb length deficiency. Other etiologies include Charcot's joint disease of the insensate foot, rearfoot trauma, tibialis posterior rupture, inflammatory arthritis, and tarsal coalitions. In rearfoot varus the heel is inverted when the subtalar joint is in neutral. When the heel is in such an inverted position, the forefoot will be inverted to the ground. For the forefoot to get to the ground in midstance phase, the subtalar joint must pronate beyond its normal range for the heel to be vertical to the ground and the forefoot to be flat on the ground. When forefoot varus is present, the forefoot is inverted to the ground when the subtalar joint with a neutral position of 0 degrees is in its neutral position. The subtalar joint must then excessively pronate for the forefoot to be flat on the ground for midstance. When this occurs, because there is no angular deviation of the heel, the heel will go into an everted position in midstance. This makes it difficult for the subtalar joint to resupinate in propulsion phase, therefore creating an unstable foot in this phase, which leads to multiple forefoot problems. Rearfoot valgus is a positional deformity where the subtalar joint is already in a valgus position. If it is 5 degrees or less, it will stay in this position in weight bearing and gait; however, if it is greater than 5 degrees, the subtalar joint will maximally pronate. In these cases the patient will be virtually ambulating out of the medial aspect of the foot with the talar head contacting the ground.

Tibia varum will cause an inverted position of the heel in the stance phase of gait. For the foot to be flat on the ground, the subtalar joint must pronate beyond normal, similar to that of rearfoot varus.

Genu valgus, on the other hand, will cause body weight to fall medial to the subtalar joint, thus causing excessive pronation with the heel being forced into valgus.

Metatarsus adductus is a condition where the metatarsals are adducted in the transverse plane. For the patient to ambulate in a forward direction, the subtalar joint must pronate to allow for unlocking of the oblique midtarsal joint, thus allowing for abduction of the forefoot. The same mechanism holds true for other internal torsional changes of the lower extremity such as internal tibial torsion, antetorsion of the hip, and retroversion of the hip.

Trauma of the calcaneus may cause a varus or valgus angulation of the calcaneus, thus resulting in excessive pronation as described earlier for rearfoot varus and valgus.

Tibialis posterior tendon rupture generally will cause a unilateral flat foot. The tibialis posterior is the major supinator of the foot, and without its action the arch will gradually flatten, leading to severe flattening of the medial longitudinal arch and severe abduction of the forefoot. It eventually may result in severe subtalar joint and midtarsal joint degenerative joint disease.

Limb length discrepancy will cause excessive pronation on the long limb side and excessive supination on the short limb side. This is an attempt to even out the limb lengths; the pronation will cause shortening of the long leg, whereas supination will cause lengthening of the short limb.

Charcot's joint disease is caused by sensory denervation and vascular abnormality of the joints, resulting in inflammation and loss of sensation of the joints of the foot. The inflammatory response leads to osteopenia, and loss of sensation leads to unchecked range of motion, resulting in massive degenerative joint disease. The most common joints of the foot to be affected are the talonavicular joint and calcaneal-cuboid joint, as well as the tarsal metatarsal joints, resulting in collapse of the medial longitudinal arch of the foot.

Inflammatory arthritides such as rheumatoid arthritis will cause osteopenia and cartilage destruction within the joints. It commonly affects the subtalar joint, resulting in severe pronation due to collapse of this joint.

Tarsal coalition, on the other hand, results in a rigid flat foot. There will be no range of motion elicited in the subtalar joint. These patients are usually seen during adolescence with foot fatigue and peroneal muscle spasm.

Equinus is a condition in which there is a lack of dorsiflexion for adequate gait. Biomechanical equinus occurs when there is less than 10 degrees of dorsiflexion. At 0 degrees the foot is maintained in a plantarflexed position known as anatomical equinus. In either case there needs to be adequate dorsiflexion of the foot and ankle as the body weight passes over the stance limb. This range of motion must be obtained from the oblique midtarsal joint. The subtalar joint must therefore pronate to allow for unlocking of the oblique midtarsal joint, leading to increased ability of the oblique midtarsal joint to dorsiflex the forefoot, which leads to adequate dorsiflexion for gait.

ASSOCIATED DISORDERS

FLEXIBLE FLATFOOT

Flexible flatfoot is a common disorder that affects children. It is the most common pediatric foot abnormality. This condition is usually noted when the child begins to ambulate (approximately 9–15 months). This condition is usually asymptomatic until the child becomes more physically active (about 5–6 years). Common symptoms of flexible flatfoot include clumsiness, anterior leg pain, arch pain, foot fatigue, and difficulty in participating in sports activities.

Physical findings include decrease in medial longitudinal arch height, valgus heel in stance and gait, abduction of the forefoot, adducto varus of the fourth and fifth toes, and normal subtalar joint range of motion. The arch may be present when non–weight bearing, and heel valgus may be reducible.

Etiologies of flexible flatfoot include forefoot varus, rearfoot varus, rearfoot valgus, equinus, metatarsus adductus, limb length inequality, and internal torsional deformities of the lower extremity.

Treatment of flexible flatfoot is both symptomatic and functional. Symptomatic treatment includes physical therapy modalities and medications; rationale for the use of these is discussed in more detail under the specific conditions caused by flatfoot. Heel stabilizers, a type of orthotic with deep heel cups and lateral and medial supports, are the treatment of choice for symptomatic and asymptomatic patients. The purpose of these is to prevent excessive pronation, thus decreasing the risk of developing clinically related syndromes by allowing the foot to function as a normal foot. Failure to relieve symptoms by conservative measures is indicative for surgical implantation of a Silastic implant into the subtalar joint; however, this is a rare occurrence.

TARSAL COALITION

Tarsal coalition is an uncommon cause of flatfoot, but it is the most common cause of rigid flatfoot. The most common tarsal coalitions are middle subtalar joint coalition, calcaneal navicular coalition, and talonavicular coalition.

Clinical Findings

Clinical findings may include all or some of the following:

- Painful legs
- Difficulty with physical activities
- Painful medial longitudinal arch
- Loss of medial longitudinal arch
- Knee pain
- Absent subtalar joint and midtarsal joint motion
- Peroneal muscle spasms
- Tenosynovitis of the anterior leg tendons
- Tenosynovitis of the tibialis posterior tendon
- Heel valgus
- Abducted forefoot
- Adductovarus of digits and hallux valgus
- Hyperkeratosis of the forefoot

Despite all the possible clinical manifestations of tarsal coalitions, these patients may remain asymptomatic until some type of traumatic event, major or trivial, sets off a clinical syndrome.

Radiographic Findings

Several radiographic findings are associated with tarsal coalitions, including:

- Increased lateral talocalcaneal angle (angle formed by the bisection of the body of the calcaneus and the body and neck of the talus visualized on lateral view.
- Visualization of the coalition itself on x-ray film.
- Talonavicular and calcaneal navicular coalitions, which are easily vi-

sualized on the appropriate views. Talonavicular coalition is best seen on the anteroposterior and lateral views, whereas the calcaneal navicular coalition is best seen on the lateral oblique view.
- It is difficult to visualize the middle talocalcaneal coalition on plain film; however, there are several associated signs, such as obliteration of the middle talocalcaneal joint, as seen on an axial calcaneal view; thickened lateral calcaneal strut; narrowed posterior subtalar joint; and beaking of the talar head.

Treatment
Treatment options for coalitions include orthotics, physical therapy for pain control, and nonsteroidal anti-inflammatory medication for pain and inflammation. In cases of peroneal muscle spasm, casting may be beneficial. In cases where conservative therapy fails to control the clinical syndromes, or the patient has frequent recurrences, surgical intervention is necessary.

TIBIALIS POSTERIOR RUPTURE AND TENOSYNOVITIS

The most common tenosynovitis associated with pronation is that of the tibialis posterior. Tibialis posterior tenosynovitis is the primary and most powerful supinator of the subtalar joint. The tibilias posterior originates from the tibia and fibula in the deep posterior compartment of the leg. It then courses distal within the leg and passes through a groove on the posterior aspect of the medial malleolus. It inserts on the navicular tuberosity, sending slips to the subtentaculum tali on the calcaneus, all cuneiforms, cuboid, and the lesser metatarsal bases.

In excessive pronation during gait the tibialis posterior tendon attempts to resupinate the foot; however, it is not powerful enough to overcome the pronatory forces and will overwork, leading to tenosynovitis. If this is allowed to continue, attenuation and degeneration of the tendon occurs, and it eventually ruptures, further worsening the flatfoot.

Clinical Findings of Tenosynovitis
Clinical findings of tenosynovitis are:

- Pain on the medial aspect of the foot with ambulation (often confused with medial ankle pain).
- Palpatory tenderness over the tendon between the medial malleolus and the navicular tuberosity. (Contraction of the tendon by plantarflexion and inversion of the foot against resistance make it more easily palpable.)
- Contraction of the tendon that may or may not be painful.
- Stretching of the tendon that may or may not be painful.
- X-ray films are usually not contributory in this condition.

Clinical Findings in Tibialis Posterior Rupture
Clinical findings in tibialis posterior rupture include:

- Gradual or increased loss of arch height, resulting in severe flattening in the medial longitudinal arch (which is usually unilateral).
- Severe abduction of the forefoot.

- Tender tibialis posterior tendon.
- A gap may be palpable. This gap may be filled in with hematoma or scar tissue, in which case no palpable gap will be felt. A palpable nodule, however, may be felt in the tendon.
- It should be noted that rupture is usually a gradual process and not sudden; therefore, the exact time of rupture may not be discernible.
- Severe heel valgus.
- Appropulsive gait.
- Extensor tendon contraction prolonged in stance.
- Decreased heel strike.
- Unstable forefoot in propulsion.
- Degenerative joint disease of the subtalar joint, talonavicular joint, and calcaneal cuboid joint may result if the rupture is long standing. This will be associated with crepitus and arthralgia.

Radiographic Findings
One may find long-standing signs of degenerative joint disease of the subtalar joint, talonavicular joint, and the calcaneal cuboid joint. Magnetic resonance imaging is also diagnostic.

Treatment of Tibialis Posterior Tenosynovitis
Treatment may include:

- Physiotherapeutic modalities such as high-volt galvanic current, pulsed ultrasound and joint manipulation.
- Corticosteroid injection into the tendon sheath. (This is ill advised because it may facilitate tendon rupture.)
- Below-knee casting.
- Orthotics.

It should be noted that whether pain control is achieved with physical therapy, manipulation or medication, the condition will be only transiently controlled unless the patient is fitted for orthotics. Support of the medial longitudinal arch is mandatory to change the pathomechanics of tibialis posterior tenosynovitis and thus decrease the overuse of the tendon, which may eventually lead to rupture. The use of orthotics will allow the tendon to function normally and not overwork to attempt to resupinate the subtalar joint in gait.

Treatment of Tibialis Tendon Rupture
Treatment includes:

- Physical therapy with orthotics. Orthotics will help support an unstable rearfoot and slow the progression of degenerative changes. Physical therapy will help maintain joint mobility and control pain.
- Rearfoot manipulation, which helps to slow the progress of degenerative joint disease and stimulate fibrocartilaginous growth, allowing for smoother joint motion.
- Reconstructive surgery. Multiple reconstructive surgical procedures have been developed for tibialis posterior rupture and are the recommended treatment of choice to prevent serious sequelae. Joint fusion is

recommended for treatment of severe, painful degenerative joint disease of the rearfoot.

PLANTAR FASCIITIS

Plantar fasciitis is the most common associated disorder of pronation. The central band of the plantar fascia is primarily responsible for symptoms. It originates from the middle calcaneal tuberosity and extends distally to the lesser metatarsal bases and then separates into deep and superficial fibers. The deep fibers attach to the plantar pads and bases of the proximal phalanges of the lesser digits, whereas the superficial fibers attach to the fat pads of the forefoot.

The pathomechanics of the pain syndrome can be explained by the Hicks windlass mechanism. The windlass consists of two components posterior and jointed in the center.

When the central axis is brought closer to the ground, the lever arm increases. Because the plantar fascia attaches to the rearfoot and the forefoot as the arch drops, or if flattening is present, there is an increase in distance or lever arm between the forefoot and rearfoot, resulting in increased tension of the plantar fascia on the medial calcaneal tuberosity. This tension results in irritation to the periosteum, leading to periosteal reaction, which leads to a heel spur.

It has been postulated in the past that the heel spur was the pain-producing agent, but it is the pull of the plantar fascia on the periosteum that leads to pain, not the spur itself. There are many cases of plantar fasciitis without the presence of a heel spur.

Clinical Findings

Clinical findings include:

- Pain occurs in the morning hours on rising from bed or after rest, which improves with a few minutes of ambulation.
- No edema, erythema, or echymosis is present.
- Tender medial calcaneal tuberosity.
- Occasionally the medial longitudinal arch is tender.
- There is pain at the medial calcaneal tuberosity with dorsiflexion of the forefoot and toes.

Radiographic Findings

A heel spur may be present but is not necessary for a diagnosis of plantar fasciitis and is usually considered a sequelae of the condition.

Treatment

Treatment includes:

- High-volt galvanic current and pulsed ultrasound. The rationale for the use of ultrasound is that of anti-inflammatory and fibroblastic effects. High-volt ultrasound controls pain and is necessary because of the contractile tissue of the first layer of plantar muscles attached to the medial calcaneal tuberosity. This may also contribute to the pain.
- Injection of corticosteroid and local anesthetic into the plantar fascia, which breaks the pain pattern, decreases inflammation. Pressure from the injection will also help to break up existing scar tissue.

- Manipulation of the joints distal to the subtalar joint, which helps to maintain mobility and proper function of the joints that the plantar fascia crosses.
- Orthotics. Orthotics are the treatment of choice, and all other treatments are only palliative. Orthotics restore proper biomechanical function of the foot and allow normal pronation while stopping abnormal degrees of pronation. They will decrease the lever arm, as well as decrease the pull of the plantar fascia on the heel. Without orthotics all other treatment methods are destined to fail because pathomechanics are still present. Orthotics are successful in 90% to 95% of cases.
- Surgical release of the plantar fascia and resection of the heel spur are a last resort when conservative care fails to relieve pain.

SINUS TARSITIS

Sinus tarsi syndrome is an often overlooked diagnosis in the foot but is seen quite commonly in patients with pronation.

The sinus tarsi is formed by groove on the dorsal surface of the calcaneus between the posterior and middle facets and a groove on the plantar surface of the neck of the talus. It courses anterolaterally to posteromedially. The sinus tarsi can be palpated as an indentation just anterior and inferior to the lateral malleolus.

The pathomechanics of the pain results from the motion of the talus in the hyperpronated foot during gait. With pronation the talus slides anteriorly, adducts, and plantarflexes. The motion results in compression of the contents of the sinus tarsi, resulting in pain.

Clinical Findings
Clinical findings include:

- Pain on the lateral aspect of the foot just distal to and inferior to the lateral malleolus. This is often confused with ankle joint pain but must be discerned for proper treatment.
- Pain primarily with ambulation that is worse after rest.
- Pain that is worse in the morning.
- Pain that is usually relieved by several minutes of ambulation.
  Radiography is usually noncontributory.

Treatment
Treatment options include:

- High-volt galvanic current and pulsed ultrasound. The purpose of pulsed ultrasound in this condition is to decrease inflammation.
- Electrical muscle stimulation is used for pain control and in certain modes may decrease inflammation.
- Corticosteroid and local anesthetic injection into the sinus tarsi will decrease inflammation of the joint, break up adhesions, and alter the pain cycle.
- Orthotics. Orthotics are the mainstay of treatment. Orthotics help control excessive pronation, which limits the anterior translation, plantarflexion, and adduction of the talus, thus decompressing the sinus tarsi. As mentioned with previous conditions, without orthotics the biome-

chanical pathomechanics will continue, resulting in recurrence of the condition. Thus, physical therapy and injection therapy are only palliative.
- Subtalar joint manipulation can be used to maintain range of motion, prevent cartilaginous degeneration, and decrease joint pressure, leading to pain control.
- Surgical evacuation of the sinus tarsi is performed when conservative care fails.

HALLUX VALGUS

Hallux valgus is defined as a lateral deviation of the great toe. It is associated with and results from a medial deviation of the first metatarsal.

Hallux valgus is usually a direct result of excessive pronation. When the subtalar joint pronates, it allows for unlocking of the oblique midtarsal joint, which allows for excessive dorsiflexion and abduction of the forefoot. The peroneus longus is now at a mechanical disadvantage to plantarflex the first ray in stance. Subsequently, ground-reactive forces overcome the actions of the peroneus longus, resulting in dorsiflexion and abduction of the first metatarsal. As a result of both soft tissue contracture on the lateral side of the first ray (adductor hallucis, lateral collateral ligament, lateral sesamoid ligaments, and the lateral joint capsule) and proprioceptive responses of the hallux, the hallux will deviate laterally and occasionally rotate in a valgus direction.

The cause of hallux valgus and contributing factors are as follows:

- Pronation.
- Genetics.
- Trauma.
- Inflammatory arthropathy.
- Shoe gear.
- Female predilection.

Clinical Findings

Clinical findings include the following:

- Prominent medial aspect of the first metatarsal head, which is often painful in shoe gear (commonly referred to as a bunion).
- Erythema and rubor over medial first metatarsal head.
- A bursa is often present over the first metatarsal head.
- The first metatarsal phalangeal joint may be tender.
- Difficulty wearing fashionable shoes.
- Positive tracking phenomena: When the hallux is placed in its normal position and dorsiflexed, a moderate to severe bunion cannot be moved purely in the sagittal plane and tracks back to its valgus position.
- Dorsiflexed first ray usually is noted when the first metatarsal has greater mobility above the second metatarsal as below it within the sagittal plane.
- Neuritis may occur because of the pressure on the nerve as it passes by the metatarsal head.

Radiographical Findings
Radiographic evaluation includes the following:

- Increased intermetatarsal angle formed by the bisection of the first and second metatarsal shafts at the intersection of these lines. The normal intermetatarsal angle is 8 to 10 degrees. In hallux valgus this angle will be increased.
- Increase in the proximal articular set angle formed by the bisection of the first metatarsal and a line drawn perpendicular to the cartilage on the articular surface of the metatarsal head. It should be less than 7.5 degrees in the normal patient.
- Increased hallux abductus angle between the bisection of the proximal phalanx and the first metatarsal. The normal angle should be less than 15 degrees.
- Increased tibial sesamoid position, which is the relative position of the tibial sesamoid to the bisection of the first metatarsal. With increasing deformity the position of the sesamoid becomes more lateral on the metatarsal.
- Dorsiflexion of the first ray in relation to the bisection of the talus on the lateral foot radiograph in a weight-bearing view.
- The first metatarsophalangeal joint should be evaluated for signs of degenerative joint disease.

Treatment
Treatment options are as follows:

- Wider shoes.
- Manipulation to maintain joint mobility, slow degenerative changes by stimulating fibrocartilaginous growth, and possibly help with pain control. It should be noted that manipulation will not reduce the deformity.
- High-volt and pulsed ultrasound to decrease inflammation, stimulate fibroblastic activity via ultrasound, and assist in pain control.
- Orthotics to slow progression of the deformity by controlling pronation and allowing normal function of the peroneus longus to plantarflex and stabilize the first ray.
- Surgical correction. This is the only method available for the reduction of a painful hallux valgus deformity. Manipulation, bracing, and exercises will not change the deformity and are essentially palliative procedures. The chiropractor in this phase of treatment is providing postoperative physical therapy via various modalities stretching exercises and manipulation.

HALLUX LIMITUS AND HALLUX RIGIDUS

Hallux limitus is a condition where there is limited range of motion of the first metatarsophalangeal joint to less than 20 degrees of dorsiflexion. Hallux rigidus is a progression of hallux limitus whereby the range of motion is less than 10 degrees of dorsiflexion.

There are several etiological factors for the development of these conditions, including trauma, pronation, rigid dorsiflexed first ray, long first metatarsal, and inflammatory arthropathy. Our discussion concentrates on pronation as a cause. Pronation, as discussed previously, causes excessive pronation of the midtarsal joint; therefore, the forefoot is unstable in the propulsive phase of the stance phase of gait. Simultaneously the peroneus longus is at a mechanical disadvantage and cannot efficiently plantarflex the first ray; therefore, ground-reactive forces overpower the peroneus longus and cause dorsiflexion of the first ray. Simultaneously in the toe-off phase of gait the first metatarsophalangeal joint needs approximately 65 degrees of dorsiflexion for smooth motion. Pure dorsiflexion of the proximal phalange on the first metatarsal head provides only 20 to 30 degrees of dorsiflexion. The remainder of the motion of the first metatarsophalangeal joint is dependent on the first ray plantarflexing to allow the base of the proximal phalange to slide over the metatarsal head. If this cannot occur, the proximal phalangeal base jams into the metatarsal head, causing limited range of motion, exostosis of adjacent joint surfaces, cartilage degeneration, and eventually advanced degenerative joint disease of the first metatarsal phalangeal joint, leading to a rigid joint.

Clinical Findings
Clinical findings include limited range of motion of the first metatarsophalangeal joint, which is usually painful at end range. Other clinical findings may include palpatory bony mass over the first metatarsophalangeal joint, overlying bursa, discoloration over the metatarsophalangeal joint, callus over the first interphalangeal joint (which occurs from rolling off the medial aspect of the foot due to decreased first metatarsophalangeal joint motion), and noticeable pronation of the foot.

Radiographical Findings
Radiographical findings include dorsiflexion of the first ray in relation to the neck of the talus, dorsal exostosis, joint narrowing, subchondral sclerosis, and periarticular osteophytes. Hallux valgus may or may not be present.

Treatment
Treatment ranges from conservative to surgical management. Conservative management includes early recognition, which can circumvent progression of the disorder. If pronation is treated via orthotics, the normal biomechanics can be restored, thus allowing proper dorsiflexion of the first metatarsophalangeal joint, preventing progression of the joint pathological conditions.

Other treatments include mobilization of the joint to stimulate fibrocartilaginous growth on the joint surface to allow for a smooth joint surface for smooth range of motion of the first metatarsophalangeal joint. Ultrasound will also assist in fibrocartilaginous growth, as well as act as an anti-inflammatory in its pulsed mode. Electrical stimulation will aid in pain control and will have an anti-inflammatory effect.

Nonsteroidal anti-inflammatory medications and corticosteroids may benefit the patient in acute flare-ups, but their effects are not long lasting.

Several surgical procedures have also been developed for the treatment of hallux limitus and hallux rigidus.

It is important to note that physical therapy and medications are only a temporary form of management, and without correction of biomechanical faults with orthotics or surgery, other treatment methods are doomed to failure.

HAMMERTOES

Hammertoe deformities are actually a group of digital flexion deformities that include hammertoes, claw toes, and mallet toes (Fig 2). A hammertoe is defined as a flexion deformity of the proximal interphalangeal joint with hyperextension of the metatarsophalangeal joint and the distal interphalangeal joint. A claw toe is a flexion deformity of the distal interphalangeal joint and the proximal interphalangeal joint. A mallet toe is defined as a flexion deformity of the distal interphalangeal joint.

Hammertoe deformities may be caused by either pronation or supination. Hammertoes occur when the flexor muscles gain a mechanical advantage over the extensors of the digit. Three theories have been postulated as to the development of hammertoes: flexor substitution, flexor stabilization, and extensor substitution.

Flexor substitution usually occurs in the supinated foot. It occurs in the late stage of the stance phase of gait. If the triceps surae are weak, the deep posterior and lateral leg compartment muscles will compensate for this weakness and fire to help plantarflex the ankle joint. In turn, they will fire late into the stance phase and cause contraction of all the toes, resulting in hammering of the digits.

Flexor stabilization is seen primarily with pronation in the late stance phase of gait. This is associated with excessive subtalar joint pronation. Excessive subtalar joint pronation, as discussed earlier, causes unlocking of the midtarsal joint, resulting in hypermobility of the forefoot. The flexor muscles fire earlier and longer in an attempt to stabilize the forefoot, sub-

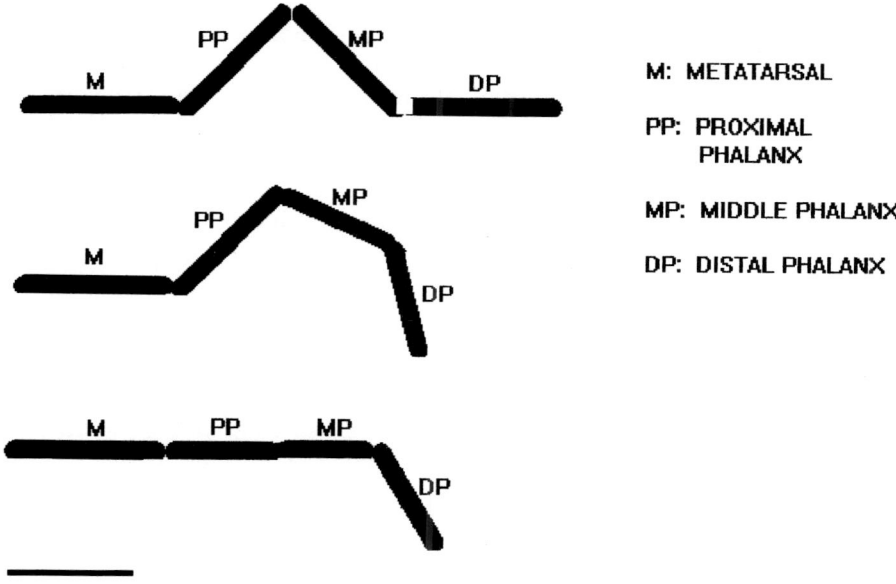

FIGURE 2.
Toe deformities.

sequently overpowering the stabilizing forces of the interosseous muscles of the digits, resulting in hammering and clawing of the digits.

Extensor substitution is seen in the swing phase of gait. This occurs with an anterior (forefoot) cavus, ankle equinus, weak lumbricales, spasticity of the extensor digitorum longus, and pain. In the swing phase of gait the extensor digitorum longus gains a mechanical advantage over the lumbricales, leading to excessive dorsiflexion of the digits in propulsion, swing phase, and heel contact. The deformity begins as a flexible deformity and then eventually becomes fixed if allowed to continue.

Clinical Findings
Clinical findings of hammertoes may include plantar hyperkeratoses beneath metatarsal heads from retrograde forces, causing prominent metatarsal heads. Hyperkeratoses occur over the interphalangeal joints both proximal and distal and at the tips of the toes. The areas of hyperkeratoses are dependent on the type of hammertoe. Hammertoes may be flexible or fixed, which can be discerned by checking range of motion of the interphalangeal joints and metatarsal phalangeal joints and pressing plantar to dorsal on the metatarsal heads. When they are flexible, the hammertoe will correct. Joint pain may be present as well. Ulceration of the skin with or without infection may occur in diabetics with neuropathy.

Radiographic Findings
Radiographic studies will show flexion deformities and degenerative changes, and hypertrophy of the phalangeal heads may be present if the deformity is long standing.

Treatment
Treatment options rarely include conservative care from a physical therapy standpoint. Joint mobilization will aid in diminishing pain and maintaining mobility and joint integrity. Ultrasound and high-volt galvanic current may help with pain and edema if they are present. Orthotics are useful in flexible deformities by restoring the normal gait pattern and decreasing abnormal pronation, thus averting the mechanism leading to fixed deformity. The most common complaint in patients with hammertoe deformities, however, is painful calluses, which can be addressed in two manners. Calluses can be debrided on regular intervals but tend to recur frequently. Because of this frequent recurrence, various surgical procedures have been developed to the bony hypertrophy, joint contractures, and calluses.

ADDUCTO VARUS OF FOURTH AND FIFTH TOES

Adducto varus of the fourth and fifth toes is a variant of hammertoes. It is an adduction of the digit at the metatarsophalangeal joint with flexion at the proximal and distal interphalangeal joints. There is also a varus rotation of the toe.

Adducto varus digits are seen in the pronated foot due to the relationship between the quadratus plantae and the flexor digitorum longus. Due to the orientation of the flexor digitorum longus, if its action is left unchecked, the pull on the toes would be one of flexion, adduction, and varus rotation. The quadratus plantae attaches to the flexor digitorum longus and functions to straighten the pull of the flexor digitorum longus on the toes. However, in the pronated foot, the distance between the quadratus plantae and the flexor digitorum longus is increased, and the quadratus plantae is at a mechanical disadvantage and therefore cannot overcome the pull on the lateral aspect of the flexor digitorum longus tendons. This results in adducto varus of the fourth and fifth toes.

Clinical Findings
One sees the deformed toes, hyperkeratoses on the dorsum of the digits, and occasionally painful joints with limited range of motion.

Radiographic Findings
Radiography will confirm bony positional changes consistent with the deformity, as well as bony hypertrophy of the proximal and middle phalanges. Hypertrophy of the middle phalange is usually present on only the fifth toe. Occasionally arthritic changes may be seen.

Treatment
Treatment protocol mirrors that of hammertoes.

ACKNOWLEDGMENTS
I would like to give my deepest gratitude to Dr. David Ward for his technical and editorial assistance.

REFERENCES

1. Barrett SL, Day SV: Endoscopic plantar fasciotomy for chronic plantar fasciitis/heel spur syndrome: Surgical technique—early clinical results. *J Foot Surg* 30:568–570, 1991.
2. Chandler TJ, Kibler WB: A biomechanical approach to the prevention, treatment and rehabilitation of plantar fasciitis. *Sports Med* 15:344–352, 1993.
3. Durrant MN, Siepert KK: Role of soft tissue structures as an etiology of hallux limitus. *J Am Podiatr Assoc* 83:173–180, 1993.
4. Gerbert J: *Textbook of Bunion Surgery*, ed 2. Mount Kisco, NY, Futura, 1991.
5. Giannestras N: *Foot Disorders: Medical and Surgical Management.* Philadelphia, Lea and Febiger, 1973.
6. Gormley J, Kuwada GT: Retrospective analysis of calcaneal spur removal and complete fascial release for the treatment of chronic heel pain. *J Foot Surg* 31:166–169, 1992.
7. McGlamry ED, Banks AS, Downey M: *Comprehensive Textbook of Foot Surgery*, ed 2. Baltimore, Williams & Wilkins, 1992.
8. Jahss MH: *Disorders of the Foot.* Philadelphia, WB Saunders, 1982.
9. Root ML, Orien W, Weed JH: *Normal and Abnormal Function of the Foot.* Los Angeles, Clinical Biomechanics, Corporation. 1977.
10. Salamao O, et al: Talocaalcaneal coalition: Diagnosis and surgical management. *Foot Ankle* 13:251–256, 1992.
11. Schoenhaus HD, Cohen RS: Etiology of the bunion. *J Foot Surg* 31:25–29, 1992.
12. Scurran B: *Foot and Ankle Trauma.* New York, Churchill-Livingstone, 1989.
13. Sobel M: Simplifying the approach to metatarsalgia. *J Musculoskeletal Med* 10:75–85, 1993.
14. Tachdjian M: *Pediatric Orthopedics*, Philadelphia, WB Saunders, vol 2, 1972.

Chiropractic Medicine for Dance

Bill Russell, M.A., M.F.A., D.C., C.C.S.P.
Post Doctoral Faculty, Logan College, Dance/Sports Injuries, St. Louis, Missouri

Working with dancers is a uniquely challenging and interesting opportunity for sports chiropractors. Dancers are subject to at least as much risk, stress, and injury as most athletes. There are probably more dancers than participants in any other single sport, yet dance medicine is just being recognized as a specialty. Until recently, dancers, who are predominantly female, have been overlooked. Gender bias against females as athletes is one of the factors responsible for the dance community being underserved.

The need for specialized dance health care is apparent. The average professional dancer has a career of only 12 years, a 9 out of 10 chance of being injured, and a 6 in 10 chance of being disabled by these injuries.[1] We as sports chiropractors have a lot to offer dancers. With our understanding of the relationship between joint biomechanics and functional strength in preventing, diagnosing, and treating injuries, we can be an invaluable asset to the dance medicine team.[2]

Dancers are complex; they are both athletes and artists. As athletes, they face many physical challenges that indicate a need for chiropractic. Dancers withstand prolonged physical stress. Professional dancers' workouts are more strenuous than many athletes, with rehearsals, classes, and performances totaling up to 50 hours per week year round. Several dance styles require extending range of motion well beyond the normal limit.

As artists, they move in a different world where beauty, spirit, and creativity are the goals; they are driven to express themselves and work beyond pain and exhaustion, beyond common sense. Consider the health care history of many dancers. As artists in a society that does not value most art, many dancers do not have health insurance. Therefore, they do not get the preventive health care they need as ordinary citizens, let alone as athletes. Many dancers have had frustrating experiences with unsuccessful or inappropriate treatments in the past, because practitioners in all traditions, chiropractors included, have only recently begun to take the needs of dancers seriously.

When working with dancers, one must understand the various movements involved to help in the development of appropriate changes in those patterns, both to prevent injuries and to enhance the performers' abilities to express themselves. This need for familiarity with the causative physical activity itself applies to all athletics, whether performing arts or sports.

Advances in Chiropractic®, vol. 2
© 1995, Mosby–Year Book, Inc.

The dance physician must understand the full spectrum of services, including physical therapy and orthopedic surgery. The physician must observe classes and performances and work in collaboration with dance masters to ensure preventive and rehabilitative support. In addition to specific recommendations for individual artists, the physician can teach classes to help dancers understand the physiological stresses incurred in performing and prevent injury.[3]

CAUSE OF INJURY

Primary cause of injury is most often overuse,[4-6] with faulty technique[7] and nonfacilitative alignment resulting from inaccurate body imaging as secondary causes. Most dance injuries are the result of a number of interrelated actions rather than a single event. Injuries are traceable to multiple microtrauma secondary to maladaptive movement patterns and nonfacilitative techniques that may have been present from the dancer's earliest training. Even with acute trauma, there may be a history of chronic problems that sets the stage for the acute injury.

The most common site of muscle injury in the dancer is the lower half of the back.[8] Rather than being caused by single trauma to the lower back muscles, it is the result of repeated microtrauma superimposed on interrelated biomechanical problems.[9,10] In many cases, dance injuries are associated with chronic somatic dysfunction of the lumbosacral spine and pelvis-related alignment problems, also characterized by unilateral or bilateral psoas shortening.

This chapter consists of background information to familiarize the physician with the etiology and epidemiology of dance injuries, and to familiarize the doctor with typical range of motion and movement patterns common to many forms of dance. I will then cover screen examination of the dancer, including proprioceptive and functional evaluation. Special emphasis will be placed on (1) Psoas insufficiency and its possible role in the development of many common injuries, and (2) treatment protocols incorporating specific orthopedic and proprioceptive testing and video evaluation specifically adapted for dance. These protocols include several procedures developed by the dance medicine community. These procedures are based on the most current research in such areas as recognition of inappropriate movement patterns (fatigue stretching),[11] proprioceptive rehabilitation using rotation disks, and Pilates' equipment and video analysis.

In the screening and treatment sections, I will focus on examination and treatment techniques unique to dance, relying on other sources to cover the more common elements. Areas covered will include evaluation of lower extremity function and its relation to dance movements; the use of video as an examination and treatment tool, concentrating on the use of basic consumer-grade equipment; and range of motion and strength examinations as they apply to dance.

This chapter will supply the physician with knowledge in the evaluation and treatment of dance injuries that can be incorporated into existing sports injuries protocols, enabling the sports physician to treat dancers more competently. These new skills can also be readily applied to the treatment of other athletes and the general population.

DANCE SCREENING EXAMINATION

When beginning to work with a dance patient, in addition to completion of a standard personal and family medical history, one must obtain a complete dance history and perform a physical examination, covering the dancer's training, chosen techniques, and injury history.[12] This dance screening examination can be used as intake with individual patients or as a preparticipation examination when one is working with dance companies or dance schools.

The dance screening examination can be very helpful to a dancer and physician due to the large amount of information that can be obtained in a relatively short period, but most dancers do not have specific dance screening examinations until after a problem is apparent. Most individual dancers do not get adequate preventive care due to inadequate health insurance or physicians who do not have the proper awareness, attitudes, and skills necessary for identifying and treating dance-related conditions.

The need for screening is especially great for local dance schools or companies; only rarely will a dance school, regional dance company, or school performing arts program have access to health professionals as consultants for the dance program, though they may screen all other athletes. With adequate screening and subsequent training modifications, many injuries may be avoided, especially with young dancers who are just beginning to develop their training habits. Dancers start very young; if they learn healthy workout habits and proper technique early, they can enjoy years of healthy dancing.[13] A chiropractor with an understanding of the needs of a dancer can have an important role in establishing this healthy foundation.

A thorough dance screening examination can be very beneficial in uncovering problems that the dancer may identify as important to the current problem; it can also be very useful in the development of a comprehensive treatment and training program.

When possible, work in conjunction with the dance instructor or the company dance master. Your relationship with the instructor or dance master can be informative and helpful in several ways. He or she can help you understand what various techniques demand from the dancer and can clarify the dancer's goals and skill levels, so that you can better support the dancer in achieving those goals. In addition, the instructor can spot potential problems as they develop and can monitor and supplement your preventive and corrective recommendations.

When the physician and the instructor are working together, the instructor can incorporate appropriate exercises[14] that relate to specific imbalances common to each style of dance, as well as specific exercises for dancers with certain conditions. Because the instructor or dance master has a great deal of influence over the dancer, he or she can strongly influence compliance to all healthy practices, including exercises you both recommend. Targeted exercises can be included throughout the day but emphasized in morning classes, because the body responds best to warm-up and flexibility work early in the day.[15]

The history form and injury form filled out by the dancer are the most important part of the screening process. The form itself should be brief and easily completed. It should contain information about all areas of the dancer's health that might affect his or her ability to dance now or in the future. It should be well organized and in a form that is easily interpreted by the dancer and his or her instructor or master. Whenever possible, dance terms should be used.[12]

PERSONAL INFORMATION

The first section should contain:

- Current address and permanent address as in the case of a student or workshop participant
- Person responsible for the dancer (parent, friend, significant other, spouse or dance teacher)
- Age, date of birth
- Current dance status (student level, company member, instructor etc.)

YOUNG DANCERS

The dancer's age is an important consideration in his or her screening and treatment. Many dancers begin to dance at a very early age, often before 5 years. One consideration with young dancers is growth spurts, which cause induced muscle shortness, because bones develop faster than muscles and tendons. Muscles also develop at different rates, which causes muscle imbalances.[16] Muscle imbalances are a contraindication to increased activity level or the learning of new skills due to the disruption of proprioceptive information from the muscles and joints involved.

Dance at a young age is not contraindicated, however; a young child simply requires careful training and monitoring. Schools and dance companies fail to stress the importance of conditioning by not requiring their dancers to take classes that will address their physical demands: strength, endurance, and correct biomechanical and aesthetic technique. The general rule is that the dancer should have been training for 5 years. Usually around the age of 11 or 12 years, depending on the development of each individual child, they will have completed growth in the feet, have developed sufficient strength for pointe, and have mastered specific preparatory skills before beginning pointe work.[16] Years and type of training are more determining factors in injury prevention than age alone. Strength and endurance are also important factors but are difficult to measure. Strength of the interosseous muscles has a greater role than strength of the plantar land dorsiflexors in the ability to maintain pointe.[17]

Young dancers place too much emphasis on increased range of motion, as in turnout. The age dancers start training can affect their ability to perform turnout. Before 11 years of age, the femoral angle is developing and can be affected by the stresses applied during dance and by careful stretching in the frog position (prone, double passé). After age 11, the femoral angle appears to be permanent, and changes are confined to the soft tissues of the hip.[2]

The older dancer, on the other hand, may experience facet impingement syndrome due to the repeated approximation of spinal joints. If forcing increased range of motion is continued, facet impingement syndrome can develop into disk problems later in the dancer's life.

MEDICAL HISTORY

A brief general medical history should cover such things as serious illnesses, recent surgeries, and menstrual history and irregularities. Excellent examples of these forms can be found in Dr. W. Ben Kibler's *The Sport Preparticipation Fitness Examination*.[18] It is common for dancers to start menses late in adolescence or to have amenorrhea due to high-energy output and low caloric intake. Amenorrhea may also be a sign of serious eating disorders.[19]

DANCE INJURY HISTORY

The screening form should cover specific dance-related injuries. This is the most important part of the form and should include the kind of injury, date, whether it is a recurrent injury, specific diagnosis, who made the diagnosis, and current status of the injury.[11] On the form, list parts of the body (back, hip, knee, ankle, foot, toe, etc.) with specific boxes for the dancer to check regarding the injuries and care received (Fig 1).

DANCE HISTORY

The final section of the form should contain a specific dance and physical activity history. Time and types of physical activities other than dance should be recorded. Regarding dance, include the number of hours spent in technique classes, rehearsal, and performance for the last 2 months and the level and type of technique practiced. Include primary and other techniques studied (e.g., African: 3 hours/day, 4 days/week; ballet; 3 hours/day, 1 day/week) and all current performance techniques.[11]

It is very common for a dancer to work primarily in one style and to perform in a completely different type of dance; for example, a dancer may teach modern dance 25 hours per week, and rehearse 10 hours per week for a jazz-based musical theater performance. When dancers are performing in styles different from their training, a common phenomenon in theater dance, it is important that they be in technique classes to counter bad technique that they may develop while performing.[20] Sudden changes in style or activity level can be a major cause of injury due to the new stresses to the body. Also, proprioceptive skills required by the new style are not fully developed.

TECHNIQUE FACTORS

Turnout

Turnout, 90-degree external rotation of the leg, is a major component of nearly all forms of dance—ballet, ethnic, and to a lesser degree modern dance.[6, 21, 22] Turnout is a complex biomechanical activity consisting of 55- to 70-degree external rotation at the hip, 10-degree external rotation at the knee, 12-degree of tibial torsion, and the remainder from abduction at the midtarsal joints (Fig 2).[1, 21, 23] With correct turnout, the midpoint of the knee-cap is aligned over the long axis of the foot, whereas the torso remains vertical, and the longitudinal arches of the foot are maintained.

With perfect turnout, the knees face directly laterally so that a straight

Name_____ Birthdate   /   /
Address_____ Height
        _____ Weight

Years of Dance Training _____   Age Started _____

Primary Status as Dancer
  ( ) Solo Performer   ( ) Principal Dancer
  ( ) Company Member   ( ) Choreographer
  ( ) Teacher/Professor   ( ) Student
      of Dance

Type of Technique Practiced   How Long
  ( ) Ballet   _____
  ( ) Modern   _____
  ( ) Jazz   _____
  ( ) Tap   _____
  ( ) Spanish   _____
  ( ) Afrocentric   _____
  ( ) Dunham   _____
  ( ) Other _____

Level of Technique Practiced
  ( ) Recreational
  ( ) Dance School Student
  ( ) College/University Student
  ( ) Instructor
  ( ) Professional

Other physical activity which you participate in and frequency
(Hrs/Week or Month) _____
_____

Number of Classes During Dunham Seminar #/Day ____ #/Week ____

INJURY HISTORY
Area Of Body Injured	Date (mo/yr)	Diagnosed no/yes/by whom	Treated no/yes/how	Recurring when
Toes				
Foot				
Ankle				
Knee				
Hip				
Pelvis				
Spine				
Shoulder				
Neck				
Elbow				
Wrist				

Are you currently being treated for any conditions (including those not listed above)? Yes / No
If yes, by whom and for what? _____
_____

FIGURE 1.
Sample dance injury history used during Dunham's technique seminars.

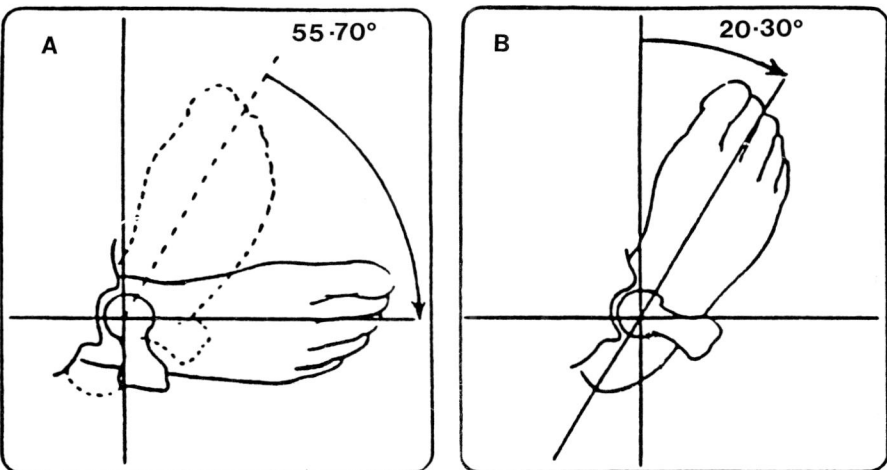

FIGURE 2.
The hip in turnout. Ninety degrees of turnout is achieved by 55 to 70 degrees of external rotation at the hip **(A)**, 10 degrees of external rotation at the knee, **(B)**, 12 degrees of tibial torsion, and the remainder from midtarsal abduction.

line can be drawn between the first and second toe of the right foot, right heel, left heel, and first and second toe of the left foot.[2] In an attempt to achieve this perfect turnout, the dancer can develop a number of improper techniques that predispose the dancer to such lower extremity problems as hallux valgus, bunion formation, hammertoe deformities, flexor hallucis longus tendinitis, and patellofemoral dysfunction.[24]

To increase external rotation at the hip and achieve maximum turnout, the dancer flexes at the hip (Fig 3),[25-28] which relaxes the anterior iliofemoral ligament, alters the orientation of the acetabulum and the femur head, and decreases the psoas length. To return to a vertical stance, the dancer must hyperextend the lumbar spine. Chronic maintenance of this hyperextended position will load the posterior compartment of the leg and increase hip flexor tightness (Fig 4).

To compensate for poor turnout, dancers may tilt the pelvis to increase external range of motion of the hip, resulting in hyperlordosis and poor body alignment, particularly of the psoas and rectus femoris. This causes restriction of hip flexion and encroachment of the innominate and the femur,[8, 25, 28-30] which results in compromised turnout.

Plié

The plié (see Fig 4) is a basic component of virtually all dance technique. Grand plié (see Fig 4) puts seven to eight times the body weight through the knee.[3] When the common plié is performed correctly, the weight is held by the psoas in a position of balance. There is a minimum of stress on the muscles of the leg and foot, and the Achilles tendon is in a state of strong stretch with the foot relaxed on the floor and the tibialis anterior maintaining a minimal amount of tension. If the dancer is holding excessive tension in the tibialis anterior (Fig 5), she or he must contract muscles that should be released. The leg muscles are supporting the

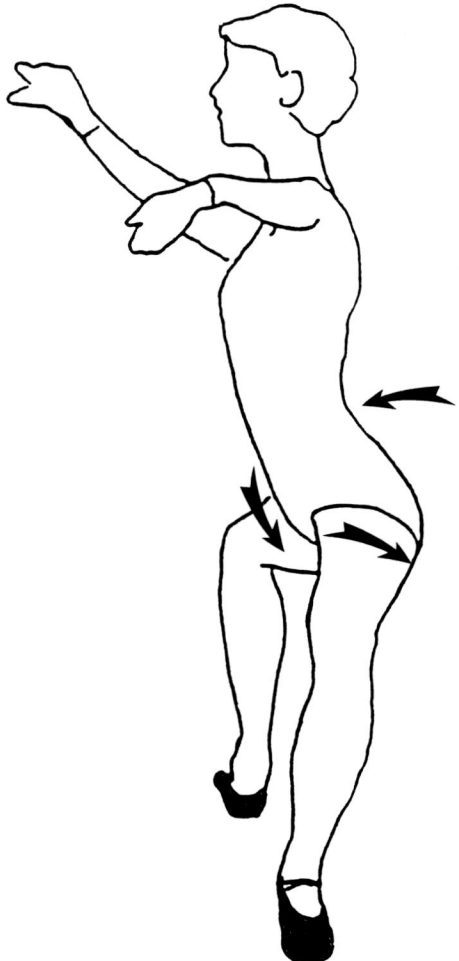

FIGURE 3.
Dancers compensating for less than 90-degree turnout will tilt the pelvis to increase external range of motion of the hip, resulting in hyperlordosis and poor alignment.

weight of the body rather than the psoas, the natural support muscle. When the anterior tibialis is contracted, it will hamper the effectiveness of the plié as the initiating movement of jumps and leaps and affect the jumps' height and distance and therefore decreasing their aesthetic appeal as well. A contracted anterior tibialis also affects the plié's function as a resilient landing, causing shock waves generated by a "hard landing" to reverberate up the leg and contributing to pariostal stress. This shock wave may be repeated hundreds of times during any given class, causing shin splints and stress fractures.[31]

Arabesque
Arabesque position, if executed improperly, results in facet impingement and spondylolysis (Fig 6).[25, 26, 32, 33] The dancer maintains a hyperlor-

Chiropractic Medicine for Dance **219**

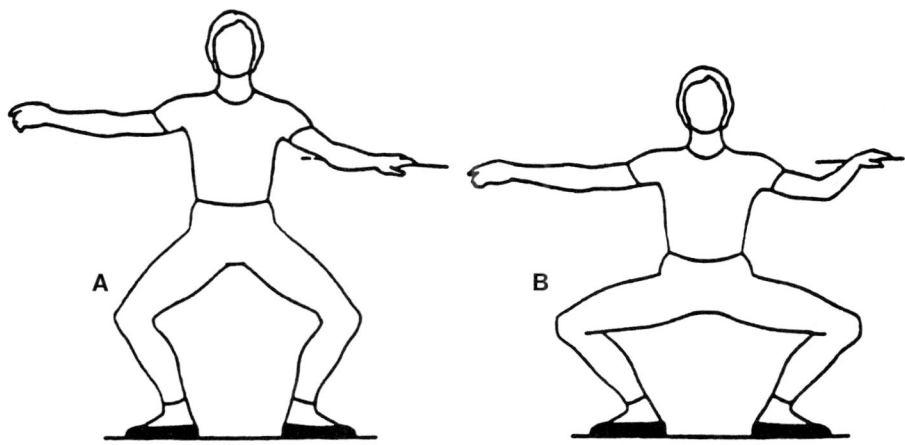

FIGURE 4.
A, Plié. B, Grand plié.

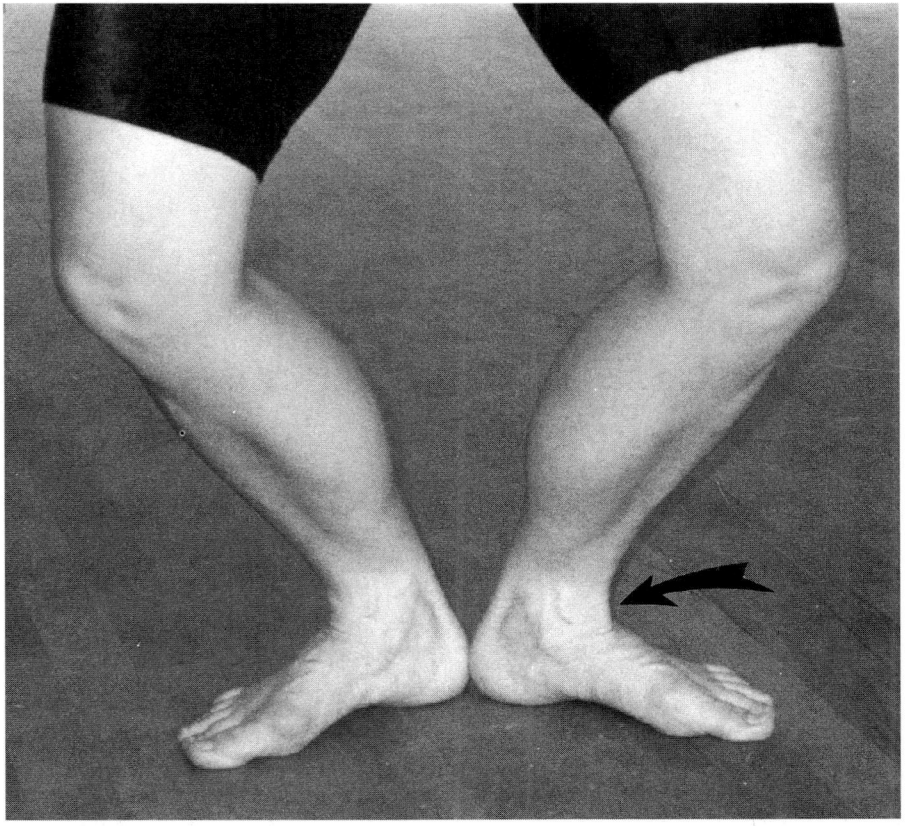

FIGURE 5.
Contracted anterior tibialis during plié.

dotic position in the presence of decreased external rotation of the hip.[26, 27, 32] With continued maintenance of the hyperlordosis and the resulting anterior tilt of the pelvis, muscle and tendon imbalances are created. The abdominals become stretched and weak, allowing the anterior hip flexors to become contracted, which decreases extension of the hip[9] and causes the dancer to increase lordosis and increase the approximation of the spinal joints.[25] The lumbodorsal fascia also becomes hypertrophic, leading to potential problems in the thoracic spine in response to the loss of flexibility. When restricted external rotation is unilateral, the dancer drops and anteriorly rotates the pelvis on that side in an effort to increase hip rotation.[10, 25, 26, 28] This causes an increase in lumbar lordotic curve and stresses the sacroiliac joint.[10, 34]

Extension

During full extension (extension in dance refers to the gesturing leg and can encompass extension and flex abduction and adduction), the dancer may have difficulty maintaining the extended or "gesturing" leg (Figs 7 and 8) without obvious tension in the quadriceps muscles as he or she attempts to lift the leg and tighten tendons around the hip socket. This prevents a graceful, stress-free extension and leads to improper positioning of the hip, correct positioning being slightly different for each individual dancer. Repeatedly performing such moves, the dancer will eventually develop "popping or snapping hip syndrome," which is believed to be caused by the contracted rectus femoris or iliopsoas tendons if the sensation is medial to the hip joint or the tensor fascia lata if the sensation is lateral to the hip joint as they slide over the hip joint. When ob-

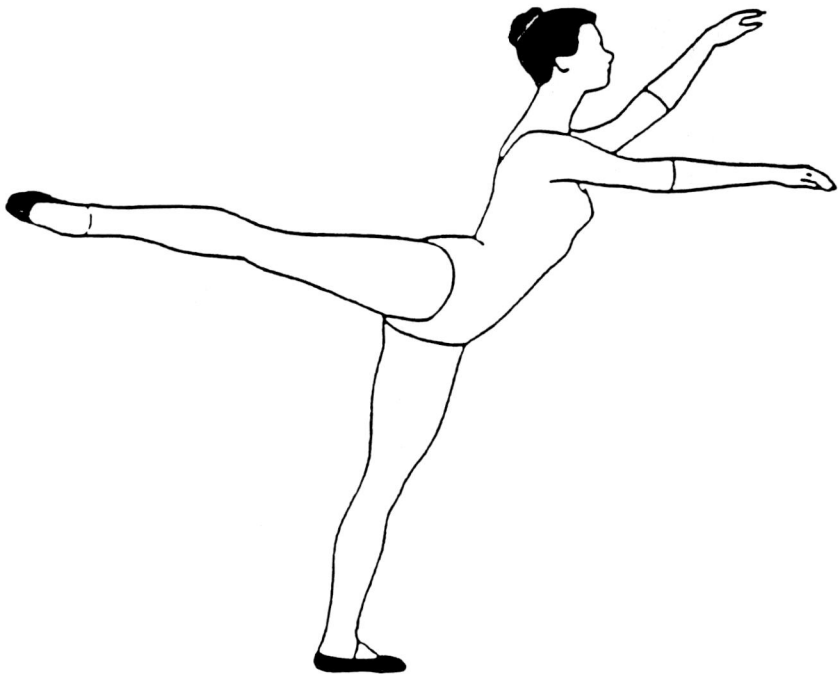

FIGURE 6.
Arabesque.

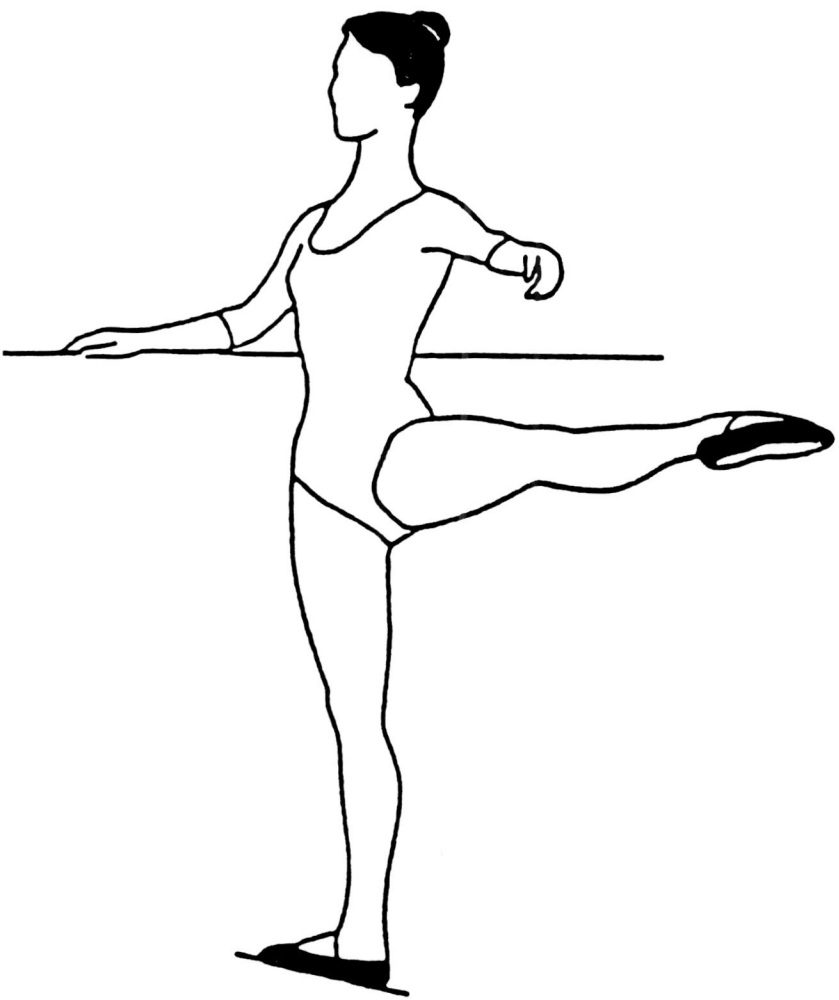

FIGURE 7.
Dancer with poor core muscle control may use quadriceps to maintain extension of the "gesturing" leg during battement.

serving the dancer performing extension during such moves as developpé and battement, you will observe that the quadriceps muscle across the top of the hip is strongly contracted. This is an indication that the superficial quadriceps is trying to take over the primary role in the lifting of the leg from the psoas rather than functioning in its normal role as a secondary flexor to the psoas. Not only is the quadriceps contracted, but the tendons that surround the hip also contract, in effect pulling the leg into the hip socket and actually restricting movement.[31]

OCCUPATIONAL FACTORS

A professional dancer's lifestyle can lead to injuries. A typical dancer may teach class 25 hours per week, take an additional 6 to 10 hours of class, log 10 hours of performance rehearsal, and perform in addition. Theater

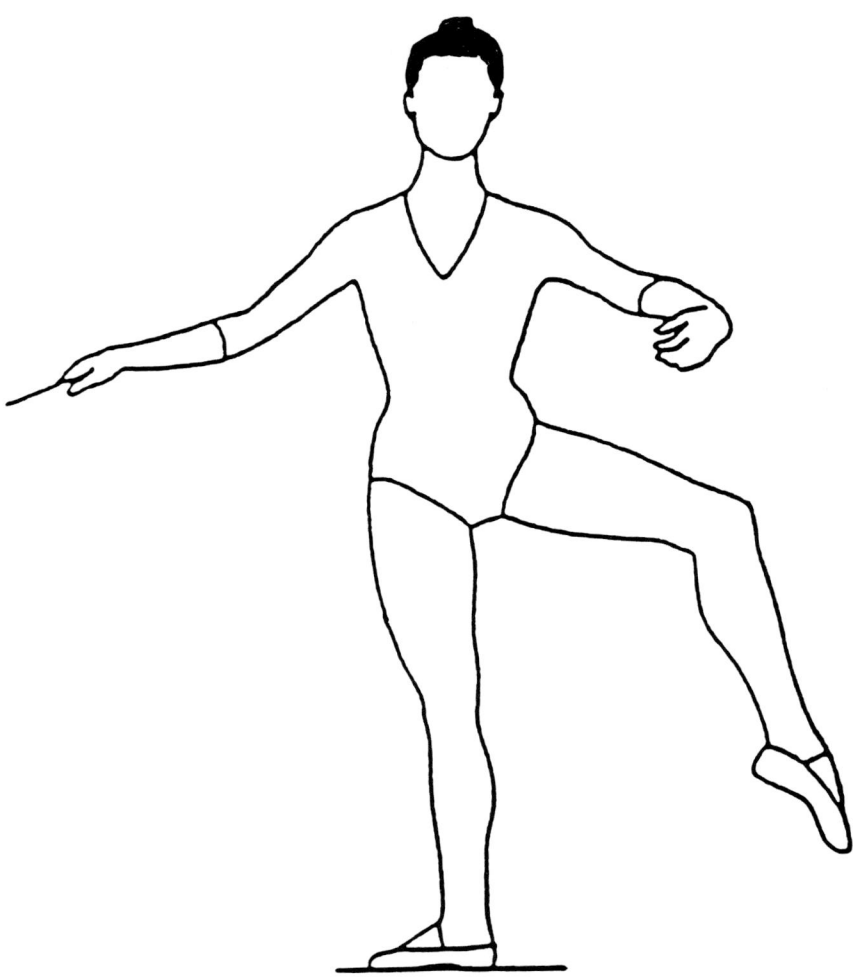

FIGURE 8.
Developpé.

dancers are under contract for six to seven 8-hour days per week of rehearsal, with 12-hour daily rehearsals during the week before the opening. A theater dancer may tour for up to 2 years in a single role that requires the same repeated movements with little time for proper cool-down or warm-up. They may be on stage for up to 1 hour before being required to perform strenuous dance movements.[20] No amount of warm-up is going to be effective under such conditions. Such a schedule sets the stage for repetitive stress injuries.

The conditions of employment can also compound the injury rate of theater dancers. They do not have workers' compensation except while employed and little time available to seek treatment when they are employed. Most theater dancers are fired if injured and have no sick leave with pay, so they may tend to continue dancing when injured or stressed. If they miss 16 consecutive shows, they are fired. If they miss 24 of 48 performances, they are fired.[20] This has the effect of causing the dancers to dance with injuries rather than have them treated while they are relatively minor and easily managed.

Professional dancers constantly increase their work loads and skill levels, learning new techniques and dances for performance. As the work loads progress, dancers become increasingly calorically deficient and dehydrated, leading to fatigue and increased rates of injury.[35] It is imperative that the dance physician understand these circumstances and work within the dancers' world. Theater dancers may also suffer injuries specific to the stage, such as injuries due to carrying props or cervical injuries due to heavy headgear often worn in theatrical dance.[20] Long hair in rows worn by some Afrocentic dancers exerts extreme forces on the neck during extremely aggressive head movement common to this style of dance.

SCREENING

During the screening examination, you will be looking at several aspects of the dancer in relation to dance in general and to the types of dance practiced: weight, height, body composition, general posture, flexibility, body type, and a general evaluation of the spine, hips, knees, ankles, and feet. During the examination, a number of factors must be considered when one is dealing with the dance population. The measurement of body composition, height, and weight is a very stressful area for the dancer and should be done with complete confidentiality by a person trusted by the dancer.[12] The person recording body composition should have experience with the equipment to ensure accurate readings. Skin calipers are the easiest to use and are as accurate as more sophisticated devices when used by a skilled practitioner.

When flexibility is tested, most commercial devices will not be adequate because most dancers are so well stretched out. Simply use a square box for the dancers to place their feet against and a ruler to measure their reach past the edge of the box.[12] Hyperflexibility is desirable in many dance styles and is essential to such styles as ballet, where average range of motion is well beyond normal. Necessary ranges of motion for ballet are 120 to 160 degrees of hip flexion (hamstring length), plus 30 degrees for hip extension (psoas length) and 60 degrees for external hip rotation.[36] Decreased joint motion in the presence of hyperflexibility leads to muscle overuse. When the dancer has decreased flexibility in soft tissue, joint movement and therefore gross movement is affected,[37] all of which leads to increased incidents of injury.

POSTURAL EXAMINATION

The postural examination as it relates to dance and the evaluation of the specific areas (spine, hips, knees, ankles, feet, and toes) are the two most valuable parts of the examination. Dancers should be dressed in two-piece swimming suits for women and trunks for men. They should also bring any orthotics or shoes worn during dance class or daily, so that you may evaluate posture with and without the orthotics. All history forms should be complete at this time, with all current, former, or recurrent injuries. To begin the examination, have the dancer stand in a "normal stance" and evaluate posture from the side and back. A postural grid or plumb line will increase the speed and accuracy of this part of the examination. The "imaginary plumb line" that is used by the mind's eye is the most practical in many screening situations because of the lack of space or resources.[12] If the circumstances allow, a great deal of valuable information can be obtained by observing the habitual postures they maintain when not performing for the examiner.

Common findings are hyperlordotic curves and anterior tilted rib cages as the dancer exaggerates what he or she perceives as correct dance posture. Scoliosis should also be looked for, especially in younger female dancers, because they are at a prime age for such problems to develop.[16] Posterior weight-bearing predisposes the dancer to calf muscle strain. Achilles tendinitis, lower extremity stress fractures, and anterior ankle impingement syndrome.[24] Anterior tilt of the pelvis either bilaterally or unilaterally is the result of iliopsoas insufficiency.[28]

Hyperextension or genu recurvatum of the knees is also common; it may even be desirable in some forms of dance. Bowlegs or genu varum are common among advanced students and professional dancers. "Rolling in" and "rolling out" (Fig 9) or "sickling" may also be seen, because they are common though inappropriate responses to trying to achieve turnout and relevé. Femoral anteversion and femoral retroversion may also be observed.[24]

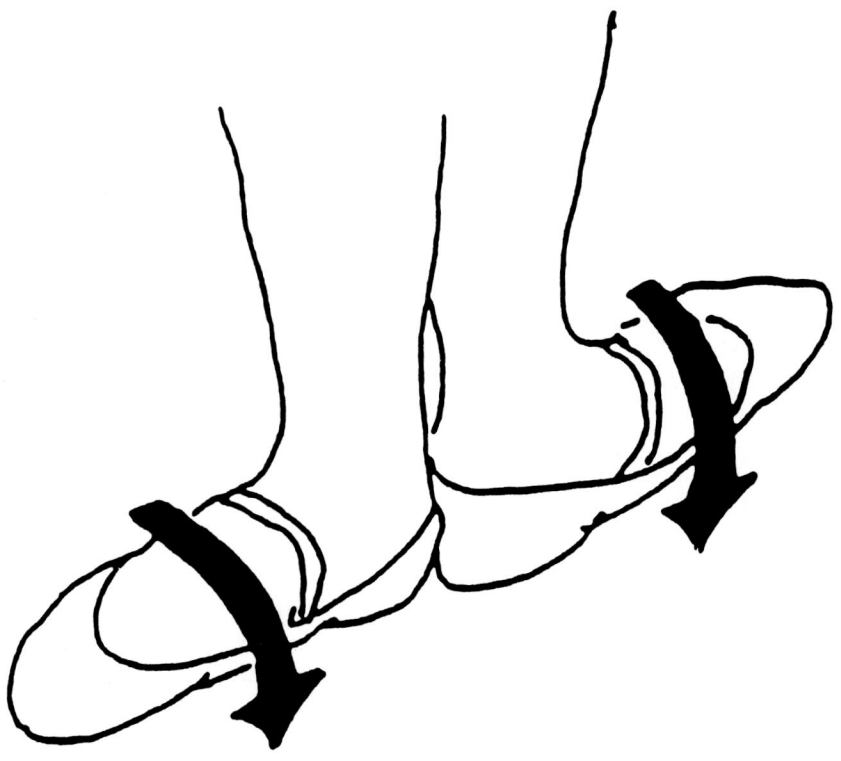

FIGURE 9.
Rolling in. The subtalar joint pronates during relevé and plié.

In addition to observing dancers in normal or parallel posture, it is important to evaluate them in turnout, a rotated hip position common in many forms of dance. If time permits, it is very helpful to evaluate them in other common postures used in their primary styles of dance (e.g., plié and relevé for ballet or flat back for Dunham).

SPECIFIC AREA EVALUATION

After the postural evaluation, each area (spine, hip, knee, ankle, foot, and toes) should be examined separately. This will help in developing a complete overall picture of the dancer's biomechanics. Though problems may occur in specific areas, they must be related to the dancer's entire biomechanical picture and professional responsibilities to develop a complete treatment program.

Skill in the evaluation of joint function and soft tissue is necessary for proper evaluation. Excellent sources for that information include *Functional Soft Tissue Examination and Treatment: The Extremities* by Warren I. Hammer[38] and *Manipulation and Mobilization* by Susan L. Edwond[39] and will not be covered in detail. In summary, a dancer's screening examination must always include activity-specific evaluation, as well as standard examination protocols. In the following section, I will discuss clinical findings common to dance.

Spine

When one is addressing the back and use of peripheral muscles, a posture common in dancers involves "pull-up," (Fig 10) pulling the rib cage up and forward, with the lumbar spine lordotic. This requires the relatively weak back muscles to maintain the upright posture rather than the large muscles on the front of the spine. From this anatomically forward and raised rib cage, the dancer tries to elevate the leg from above by initiating the movement from the rib cage rather than the psoas, imposing even greater stress to the lumbar and thoracic spine and increasing the potential of hypertrophy of the back muscles. By observing the dancer from the side and palpating the muscles of the back as they perform basic movements such as plié and developpé, you can instruct the dancer to release the rib cage, using your hands to gently reposition the rib cage into proper vertical alignment while supplying tactile information that helps the dancer locate and relax the muscles of the back[25] and chest that are being used to maintain this posture.[31]

Another manifestation of "tight back" is caused by lordotic spine (see Fig 10).[14] In response to the stresses applied to the articular pillars during hyperextension-hyperflexion, such problems as spondylolysis and facet impingement syndrome.[25, 40] may occur. Spondylolysis is most commonly seen in adolescent female dancers[8, 25, 26, 41, 42] and progresses to spondylolisthesis in the presence of excessive pull by short psoas muscles.

Lumbopelvic dysfunction is related to problems of the sacroiliac and apophyseal joints. Hyperextension in the lumbopelvic region results in musculature hypertrophy and disruption of lower extremity muscle balance, all of which increase dancers' use of maladaptive movement patterns and the incidence of cumulative microtrauma.[24]

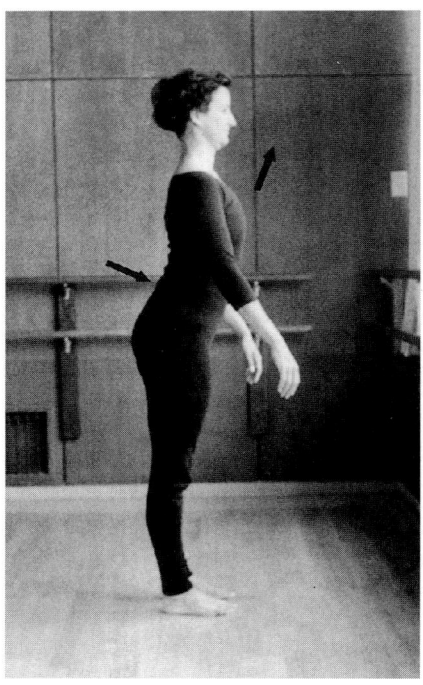

FIGURE 10.
Pull up. Pulling the rib cage up and forward, with the lumbar spine lordotic (Courtesy of Susanne Grace, Durning Feet Dance, St. Louis.)

Forced turnout in the presence of short psoas muscles can also lead to sartorius tendinitis around the hip when the dancer uses the sartorius to overcome tight internal rotators of the hip[6, 27] during developpé.[22, 33] In developpé (see Fig 8), the leg is lifted off the floor and externally rotated (see Fig. 14). Tendinitis can develop in the superficial anteriorly tilted hip. When the gluteal and piriformis muscles are used to force turnout, deep gluteal pain from gluteal/piriformis tendinitis[6, 23, 26] can develop, with occasional development of secondary sciatica.[6, 27] In my own practice, I have found that in dance styles that concentrate on internal rotation of the hip, trochanteric bursitis can be a problem, especially for dancers whose training has been primarily ballet, with its emphasis on externally rotated hip and femoral neck retroversion.

Knee

ROLLING IN.—Rolling in (see Fig 9) has a detrimental effect on the knee and the muscles related to its stability.[21, 41] During dorsiflexion, the subtalar joint pronates, increasing the degree[1, 40, 43] and speed[43] of internal tibial rotation present during knee flexion,[24, 43] a necessary component of plié. These movements prevent the knee from achieving final lockout phase during extension[44] and place excessive stress and shear on the medial meniscus.[23, 26, 32, 43] The tibia also exerts a medial force on the patellar tendon and the iliotibial band, medially displacing the patella and increasing the Q angle,[21, 23, 27] resulting in anterior knee pain syndrome[27, 34, 45] and patellofemoral dysfunction.[23, 26, 43] The increased stress on the iliotibial band is associated with an increase in iliotibial band syndromes.[24, 46, 47] The medial displacement of the patella, which decreases its functional ability, causes loss of strength and muscle weakness problems. Full extension is painful and avoided, leading to vastus medialis atrophy. This muscle is activated only during the last 15 degrees of extension,[26] increasing instability of the knee, and contributing to medial colateral ligament problems.[23, 26, 32, 43]

SCREWING THE KNEE.—Another maladaptive technique is screwing the knee (Fig 11). The dancer flexes the knee, which increases tibial torsion by an additional degree,[1, 43] and then places the foot in maximum external rotation. With the foot fixed in this position, the dancer extends the knee,

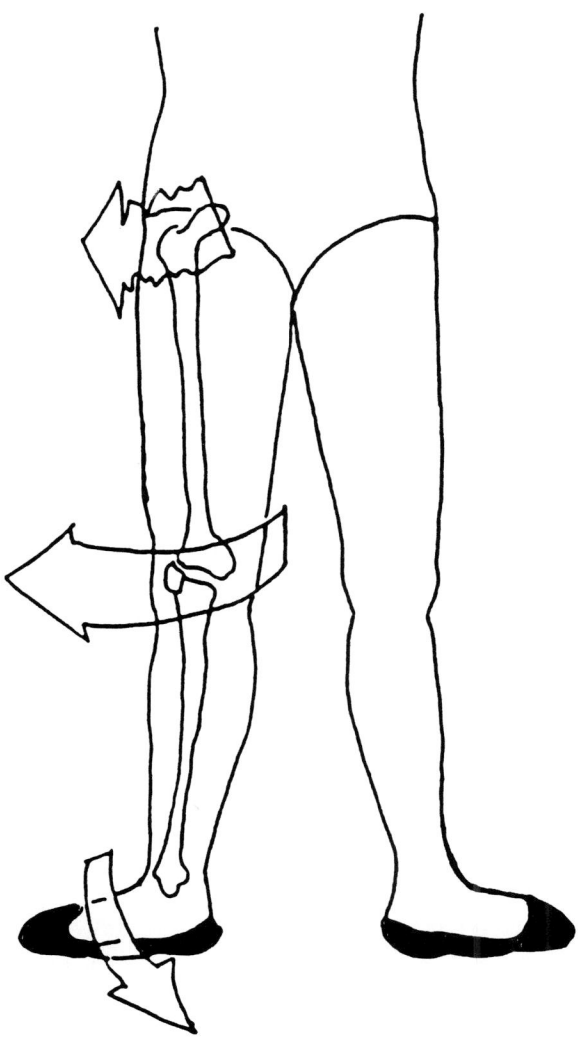

FIGURE 11.
Screwing the knee.

inducing rolling in and exerting excessive stress and shear forces at the knee,[10, 32] which causes the same types of problems as discussed previously.

Ankle

To compensate for decreased dorsiflexion at the talotibial joint, the dancer develops a maladaptive movement pattern to achieve a perceived increase in dorsiflexion. When the dancer pronates the midfoot, abducts the forefoot, and hyperflexes at the midtarsal joint, the plantar fascia is stretched and the midtarsal joints are flexed. When repeated over time, this maladaptive movement pattern develops into anterior impingement syndrome.[43, 48]

During plié, in the presence of tight triceps surae (equinus), the Achilles tendon acts to invert the calcaneus, which increases its varus tilt and possible rotary motion.[43, 44, 48–50] The peroneus, a rear foot evertor during dorsiflexion,[1, 49] opposes the Achilles tendon, creating muscle imbalance between the peroneus and the triceps surae, further reducing these muscles' shock-absorbing capabilities[21] and predisposing the dancer to peroneal tendinitis[51] and stress fractures of the fibula.[1, 44]

Another improper technique dancers may use to overcome decreased turnout is rolling in (see Fig 9) the foot while in first through fifth position (Fig 12) and during plié and demiplié.* This compensatory movement causes excessive motion around the subtalar joint.[45] The calcaneus

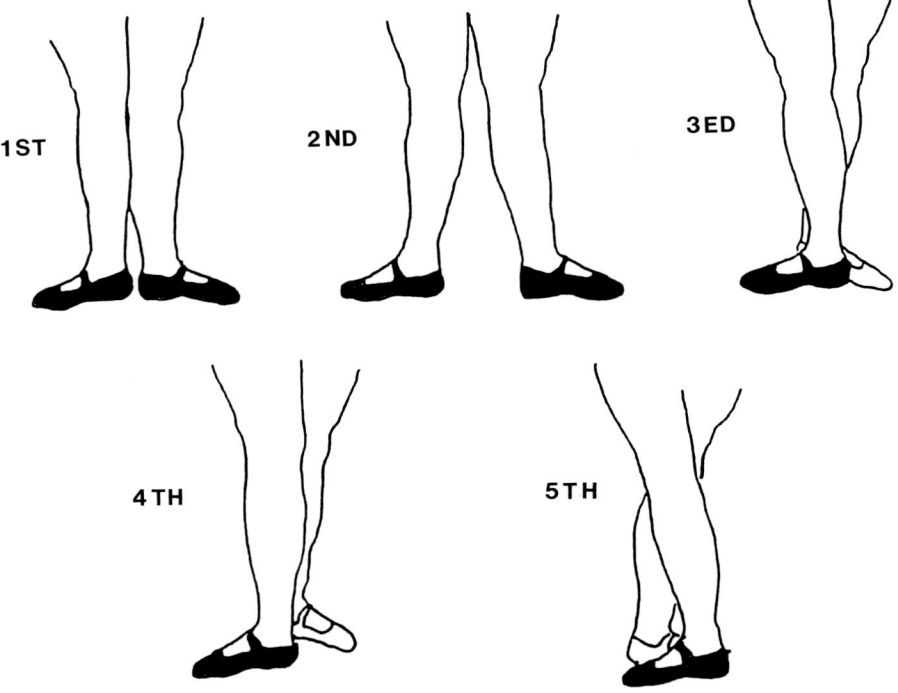

FIGURE 12.
During first through fifth positions, external rotation of the hip is characteristic.

everts and the subtalar pronates, allowing a parallel relationship to develop between the calcaneocuboid and the talonavicular joints. This unlocks the arch structure and allows it to collapse, placing stretch on the plantar fascia and stressing the midtarsal joint,[43, 49] with the potential development of anterior impingement syndrome,[1, 26, 48] plantar fasciitis,[21, 42] and heel spurs.[43] The medial metatarsals are forced to carry more of the weight, causing an increase in metatarsal stress fractures[26, 31, 52, 53] and metatarsophalangeal joint capsulitis.[27, 40, 43, 52] The first ray becomes hypermobile, abducting and internally rotating[23, 27] and causing flexor hallucis longus tendinitis[21, 25, 50, 52] (the most common tendinitis in dancers),[29, 42] trigger toe,[23, 28, 50, 54] and bunions.[4, 23, 40, 44]

A number of other injuries are associated with consecutive repetitive motion and sudden and major increases in training intensity or environment. Achilles tendinitis is one of the most common. Another common injury is "shin splints," a term that covers a large number of problems. The condition is the result of cumulative microtrauma aggravated by repeated jumping and dancing on demipointe, all common movements in Afrocentric and modern dance. It is also common to inexperienced dancers or experienced dancers with ridged cavus feet or pronation problems.[24] Shin splints can start in one leg but are commonly bilateral.

Posterior weight shift and the resulting hypertrophy of the calf muscles[26, 55] increases the probability of repeated microtrauma[43] and decreases accessory motion in the talotibial joint,[40] primarily dorsiflexion, an essential component of demiplié and plié (see Fig 4).[33] Posterior weight shift predisposes the dancer to Achilles tendinitis[42] and triceps surae strain. With atrophy, the calf muscles' shock-absorbing ability is compromised, increasing lower extremity stress fractures, particularly of the tibia.[4, 40, 44] Because weight is shifted to the heels, the intrinsic muscles of the forefoot lose their ability to grip the floor and become weak; the stirrup muscle attempts to compensate and becomes overdeveloped; and during plié, the toes hammer in an attempt to grip the floor.[30, 52]

Foot

Symptoms of flexor hallucis longus tendinitis include painful and restricted plié, pain on pointe and a sensation of grinding, particularly in grand plié and relevé. The dancer will often complain that "it gets stuck and then snaps, and the more I work it, the worse it gets." This is the most common tendinitis found in dancers but is very rare in other forms of athletics.[42]

When evaluating the feet, note development and location of bunions as an important indicator of alignment and muscle balance problems. Note the mobility, alignment, strength, and stability of the toes in all postures. Especially note the first ray, due to its effect on total lower extremity stability during many common dance movements.[24] First ray hypermobility can also contribute to such problems as posterior impingement,[1, 5, 56–58] anterior impingement,[4, 38, 59] peroneal tendinitis,[1, 10, 42, 61] posterior tibial tendinitis, fracture of fifth metatarsal,[25] and fibular stress fracture.[1, 43] Because hypermobility decreases foot stability during plantar flexion[26, 32, 49, 50] in pointe, demipointe, and relevé (Fig 13), the first

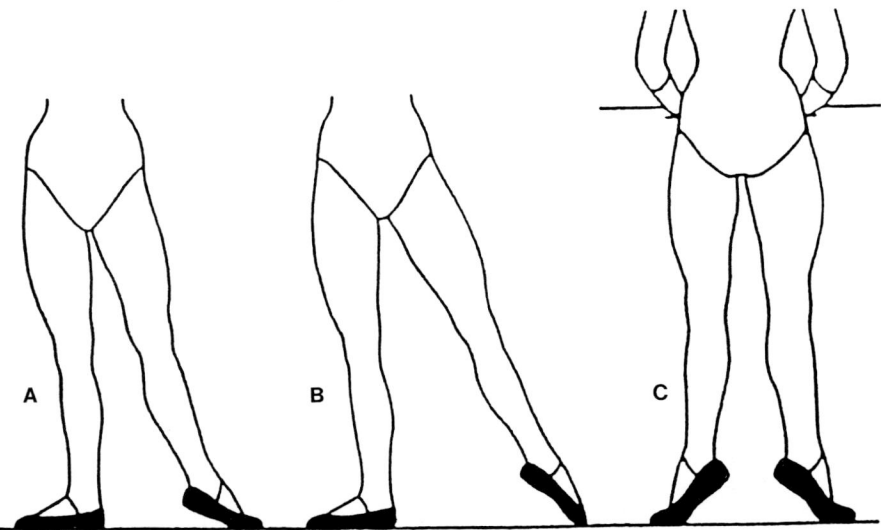

FIGURE 13.
A, Demipointe; B, pointe, and C, relevé.

ray's ability to support the medial column of the foot is also compromised.[43, 52] In addition, Achilles tendinitis is possible because the medial aspect of the tendon is stretched by the eversion of the calcaneus.[23, 27]

SCREENING CONCLUSION

When the examination is completed and an evaluation has been made, the practitioner must recommend an appropriate strengthening and stretching program to correct the imbalances identified. It is important to have a conference with each dancer and explain the findings and the importance of correcting any problems and help the dancer understand the goals and components of any rehabilitation that may be necessary. This should be done in cooperation with whoever is responsible for their training to ensure consistent support of the rehabilitation during workouts.[12]

PSOAS INSUFFICIENCY SYNDROME

Of specific interest to any practitioner in the dance injury field are the lumbosacral area and the psoas muscles in particular because of their direct effects on the biomechanics of the lower extremity and on the ability of the dancer to perform many movements necessary in dance. The psoas muscles originate from the body's intervertebral disk and transverse processes of T-12 through L-5, extending distally anteriorly and slightly laterally. They run anterior to the hip joint and insert into the lesser trochanter; enervation is supplied by lumbar nerves I through V. Psoas insufficiency can affect the movement patterns of dance directly, restricting external rotation of the hip and causing a general posterior shift in weight bearing.[25] Restricted external rotation of the hip leads to additional maladaptive movement patterns such as hyperextension of the lumbosacral joint complex.[24]

Psoas muscles are some of the strongest muscles of the body, responsible along with the triceps equinus for maintaining static upright posture. The psoas, in conjunction with the triceps surae, are the only muscles that show electrical activity during erect posture.[6] The psoas muscles act as paired muscles with the lower extremities to flex the trunk at the hip. They also extend the pelvis on the spine and pull the lumbar vertebrae anteriorly, which increases lordosis. The psoas anteriorly rotates the pelvis and laterally flexes and rotates the lumbar vertebrae on the ipsilateral side.[6, 25, 26, 28]

When acting on a non-weight-bearing leg, the psoas, due to its polyanthroidal nature, is the primary flexor of the hip.[6, 22] It is also an abductor and limited external rotator of the hip. With the lower extremity fixed and in conjunction with the external hip rotator, the psoas rotates the pelvis externally on the hip, which advances the pelvis on the opposite side during the swing phase of gait and makes the psoas an internal rotator of the hip.[26, 28] Thus, a tight psoas restricts weight-bearing turnout (external rotation), particularly at end range.[13]

The dancer may complain of pain in any of the areas previously mentioned. Regardless of the area of chief complaint, when questioned, the dancer will usually admit to pain or difficulty during battement (see Fig 15), developpé, and forward extensions.[26, 28] He or she may also have difficulty stretching over the involved side while sitting in second position.[28] Arabesque extension to the rear will be painful and lower on the involved side. There may also be a history of vague intermittent knee pain, particularly at the bottom of a grand plié or when the weight-bearing leg is fully extended.[25, 26, 28]

During the dance screening examination, the following signs will be noted in the presence of psoas insufficiency syndrome:

1. Restricted sacroiliac motion on the side of primary involvement
2. Anterior tilt of the pelvis, unilateral or bilateral
3. Positive forward flexion test (Fig 14)
4. Lumbar scoliosis convex on the side of the predominant psoas contracture
5. Positive Michele's test result (Fig 15) more pronounced on the side of the primary dysfunction[25, 26, 28]
6. Restricted flexion and extension at hip joint
7. Trigger points at psoas motor points
8. Positive Ober's test result, often bilateral[25, 26, 28, 46, 47]
9. Hyperlordosis, except in the few cases where the body is pitched forward and flexed at the hip
10. Weak abdominal muscles and tight hamstrings
11. Foot pronation, possibly bilateral
12. Decreased external hip rotation

Relief of pain, even temporarily, and increased range of motion after psoas stretching are probably the most important indicators of psoas insufficiency syndrome.[25, 26, 28]

Psoas insufficiency and its restriction of external rotation of the hip is a major cause of maladaptive technique as the dancer attempts to achieve perfect turnout.[21, 25, 26, 28, 44] The ability to achieve turnout is controlled by a number of factors: angle of anteversion, orientation of acetabulum, elasticity of hip capsule, and flexibility of hip muscles (see Figs 6 and 7).[21, 22, 44] To overcome a lack in any one of these, dancers resort to a number of compensatory techniques such as flexion at the hip,[10, 13, 25] rolling in pronation of the foot,[4, 21, 27] and excessive rotation of the knee,[21, 25, 26, 28] all of which can compound psoas insufficiency.

In the presence of unilateral psoas insufficiency, there is a downward and interior pull on the pelvis in the ipsilateral side. This loads the hamstrings and gluteus maximus, tightening the piriformis and loading the iliotibial hands primarily on the contralateral side and causing excessive stress in the sacroiliac joint.[10, 26, 28, 32] Acting on the lumbothoracic spine, the one-sided psoas pull increases scoliosis on the side of shortening and rotates the vertebral bodies in the opposite direction.

Bilateral psoas insufficiency causes an increase in extension of the pelvis on the spine, increased lordosis, and slight flexion at the hip, which shifts the center of gravity anteriorly. The abdominals become stretched and weak, decreasing the effectiveness of the hamstrings and the gluteus muscles as flexors of the pelvis and inhibiting the gluteus maximus as an external rotator of the hip. To compensate for the anterior displacement of the center of gravity, the dancer shifts weight to the heels, loading the posterior compartment and impairing the purchase of the forefoot muscles.[26, 28] External rotation of the hip is restricted by the tight psoas, and forward flexion is restricted by the hamstrings and gluteal muscles (see Fig 3). Psoas tightness also compromises backward movement because of (1) concentric flexor contraction and bony impingement of the apophyseal joint and (2) spinous processes resulting from hyperlordosis

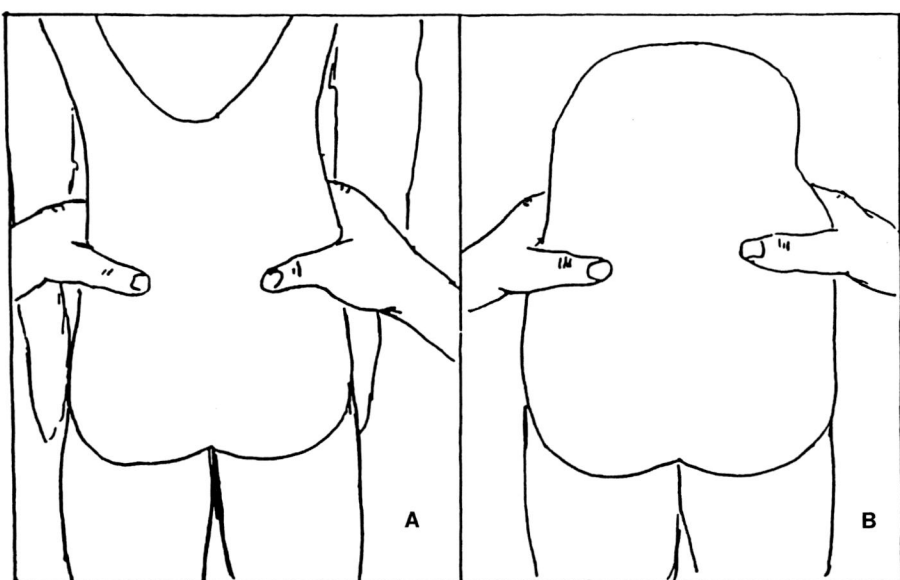

FIGURE 14.
Forward flexion test. **A,** Beginning position; **B,** positive forward flexion test, short psoas in low side (*arrow*).

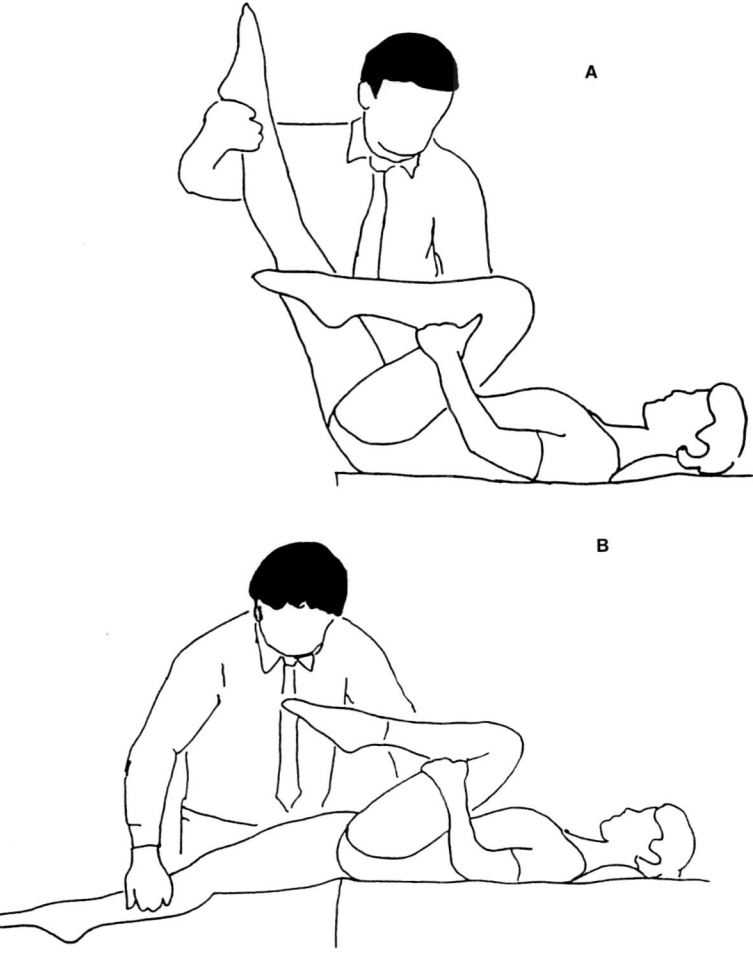

FIGURE 15.
Michele's test. **A,** Beginning position; **B,** marked psoas tightness if less than 30-degree extension. Psoas stretch may be applied in this position (modified Michele's test).

and pelvic extension. With abdominal muscles stretched and weakened, the anterior compartment of the thigh takes over the lifting of the leg, resulting in muscular hypertrophy. Muscular hypertrophy compromises muscle balance between hamstrings and quadriceps with increased instability of the effected joints,[13, 21, 55] particularly the knees.[40, 41]

TREATMENT OF DANCE INJURIES

To successfully treat and manage common dance injuries, one must treat the underlying maladaptive movement patterns. A program of stretching (see Fig 15, B), strengthening of the core muscles (psoas and abdominals), and manual manipulation[25, 26, 28] must be combined with postural and kinesthetic reeducation and visualization techniques to correct the underlying somatic dysfunction, reestablish facilitative movement patterns,[28, 38, 50] and break the chain of injury.

To maintain these corrections, dancers must use active stretching and strengthening exercises. Most important, they must replace maladaptive patterns with new facilitative movement through the use of repatterning techniques such as Alexander, Bartenof, and Pilates. By taking these steps, the dancer can avoid the trap of chronic reinjury and possible early retirement from dance.

Be careful not to name conditions by structure because of the danger of pigeon-holing the dancer's symptoms as a single condition rather than as a manifestation of a series of imbalances and maladaptive movements. It is necessary to treat the entire dancer—the structural body, the functional requirements of the movement style of the individual dancer, and the needs of expressiveness implicit to the arts.

REHABILITATION OF THE INJURED DANCER

Most dance-related problems are multifaceted. Of primary concern is the restoration of normal alignment through the use of manipulation and appropriate stretching and strengthening techniques. In the presence of chronic injury, the restoration of proper proprioceptive function is also necessary.[21, 59] Acupuncture can be beneficial in acute conditions and is especially valuable in reduction of swelling.[24] Among the most useful techniques in treating the overuse injuries common to dance is active release technique developed by Dr. Michael Leahy.[60]

Changing foot mechanics with *orthotics* is a controversial practice because of the inability to duplicate these orthotic corrections in dance shoes or bare feet. For some techniques such as ballroom, shoes are designed to enhance the dancers' awareness of the floor, and orthotics would interfere. Ballet uses a minimal shoe, the design of which is determined by years of tradition. Most modern dance is performed barefooted.[61] Many practitioners believe that to use orthotics when they can be used only in street shoes will alter dancers' proprioception and lead to further injury when they are on the dance floor.[62] When the biomechanics need to be corrected as part of a comprehensive treatment plan, appropriate taping techniques should be taught to the dancer for use while dancing.[6] During early phases of rehabilitation, athletic tape or Aircasts are useful in restricting unwanted movement and should be used on and off the dance floor. *Athletic tape* to restrict movement is not good for later phases of rehabilitation. The tape stretches as the dancer performs the wide range of foot and ankle motion necessary for many dance movements, offering little or no support, or restricts movement to such a great extent that the dancer will not wear it. When some support during later stages of rehabilitation is indicated, elastic self-gripping type of tapes are recommended for a better use-compliance rate and shorter learning curve for self-application.

New shoe designs by Gaynor Minden, Inc. of New York City which use new high-tech materials such as heat-moldable shanks, shock-absorbing materials, and insert kits allow the dancer to custom fit a dance shoe without a long break-in period. But these shoes are relatively new, and little research is available to determine if they are effective in correcting foot problems or even if dancers will wear them, because they are a departure from tradition, which is a very strong force in the dance world.

To treat problems related to inefficient or inappropriate use of the psoas and of the deep core muscles, the dancer must thoroughly strengthen these muscles and become sensitized to their proper use. Recommended exercises include those by Ruth Soloman,[63] as demonstrated in her videotape *Anatomy as a Master Image in Training Dancers* and in *Dance Longer Dance Stronger* by Andrea Watkins and Priscilla Clarkson.[14]

For the dancer to effectively perform "extension," the psoas must be the primary mover, initiating the movement from the core and allowing the more superficial muscles to be secondary muscles of extension. To achieve this, the physician must encourage the dancer to release the tendons of the hip socket during extension. Have the dancer reproduce positions that incorporate extension such as developpé (see Fig 8) or second position (see Fig 12), and palpate the tendons around the hip socket such as the rectus femoris and the iliacus. In chronic cases, the dancer may attempt to hold the hip in position with the tensor fascia lata and the gluteal muscles, causing even greater inhibition of movement. The dancer may begin to feel a sensation of grinding and popping or snapping sounds on the inside of the hip socket as the contracted rectus femoris or iliopsoas tendon moves across the head of the femur and/or on the outside of the hip as the tensor fascia lata slide across the head of the femur.

STRETCHES

Many stretching techniques are available, and all can be of value in the treatment of dance injuries. Stretches that address the problems unique to each style of dance and each individual dancer should be incorporated into any rehabilitation program in conjunction with a strengthening program that addresses the instability of hypermobile joints. If these two elements are not addressed together, the practitioner will only be trading one set of injuries for another.

Proprioceptive neuromuscular facilitation (PNF)[64] is a system of stretching techniques that uses the agonist-antagonist muscles and the body's reflex response to improve muscle function and range of motion.[65,66] PNF patterns replicate movements commonly used during specific dance techniques and styles.[15]

PROPRIOCEPTIVE REHABILITATION

When a dancer is injured, every part of the body is affected by or affects the injury or dysfunction. To return the dancer to the preinjury state, one must be aware of the factors that contribute to the cause and its repair. (1) the structure and function of the physiological joint complex, (2) how the injury interfaces with the locomotive system, and (3) the injury's effect on the body's proprioceptive systems. Successful rehabilitation of the proprioceptive system requires a basic understanding of its structure and function. Structurally the proprioceptive system consists of specialized sensory receptors that respond to:

- Movement of the joint via pacinian corpuscles (which respond to acceleration and deceleration), and nerve endings (which resemble Golgi's tendon organs, which respond to strain and reflex inhibition)
- Contraction of the muscles and tendons through the Golgi tendon organs (which are affected by tension and muscle spindles, which are affected by stretch)
- Changes in interarticular pressure, probably through special encapsulated nerve endings[49, 65, 68, 69]

STRUCTURE AND FUNCTION

To effectively treat the proprioceptive system, one must understand the structures involved, such as ligaments, muscles, tendons, joint capsules, and fascia, and cause of damage to its receptors, including trauma, inflammatory, aging, joint dysfunction, and decreased stimulation.

The function of the proprioceptive system is to allow dancers to perform properly coordinated movement through the reflex action and to give them their kinetic sense (position in space).[70] This makes possible the coordination, tuning, and delicate balance[65] necessary for dancer's artistic expression and injury prevention. Proprioception is the key communication link between the central nervous system and the kinetic chain. If that communication is not available or is inaccurate, inappropriate movement and injury may occur.[70]

COMMON CAUSES OF INJURY

Common causes of injury to the proprioceptive receptors (pacinian corpuscles, Golgi's tendon organs, muscle spindles, etc.) are:

1. Joint and bone trauma
- Ankle strain, ligament stretching or rupture
- Joint dysfunction, lack of joint play
- Fractures from stress, compression, or tension forces
2. Acute and chronic inflammation
- Acute or chronic tendonitis due to improper joint function
- Acute or chronic tendonitis due to improper muscle balance
- Supermaximal muscle loading when unprepared to accept it
3. Immobilization
- Decreased mechanoreceptor feedback from previous injuries not properly rehabilitated
- Decreased nutritional flow
- Improper sense receptor functioning or inappropriate muscle firing
4. Increasing age
- Decreased nutrition to cartilage
- Degeneration of cartilage
- Absence of adequate mechanical stimulation of tissue[71]

Proprioceptive rehabilitation focuses on facilitating the body's sense of itself in space through the use of specially developed maneuvers and specifically designed equipment (tilt board, biomechanical ankle platform system (BAPS) board, oscillating board, rotator disks) for reconditioning the locomotive system in relation to spacial sense and proper alignment. In the final stages of rehabilitation, the focus shifted to performance of dance-specific skills and exercises to redevelop the skills that the dancer needs to return to a normal dance and performance schedule without reinjury.

Proprioceptive rehabilitation is a process of taking the patient from less to more

- Decreased mobility to increased mobility
- Decreased intensity of activity to increased intensity of activity
- Decreased strength to increased strength

This progression is accomplished with the use of specially developed maneuvers, specifically designed equipment, motion skill development activities, and, finally, a regime of dance-specific movements, with a gradual return to a normal rehearsal schedule and performance schedule. This progression should be carried out in conjunction with an appropriate stretching/strengthening program[72] and proper joint mobilization/manipulation[36, 37] to ensure maximal functional capability of the physiological joint as the program progresses.

DANCE-SPECIFIC MOVEMENT

Dance-specific movement is necessary for the redevelopment of movement patterns. Different dance styles require different types of movement. After injury, it is necessary to reestablish body and mind communication specific to each style of dance. Proper movement patterns must be redeveloped and inappropriate patterns unlearned. During this phase of rehabilitation, video can be a very useful tool in establishing kinesthetic sense in the dancer through the addition of visual stimulus.

When a dancer is injured, the entire body is affected, including the proprioceptive system. By rehabilitating this system as a part of a comprehensive rehabilitation plan, one reduces the chance of reinjury or chronic dysfunction. A progressive rehabilitation program begins with low-intensity activity and gradually increases in difficulty. Components include starting the patient out on stable surfaces, progressing to unstable surfaces to develop kinesthetic sense, adding activities designed to develop functional motor skills, and concluding with dance-specific activities to reestablish effective movement patterns and proper kinesthetic awareness.[73] Gradually introducing the dancer to a normal performance schedule will give the dancer the greatest opportunity to return to a free, long, productive, and injury-free dance career.

PROPRIOCEPTIVE TESTING

Before the following tests are performed, the patient should be free of swelling and pain in the injured joint if possible and be able to bear full weight on the injured limb. Because of the chronic nature of many dance injuries and the accompanying swelling, it is not always possible to wait

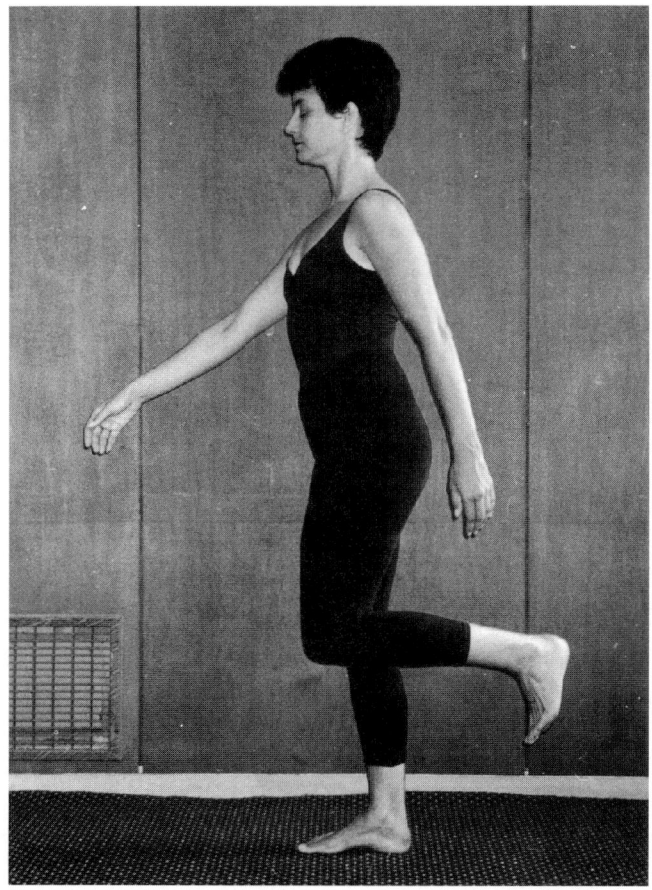

FIGURE 16.
Modified Romberg test. (Courtesy of Susanne Grace, Durning Feet Dance, St. Louis.)

for the effected joint to be free of swelling. The two most common tests used to determine proprioceptive function are:

- Modified Romberg test in which the patient balances, standing on injured foot, first with eyes open, then with eyes closed (Fig 16). The test result is considered positive if the patient cannot maintain this position for 1 minute with eyes closed.[71]
- Parallel position test, in which the patient's eyes are closed, and the ankle is placed in various positions using minimal tactile input. The patient is then asked to mirror the position by holding the palm of the hand parallel to the plantor surface of the foot. This test result is considered positive if the foot and hand are more than 10 to 15 degrees off parallel. This could indicate injury to the proprioceptive system.[67, 74]

There have also been a number of recent studies using stabilometry[75–77] in which the patient's equilibrium is evaluated electronically using such instruments as a Kistler force plate and a computerized strain gauge force plate[68] to measure swaying motion. It may be possible in the future to use such instrumentation to differentiate specific areas of dysfunction or injury and to help to develop individual rehabilitation programs.

SPECIAL MANEUVERS

The following maneuvers are performed with the patient standing on level floor to reestablish the initial kinesthetic sense and proper alignment:

1. One leg stand (see Fig 16)
- Stand on one leg with eyes closed for 1 minute (modified Romberg test).
- Stand on one leg, swinging arms back and forth for 1 minute.
- Stand on one leg, moving opposite leg into abduction, adduction, flexion, extension, and circumlocution. Repeat six to eight times.[78]
2. Advance one leg stand (Fig 17)
- While standing on one leg, rise onto toes while abducting opposite leg

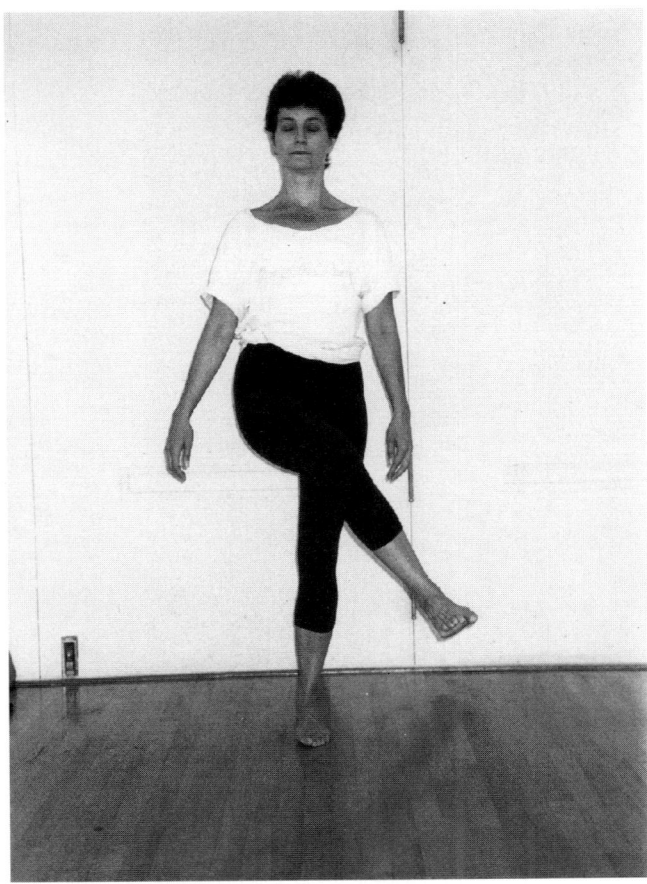

FIGURE 17.
Advanced one leg stand. (Courtesy of Susanne Grace, Durning Feet Dance, St. Louis.)

and plantar flexing foot. Then lower heel to floor while adducting opposite leg and dorsiflexing the foot. Repeat six to eight times.
- To improve resistance and stability, add elastic band between weight-bearing ankle and stationary object.[71]
3. Standing with ball (Fig 18)
- Hold onto a stationary object for support. Stand on a raised platform, and place a tennis ball between the medial malleoli. First raise up onto the balls of the feet, then lower back down to the level of the forefoot. Now lower to below the level of the forefoot. The rhythm of this exercise can be changed to improve strength, coordination, and muscle tone.[71]
4. Balance on towel (Fig 19)
- Roll up a small towel. Place under one foot and balance. Progress from using a stable support to unsupported.[79] A variation of this can be done by substituting a 6 by 4 by 12 in. block of foam rubber for the towel.[80]

PROPRIOCEPTIVE REHABILITATION EQUIPMENT

Such equipment as the tilt or wabble board, BAPS board, and minitrampoline[81] are common to rehabilitation. Equipment less familiar to practi-

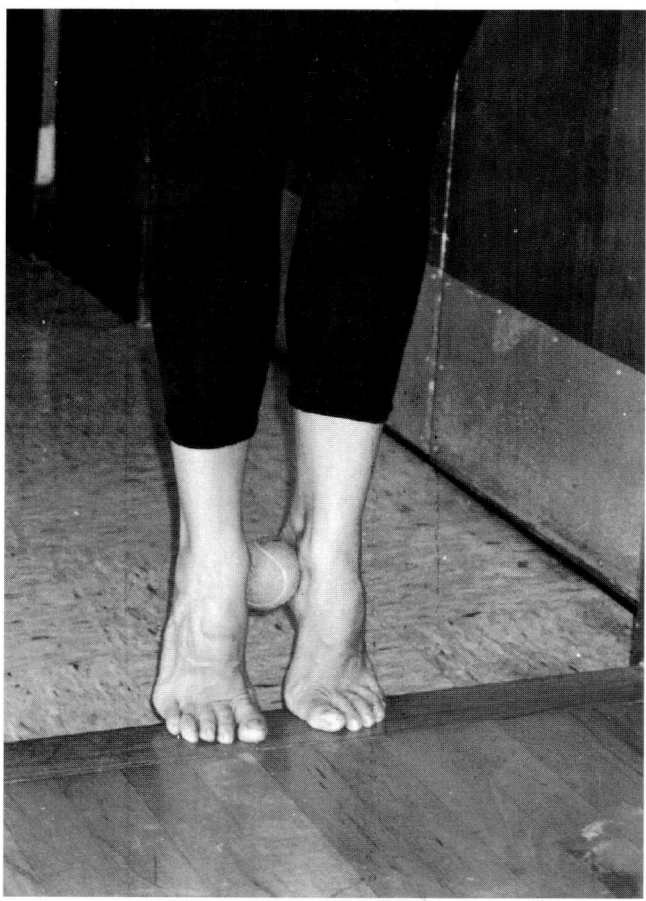

FIGURE 18.
Standing with ball.

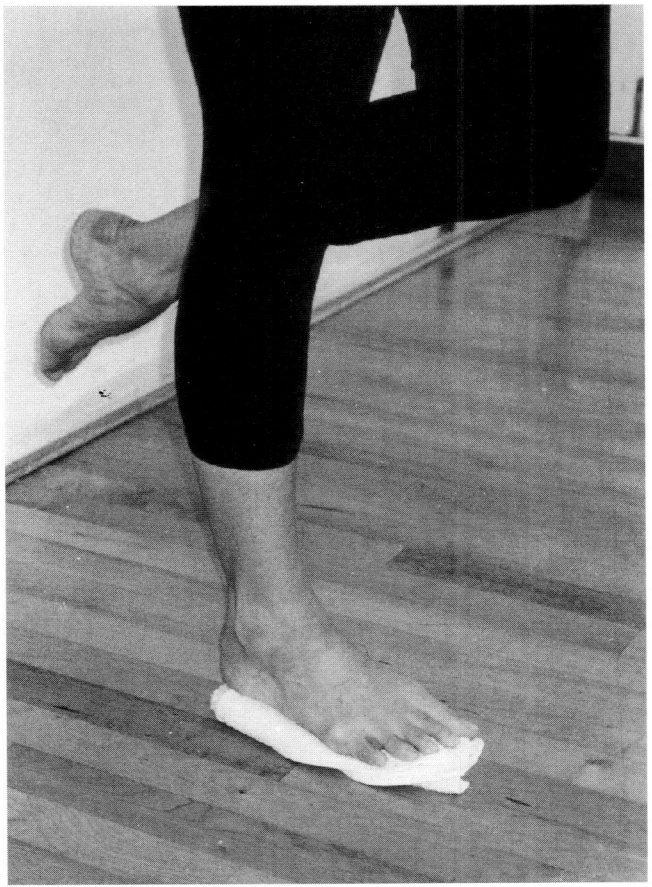

FIGURE 19.
Balance on towel.

tioners are rotator disks (Fig 20),[37] which are rotating platforms mounted on ballbearings. Rotator disks allows the dancer to retrain muscle balance and proprioception while performing common dance movements (see Fig 13).

Rotator disks are ¾-in. plywood disks mounted to ballbearing plates, which allow weight-bearing rotation to take place without the effect of friction. The disks establish a fixed center to measure rotation, making the measurement of weight-bearing rotation and charting of changes easier and more accurate. As a tool for rehabilitation, the disks transfer the imbalanced forces that are generated by improper technique into rotation. By giving a physical response to the imbalances generated during inappropriate technique, one can more easily visualize the movement, increasing the proprioceptive input,[15] as dancers train to maintain balanced technique. As their skill level increases, Theraband and Theratubing can be used, requiring the dancer to maintain centered movement against external forces.[37]

1. Tilt or wabble board (Fig 21)
   - Balance front to back with eyes open for 2 minutes.
   - Balance front to back with eyes closed for 2 minutes.

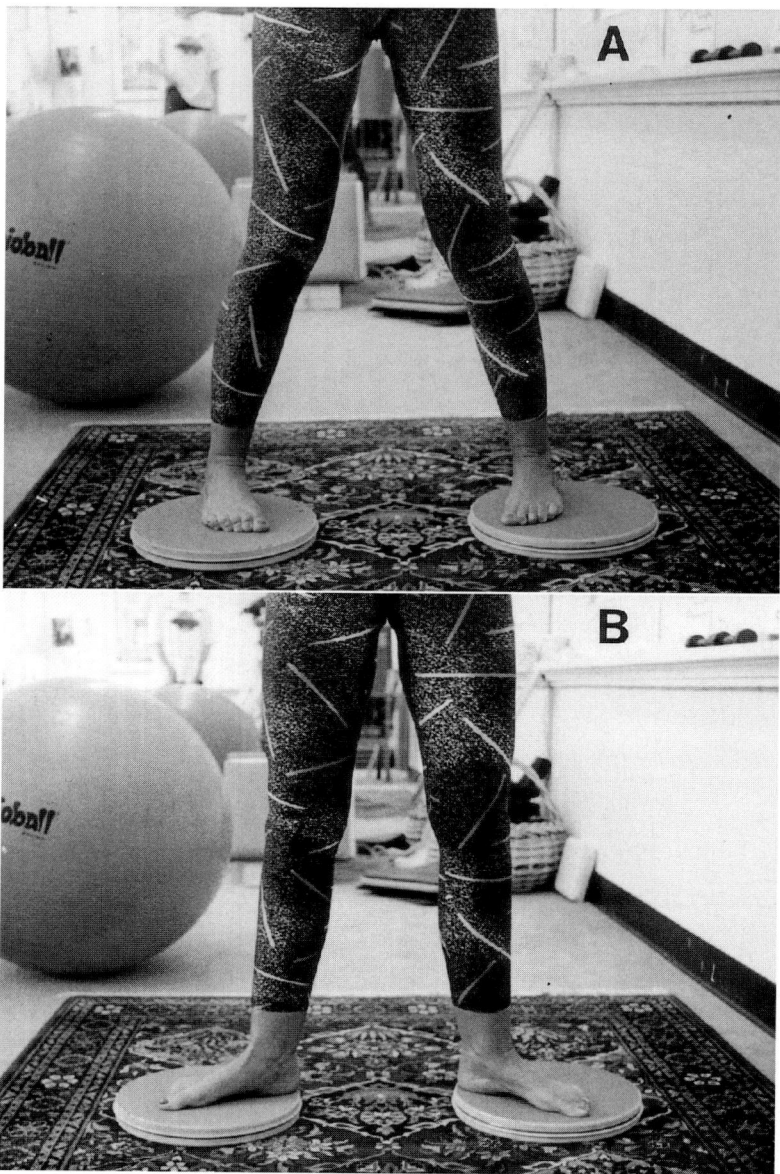

FIGURE 20.
Rotator disks. **A,** Parallel position; **B,** turnout position.

- Balance side to side with eyes open for 2 minutes.
- Balance side to side with eyes closed for 2 minutes.[81, 82]
2. Round balance board (Fig 22)
    - Stand with one foot in the center of the board.
    - Rotate board clockwise for 2 minutes and then counterclockwise for 2 minutes, keeping the edge of the board in contact with the floor throughout the exercise.
    - Weights may be added to the platform to increase stress to specific structures.[65, 71, 83]

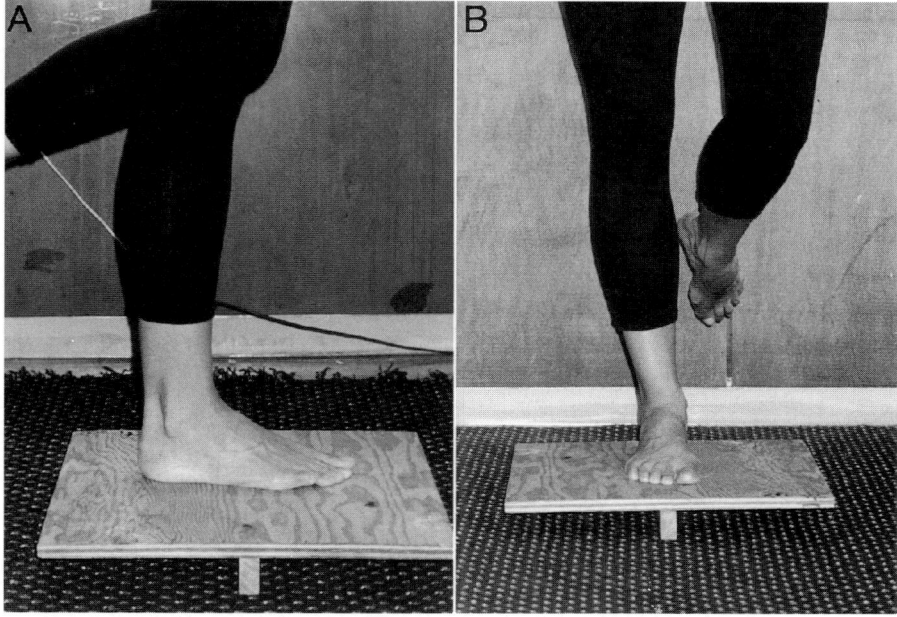

FIGURE 21.
Tilt or wabble board. **A**, Front to back; **B**, side to side.

3. Oscillating board (Fig 23)
    - 30 by 10 in. board balance on a 1¾-in. dowel.
    - Place board on dowel. Stand with both feet on board and balance.
    - Gradually roll the board from side to side while maintaining balance.
    - Begin holding onto a stationary object and progress to unsupported.[81]
4. Minitramp (Fig 24)
    - Standing on one foot, put the other leg through hip extension, hip flexion, leg extension, abduction, adduction, circumvention, and one-legged squats.[81]
5. Rotator disks (see Fig 20)
    - Use 2 12-in.-diameter, ¾-in. plywood disks mounted on ball bearings.
    - Perform turnout and parallel exercises.
    - Perform developpé.
    - Perform arabesque.
    - Weight-bearing movement that is common to specific dance styles.[84]

MOTOR DEVELOPMENT SKILLS EXERCISES

Motor development skills exercises are for evaluation[65] and redevelopment of specific motor skills necessary for the dancer to safely return to activity.[85] One example is the "ballet rehab class" taught by Richard Gibb, M.D., for the San Francisco Ballet,[3] which incorporates PNF exercises, strengthening, and stretching into a traditional ballet barre class as part of a prescribed rehabilitation class for injured company members.

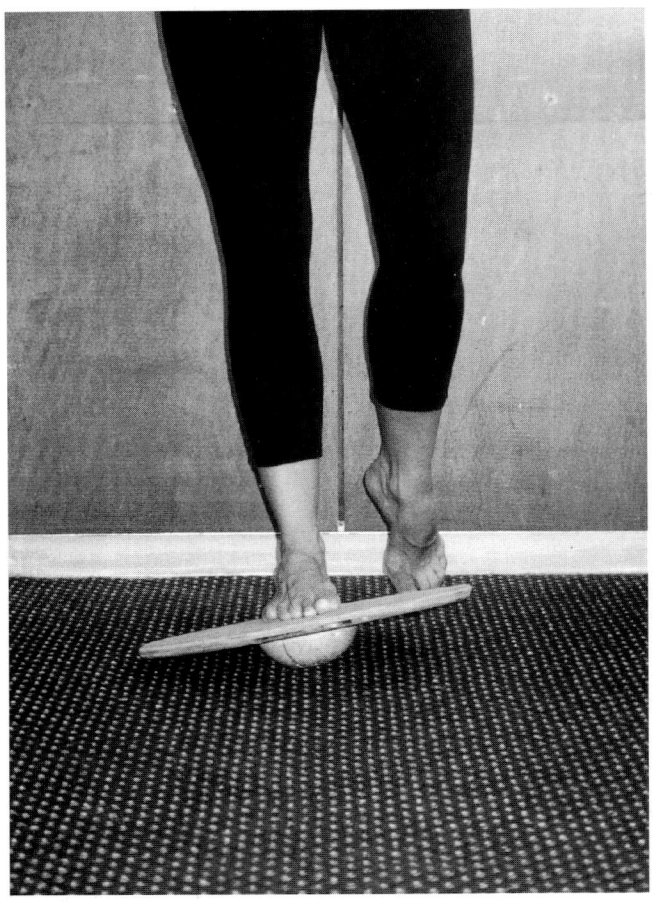

FIGURE 22.
Biomechanical Ankle Platform System (BAPS) board.

BODY THERAPIES

Body therapy systems focus on muscle control at the proprioceptive level, facilitating reeducation and repatterning for the purpose of restoring more efficient fluid motion of the body. Some familiar examples are Alexander, Ideokenesis, and Laban. For a more complete description of individual body therapies, refer to the Meyers chapter on perceptual awareness in *The Dancer as Athlete*.[86]

Pilates' Technique

Pilates' technique is a system of conditioning exercises that is common to the dance rehabilitation world. It was developed by Joseph Pilates in the 1920s.[87] Pilates' technique combines principles common to Eastern disciplines (Qi Gong, Tai Chi, Aikido), which concentrate on the blending of the body and mind and focus on the development of increased centeredness and flexibility with Western methods of physical training that focus on dynamic and kinetic activities and emphasize motion, muscle tone, and strength, which can lead to increased muscle imbalances and increased injury.[88]

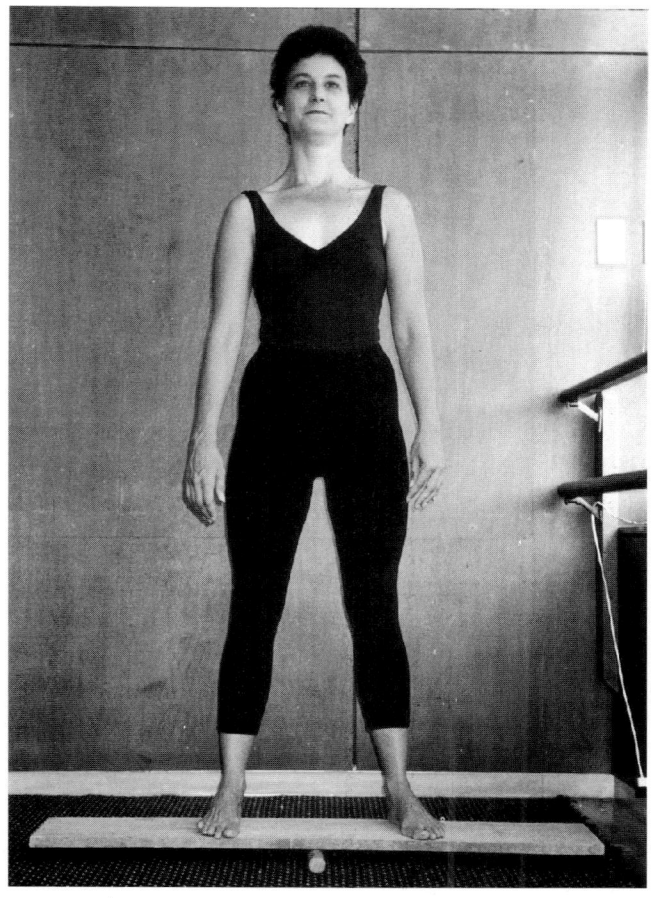

FIGURE 23.
Oscillating board. (Courtesy of Susanne Grace, Durning Feet Dance, St. Louis.)

Many of the Pilates exercises are performed on the reformer (Fig 25). The reformer uses springs for variable resistance attached to a horizontally sliding bed.[89] The reformer is used extensively by dance medicine rehabilitation centers throughout the world, including the Israel Dance Medicine Center in Tel-Aviv, Israel, Dance Medicine Center for Sports Medicine at St. Francis Memorial Hospital, San Francisco, and Westside Dance/Physical Therapy, New York.[89]

The advantage to Pilates in the rehabilitation of dancers is that it allows them to combine stretching and strengthening exercises with proprioceptive rehabilitation by enabling them to reproduce specific dance movements against variable resistance. Using the reformer as part of an injury rehabilitation program has been shown to allow the dancer to work in demiplié with significant decrease in caudally directed force at the knee by allowing the dancer to work in a stable position under controlled loads.[89] By reproducing common dance positions on the reformer and other Pilates-based equipment such as the trapeze (Fig 26), the dancer is able to retrain the proprioceptive system while simultaneously improving strength and flexibility, redeveloping the necessary

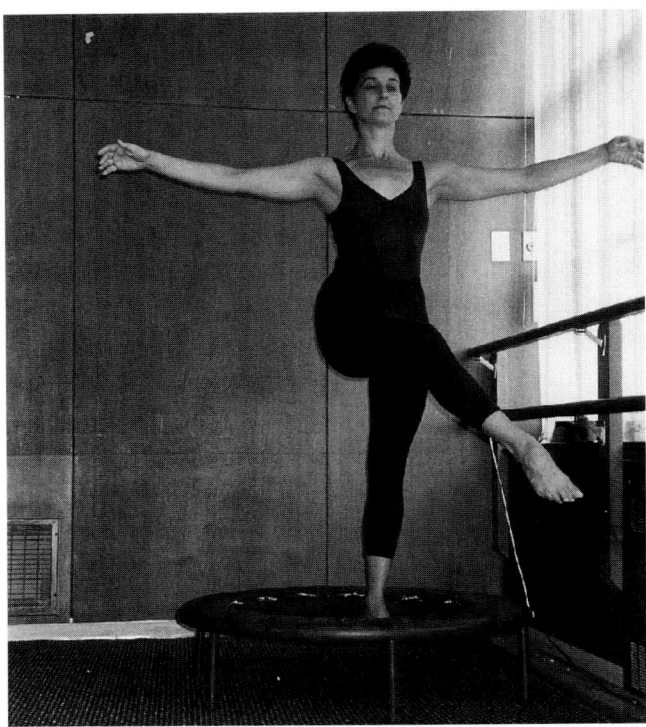

FIGURE 24.
Mine tramp. (Courtesy of Susanne Grace, Durning Feet Dance, St. Louis.)

skills and proper alignment necessary to return to a normal dance performance schedule.[83]

VIDEO AND DANCE INJURIES

Video is valuable, both as a diagnostic tool and as a way to demonstrate inappropriate movement to the dancer. Dr. Emil Pascarelli considers the video camera to be his most important diagnostic tool for the evaluation of repetitive strain injury at Kathryn and Gilbert Miller Health Care Institute for Performing Artists in New York City.[90] With video the practitioner is able to detect inappropriate movement patterns that are responsible for the majority of injuries in dance. Video allows you to look at movement as individual moments in time and to evaluate changes in movement that take place over time. As a tool for rehabilitation, it can relay information to the dancer using a language that they intimately understand, movement.

Video can be a powerful tool in the evaluation and preventive and rehabilitative treatment of dancers. With video, tendencies that lead to movement that is aesthetically unpleasing, and from a medical point of view potentially harmful, are readily apparent because they visibly influence the contour of the body. Inefficient movements are apparent with video observation; movement is inefficient specifically when it is initiated by the muscles of the periphery (muscles that lie near the surface of the body and are highly visible). Movement that is initiated from the deep core muscles and specifically from the psoas system, which connects the anterior of the spine to the thigh, is stronger, more balanced, and appears more centered.[31]

When the chiropractor's trained ability at postural analyses is combined with stop-motion and slow-motion video to observe the balance and kinetic flow of the dancer, it allows us to evaluate function in a way that is not possible with static testing. By observing dance movement in sequence, frame by frame, one can observe small variations in movement that would not be possible in real time, making it possible to evaluate very fine movement and make critical corrections to reduce such repetitive stress injuries as tenosynovitis and periostitis, which are common to dance.

Video is extremely valuable when dancers are evaluated over time. By videoing a dancer during a class, usually for 1 to 1½ hours, you can observe changes that take place because of muscle fatigue. The dancer's technique can deteriorate as muscles fatigue. One example would be a turnout that starts out well balanced and correct and then deteriorates into placement of the foot first and screwing of the knee as the hip rotators fatigue and are not able to function appropriately. Another response to fatiguing muscles is that the dancer drops into quick ballistic stretches and then hangs on the effected joints at their physicalogical limits.[11]

When used as part of rehabilitation, video can have a profound effect on changing the way the dancer moves. When a dancer moves, that move-

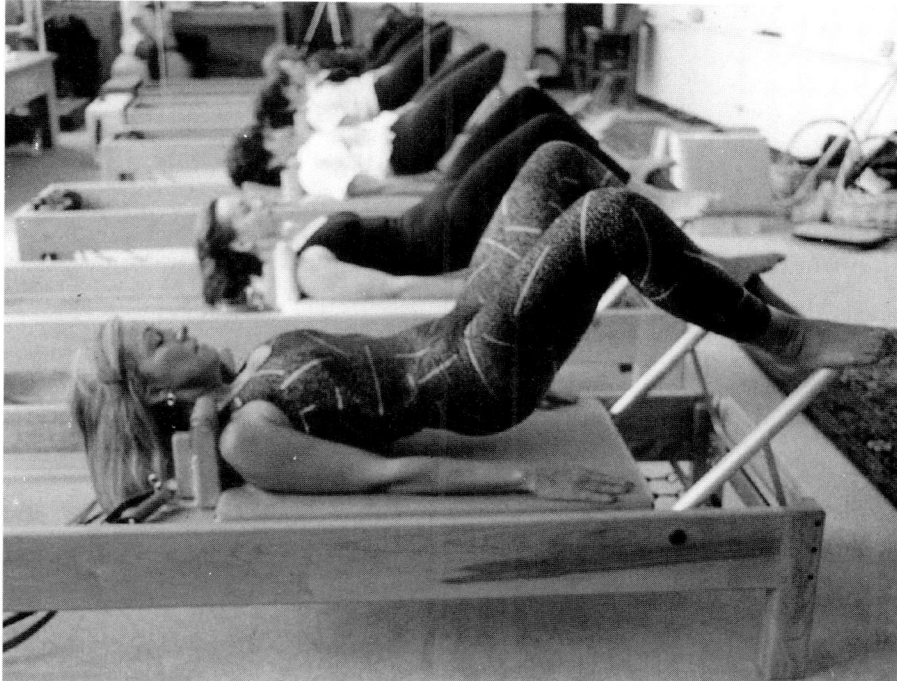

FIGURE 25.

Reformer. Dancer is performing relevé type of exercises with external rotation of the hip. (Courtesy of Karen Prechtl, Karen Prechtl Fitness, St. Louis.)

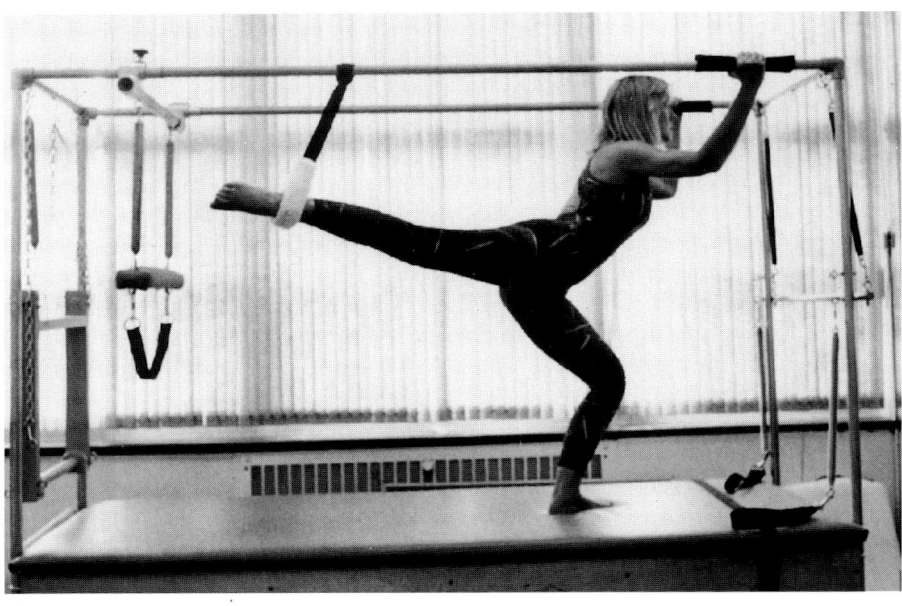

FIGURE 26.
Trapeze. Dancer is reproducing common dance positions. (Courtesy of Karen Prechtl, Karen Prechtl Fitness, St. Louis.)

ment is being initiated in the cerebral cortex as the initial formation of an impulse, or "idea," to move. This idea of movement changes from a memory to the movement through a complex set of neuronal impulses that eventually reach the appropriate muscle groups, and the idea becomes movement.[15] When this system breaks down because of a distortion of the proprioceptive information being fed into the system, the idea of the movement and the movement are no longer the same. When we rehabilitate the proprioceptive system, we are facilitating the neurological input to match the idea of the movement through controlled exercises. Video gives us another tool to introduce visual information, one of the primary sources of proprioceptive information[15] into this process. When dancers are shown a video of themselves performing an inappropriate movement, one that does not match the ideal, their conscious awareness changes. They can match the visual image of the inappropriate movement, the inappropriate idea, with the physical sensation of that movement. This makes it easier for them to recognize their compensatory movements and alter them to match their true intent. When the dancer visualizes the intended movement correctly, the cerebral cortex can form the idea and initiate the movement, with the final result being a movement that matches the intended idea and one that will keep the dancer dancing longer and stronger.

Equipment necessary for video analysis of sufficient quality for a clinical situation is very minimal. Most analyses can be done with consumer-grade equipment. The basic equipment needed is a camcorder, tripod, and video deck. The camcorder can be any of the commercially available formats; VHS, S-VHS, or Hi8, although S-VHS and Hi8 will give you a higher-quality image. Tripods should have floating heads and be heavy duty enough to be stable while shooting. Any quality brand of videotape recorder that is the same format as your camcorder and has four heads will be able to supply slow-motion and stop-frame images. A number of multimedia computers have the capability to produce slow-motion and stop-frame imaging as well.

CONCLUSION

In dance most injuries are the result of faulty technique. The majority are caused by maladaptive movement patterns related to inappropriate body imaging and compensation for biomechanical limitations such as restricted external rotators. Although the most common site of muscular injury in the dancer is the lower half of the back, the majority of dance injuries are of the lower extremity and the result of repeated overload leading to microtrauma (repetitive stress injury), all of which have been superimposed on multiple interrelated biomechanical factors. To successfully treat these problems, you must examine the biomechanical relationship between the cumulative microtraumatic injuries found most often in dance (stress fracture, ankle impingement syndrome, Achilles tendinitis, flexor hallucis longus tendinitis, patellofemoral dysfunction), and psoas insufficiency and the lumbopelvic dysfunction.

To gain the confidence and cooperation of the dancer, the dance physician must be trusted in terms of both ability and attitude. You must demonstrate not only that you have the skills to diagnose and treat but that you understand and appreciate the world of the dancer. Many dancers have become suspicious of health care providers who do not understand their challenges and dreams. It is all too common for a dancer to be told to stop doing a movement essential to the dance technique that they practice rather than how to correct the inappropriate movement patterns and thereby improve their ability to perform what is required of them and still remain injury free.

Many professional dancers require ongoing preventive or rehabilitation treatments to maintain their dance regimen, and amateur dance students benefit from our services as well. One of the most important groups that need our skills is local dance schools. By working with young dancers before they develop inappropriate movement patterns that lead to bad technique and injury, we can help them excel in dance to the full potential by reducing their injuries and giving them a basic level of health care that will benefit them throughout their career.

As chiropractors, we can effectively treat dancers as part of a team of dance medicine practitioners (orthopedists, physical therapists, dance instructors, etc.) and return them to dance safely, enabling them to continue expressing themselves. The dance physician must accept that the dance environment is far from the chiropractic ideal. Dancers and instructors fear that change in training will affect their technique and the quality of performance, making them reluctant to change the way they do things. This makes incorporating knowledge from dance research into training difficult to do because of technique and performance overlay.[3]

To work with dancers and understand the causes of their injuries, you must watch and watch and watch. Take classes in the style that most interests you; most instructors will be happy to have you there. Become familiar with the biomechanics of the style and understand the interrelation of body parts and their actions to one another. Most important, remember that your goal is to help the dancer perform more efficiently and ultimately better realize his or her desire to express creativity through movement.

ACKNOWLEDGMENT

I would like to thank Joyce Chaney for contributing her editorial skills, Susanne Grace of Burning Feet Dance, St. Louis, for her assistance with the exercise photographs, and Karen Prechtl of Karen Prechtl Fitness, St. Louis, for the use of her Pilates Studio.

REFERENCES

1. Stephens RE: The etiology of injuries in ballet, in Ryan A, Stephens RE (eds): *Dance Medicine.* Chicago, Pluribus Press, 1987, pp 16–50.
2. Clippinger-Roberton K: Biomechanical considerations in turnout in Solomon R, Minton RS, Solomon J (eds): *Preventing Dance Injuries: An Interdisciplinary Perspective.* Reston, Va, American Alliance for Health, Physical Education, Recreation, and Dance, 1990, pp 75–102.
3. Gibb R: Ballet rehab class. Paper presented at the Fourth Annual Conference of the International Association for Dance Medicine and Science, San Francisco, 1994.
4. Hardaker WT: Medical considerations in dance training for children. *Am Fam Physician* 3:93–99, 1987.
5. Howse AJG: Posterior block of the ankle joint in dancers. *Foot Ankle* 3:81–84, 1989.
6. Sammarco GI: The dancer's hip. In Ryan AS, Stephens RE (eds): *Dance Medicine.* Chicago, Pluribus Press, 1987, pp 220–242.
7. Howse JE: Disorders of the great toe in dancers. *Clin Sports Med* 2:499–505, 1983.
8. Wheeler LP: Common musculoskeletal dance injuries. *Chiropr Sports Med* 1:17–23, 1987.
9. Micheli LI: Back injuries in dancers. *Clin Sports Med* 2:473–489, 1983.
10. Sammarco GI: Diagnosis and treatment in dancers. *Clin Orthop* 187:176–187, 1984.
11. Batson G: Spinal hypermobility in the dancer: Implications for conditioning. *Kinesiology and Medicine for Dance* 14:39–56, 1992.
12. Plastino JG: Physical screening of the dancer: General methodologies and procedures, in Solomon R, Minton RS, Solomom J (eds): *Preventing Dance Injuries: An Interdisciplinary perspective.* Reston, Va, American Alliance for Health, Physical Education, Recreation, and Dance, 1990, pp 155–176.
13. Micheli LJ, Solomon R: Training the young dancer, in Ryan A, Stephens RE (eds): *Dance Medicine.* Chicago, Pluribus Press, 1987, pp 51–72.
14. Watkins A, Clarkson PM: *Dance Longer Dance Stronger: A Dancer's Guide to Improving Technique and Preventing Injury.* Pennington, NJ, 1990, pp 251–254.
15. Stephens RE: The Neuroanatomical and Biomechanical Bases of Flexibility Exercises in Dance, in Solomon R, Minton RS, Solomon J (eds): *Preventing Dance Injuries: An Interdisciplinary Perspective.* Reston, Va, American Alliance for health, Physical Education, and Dance, 1990 pp 271–292.

16. Howse AG: The young ballet dancer, in Ryan A, Stephens RE (ed): *Dance Medicine: A Comprehensive Guide*. Chicago, Pluribus Press, 1987, pp 107–114.
17. Solomon R, Micheli L, Ireland ML: Physiological assessment to determine readiness for pointe work in ballet students. *Impulse* 1(1):21–38, 1993.
18. Kibler WB: *The Sport Preparticipation Fitness Examination*. Champaign, Ill, Human Kinetics, 1990, pp 5–14.
19. Vincent LM: *Competing with the Sylph*. Kansas City, Kan. Andrews and McMel, 1979, p 9.
20. Weiss DS: Musical theater ("Broadway") dance. Paper presented at the Fourth Annual Conference of the International Association for Dance Medicine and Science, San Francisco, 1994.
21. Hardakee WT, et al: The pathogenesis of dance injury, in Shell CG (ed): *The Dancer as Athlete*. 1984 Olympic Scientific Congress Proceedings, Champaign, Ill, Human Kinetics, 1986, pp 11–30.
22. Sammarco GI: The dancers hip. *Clin Sports Med* 2:485–498, 1983.
23. Hamilton WG: Physical prerequisites for ballet dancers. *J Musculo Med* 11:61–66, 1986.
24. Russell B: A study of lumbopelvic dysfunction psoas insufficiency and its role as a major cause of dance injury. *Chiro Sports Med* 5:9–17, 1991.
25. Backrach RM: Diagnosis and management of dancer injuries to lower back: An osteopathic approach, in Shell CG (ed): *The Dancer as Athlete*. 1984 Olympic Scientific Congress Proceedings, Champaign, Ill, Human Kinetics, 1986, pp 83–90.
26. Backrach RM: The relationship to low back/pelvic somatic dysfunction. *Orthop Rev* 17:1037–1043, 1988.
27. Garrick JG: *Turn-out and its relationship to injury*. Paper presented at the Second Annual Dance Medical Symposium Proceedings, Irvine, Calif 1989.
28. Bachrach RM: Injuries to the dancers spine, in Ryan AJ, Stephens RE (eds): *Dance Medicine*. Chicago, Pluribus Press, 1987, pp 213–266.
29. Rooere GD: Musculoskeletal injuries in theatrical dance students. *Am J Sports Med* 11:195–198, 1983.
30. Washington EL: Musculoskeletal injuries in theatrical dancers: Site frequency and severity. *Am J Sports Med* 6:75–98, 1978.
31. Solomon R: In Search of more efficient dance training, in Solomon R, Minton RS, Solomon J (eds): *Preventing Dance Injuries: An interdisciplinary perspective*. Reston, Va, American Alliance for Health, Physical Education, Recreation, and Dance, 1990, pp 191–222.
32. Backhouse KM: Medicine and ballet. *Trans Med Soc Lond* 1980–1981 97:51–52.
33. Hammand SN: *Ballet Basics*, ed 2. Mountain View, Calif, Mayfield, 1984, pp 62–104.
34. Marymont IV: Exercise-related stress reaction of the sacroiliac joint. *Am J Sports Med* 11:320–323, 1986.
35. Vincent LM: Dancers and the war with water and salt. *KMFD* 12:40–49, 1990.
36. Clippinger-Robertson K: Flexibility in dance. *Kinesiology and Medicine for Dance* 12:1–16, 1990.
37. Molnar M: Results of biomechanical foot and ankle examination on professional ballet students. Paper presented at the Fourth Annual Conference of the International Association for Dance Medicine and Science, San Francisco, 1994.
38. Hammer WL: *Functional Soft Tissue Examination and Treatment by Manual Methods: The Extremities*. Gaithersburg, Md, Aspen, 1991.
39. Edmond SL: *Manipulation Mobilization: Extremity and Spinal Techniques*. St Louis, Mosby, 1993.

40. Tectz CC: Sports medicine concerns in dance and gymnastics. *Pediatr Clin North Am* 29:399–421, 1982.
41. Hall SJ: Mechanical contribution to lumbar stress injuries in female gymnasts. *Med Sci Sports Exerc* 18:S99–602, 1986.
42. Rouere GD: Low back pain in athletes. *Physician Sports Med* 15:105, 1987.
43. Keavitz SR: Biomechanical implications of dance injuries. In Shell CG (ed): *The Dancer as Athlete*. Paper presented at the 1984 Olympic Scientific Congress Proceedings. Champaign, Ill, Human Kinetics, pp 43–52, 1984.
44. Ryan A, Stephens RE: The epidemiology of dance injuries, in Ryan A, Stephens RE (eds): *Dance Medicine: A Comprehensive Guide*. Chicago, Pluribus Press, 1987, pp 3–15.
45. Garrick JG: Anterior knee pain. *Physician Sports Med* 17:75–84, 1989.
46. Reid DC: Lower extremity flexibility pattern in classical ballet dancers and their correlation to lateral hip and knee injuries. *Am J Sports Med* 15:347–352, 1987.
47. Grady JF: Iliotibial band syndrome. *J Am Podiatric Med Assoc* 76:558–561, 1986.
48. Kleiger B: Anterior tibiotalar impingement syndromes in dancers. *Foot Ankle* 3:69–73, 1982.
49. Dercheid GL: Rehabilitation of the ankle. *Clin Sports Med* 4:527–544, 1985.
50. Hamilton WG: Stenosing tenosynovitis of the flexor hallucis longus tendon and posterior impingement upon the os trigonum in ballet dancers. *Foot Ankle* 3:74–80, 1982.
51. Hamilton W: Sprained ankles in ballet dancers. *Foot Ankle* 3:99–102, 1982.
52. Sammarco GI: Forefoot conditions in dancers: I. *Foot Ankle* 3:85–92, 1982.
53. Picone JV, Acute/chronic ankle sprain a case study. *Chiropr Sports Med* 3:74–80, 1989.
54. Sammarco GI: Forefoot conditions in dancers: II. *Foot Ankle* 3:93–98, 1982.
55. Baratta R: Muscular coactivation. *Am J Sports Med* 16:113–122, 1988.
56. Johnson RP: The os trigonum syndrome. *J Trauma* 24:xx, 1984.
57. Micheli LI, Ireland ML: Prevention and management of calcaneal apophysitis in children: An overuse syndrome. *J Pediatr Orthop* 7:34–38, 1987.
58. Quirk R: Talar compression syndrome in dancers. *Foot Ankle* 3:65–68, 1982.
59. Stoller SM: A comparative study of the frequency of anterior impingement exostosis of the ankle in dancers and nondancers. *Foot Ankle* 4:201–203, 1984.
60. Leahy PM: *Video Active Release Techniques*. Colorado Springs, Colo, Video Colorado Springs Company, 1993.
61. Spilken TI: *The Dancer's Foot Book*, Pennington, NJ, Princeton Books, 1990.
62. Novella T, Hamilton WG, Marchall P, et al: Multidisciplinary approaches to the evaluation and treatment of the foot. Paper presented at the Third Annual Conference of the International Association for Dance Medicine and Science, San Francisco, 1994.
63. Solomon R: *Anatomy as a Master Image in Training Dancers*. Video, Santa Cruz, University of California, 1988.
64. Knott M, Voss DE: *Proprioceptive Neuromuscular Facilitation: Patterns and Techniques*, ed 3. New York, Harper & Row, 1985.
65. Long PL: Rehabilitation and return to activity after sports injuries. *Primary Care* 11:137–150, 1984.
66. Nagrin D: *How to Dance Forever*. New York, William Morrow, 1989, pp 139–141.
67. Dercheid GL, Brown WS: Rehabilitation of the ankle. *Clin Sports Med* 4:527–544, 1985.

68. Fridem R: A stabilometric technique for evaluation of lower limb instabilities. *Am J Sports Med* 17:118–122, 1989.
69. Baro K: *The Human Nervous System*. New York, Harper & Row, p. 67, 1983.
70. Molnar M: Rehabilitation of the injured dancer, in Ryan A, Stephens RE (eds): *Dance Medicine: A Comprehensive Guide*. Chicago, Pluribus Press, 1987, pp 302–320.
71. Molnar M: Rehabilitation of the injured ankle. *Clin Sports Med* 7:193–204, 1988.
72. Andrews JR, Harrelson GL: *Physical Rehabilitation of the Injured Athlete*. Philadelphia, WB Saunders, 1993.
73. Dunn J: *Dance science: An overview*. Lecture notes from the Mid-America Dance Network Conference, 1989.
74. Wyke B: The neurology of joints. *Ann R Coll Surg Engl*, 41:25–50, 1967.
75. Sahistrand T: Postural equilibrium in adolescent idiopathic scoliosis. *Acta Orthop Scand* 49:314–365, 1980.
76. Tropp H: Stabilometry in functional instability of the ankle and its value in predicting injury. *Med Sci Sports Exerc* 16:64–66, 1984.
77. Tropp H: Stabilometry in functional and mechanical instability of ankle joint. *Int J Sports Med* 6:180–182, 1985.
78. Baldini J: Management and rehabilitation of ligamentous injuries to the ankle. *Sports Med* 4:364–380, 1987.
79. Hazel RH: *Biomechanics and pathomechanics of leg ankle and foot sports injury and physical fitness program*. Postgraduate Program, St Louis, Logan College, 1989.
80. Nash J: Personal communication, 1994.
81. Picone JV: Acute/chronic ankle strain: A case study. *Chiropr Sports Med* 3:112–117, 1989.
82. Leaman S: Treatment of sprained ankles by physiotherapists at professional soccer clubs. *Arch Emerg Med* 5:177–179, 1988.
83. Mitch LO: Rehabilitation exercises following inversion ankle sprains. *J Am Podiatr Med Assoc* 76:577–581, 1986.
84. Molnar M: Alternative training for dancers. Paper presented at the Third Annual Conference of the International Association for Dance Medicine and Science. San Francisco, 1993.
85. Russell B: Proprioceptive rehabilitation in dancers' injuries. *Kinesiology and Medicine for Dance* 14:39–56, 1992.
86. Meyers M: Perceptual awareness in integrative movement behavior, in Shell CG (ed): *The Dancer as Athlete*. Champaign, Ill, Human Kinetics, 1986, pp 1963–1986.
87. Larkham E: Dance medicine rehabilitation protocols and conditioning programs using apparatus based on designs by Joseph Pilates. Paper presented at the Third Annual Conference of the International Association for Dance Medicine and Science, San Francisco, 1994.
88. Parrott AA: The effects of Pilates technique and aerobic conditioning on the aesthetic quality of a dancer. *Kinesiology and Medicine for Dance* 15:45–64, 1993.
89. Fitt S, Sturman J, McClain-Smith S: Effects of Pilates-based conditioning on strength, alignment, and range of motion in university ballet and modern dance majors. *Kinesiology and Medicine for Dance* 16:36–35, 1993–1994.
90. Wolkomir R: When the work you do ends up costing you an arm. *Smithsonian* 25:90–101, 1994.
91. Dunn J: Development in dance medicine and science: The professional environment. Paper presented at the Fourth Annual Conference of the International Association for Dance Medicine and Science, San Francisco, 1994, pp 761–764.

Depressive Disorders, Prevalence, Assessment in, and Impact on the Primary Care Setting

Alan B. Korbett, D.C., D.O., D.A.B.C.O., C.C.S.P., D.A.C.A.N.
PGY III Psychiatry Resident/House Staff, Department of Psychiatry, University of Iowa Hospitals and Clinics, Iowa City, Iowa

More than 1 million individuals worldwide have a depressive disorder of some form and severity. Over the past 20 years strides in the elucidation of the pathophysiological and psychological etiologies of and treatment of mood disorders have been attained. Technological advances in brain imaging, psychopharmacology, and psychotherapeutic techniques have been made relative to the assessment and therapeutics of mood disorders. Amid all of these advancements toward the solving of the depressive disorder riddle, a key component of the equation has eluded consideration: the appreciation of mood disorders' prevalence in the primary care setting and the necessity of the primary care practitioner to be alert and vigilant of the inclusion of psychiatric illness, especially mood disorders, in his or her differential diagnosis either as a concurrent, comorbid, or primary condition.

The objective of this work is to bring to the forefront the pervasiveness of mood disorders, with emphasis on depressive disorders. My goal is to facilitate the appreciation of psychiatric diagnostics as a integral part of the total patient assessment. The clinical assessment of the heart is not within the exclusive domain of cardiology but is an essential component of the general physical examination, nor is the assessment of the mental status examination (MSE) and consideration of concurrent or primary psychiatric illness the exclusive property of psychiatry; it also needs to be integrated into each patient's assessment.

HISTORICAL PERSPECTIVE OF MENTAL ILLNESS

The recognition of mental illness as a discrete entity dates back to antiquity. One of the most dated medical documents, the Eber papyrus, composed approximately 1900 B.C., refers to depression. The chronological progression of civilization embraced a wide array of philosophical attitudes as to the basis of mental illness.

During the classical period the etiologies of mental illness were diverse. Hippocratic philosophy perceived mental illness as derived from the brain; galenian philosophy posed the cause to be the result of imbalance of bodily fluids. Others espoused an "organ theory," attributing specific illnesses to abnormalities of specific organs. For example, hysteria was the result of a wandering uterus. Although many positions were maintained during the classical period, the common thread of mental illness being seated in the physical domain separate from mind, soul, or spirit connected all schools. During the medieval period mental illness was ascribed to as being of spiritual rather than physical aberration. The church and theologians often administered "treatment," and medieval principles were still evident into the 18th century, such as the Salem, Massachusetts witch trials in the United States. During the Renaissance the foundation of modern psychiatry was laid with the reemergence of mental illness as a physically rooted aberration. As psychiatry evolved, two models moved to the forefront: the biological model and the psychodynamic model. The biological model attempts to define a patient's mental illness by signs and symptoms of a recognized disorder, whereas the psychodynamic model focuses on the understanding of the patient's complaint as it relates to familial or life experiences.

DEVELOPMENT OF THE DIAGNOSTIC AND STATISTICAL MANUALS OF MENTAL DISORDERS

Historically the forging of the present-day psychiatric discipline was shaped and molded by the numerous difficulties encountered and overcome. The clinical signs and symptoms of mental illness may manifest in a vast spectrum of emotional, behavioral, or cognitive abnormalities. This posed a formidable problem as to classification and categorization. Psychiatric training and diagnostic practices were varied, reflecting the diversity of philosophies that directed the individual schools. The individuality and lack of unity among the schools became apparent during World War II as clarity of communication in the clinical setting became a prominent obstacle, hampering patient care and impeding the development of the psychiatric profession. After the close of World War II, the American Psychiatric Association (APA) convened a task force that produced the *Diagnostic and Statistical Manual of Mental Disorders (DSM-I)* published in 1952, which focused on clinical utility. The DSM-I contained a glossary of descriptions of diagnostic categories and specified symptoms necessary to make a given diagnosis. The DSM-I was revised in 1968 to reflect the mental disorders section of the eighth revision of the *International Classification of Diseases* published by the World Health Organization (WHO), to which the APA consultants had contributed. The DSM has since undergone three more revisions: DSM-III, published in 1980; DSM-III-R, published in 1987; and DSM-IV, published in 1994. Notably DSM-III was a major departure from prior DMSs; it provides a medical nomenclature for clinicians and empirical research by including explicit diagnostic criteria, a multiaxial system, and a descriptive approach. The design of DSM-III established the framework for today's diagnostic parameters.

USE OF DSM-IV

The DSM-III, DSM-III-R, and DSM-IV are based on a multiaxial assessment system; each axis encompasses a different focus of clinical information. The DSM-IV subscribes to a five-axis system; the first three axes constitute the official diagnostic assessment.

DEFINING AXES I TO V

Axis I refers to *clinical syndromes and other conditions that may be a focus of clinical attention*,[1] which include:

- Disorders usually first diagnosed in infancy, childhood, or adolescence (excluding mental retardation)
- Delirium, dementia, and amnesic and other cognitive disorders
- Mental disorders due to general medical conditions
- Substance-related disorders
- Schizophrenia and other psychotic disorders
- Mood disorders
- Anxiety disorders
- Somatoform disorders
- Factitious disorders
- Dissociative disorders
- Sexual and gender identity disorders
- Eating disorders
- Sleep disorders
- Impulse-control disorders
- Adjustment disorders
- Other conditions that may be a focus of clinical attention[1]

Axis II is used for the coding of *personality disorders*, which are defined by particular personality traits that become inflexible and maladaptive, resulting in functional impairment or subjective distress. The 10 domains of personality disorders are arranged into three clusters: *Cluster A* disorders are symptomatically related to psychotic disorders (i.e., paranoid personality), *Cluster B* relates to "acting out" personality disorders (i.e., histrionic), and *Cluster C* personality disorders are hallmarked by fearfulness or anxiety (i.e., obsessive-compulsive personality). Also included in axis II is *mental retardation*.

Axis II includes[1] the following:

- Paranoid personality disorder
- Schizoid personality disorder
- Schizotypal personality disorder
- Antisocial personality disorder
- Borderline personality disorder
- Histrionic personality disorder
- Narcissistic personality disorder
- Avoidant personality disorder
- Dependent personality disorder

- Obsessive-compulsive personality disorder
- Personality disorder not otherwise specified
- Mental retardation

Axis III is used for coding current medical conditions. Axis III allows medical conditions to be considered in terms of the relationship to the psychiatric disorder (i.e., hypothyroidism and "myxedema madness") and medication interaction (i.e., Parkinson's disease and haloperidol). General medical conditions recorded on Axis III include[1]:

- Infectious and parasitic diseases
- Neoplasms
- Endocrine, nutritional, and metabolic diseases and immunity diseases
- Diseases of the blood and blood-forming organs
- Diseases of the nervous system and sense organs
- Diseases of the circulatory system
- Diseases of the respiratory system
- Diseases of the digestive system
- Diseases of the genitourinary system
- Complications of pregnancy, childbirth, and the puerperium
- Diseases of the skin and subcutaneous tissue
- Diseases of the musculoskeletal system and connective tissue
- Congenital anomalies
- Certain conditions originating in the perinatal period
- Symptoms, signs, and ill-defined conditions
- Injury and poisoning

Axis IV is used for the coding of the severity of psychosocial or environmental stressors that may contribute to or exacerbate the psychiatric illness. Axis IV *psychosocial and environmental problems* include[1]:

- Problems with primary support groups
- Problems related to the social environment
- Educational problems
- Occupational problems
- Housing problems
- Economic problems
- Problems with access to health care services
- Problems related to interactions with the legal system or to crime
- Other psychosocial and environmental problems

Axis V allows for the *prognostication of outcome* relative to the overall level of function and "psychological health" based on the parameters of psychological, social, and occupational function of the client. The *Global Assessment Function (GAF) Scale*, scored from 0 to 100 (100 reflecting minimal or absence of symptoms), is the instrument-defining axis V. The GAF scale may be used to reflect a relative chronological period (e.g., time of admission or time of discharge). Scores are used as follows[2]:

- 100–91—Superior functioning in a wide range of activities; life's problems never seem to get out of hand; is sought out by others because of his or her many positive qualities; no systems.
- 90–81—Absent or minimal symptoms; good functioning in all areas; interested and involved in a wide range of activities; socially effective; generally satisfied with life; no more than everyday problems or concerns.
- 80–71—If symptoms are present, they are transient and expectable reactions to psychosocial stressors; no more than slight impairment in social, occupational, or school functioning.
- 70–61—Some mild symptoms or some difficulty in social, occupational, or school functioning but generally functioning pretty well.
- 61—Has some meaningful interpersonal relationships.
- 60–51—Moderate symptoms or moderate difficulty in social, occupational, or school functioning.
- 50–41—Serious symptoms or any serious impairment in social occupational, or school functioning.
- 40–31—Some impairment in reality testing or communication or major impairment in several areas, such as work or school, family relations, judgment, thinking, or mood.
- 30–21—Behavior is considerably influenced by delusions or hallucinations or serious impairment in communication or judgment or inability to function in almost all areas.
- 20–11—Some danger of hurting self or others or occasionally fails to maintain minimal personal hygiene or gross impairment of communication.
- 10–1—Persistent danger of severely hurting self or others, persistent inability to maintain minimal personal hygiene, or serious suicidal act with clear expectation of death.
- 0—Inadequate information.

DIAGNOSTIC CODING

The purpose of diagnostic coding is to facilitate data collection, retrieval, statistic data compilation, and reporting. The coding system used in the United States relative to DSM-IV is compatible with the codes of the *International Classification of Diseases, Ninth Revision* in the clinical modifications (ICD-9-CM) section for mental disorders developed by the WHO. The following is an example of diagnostic coding pertaining to the five axes:

	Diagnostic code	DSM-IV Nomenclature
Axis I	294.xx	Major depressive disorder (MDD)
Axis II	Diagnostic code 301.6	DSM-IV nomenclature Dependent personality disorder
Axis III	ICD-9-CM code 244.9	ICD-9-CM nomenclature Hypothyroidism
Axis IV	Stressful work schedule	
Axis V	GAF = 55 (current)	

MOOD DISORDERS

The distinguishing feature of the mood disorders is the disturbance to mood, which is defined as disturbances involving emotional, cognitive behavioral, and somatic regulation. The domain of mood disorders is descriptively divided into mood episodes, the mood disorder, and the specifier.

The *mood episodes* (e.g., major depressive episode and manic episode) unto themselves are not coded as separate entities but serve as a foundation for disorder diagnosis. Each specific mood episode has distinguishing signs and symptoms to fulfilling minimal diagnostic criteria. The diagnosis of the mood disorder in most cases includes in its criteria the inclusion or omission of the mood episode. The final descriptive element is the specifier, which characterizes the most recent episode or the course of recurrent episodes (i.e., mild, moderate, severe, in partial remission, in full remission, or history of).

The mood disorder categories encompass (1) *Depressive disorders*, which include MDD, dysthymic disorder, and depressive disorder not otherwise specified; (2) *bipolar disorders*, which include bipolar I disorder, bipolar II disorder, cyclothymia, and bipolar disorder not otherwise specified; (3) *mood disorders caused by a general medical condition*; (4) *substance-induced mood disorder*; and (5) *mood disorder not otherwise specified*. Depressive disorders are the primary focus of this discussion due to their incidence, prevalence, and treatment outcome.

DEPRESSION

Depression and its failure to be diagnosed has been recognized as one of the largest problems in the primary care setting. Due to the magnitude and the socioeconomic impact of depression, Congress has targeted depression as one of the initial conditions for the development of guidelines by a select panel with the support of the Agency for Health Care Policy and Research (AHCPR). The objective of the panel (Depressive Guideline Panel) was to develop a document *(Clinical Practice Guidelines: Depression in Primary Care)* for the primary care physician for assessment and treatment of psychiatric problems.

The statistics relative to depressive disorders bear witness to the magnitude of this disorder: Approximately one in every eight persons may require treatment for depression at some point in his or her life. Major depression has an annual prevalence of 5% and a lifetime prevalence of 20% in the general population (7% to 12% for males and 20% to 25% for females), and fewer than one third will be accurately diagnosed and treated.[3] In western industrialized nations, the point prevalence for MDD is 2.3% to 3.2% among males and 4.5% to 9.3% among women. MDD is present in approximately 4% to 6% of the primary care outpatient population, and milder forms of depression are present in 6% to 14% of said population.[4] It is estimated that greater than 60% of suicides are attributed to MDD. Forty-three percent of patients with MDD have a lifetime history of one or more psychiatric conditions other than affect disorders.[5] Clinically significant depressive symptoms are present in 12% to 36% of patients with concurrent medical conditions.[6]

The socioeconomic impact of depressive disorders is evident; studies have demonstrated that individuals diagnosed with depressive disorders place a greater demand on medical services and economic resources in general,[7] accruing up to five times as many disability days,[8] requiring activity restrictions,[9] and incurring a greater number of accidental deaths.[10] The total cost of mood disorders nationally inclusive of such direct charges as hospitalizations, institutionalizations, and physician visits and such indirect charges as lost productivity[11] is estimated to be 43.7 billion dollars annually.[12] It is imperative that primary care practitioners become diagnostically aware and initiate therapeutic intervention to impact on the detrimental personal, social, and economic consequences of depressive disorders.

Defining Depressive Disorders

To be able to entertain a differential diagnosis, one must first be familiar with the defining signs and symptoms. The criteria defining a major depressive episode involve fulfilling inclusionary and exclusionary parameters, as well as those for single episode and recurrent MDD and dysthymic disorder.

DIAGNOSTIC CRITERIA FOR MAJOR DEPRESSIVE EPISODE.[1]

1. Five or more of the following symptoms have been present during the same *two-week period* and represent a change from previous functioning, and at least one of the symptoms is either (1) depressed mood or (2) loss of interest or pleasure. Note: Do not include symptoms that clearly are the result of general medical conditions, mood-incongruent delusions, or hallucinations.
    a. Depressed mood most of the day, nearly every day, as indicated by either subjective report (e.g., feels sad and empty) or observation made by others (e.g., appears tearful). Note: Children and adolescents may have an irritable mood.
    b. Markedly diminished interest or pleasure in all or almost all activities most of the day, nearly every day (as indicated by either subjective accounts or observations made by others).
    c. Significant weight loss when not dieting or weight gain (e.g., a change of more than 5% of body weight in 1 month) or decrease or increase in appetite nearly every day. Note: In children, consider failure to make expected weight gains.
    d. Insomnia or hypersomnia nearly every day. Insomnia may manifest as *initial insomnia*, in which the individual has difficulty falling asleep; *middle insomnia*, in which the individual awakens in the middle of the night, is awake for 1 to 2 hours, and eventually returns to sleep; and *terminal insomnia*, in which the individual awakens early (generally several hours before their habitual awakening hour) and is unable to return to sleep. Terminal insomnia is a hallmark feature of depression.
    e. Psychomotor agitation or retardation nearly every day (observable by others, not merely subjective feelings of restlessness or being slowed down).
    f. Fatigue or loss of energy nearly every day.

g. Feelings of worthlessness or excessive or inappropriate guilt (which may be delusional) nearly every day (not merely self-reproach or guilt about being sick).
h. Diminished ability to think or concentrate or indecisiveness nearly every day (either by subjective account or as observed by others).
i. Recurrent thoughts of death (not just fear of dying), recurrent suicidal ideations without a specific plan, or a suicide attempt or a specific plan for committing suicide.
2. The symptoms do not meet the criteria for a mixed episode.
3. The symptoms cause clinically significant distress or impairment in social, occupational, or other important areas of function.
4. The symptoms are not the result of direct physiological effects of a substance (e.g., a drug of abuse, a medication) or a general medical condition (e.g., hypothyroidism).
5. The symptoms are not better accounted for by bereavement (e.g., after the loss of a loved one), or the symptoms persist for longer than 2 months or are characterized by marked functional impairment, morbid preoccupation with worthlessness, suicidal ideations, psychotic symptoms, or psychomotor retardation.

Diagnostic Criteria for 296.2x Single Episode MDD.[1]

1. Presence of a single major depressive episode.
2. The major depressive episode is not better accounted for by schizoaffective disorder and is not superimposed on schizophrenia, schizophreniform disorder, delusional disorder, or psychotic disorder not otherwise specified.
3. There has never been a manic episode, a mixed episode, or a hypomanic episode. Note: This exclusion does not apply if all the manic-like, mixedlike, or hypomanic-like episodes are substance or treatment induced or are the results of the direct physiological effects of a general medical condition. Specify (for current or most recent episode):

- Severity/psychotic/remission specifiers
- Chronic
- With catatonic features
- With melancholic features
- With atypical features
- With postpartum onset

Diagnostic criteria for 296.3x Recurrent MDD.[1]

1. Presence of two or more major depressive episodes. Note: To be considered separate episodes, there must be an interval of at least two consecutive months in which criteria are not met for major depressive episode.
2. The major depressive episode is not better accounted for by schizoaffective disorder and is not superimposed on schizophrenia, schizophreniform disorder, delusional disorder, or psychotic disorder not otherwise specified.
3. There has never been a manic episode, a mixed episode, or a hypo-

manic episode. Note: This exclusion does not apply if all the maniclike, mixedlike, or hypomanic-like episodes are substance or treatment induced or are caused by the direct physiological effects of a general medical condition.

Specify (for current or most recent episode):

- Severity/psychotic/remission specifiers
- Chronic
- With catatonic features
- With melancholic features
- With atypical features
- With postpartum onset

Specify:

- Longitudinal course specifiers (with and without interepisode
- recovery)
- With seasonal pattern

Major depressive episode *specifiers* for current or most recent episode (which pertain to both single episode and recurrent episode MDD) have clinical significance defining the subgroups by their essential features, as well as having diagnostic implications. The specifier may also have treatment and prognostic implications. Specifiers indicative of severity, remission, and psychotic features can be coded in the second place to the right of the decimal (xxx.x1) for most mood disorders. Each specifier has well-delineated criteria cited in the DSM-IV to which readers may refer.

DIAGNOSTIC CRITERIA FOR 300.4 DYSTHYMIC DISORDER.[1]

1. Depressed mood for most of the day, for more days than not, as indicated by either subjective account or observation by others, for at least 2 years. Note: In children and adolescents, mood can be irritable, and duration must be at least 1 year.
2. Presence, while depressed, of two or more of the following:
   a. Poor appetite or overeating.
   b. Insomnia or hypersomnia.
   c. Low energy or fatigue.
   d. Low self-esteem.
   e. Poor concentration or difficulty making decisions.
   f. Feelings of hopelessness.
3. During the 2-year period (1 year for children or adolescents) of the disturbance, the person has never been without the symptoms in criteria 1 and 2 for more than 2 months at a time.
4. No major depressive episode has been present during the first 2 years of the disturbance (1 year for children or adolescents); in other words, the disturbance is not better accounted for by chronic MDD or by MDD in partial remission.
   Note: There may have been a previous major depressive episode, provided there was full remission (no significant signs or symptoms

for 2 months) before development of the dysthymic disorder. In addition, after the initial 2 years (1 year for children or adolescents) of dysthymic disorder, there may be superimposed episodes of MDD, in which case both diagnoses may be given when the criteria are met for a major depressive episode.
5. There has never been a manic episode, a mixed episode, or a hypomanic episode, and criteria have never been met for cyclothymic disorder.
6. The disturbance does not occur exclusively during the course of a chronic psychotic disorder, such as schizophrenia or delusional disorder.
7. The symptoms have not resulted from the direct physiological effects of a substance (e.g., a drug of abuse, a medication) or a general medical condition (e.g., hypothyroidism).
8. The symptoms cause clinically significant distress or impairment in social, occupational, or other important areas of functioning.

Specify if:

- Early onset (if onset is before age 21 years).
- Late onset (if onset is age 21 or older).

Specify (for most recent years of dysthymic disorder):

- With atypical features.

DETECTING AND DIAGNOSING MOOD DISORDERS

The *Clinical Practice Guidelines (Depression in Primary Care)* have enumerated steps for the detection and treatment of depressive conditions. These steps have been adapted as a reference for the logical progression of patient assessment and a platform for clinical understanding.

Maintain a High Index of Suspicion and evaluate Risk Factors

Clinical clues that heighten the index of suspicion of the presence or history of depressive disorder, especially in individuals less than age 40 include complaints of *pain* (headache or abdominal), *anhedonia* (low energy or reduced capacity for pleasure or enjoyment), *sexual complaints* (functioning or desire), and *altered mood* (e.g., apathy, irritability, or anxiety in presence or absence of overt sadness). Additional risk factors for depression are:

1. Prior history of depression. The experiencing of a single episode of major depressive episode is associated with a 50% chance of a subsequent episode, 70% chance with two episodes, and 90% chance with three or more episodes over a lifetime for recurrent depression.[13]
2. Family history of depressive disorder. An individual who develops MDD before age 20 has a greater familial morbidity for depression.
3. Prior suicide attempts.
4. Female gender.[14,15]
5. Age of onset less than 40.
6. Postpartum period.

7. Medical comorbidity.
8. Lack of social support.
9. Stressful lifestyle.
10. Current alcohol or substance abuse.

Suicide is of particular concern for individuals with mood disorders. The assessment and recognition of suicidal risk factors impact greatly on the management and safety issues of the individual with mood disorders. *Suicide risk factors* can be arranged into the domains of *psychosocial and clinical risk factors, historical* and *diagnostic*. Psychosocial and clinical risk factors include hopelessness, white race, male gender, advanced age, and living alone. The history of prior suicide attempt, family history of suicide attempt, or family history of substance abuse also should alert the practitioner to concerns of suicide. Individual diagnosed with a general medical illness, such as cerebral infarction, dementia (cortical and subcortical disorders) diabetes, myocardial infarction, malignancy, psychosis, and substance abuse, are statistically recognized as a population at greater depressive disorders risk requiring clinical inquiry.

Detect Depressed Symptoms With Clinical Interview or Self-Report Questionnaire

The evaluation of depression can be sought by direct clinical interview with the client, administration of self-report questionnaires, and history provided by a spouse or knowledgeable other. The clinical work-up for psychiatric evaluation follows the traditional Lawrence Weed Problem-Oriented Medical Information Systems model of subjective, objective, assessment, and plan formula with modification for psychiatric adaptation. The *subjective* section is subcategorized into chief complaint, history of present illness, past medical history, past psychiatric history, social history, family history, and review of systems. The *objective* section subcategories include physical examination, MSE, laboratory tests, and adjunctive testing (e.g., imaging and electrodiagnostics). The assessment section focuses on the five axes. The plan section addresses further assessment, testing, and treatment considerations.

The MSE is the cornerstone of the psychiatric evaluation. It is conducted as an integrated assessment in which information from the entire interview, examination, and specific testing is formulated. The MSE is an assessment of the individual's current mental status. The MSE provides insight into the emotional, behavioral, and cognitive status of the individual.

The MSE can be divided into topical features to which the examiner may direct his or her focus and attention. The MSE includes the assessment of appearance, attitude, psychomotor activity, mood, affect, speech, language, thought process, thought content, perception, cognition, insight, and judgment. Due to the scope of this chapter, a treatise on the MSE is not the goal but a working understanding specifically related to depressive disorders. As in any examination, the development of a structured organization of the MSE is inherent to avoid omissions and diagnostic misadventure.

Appearance focuses on the patient's physical characteristics (e.g., bodily habitus, dress, grooming, hygiene, apparent age, level of conscious ness, and eye contact), which may provide insight into the patient's mood, awareness of self, motor integrity, general physical health, thought content, and thought processing.

Attitude reflects the relationship between the patient and the examiner, as well as the patient's response to the interview process. The examiner summarizes observation made during the course of the interview, such as tone of voice, attentiveness, and evasiveness in response. Descriptive terms of the patient's general demeanor, such as cooperative, hostile, guarded, and suspicious, are commonly employed to denote attitude.

Psychomotor activity refers to the posture, position, and the motor presentation of the client, which may reflect the patient's mood, energy level, muscle strength, or coordination. The focus of the MSE is to note abnormalities of the excess, repetition, or paucity of activity or behavior. Consideration of hyperkinesia, bradykinesia, mannerisms, or aberration of movements may provide insight to physical etiologies of illness, drug side effects, or psychiatric etiologies.

The individual with depression may have any manifestation of the spectrum of psychomotor activity from psychomotor agitation to psychomotor retardation. The client with psychomotor agitation may appear fidgety or may constantly be in motion. The examiner may observe hand wringing, scratching, nail biting, frequent postural reposition, crossing-uncrossing of legs, or any host of stereotypical or repetitive motor activities. The individual with depression exhibiting psychomotor agitation typically denies depressive signs and symptoms and instead complains of being tense and irritable. Conversely, the psychomotor retarded individual with associated depression typically has slowing of movements, speech, and thought processing. Such individuals complain of decreased energy and of being easily fatigued; often they will sit for hours without speaking with minimal movement or gesturing and expressing a sad or blank facies.

Mood is a descriptive term reflecting the patient's predominant internal feelings at a given time; it is the patient's *subjective* interpretation. The patient may use descriptors such as euthymic, dysphoric, euphoric, angry, apathetic, or apprehensive and their synonyms to relate his or her mood. Using a gradation scale of 1 to 10 (1 being the worst and 10 being the best ever experienced) may help the patient express his or her mood in more precise terms. The individual with depression may express his or her mood in any number of terms that equate to being low, citing feelings of worthlessness, hopelessness, and despair. He or she may express feelings of guilt over an actual or imagined event. If the event is actual, it is often perceived magnified and out of factual proportions. The individual with depression often feels the situation is unable to be rectified or improved, and that he or she does not deserve it to be.

Affect reflect the objective, moment-to-moment changes of the patient's emotional state as perceived by the examiner. Parameters of affect address gradations of appropriateness, congruence, intensity (blunt to overly dramatic), mobility (constricted to labile), range (full to restricted), and reactivity. A "normal" individual displays a variety of affects relative to the theme of conversation and changes in the external environment. The individual with depression may have various aberrant affects such as incongruent, flat, blunted, or constricted, *objectively* defined by the examiner.

The neurological, psychiatric, and clinical considerations of *speech and language* greatly exceed the scope of this passage, and the depth of discourse is vastly disproportionate to the clinical significance for differential diagnoses. Aberrances of speech and language performance may be attributed to central nervous system etiologies (stroke, trauma, space-occupying mass, infection, etc.), as well as a variety of psychiatric conditions (e.g., mania, dementia, delirium, schizophrenia, and anxiety). The presence of a language disorder does not exclude the concurrent existence of a psychiatric disorder. Therefore, it is important to be able to recognize and describe the specifics of speech and language as part of the MSE.

The assessment of language function requires the evaluation of fluency of speech, repetition, comprehension, naming, writing, reading, prosody, and quality of speech. *Fluency* can be assessed by noting the client's spontaneous speech for substantive content, grammatic integrity, clarity of articulation, evidence of latency, or the paucity or excess of words. Disorders of language fluency may be defined as *fluent* (e.g., Wernicke's aphasia) or *nonfluent* (e.g., Broca's aphasia).

Repetition may be assessed by having the client repeat spoken words or phrases, initially monosyllabic words, then multisyllabic words, progressing to short phrases, next advancing to simple sentences, and ending with the repetition of sentences with complex syntax. The ability of the clients to repeat appropriately may aid the examiner's differential diagnosis of various psychiatric disorders and of the various types of aphasias.

Comprehension may be assessed by having the client execute increasingly complex sets of commands. Initially, single-stop commands such as "touch your nose" should be directed, progressing to two-step and finally three-step commands such as "take a piece of paper with your right hand, fold it in half, then place it on the bed." Comprehension should also be assessed by the evaluation of abstract or conceptual thinking. The interpretation of proverbs "a rolling stone gathers no moss" or resolving of sentences involving comparisons and relationship concepts "If you purchase a 35-cent newspaper and give the storekeeper a 1-dollar bill, which coins do you receive as change?" provides insight as to integrity or impairment of comprehension. Aberrances of comprehension may also assist the examiner's differential diagnosis of various psychiatric disorders and of the various types of aphasias.

There are a number of instruments and methods to evaluate the client's *naming* ability. Confrontational naming is a commonly used method whereby the examiner points to an object (e.g., a watch) and asks the client, "What is this called?" The examiner will also ask the client to name specific parts of the object, such as watchband, crystal, and hands. Another method to evaluate naming is to ask the client to generate a list of items from a particular category, such as things from a grocery store, or to name items beginning with a particular letter, such as things that begin with the letter "C" (e.g., coins, cotton, coat, and candy). "Normal" individuals can generate 20 words or items in 60 seconds.

Writing is assessed on an increasingly complex task performance evaluation. The client is initially instructed to write something familiar such as his or her address, then instructed to copy a sentence or a design, and finally to write a sentence of his or her choice. Writing difficulties may reflect a number of disorders, including aphasia, movement disorders, and visual-spatial deficits. *Reading* may be evaluated by instructing the client to read aloud from a text or newspaper. The ability to accomplish this task suggests the gross integrity of the phonological output system. Comprehension may be evaluated at this time by asking the client to describe what he or she just read. The client should also be instructed to read a passage silently and his or her comprehension then assessed. The ability to comprehend silent vs. aloud reading suggests differing aphasia diagnoses.

Prosody refers to the speech quality of rate, rhythm, amount, and intonation of words and phrases, as well as the reflection of intonation to the meaning of the words, phrases, or sentence. The evaluation of the quality of speech (e.g., pitch, loudness, loquacity, phonation, articulation, or evidence of dysarthria) may suggest a number of possible etiologies. The aberrances of the quality of speech must be considered in total of the examination for clinical and diagnostic implications. The prototypical speech of a psychomotor retarded individual with depression is marked by slow, monotonous, brief, and laconic replies.

The clinical assessment of *thought content* and *processing* is a critical element in the assessment of the patient's psychiatric status. Thought processes and the thoughts of the patient cannot be actually known by the examiner, but an inferred appreciation can be gained by the patient's spoken language or writing. The assessment of the patient's organization, flow, and production of thoughts are areas to focus on. An individual devoid of abnormal thought processing exhibits coherent thoughts that are clear, logical, understandable, and easily followed. A plethora of categories and subcategories exist to describe the various altered thought content and processing, which are associated with or are hallmarks of specific psychiatric diagnoses. The individual with depression spans the gamut of aberrant thought content and processes, often reflecting the severity of the disorder. These individuals may exhibit disorders of thought connectedness, organization, or other specific thought peculiarities. Individuals with mild depression may exhibit *perseveration* (persistent repetition of words, ideas, or phrases, usually out of context and mechanically fashioned) or *thought blocking* (arrest of thoughts in midsentence, accompanied by a pause, then resumed with a new unrelated topic). Severe depression can be of a psychotic depth, manifesting as delusional thoughts (delusions are an abnormality of thought content) and hallucinations (hallucinations are perceptual disturbances). The delusional thoughts of an individual with depression are often persecutory, nihilistic, or somatic in content. Individuals with depression may think about suicide and death. It is a misnomer that the inquiring of suicide places the individual at risk by "putting thought" into their head. To the contrary, it allows the individual to express concerns and provides noninjurious interventions and alternatives. It also allows the practitioner to assess the level of intervention that may be required to protect the patient's safety.

The assessment of *cognition* involves the examination or orientation, attention and concentration, registration and memory, constructional and visual-spatial ability, and abstraction and conceptualization. The Mini-MSE is one of the most commonly and widely used screening test of cognitive function. A maximum score of 30 can be achieved; a score of 24 or less indicates cognitive dysfunction (Fig 1). The individual who is clinically depressed may have greatest deficit in the area of attention.

Assessment of *insight* and *judgment* requires the appreciation of the relationship of insight and judgment. Insight is the awareness and knowledge of internal and external realities. Insight is the ability to examine the multiplicities of viewpoints, dimensional aspects, and consequences that precedes the formulation of an opinion or judgment. Insight is influenced by defense mechanisms and personality. Judgment presupposes adequate insight, intact cognition, appreciation of impact and consequences, as well as cultural and societal factors. The individual with a depressive disorder may find his or her insight and judgment impaired by the vegetative and negative, pessimistic, guilt feelings, and low self-image.

REPRESENTATIVE VIGNETTE OF CLIENT HISTORY

Sue Green is a 45-year-old married woman. She is admitted to the local emergency room on her birthday with suicidal ideations and a plan. Mrs. Green relates that she has been thinking of taking an overdose of nonprescription sleeping pills. Mrs. Green relates that 2 months ago her husband of 25 years told her of an affair he was having and that he had filed for a divorce. He has moved out of their house and has not spoken with her since. Mrs. Green has been a homemaker for the past 25 years. Her children are grown and attend college out of state. She has spent most of her life attending the needs of her family and has developed few out-of-home interests or friends. For the past 2 months she reports difficulty getting to sleep and after only a few hours waking, not being able to return to sleep. She also reports poor appetite, a 6.8-kg weight loss, poor concentration, loss of motivation and energy, and feelings of worthlessness. Mrs. Green relates continuous thoughts of the divorce being her fault, she has been a failure as a wife, and she deserves what is happening to her. Mrs. Green states she feels helpless and alone.

Mrs. Green has no prior psychiatric history, no active medical problems and no history of alcohol or illicit drug abuse. She is currently not taking any prescription medications; her only medication is the nonprescription sleeping pills.

REPRESENTATIVE MSE OF VIGNETTE

Appearance, Attitude, and Psychomotor Activity.—The patient appears to be her stated age, her clothing is disheveled, and she is not wearing makeup. She is moderately psychomotor retarded; her face is expressionless, and she sits slumped in a chair. Her eye contact is limited; her eyes predominately cast down to the floor. She is cooperative with the interviewer.

Mood and Affect.—The patient states her mood to be "depressed," rating her mood as 3/10, and expresses feelings of hopelessness. Her affect is blunted, with reduced range and is nonreactive.

	Score	Points

Orientation

1. What is the
   - Year? — 1
   - Season? — 1
   - Date? — 1
   - Day? — 1
   - Month? — 1

2. Where are we?
   - State? — 1
   - County? — 1
   - Town or city? — 1
   - Hospital? — 1
   - Floor? — 1

Registration

3. Name three objects, taking 1 second to say each. Then ask the patient all three after you have said them. Give 1 point for each correct answer. Repeat answers until the patient learns all three. — 3

Attention and calculation

4. Serial 7's: $\overline{}$, $\overline{93}$, $\overline{86}$, $\overline{79}$, $\overline{72}$, $\overline{65}$
   Alternate: Spell WORLD backwards. — 5

Recall

5. Ask for the names of three objects from question no. 3. Give 1 point for each correct answer. — 3

Language

6. Point to a pencil and a watch. Have the patient name them as you point. — 2

7. Have the patient read "No ifs, ands, or buts." — 1

8. Have the patient follow a three-stage command. "Take the paper in your right hand, fold the paper in half, put the paper on the floor." — 3

9. Have the patient read and obey the following: "Close your eyes." — 1

10. Have the patient write a sentence of his or her own choice. (The sentence should contain a subject and an object and should make sense. Ignore spelling errors. — 1

11. Enlarge a design to 1.5 cm per side and have the patient copy it. Give 1 point if all sides and angles are preserved and if the intersected sides form a quadrangle. — 11

Total: 30

FIGURE 1.

Mini MSE. (From Folstein MF, Folstein SE, McHugh PR: *J Psychiatry Res* 12:189–198, 1975. Used by permission.)

Speech and Language.—Her speech is fluent, rate is decreased, and there are marked prolonged latency and pauses. Occasionally she has word-finding difficulties.

Thought Content, Processing, and Perception.—The patient has active suicidal ideation and plan. She states feelings of hopelessness and worthlessness. She denies homicidal ideations, hallucinations in any modalities, or delusional thoughts. Content is centered on low self-image and feelings of abandonment.

Cognition.—The patient is oriented times three (self, place, time). She has mild short-term memory deficit, with two out of three object recall after 5 minutes. She demonstrated attention deficit on the Symbol Digit Test with a digit span forward of 6 and 3 backward. The patient scored 24/30 on the Mini-MSE.

Insight and Judgment.—Insight is impaired by depressive symptoms of hopelessness, worthlessness, and despondence. Judgment is impaired as evidenced by suicide ideations.

The primary care physician also has several instruments available for clinician-directed interviews specifically focused toward the assessment of depressive disorders: the Hamilton Rating Scale for Depression, Montgomery-Asberg Depression Rating Scale, the Inventory for Depressive Symptomatology–Clinician Rated, and the Bech-Rafaelsen Depression Scale.

Self-reporting scales such as the Beck Depression Inventory, the Zung Self-Reporting Depression Scale, the General Health Questionnaire's Depression Subscale, and Center for Epidemiological Studies–Depression Scale help to identify potentially depressed individuals. These instruments have not been extensively applied in the primary care setting, and they are not very specific. Therefore, practitioners should not use these instruments exclusively as the basis for diagnosing depressive disorders. These instruments do serve to heighten the practitioner's suspicion and focus the need for a clinical interview.[16] All of the prior instruments produce false-positive results 25% to 40% of the time.[16] A recently developed instrument called Prime-MD provides clinicians an evaluation guide for mood, anxiety, alcohol abuse, and eating and somatoform disorders. The client initially completes a questionnaire. The clinician then follows a decision-making algorithm interview developing the differential diagnosis.

Define the Mood Syndrome (by Clinical History, Interview, or Report by Spouse or Significant Other)

The differential diagnoses of the primary mood disorders of MDD, bipolar disorder, dysthymic disorder, MDD in partial remission, and depressive disorder not otherwise specified can be delineated based on the following decision-making algorithm (Fig 1). First, for any of the prior noted disorders to be considered, the complaint of either sad, low mood, or loss of interest/pleasure (anhedonia) must be present. Second, the individual has experienced five of the nine symptoms of the criteria of major depressive episode, currently or in the past. Third, the individual has experienced a prior manic episode. Finally, symptoms (not sufficient to meet criteria of MDD) have persisted for more than 2 years. These factors need to be elucidated for rendering a clinical diagnosis (Fig 2).

Evaluate the Patient with a Complete Medical History, Physical Examination, and Laboratory and Supportive Tests

Ascertaining the medical history and conducting the physical examination essentially do not vary regardless of the patient. Some special considerations of laboratory and adjunctive tests with specificity to depressive disorders warrant mention.

The use of laboratory diagnostics as in any assessment should have a rational basis for selection and conduct. Clinical investigation is being conducted relative to laboratory tests with high specificity for depressive disorders. Thyrotropine-releasing hormone stimulation test, dexamethasone suppression test, and sleep electroencephalograms[17] are being evaluated as to their capability to identify biological abnormalities characteristic of depression. The use of the aforementioned test are not indicated for routine screening of depressive disorders due to their lack of specificity and their lower sensitivity in the less severely ill.

It is essential to keep in perspective that laboratory tests are used to *assist* in the differential diagnosis. Epidemiological studies in the general population suggest that previously unrecognized laboratory abnormalities are present in 0.8% to 4.0% of the general population.[18] It should also be kept in mind that a significant portion of these abnormalities are predictable based on clinical assessment[19] or represent false positives. Selection and ordering of laboratory tests should be tempered by the characteristics of the population being served (e.g., age, gender, and race) and, more specifically, the patient's clinical signs and symptoms.

Questions have also been raised concerning the use of psychological tests. In general the use of psychological and neurophysiological tests are

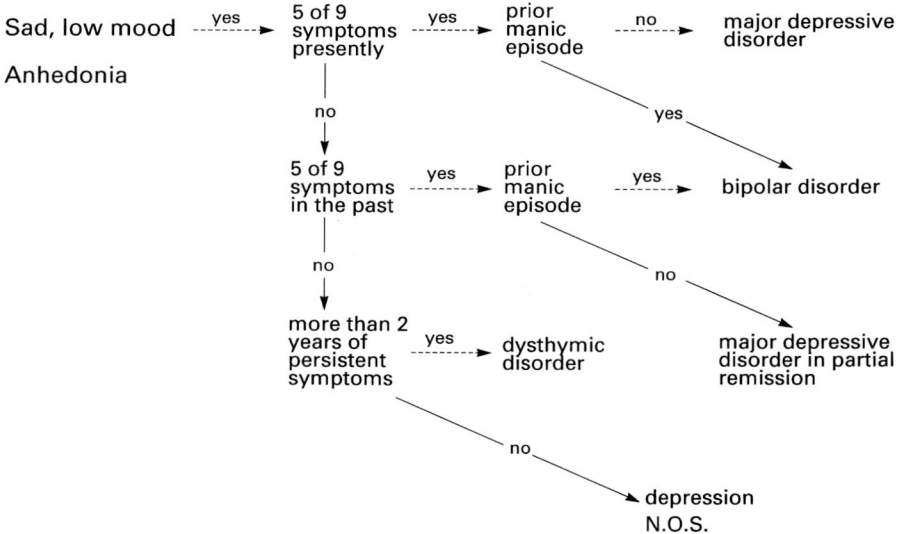

FIGURE 2.
Decision-making algorithm for various mood syndromes.

not recommended for routine screening in the depressive disorder population. The use of such instruments as the Minnesota Multiphasic Personality Inventory (MMPI), Symptoms Checklist 90, and the Million Clinical Multiaxial Inventory may assist in substantiating a diagnosis; they do not independently render the diagnosis. A concurrent nonpsychiatric medical condition can skew the test results of a patient being evaluated for depression. Therefore, tests such as the MMPI should not be used as the sole determinant of a depressive disorder diagnosis. Psychological tests may help direct a differential diagnosis, but like laboratory tests, they should not be used as a routine screening instrument or administered for all differential diagnostic situations.

Define Potential Known Causes of Mood Symptoms and Treat the Potential Causes

A number of conditions may be associated with mood symptoms or major depressive episodes: substance abuse, concurrent medications, general medical disorders, causal nonmood psychiatric disorders, and grief reactions. Each of these associations must be considered when an individual is evaluated for depression for proper clinical intervention to be administered.

Alcoholism and major depressive disorder are distinct and separate clinical entities. Studies assessing the relationship of individuals with primary depression developing alcoholism reveal that alcoholism is rarely a consequence of depression. The prevalence of alcoholism in individuals with primary depression is approximately that of the general population.[20, 21] Conversely, studies have supported a relationship between alcoholism and the development of depression. Ten percent to 30% of alcoholic individuals develop depression.[22] Evidence suggest that women may have a greater tendency than their male counterparts to develop depression as a consequence of prolonged drinking, and daughters raised by alcoholic biological parents are more likely to develop depression as adults.[23, 24] Adoption studies provide evidence of the independent transmission of depression and alcoholism, thus refuting the notion of familial aggregation between alcoholism and depression.

Concerning *concurrent medications*, a variety of medications have been reported to cause or to be associated with mood symptoms or mood disorders as side effects. Idiosyncratic reactions to medications do occur: clinical judgment should dictate whether a medication should be changed or discontinued based on medical indications. Select medications such as reserpine, glucocorticoids, and anabolic corticosteroids have been associated with de novo development of depression as a side effect. Other therapeutic agents such as histamine$_2$ receptor blockers (cimetidine and ranitidine), anticonvulsants (phenobarbital and carbamazepine), and antihypertensives (propranolol) have been implicated by case reports. It is evident that concurrently used medications should be suspect in a individual with depressive symptoms.

The DMS-IV coding of 293.83 *Mood Disorder Due to a General Medical Condition* is distinguished by the prominent and persistent disturbance of mood attributed to the direct physiological effect of the medical condition. Subtypes of mood disturbance episodes may be used to indicate predominant symptoms in the absence of full mood disorder criteria being met. The subtype designations are as follows: with depressive features, with major depressive-like episode, with manic features, and with mixed features, each subtype having its own qualifying criteria.

Clinically significant depressive symptoms are present in 12% to 36% of individuals with another nonpsychiatric general medical condition. To properly treat the diagnosed depression occurring concurrently with a general medical condition, one must answer the following questions:

1. Is the general medical disorder biologically causative of the depression based on history, physical examination, and laboratory findings?
2. Did the general medical disorder trigger the onset of the depression in an individual genetically vulnerable to depressive disorders?
3. Did the general medical disorder psychologically trigger the depression as a reaction to the anticipated morbidity and the prognosis of the medical disorder?
4. Are the general medical disorder and the depression causally related? It is important to identify the relationship of depression and the general medical disorder because it will dictate the prioritization of treatment intervention. In other words, treat the general medical disorder, and if after stabilization the depression persists, treat the depression. Treat the general medical disorder while supportive therapies and medications treat the depression or initiate specific treatment for the general medical disorder and the primary mood disorder as two distinct entities.

The presence of one psychiatric disorder does not preclude a second disorder from manifesting. Depression may also occur with other causal nonmood psychiatric disorders such as anxiety disorders, eating disorders, obsessive-compulsive disorders, somatization disorders, and personality disorders, which impact on morbidity, treatment, and mortality.

Panic disorder is present in up to 20% of individuals with MDD seen in an ambulatory treatment setting. As to which disorder occurred initially, the panic disorder precedes the MDD in approximately 50% of these individuals.[25, 26] The association of panic disorder with MDD has significant clinical implication; depressed individuals with associated panic attacks have a more severe depressive illness and are less likely to recover during a 2-year follow-up compared with those with depression only[27]; the lifetime suicide attempt rate for individuals with both panic disorder and MDD is greater than two times that of panic disorder without MDD.[28]

The impact of *eating disorders* must also be considered when one is assessing depressive symptoms. Up to 75% of individuals with eating disorders have a lifetime history of MDD. One third to one half of individuals with eating disorders (anorexia or bulimia) suffer MDD concurrently. The incidence and prevalence of anorexia nervosa have not been determined in the general population, but data suggest a 0.5% to 1.0% prevalence in females of late adolescence to young adulthood age. Little is known of the prevalence of bulimia nervosa in the general population; available data suggest that 1% to 3% of young women will develop full blown symptoms of bulimia nervosa and that a higher percentage will engage in activities placing them in a subthreshold classification. Individuals experiencing undernutrition from a variety of etiologies often exhibit depressive symptoms, which usually improve with weight gain; therefore, weight restoration is usually the initial targeted treatment when both eating disorders and depressive disorders are present.

The presence of *somatization disorder* can obscure and may contribute to the misdiagnosis of psychiatric illness in the primary care setting.[29] Studies have revealed that 50% to 70% of primary care patients with psychiatric illness (primarily mood disorders) have somatic complaints.[30] Studies have also conversely demonstrated that pain symptoms occurred in approximately 60% of patients with MDD of the group studied.[31] Medical review of symptoms reveal that patients with two pain complaints were six times more likely and patients with three pain complaints were eight times more likely to have a clinical depression than patients with a single complaint.[32] Due to the circular relationship of depression and somatic complaints, it has been found that treatment of the major depressive disorder in individuals with MDD and somatic complaints usually results in complete relief of the pain complaint.

Personality disorders that occur with depressive disorders may have negative effects on the natural course and treatment response of the latter. Studies have demonstrated that individuals with personality disorders have their initial depressive episode at an earlier age; their depressive symptoms were more severe; they experienced more frequent and longer depressive episodes; and they have poorer short-term recovery with both antidepressant medications and psychotherapy, as well as greater residual symptoms at later follow-up.[33, 34] Borderline personality disorder appears to account for the larger proportion of the general negative effects of personality disorders on the outcome of depression. Individuals with depression with comorbid borderline personality disorder have a poorer social outcome and higher level of residual symptoms at both 4- and 7-year follow-ups.[35] There are insufficient data of the incidence of personality disorders in the primary care setting to identify prevalence, but an estimate of community prevalence of borderline personality disorder is 0.2%.[36]

Reevaluate for Mood Syndrome
If the individual continues to have depression after treatment of the associated psychiatric, general medical disorders, or substance abuse disorders, treat the depression as a primary mood disorder.

Develop a Treatment Plan
Once diagnosed, depression can almost always be successfully treated. The efficacy of treatment rest on accurate diagnosis. The treatment of depressive disorders can be arranged into five categories: medication, psychotherapy, combination of medication and psychotherapy, electroconvulsive therapy, and light therapy. Medication and psychotherapy are the principal treatment choices for uncomplicated, nonpsychotic MDDs. Whichever treatment modality is selected, a sufficient trial period is required to assess the individual's response to said treatment. A recommended trial period of 4 to 6 weeks for medications or 6 to 8 weeks for psychotherapy is required to evidence a partial response. Recommended

parameters concerning medication therapy generally note if the patient fails to respond by 6 weeks or only partially responds by 10 to 12 weeks other treatment options should be considered. These parameters also pertain to application of psychotherapy alone; failure of response by 6 weeks or only partial response by 12 weeks suggests the initiation of a trial of medication.

Psychopharmacological treatment is a three-phase process: acute treatment, continuation treatment, and maintenance treatment. The goal of *acute treatment* is to remit the current depressive episode's signs and symptoms and to restore psychosocial and occupational function. Attaining these objectives of the acute phase constitutes a *remission*. When a remission is attained, the patient should be seen two to three times over the next 6 to 12 months to monitor for relapse. Improvement or only partial remittance is referred to as a *response*. The return of symptoms of the current depressive episode within a 6-month period from remission is known as a *relapse*. The purpose of *continuation treatment* is to prevent relapse. *Recovery* is achieved when the patient has been asymptomatic for 4 to 9 months after the remission of the depressive episode. Premature termination of medication is associated with approximately a 25% relapse rate within 2 months.[37] Continuation treatment may be stopped once recovery is attained. *Maintenance treatment* is directed toward patients who experience recurrent depressive episodes. The objective of maintenance treatment is to prevent recurrence, which may require lifetime intervention.

The impetus to diagnose and treat depressive disorders may be founded in the humanitarian consciousness to relieve the individual suffering and that of those in acquaintance or, if motivated, from a pragmatic perspective to impact on the social and economic consequences. Studies have demonstrated that effective treatment of depressive disorders results in remission of symptoms and improvement of interpersonal, marital, and occupational function.[38] There is also reduced potential of suicide and reduction in excessive health care use and cost.[39] Reduced disability from concurrent general medical conditions and improvement in long-term outcome[40] are also realized by effective treatment of depressive disorders.

CONCLUSION

The statistics and data presented in this chapter reflect the impact of mood disorders, particularly depressive disorders, seen in the primary care setting of the allopathic and osteopathic professions. It may easily be extrapolated that these statistics hold true for the chiropractic setting. At the present time this is only an assumption, and efforts are being directed to ascertain these data. If client populations are homogeneous, we must become more cognizant of psychiatric disorders in the chiropractic setting.

REFERENCES

1. American Psychiatric Association: *Diagnostic and Statistical Manual of Mental Disorders*, ed 4. Washington, DC, American Psychiatric Association, 1994.

2. Endicott J, Spitzer RL, Fleiss JL, et al: The Global Assessment Scale: A procedure for measuring severity of psychiatric disturbance. *Arch Gen Psychiatry* 33:766–771, 1976.
3. Magruder-Habib K, Zung WWK, Feussner JR, et al: Management of general medicine patients with symptoms of depression. *Gen Hosp Psychiatry* 11:201–206, 1989.
4. Barrett EJ, Barrett JA, Oxman TE, et al: The prevalence of psychiatric disorders in a primary care practice. *Arch Gen Psychiatry* 45:1100–1106, 1988.
5. Sargeant JK, Bruce ML, Weissman MM: Factors associated with 1-year outcome of major depression in the community. *Arch Gen Psychiatry* 47:519–526, 1990.
6. Schulberg HC, Saul M, McClelland M, et al: Assessing depression in primary medical and psychiatric practices. *Arch Gen Psychiatry* 42:1164–1170, 1985.
7. Regier DA, Heirschfeld MA, Goodwin FK, et al: The NIMH depression awareness, recognition and treatment program: structure, aims and scientific basis. *Am J Psychiatry* 145:1351–1357, 1988.
8. Broadhead WE, Blazer DG, George LK, et al: Depression, disability days, and days lost from work in a prospective epidemiologic survey. *JAMA* 264:2524–2528, 1990.
9. Wells KB, Golding JM, Burnam MA: Psychiatric disorders in a sample of the general population with and without chronic mental conditions. *Am J Psychiatry* 145:976–981, 1988.
10. Wells KB: *Depression as a Tracer Condition for the National Study of Medical Care Outcomes—Background Review.* Santa Monica, Calif, Rand, 1985.
11. Wells KB, Stewart A, Hays RD, et al: The function and well-being of depressed patients: Results from the Medical Outcome Study. *JAMA* 262:914–919, 1989.
12. Greenberg PE, Stiglin LE, Finkelstein SN, et al: The economic burden of depression in 1990. *J Clin Psychiatry* 54:405–418, 1993.
13. NIMH Consensus Development Conference Statement: Mood disorders: Pharmacologic prevention of recurrences. *Am J Psychiatry* 142:469–476, 1985.
14. Wittchen H, Essau CA, Von Zerssen D, et al: Lifetime and six month prevalence of mental disorders in the Munich follow up study. *Eur Arch Psychiatry Clin Neurosci* 241:247–258, 1992.
15. Weissman, Bland R, Joyce PR, et al: Sex differences in rates of depression: Cross-national perspectives. *J Affective Disord* 29:77–84, 1993.
16. Coulehan JL, Schulberg HC, Block MR: The efficiency of depression questionnaires for case finding in primary medical care. *J Gen Intern Med* 4:542–547, 1989.
17. Rush AJ, Cain JW, Raese J, et al: Neurobiological bases for psychiatric disorders, in Rosenberg RN (ed): *Comprehensive Neurology.* New York, Raven Press, 1991, pp 555–603.
18. Korvin CC, Pearce RH, Stanley J: Admission screening: Clinical benefits. *Ann Intern Med* 83:197–203, 1975.
19. Dolan JG, Mushlin AI: Routine laboratory testing for medical disorders in psychiatric inpatients. *Arch Intern Med* 145:2085–2088, 1985.
20. Deykin EY, Levy JC, Wells V: Adolescent depression, alcohol and drug abuse. *Am J Public Health* 77:178–182, 1987.
21. Hasin DS, Grant BF, Endicott J: Lifetime psychiatric comorbidity in hospitalized alcoholics: Subject and familial correlates. *Int J Addict* 23:827–850, 1988.
22. Petty F: The depressed alcoholic: Clinical features and medical management. *Gen Hosp Psychiatry* 14:458–464.
23. Goodwin DW, Schulsinger F, Knopf J, et al: Psychopathology in adopted and

nonadopted daughters of alcoholics. *Arch Gen Psychiatry* 34:1005–1009, 1977.
24. Goodwin DW, Schulsinger F, Hermansen L, et al: Alcohol problems in adoptees raised apart from alcoholic biological parents. *Arch Gen Psychiatry* 28:238–243, 1973.
25. Vollrath M, Koch R, Angst J: The Zurich study: IX. Panic disorders and sporadic panic: Symptoms, diagnosis, prevalence, and overlap with depression. *Eur Arch Psychiatry Neurol Sci* 239:221–230, 1990.
26. Kanton W, Vitaliano P, Russo J, et al: Panic disorder: Epidemiology in primary care. *J Fam Pract* 23:233–239, 1986.
27. Coryell W, Endicott J, Andreasen NC, et al: Depression and panic attacks: The significance of overlaps reflected in follow-up and family study data. *Am J Psychiatry* 145:293–300, 1988.
28. Johnson J, Weissman MM, Klerman GL: Panic disorders, comorbidity, and suicide attempts. *Arch Gen Psychiatry* 47:805–880, 1990.
29. Bridges KW, Goldberg DP: Somatic presentation of DSM-III psychiatric disorders in primary care. *J Psychosom Res* 29:563–569, 1985.
30. Kanton W: The epidemiology of depression in medical care. *Int J Psychiatry Med* 17:93–112, 1987.
31. Magni G, Schifano F, de Leo D: Pain as a symptom in elderly depressed patients: Relationship to diagnostic subgroups. *Arch Psychiatry Neurol Sci* 235:143–145, 1985.
32. Dworkin SF, von Korff M, LeResche L: Multiple pains and psychiatric disturbances. *Arch Gen Psychiatry* 47:239–244, 1990.
33. Ionescu R, Popescu C: Personality disorders in students with depressive pathology. *Neurol Psychiatry (Bucur)* 27:45–55, 1989.
34. Black DW, Bell S, Hulbert J, et al: The importance of axis II in patients with major depression: A controlled study. *J Affective Disord* 14:115–222, 1988.
35. Pope HG, Jonas JM, Hudson JI, et al: The validity of DSM-III borderline personality disorder: A phenomenologic, family history, treatment response, and long term follow-up study. *Arch Gen Psychiatry* 30:23–30, 1983.
36. Weissman MM, Myers JK: Psychiatric disorders in a US urban community: The use of Research Diagnostic Criteria to a resurveyed community sample. *Acta Psychiatr Scand* 62:99–111, 1980.
37. Maj M, Veltro F, Pirozzi R, et al: Patterns of recurrence of illness after recovery from an episode of major depression: A prospective study. *Am J Psychiatry* 149:795–800, 1992.
38. DiMascio A, Weissman MM, Prusoff BA, et al: Differential symptom reduction by drugs and psychotherapy in acute depression. *Arch Gen Psychiatry* 36:1450–1456, 1979.
39. McDonnell-Douglas Employee Assistance Program Studies 1989 and 1990. St Louis, McDonnell-Douglas.
40. von Korff M, Ormel J, Kanton W, et al: Disability and depression among high utilizers of health care: A longitudinal analysis. *Arch Gen Psychiatry* 49:91–100, 1992.

Conservative Management of Shoulder Injuries in Athletes

Tom Hyde, D.A.C.B.S.P
Executive Director, American Chiropractic Association Council on Sports Injuries and Physical Fitness, Miami, Florida

Margaret Karg, D.C., C.C.S.P.
Private Practice, Belmont, Massachusetts

John Danchik, D.C., C.C.S.P.
Private Practice, Belmont, Massachusetts

Injuries to the shoulder in athletes vary from rotator cuff disorders to fractures, dislocations, overuse syndrome, and everything in between. This chapter will cover a brief anatomy of the shoulder, discuss the biomechanics involved in several sports, discuss the more common injuries seen in athletes, discuss orthopedic testing for differential diagnosis, and finish with conservative management approaches. Although shoulder injuries are very common in athletes involving over-hand activities such as tennis, pitching, and throwing, other sports may also contribute to disorders of the shoulder. These sports include hockey, football, golf, wrestling, skiing, rodeo, volleyball, and rugby.

The shoulder joint complex consists of several joints and serves to connect the upper extremity to the axial skeleton. To better understand the shoulder and injuries sustained, one must understand the anatomy and the biomechanics of movement within this complex structure. This better understanding of anatomy and biomechanics should aid the clinician in an attempt to prevent injuries by careful observation of the athlete in motion and reducing the recovery time by use of sound conservative management when surgery is not an option.

HISTORY

It is crucial to obtain a complete and thorough history from an athlete with any shoulder injury. The history should include the date of the injury and mechanism of injury, ability to abduct, adduct, and internally and externally rotate the shoulder. Is the pain secondary to trauma or insidious in onset? Is there a history of prior surgery or prior injury? Has the athlete suffered a recent infection? Is he or she currently taking any medication of any type for any condition? Does the medication taken reduce the symptoms? Does the pain awaken the athlete at night? Can the patient lie on the affected shoulder? Are there any signs of radiating pain into the extremity? Is the pain aggravated or relieved by activity? Is the pain increased with coughing, sneezing, and bowel movements? What are the age and sex of the patient? Is the athlete a novice, professional, or intermediate-level participant? Has the athlete altered the position he or she has previously been assigned to play or changed any other biomechanics related to that particular sport. Which activities aggravate and which activities reduce the athlete's symptoms? Has the athlete recently run a fever? Has the athlete undergone weight loss? Has the athlete noted any deformity, edema, or heat or cold sensations of the shoulder or upper extremity? A thorough family history and past history should also be taken.

ANATOMY

The shoulder joint complex is composed of four joints: the sternoclavicular, the acromioclavicular, the glenohumeral, and the scapulothoracic.[1-3] In contrast to the four joints just listed, Calliet[4] lists seven joints comprising the shoulder girdle. These joints consist of the glenohumeral, suprahumeral, acromioclavicular, scapulocostal, sternoclavicular, costosternal, and costovertebral. For the purposes of this chapter, the discussion is limited primarily to the first four joints listed.

STERNOCLAVICULAR JOINT

The sternoclavicular joint is composed of the medial end of the clavicle and its articulation with the sternum at the clavicular notch, together with the first costal cartilage. A fibrous capsule, along with several ligaments and the articular disk, complete the sternoclavicular joint. Ligaments of the sternoclavicular joint include the anterior sternoclavicular, posterior sternoclavicular, interclavicular, and costoclavicular. The articular disk is flat, almost circular, and lies between the sternum and clavicular surfaces attached superiorly to the superoposterior border of the clavicular articular surface and below to the first costocartilage near the sternal junction.[5]

ACROMIOCLAVICULAR JOINT

The acromioclavicular joint is composed of the lateral end of the clavicle and the acromion process of the scapula, the acromioclavicular ligament and the coracoclavicular and articular disk, and a fibrous capsule. The coracoclavicular ligament and coracoclavicular disk, connect the clavicle to the coracoid process on the scapula. This connection occurs via the trapezoid and conoid ligaments. Both the coracohumeral and acromioclavicular ligaments also attach to the conoid process.[5] The quadrangular space is occupied by the axillary nerve in the posterior humeral circumflex artery. This space is bordered superiorly by the teres minor, medially by the humerus, laterally by the lateral head of the triceps muscle, and inferiorly by the teres major muscle.

GLENOHUMERAL JOINT

Movement of the shoulder centers around the glenohumeral joint. This joint has also been referred to as the scapulohumeral joint or the shoulder joint.[4] The glenohumeral joint is incongruous. The glenoid portion of the joint is very shallow with a concave surface that articulates with the humeral head, therefore constituting an incongruous joint with dissimilar surfaces. This does not allow seating of the convex portion of the joint within the shallow concave glenoid articulation, ultimately resulting in an unstable joint.[4]

Glenoid Labrum

The glenoid labrum lines the rim of the glenoid cavity. It has most recently been described as a redundant fold of capsular tissue with a minimal fibrocartilizing component near its transitional zone.[1] The glenoid fossa faces slightly anterior, lateral, and superior. The long head of the biceps attaches to the superior aspect of the glenoid fossa, invaginating the capsule but not entering the synovial cavity. This configuration allows the biceps tendon to remain intracapsular but extrasynovial.[3]

Glenohumeral Ligaments

The three ligaments associated with the glenohumeral joint are superior, middle, and inferior ligaments. A foramen exists between the superior and middle glenohumeral ligaments known as the *Foramen of Weitbrecht*. The coracohumeral ligaments lie superior to connecting the coracoid process, the humerus. The glenohumeral joint depends on strong muscles rather than bones or supporting ligaments for its support. The rotator cuff group functions to pull the humerus down into the lower aspect of the glenoid cavity.[4]

SCAPULOTHORACIC ARTICULATION

Although not a true joint, the scapulothoracic articulation is characterized by riding of the scapular on the posterior surface of the thoracic cage.[1]

SHOULDER BURSAE

Several bursae are located around the shoulder. An inflammation of the bursa, resulting in bursitis, can severely limit the ability to abduct the arm. Bursae of interest around the shoulder include the subcoracoid, subacromial, subdeltoid, and scapulothoracic. Bursae are located in areas subject to friction. They may lie between tendon and bone, muscle and tendon, tendon and tendon, ligament and bone, or any other structures subject to stress and friction.

ROTATOR CUFF

The rotator cuff muscles consist of the supraspinatus, infraspinatus, teres minor, and subscapularis. These muscles serve as rotators. With combined action of the deltoid, they aid in abduction. The origin of the supraspinatus muscle is along the supraspinatus fossa of the scapula. It then traverses laterally, moving under the coracoacromial ligament to attach to the greater tuberosity of the humerus. The infraspinatous muscle has its origin from the infraspinatus fossa on the scapula directly below the spine of the scapula. It continues laterally, inserting just inferior to the attachment of the supraspinatus muscle on the greater tuberosity of the humerus. The teres minor muscle originates from the lateral border of the scapula. It extends laterally and superiorly, inserting on the humerus below the attachment of the infraspinatus muscle at the greater tuberosity. The tendons of these three muscles merge just before their insertion into the greater tuberosity, becoming a single tendon. The subscapularis muscle arises from the anterior surface of the scapula. It then passes laterally, attaching to the lesser tuberosity of the humerus. As the subscapularis passes anterior to the shoulder joint, it is separated from the neck of the scapula by bursae. Innervation of rotator cuff muscles arise from C-4 through C-6.[4]

Other muscles of the shoulder attached to the scapula consist of the trapezius, rhomboid major and minor, serratus anterior, and levator scapula. The trapezius muscle is a very large muscle, with a triangular shape arising along the superior nuchal line and the external occipital protuberance, as well as the spinous processes of C-1 through T-12. Portions of the upper fibers run obliquely downward, inserting along the distal third of the clavicle. The fibers of the middle trapezius originate from the lower cervical and upper thoracic region, extending laterally and inserting into the acromion. Fibers from the lower thoracic spinous processes extend laterally and upward, inserting into the spine of the scapula. The rhomboid muscles lie deep to the trapezius muscle. The rhomboid minor originates from the spinous processes of C-7 and along the thoracic vertebrae, as well as portions of the supraspinatus ligament. Its insertion is near the medial aspect of the spine of the scapula. The rhomboid major originates from the spinous processes of T-2 through T-5, as well as their supraspinatus ligaments, inserting just inferior to the rhomboid minor along the medial border of the scapula. The serratus anterior originates along the outer surface of the first eight ribs, following the curvature of the ribs, inserting along the medial aspect of the scapula on its costal surface. The superior muscle fibers of the serratus anterior attach to the medial border of the scapula, whereas the fibers of the lower portion insert into the inferior angle of the scapula. The levator scapula has its origin from the posterior tubercles of the transverse processes of C-1 through C-4, inserting into the superior angle of the scapula along its medial border. The trapezius muscle is innervated by the spinal accessory nerve, the rhomboids by the dorsal scapular nerve, the serratus anterior by the long thoracic nerve, and the levator scapulae by the cervical plexus with an occasional innervation from the dorsal scapular nerve.[3]

VASCULAR SUPPLY TO THE SHOULDER

The majority of blood supplied to the shoulder is via the axillary artery. The axillary artery then becomes the brachial artery, giving rise to the radial and ulnar arteries at its terminal branches. The six main branches of the axillary artery are the superior thoracic, thoracoacromioclavicular, lateral thoracic, subscapularis, and anterior and posterior circumflex humeral arteries. Numerous other small branches provide circulation to the various structures of the shoulder.

VENOUS SUPPLY

The primary venous supply to the shoulder complex is by the axillary, basilic, and cephalic veins.[3] Assessment of injuries of the shoulder must always include a vascular and neurological component.

BIOMECHANICS

Motion of the shoulder is said to take place in three patterns: elevation, internal rotation, and external rotation.[1] During movement of the shoulder, it is imperative that normal scapulohumeral rhythm is present. This movement also includes movement of the clavicle. From 0 to 30 degrees of scapular rotation, the clavicle also elevates 30 degrees. From 30 to 60 degrees of scapula rotation, the clavicle does not elevate further but rotates along its long axis so that the distal portion moves upward and forward because of the S shape of the clavicle.[6]

ELEVATION

Scapular elevation should occur through a 180-degree arc. However, it has been shown that men and women on average are limited to 167 and 171 degrees of elevation, respectively.[1]

INTERNAL AND EXTERNAL ROTATION

Both of these rotations occur mainly at the glenohumeral joint. The maximum mark of rotation is 180 degrees with the arm at the side, with 108 degrees of external rotation and 71 degrees of internal rotation. If the arm is abducted to 90 degrees, the maximum arc then becomes 120 degrees, with internal rotation comprising the greatest component.[1]

HORIZONTAL FLEXION AND EXTENSION

The maximum arch is 180 degrees for horizontal flexion and extension, 135 degrees for anterior flexion and extension, and 45 degrees for posterior flexion and extension.[1]

The downward and medial pull of the rotator tendons balanced with the upward and outward pull of the deltoid during shoulder elevation is known as *force couple*. The force couple causes the humeral head to turn about its axis, creating a gliding motion at its point of contact on the glenoid surface. The inability of any of the four rotator cuff muscles or deltoid muscle to function normally results in an abnormal relationship at the shoulder joint, ultimately leading to the potential of subluxation or other forms of shoulder impairment.[1]

ORTHOPEDIC EXAMINATION

The examination begins with visualization comparing structures bilaterally. Visualization should include bilateral comparison, noting any asymmetries, atrophy, or hypertrophy, sign of deformity, edema, coloration, sulcus sign, and signs of prior surgery. Next, range of motion should be examined, comparing the injured side with the noninjured side (Table

1). The shoulder ranges of motion are abduction, 170 to 180 degrees; forward flexion, 160 to 180 degrees; extension, 50 to 60 degrees; adduction, 50 to 75 degrees; internal rotation, 90 degrees; external rotation, 90 degrees; horizontal abduction/adduction, 130 degrees; circumduction, 200 degrees; lateral rotation, 80 to 90 degrees; and medial rotation, 60 to 100 degrees. Movement should also be examined via Appley's scratch test (Fig 1), whereby the patient attempts to touch the fingers of each hand behind his or her back, performing the movement necessary to comb the hair and reaching behind to place a wallet in the pocket with each hand.

Orthopedic testing of the shoulder can be divided into anterior shoulder instability, posterior shoulder instability, inferior and multidirectional shoulder instability, specific tests for specific joints, neurological testing, vascular testing, and assessment of joint play. Tests for anterior shoulder instability include the anterior drawer test of the shoulder, Protzman's test for anterior instability, anterior instability test, Rockwood test for anterior instability, Rowe test for anterior instability, fulcrum test, apprehension (crank) test for anterior shoulder dislocation, and cluck test. Tests for posterior shoulder instability include the posterior drawer test of the shoulder, Norwood stress test for posterior instability, jerk test, push-pull test, and posterior apprehension test. Tests for interior and multidirectional shoulder instability include the test for inferior shoulder instability (sulcus sign), Feagin test, and Rowe test for multidirectional instability. Tests for specific shoulder joints include the acromioclavicular shear test. Tests for muscles/tendon pathology include Yergason's test, Speed's test (biceps for straight arm test), drop arm test, Ludington's test,

TABLE 1.
Muscle Action at the Shoulder*

Abduction	Deltoid, supraspinatus (primary), infraspinatus, subscapularis, teres minor (secondary)
Adduction	Pectoralis major, latismus dorsi, teres major subscapularis
Forward elevation	Deltoid (anterior fibers), pectoralis major (clavicular fibers), coracobrachialis, extension deltoid (posterior fibers), teres major, teres minor, latismus dorsi, pectoralis major (sternocostal fibers), triceps (long head)
Horizontal abduction	Deltoid (posterior fibers), teres major, teres minor, infraspinatus
Horizontal adduction	Pectoralis major, deltoid (anterior fibers)
Medial rotation	Pectoralis major, deltoid (anterior fibers), latismus dorsi, teres major, subscapularis
Lateral rotation	Infraspinatus, deltoid (posterior fibers), teres minor
Elevation of scapula	Trapezius (upper fibers), levator scapula, rhomboid major, rhomboid minor

*From Magee DJ: *Assessment*. Philadelphia, WB Saunders, 1992. Used by permission.

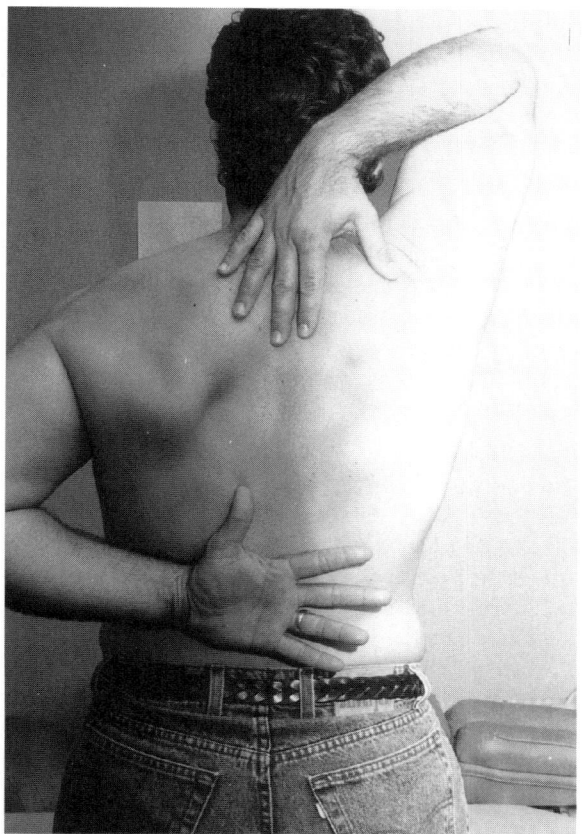

FIGURE 1.
Appley's scratch test.

supraspinatous test, impingement test, Hawkins-Kennedy impingement, Gilchrest sign, Lippman test, Heuter's sign, and pectoralis major contracture test. Neurological tests include upper limb tension (brachial plexus tension) test and Tinel's sign (at the shoulder). Vascular tests include Allen's test, Wright's test or maneuver, Adson's maneuver, Halstead's maneuver, costoclavicular syndrome test, Roos' test, and provocative elevation Test.

ANTERIOR SHOULDER INSTABILITY TEST

Anterior Drawer Test

The anterior drawer test is performed with the patient lying supine while the examiner places the hand of the affected shoulder in the examiner's axilla region, holding the patient's hand with the arm to relax the patient. The patient's scapula is stabilized with the examiner's opposite hand while pushing the spine and the scapula forward with the index and middle fingers. Counterpressure is exerted by the examiner's thumb on the coracoid process of the patient. The examiner's hand stabilizes the patient's hand around the patient's relaxed upper arm, drawing the humerus forward. The shoulder is tested in abduction between 80 and 120 degrees, forward flexed position between 0 and 20 degrees, and laterally rotated between 0 and 30 degrees. A click or apprehension on behalf of the patient may be present. This test is compared with the contralateral side. A positive test result indicates anterior instability.[7]

Protzman's Test for Anterior Stability
The examiner abducts the patient's arm to 90 degrees while in the seated position and supports the arm against the examiner's hip. The anterior aspect of the head of the humerus is palpated by the examiner with the opposite hand deep in the patient's axilla. The humeral head is then pushed anteriorly and inferiorly by the examiner. Pain indicates abnormal anterior inferior movement, positive for anterior instability.[7]

Anterior Instability Test
The examiner stands behind the patient's shoulder to be tested as the patient sits. The examiner's hand is placed over the shoulder so that the index finger is over the head of the anterior humerus and the middle finger is over the coracoid process. The thumb is placed over the posterior humerus while the other hand grasps the patient's wrist while carefully abducting and externally rotating the arm. The finger palpating the anterior humeral head may move forward with this movement. If this happens, the test result is positive for anterior instability, indicating a positive test result for anterior instability.[7]

Rockwood Test for Anterior Instability
The patient is seated with the examiner standing behind the involved shoulder. The examiner laterally rotates the shoulder while abducting the arm to 45 degrees. This procedure is repeated at 90 and 100 degrees. A positive test result represents anterior instability.[7]

Rowe Test for Anterior Instability
The Rowe test is performed with the patient supine, placing the hand of the involved side behind the head. While extending the athlete's arm, the examiner places a clenched fist over the posterior humeral head and pushes up. Apprehension is indicative of a positive test result.[7]

Fulcrum Test
The fulcrum test is performed with the athlete supine and the arm abducted to 90 degrees. The examiner then places one hand under the glenohumeral joint, using this as a fulcrum. The athlete's arm is extended and laterally rotated over the fulcrum. Apprehension indicates a positive test result for anterior instability (Fig 2).[7]

Apprehension (Crank) Test for Anterior Shoulder Dislocation
The athlete's shoulder is abducted 90 degrees and externally rotated by the examiner. Apprehension is indicative of a positive test result. This test should be performed slowly to avoid the possibility of dislocating the shoulder. In external rotation, once a position of apprehension is noted, the examiner may be able to apply posterior stress to the arm (relocation test), causing the athlete to lose apprehension, allowing further external rotation before apprehension returns.[7]

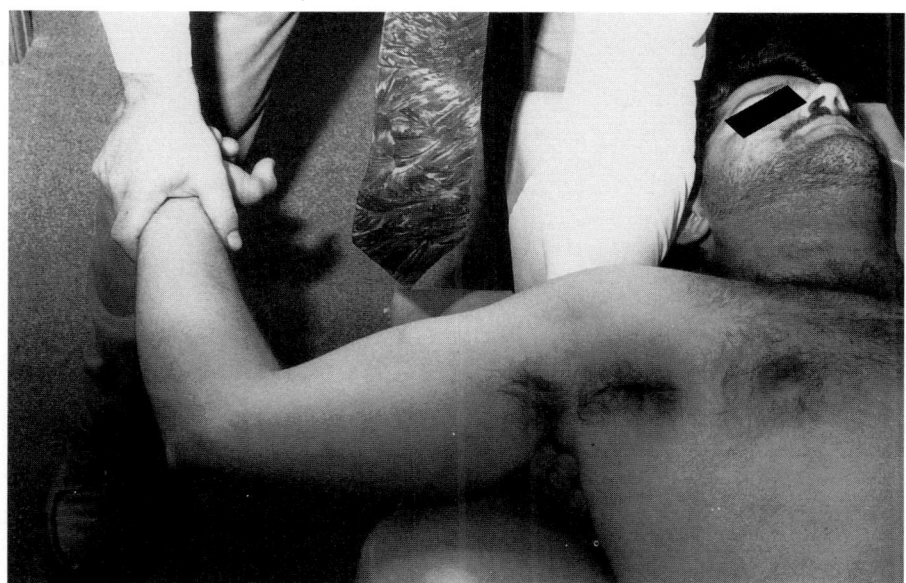

FIGURE 2.
Fulcrum test.

Clunk Test
The clunk test is used to locate a tear of the glenoid labrum. The test is performed with the athlete lying supine while the examiner places one hand on the posterior aspect of the shoulder directly over the humeral head. The examiner's opposite hand holds the humerus at the elbow. The arm is then fully abducted over the athlete's head. The humeral head is pushed anteriorly and simultaneously externally rotated. A clunk or grinding noise constitutes a positive test result. The test may also cause apprehension indicative of anterior instability (Fig 3).

POSTERIOR SHOULDER INSTABILITY TESTS

Posterior Drawer Test
The posterior drawer test is performed with the athlete lying supine while the examiner grasps the proximal forearm of the athlete in one hand, flexing the elbow to 120 degrees and the shoulder to 80 to 120 degrees of abduction, coupled with 20 to 30 degrees of forward flexion. The examiner's opposite hand stabilizes the scapula by placing the index and middle fingers on the spine of the scapula and thumb on the coracoid process. The forearm is then internally rotated and forward, flexed 60 to 80 degrees, while the thumb of the other hand is removed from the coracoid process and the head of the humerus is pushed posteriorly. Typically this test is pain free; however, the patient may exhibit apprehension, indicating posterior instability.[7]

Norwood Stress Test for Posterior Instability
The Norwood stress test is performed with the athlete supine and the shoulder abducted between 60 and 100 degrees. The arm is then exter-

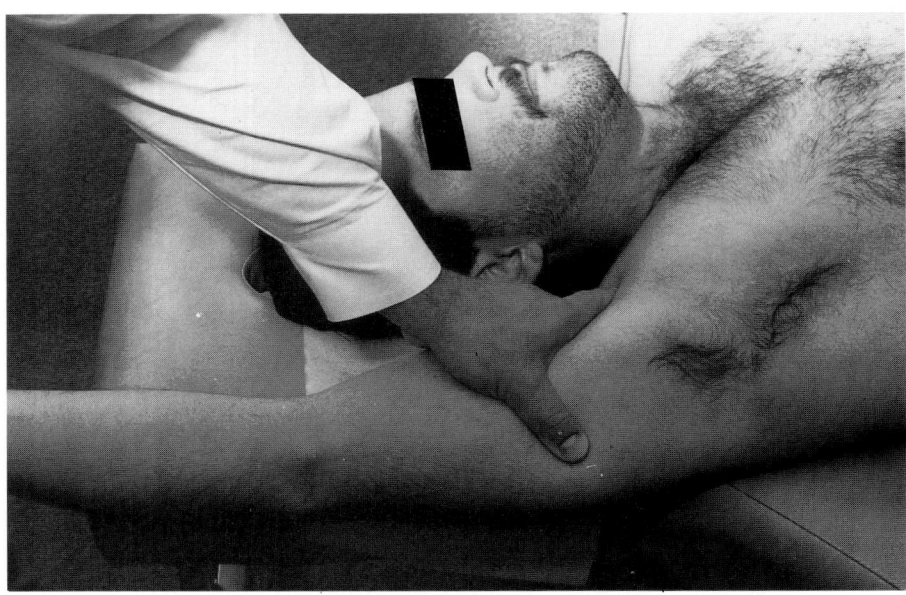

FIGURE 3.
Clunk test.

nally rotated to 90 degrees with the elbow flexed to 90 degrees with the arm horizontal. The scapula is stabilized with one hand while the posterior humeral head is palpated with the fingers and the upper limb is stabilized with the opposite hand by holding the forearm and elbow at the elbow. The arm is then brought into forward flexion with the elbow being pushed posteriorly along the long axis of the humerus. A positive test result is indicated by a posterior slipping of the humeral head in relation to the glenoid. Again, care should be taken not to sublux or dislocate the athlete on testing. A clicking may be present during this testing procedure.[7]

Jerk Test

The jerk test result is positive for recurrent posterior instability and is performed with the athlete sitting, the shoulder internally rotated and forward flexed 90 degrees. The athlete's elbow is held by the examiner with axillary loading of the humerus in a proximal direction. Maintaining axial loading, the examiner then moves the arm horizontally across the body. As this maneuver proceeds, a sudden jerk may be felt as the humeral subluxes from the back of the glenoid. As the arm is returned back to its original position at 90 degrees, the head of the humerus may reduce, producing a second jerk.[7]

Push Pull Test

The push pull test result is positive for posterior instability and is performed with the athlete supine. The athlete's arm is held at the wrist while the shoulder is abducted to 90 degrees, followed by forward flexion of 30 degrees. The examiner then places the other hand over the humerus near the humeral head. When the examiner pushes up on the arm at the wrist and simultaneously pushes down on the humerus with the other hand, 50% posterior translation is possible. If greater than 50% translation exists or the patient becomes apprehensive, the test result is positive.[7]

Posterior Apprehension Test
The posterior apprehension test result is positive for posterior dislocation and is performed by having the athlete's shoulder forward flexed and internally rotated by the examiner. The posterior force is applied to the athlete's elbow, with a positive result indicated by a look of apprehension. The test may also be performed with the shoulder at 90 degrees abduction while the examiner palpates the head of the humerus with one hand while the other hand applies a posterior force to the humeral head. Greater than 50% posterior movement is indicative of posterior instability. A clunk may be heard when this maneuver is performed.[7]

OTHER TESTS

Sulcus Sign
This test result is positive for inferior instability and is performed by having the athlete standing with the arm to be tested at the athlete's side. The athlete's forearm below the elbow is held by the examiner, and the arm is pulled distally.[7] The presence of an indentation just inferior to the glenohumeral joint connotes a positive sulcus sign.

Feagin Test
The Feagin test result is positive for anteroinferior instability and is performed with the athlete standing, shoulder abducted by 90 degrees. The elbow is extended resting on top of the examiner's shoulder. The examiner then clasps both hands over the midhumerus as the humerus is pushed down and forward. Apprehension of the patient to perform this test represents a positive test result (Fig 4).[7]

Rowe Test for Multidirectional Instability
The Rowe test may be used to determine anterior and posterior instability. It is performed by having the athlete stand with 45 degrees of forward flexion at the waist. The arms hang in a relaxed fashion while the examiner places one hand over the shoulder with the index and middle finger placed over the anterior aspect of the humeral head while the thumb is placed over the posterior aspect of the humeral head. At this point the examiner pulls the arm slightly down. The humeral head is then pushed anterior with the thumb while the arm is extended to 20 to 30 degrees, testing for anterior instability. The humeral head is pushed posteriorly with the index and middle fingers while the arm is flexed at 20 to 30 degrees, testing for posterior instability. With increased traction a sulcus sign may be present.[7]

Acromioclavicular Shear Test
The acromioclavicular shear test result is positive for acromioclavicular abnormalities and is performed with the athlete sitting. The examiner then cups the hands over the deltoid muscle with one hand on the clavicle and one hand on the spine and scapula and squeezes the heels of the

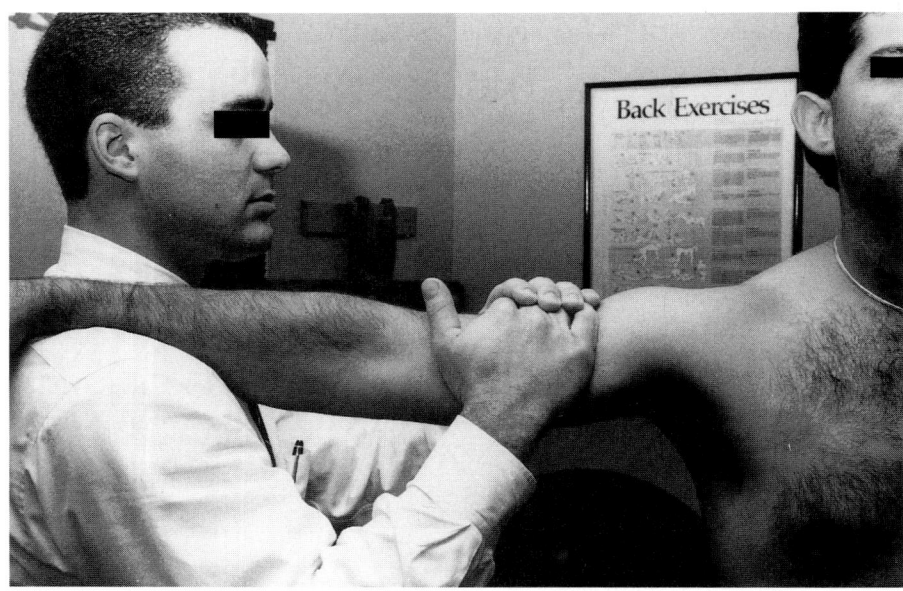

FIGURE 4.
Feagin test.

hands together. Pain or abnormal movement felt in the acromioclavicular joint represents a positive test result.[7]

Yergason's Test

Yergason's test is indicative of biceps tendinitis and is performed with the patient's elbow flexed to 90 degrees and stabilized against the body. The forearm is pronated while the examiner resists supination and the athlete laterally rotates the arm against resistance.[7]

Speed's Test

Speed's test result is positive for biceps tendinitis and is performed with the examiner resisting shoulder forward flexion with the athlete's forearm supinated with the arm in a completely extended position. Pain and tenderness in the bicipital groove represents a positive test result.[7]

Drop Arm Test

The drop arm test result is positive for tearing of the rotator cuff complex and is performed with the examiner abducting the athlete's shoulder 90 degrees, then slowly lowering the arm to the side. Should there be severe pain or if the patient is unable to return the arm to the side, the test result is positive (Fig 5).[7]

Ludington's Test

A Ludington's test positive test result is indicative of a rupture of the long head of the biceps tendon and is performed with the patient clasping both hands on top of the head. The patient then alternates, contraction and relax action of each bicep muscle. During this procedure the examiner palpates the biceps tendon. The tendon will not be felt on the side of rupture during this procedure (Fig 6).[7]

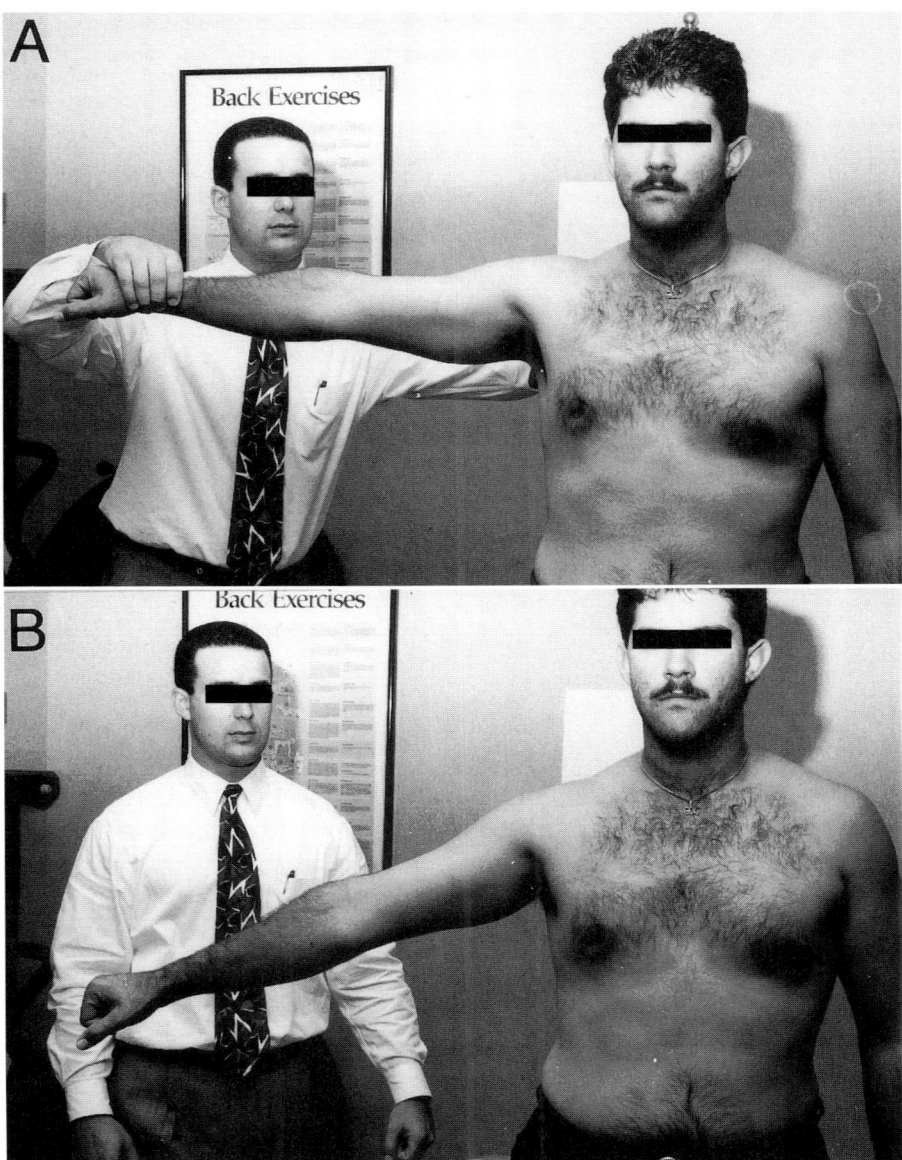

FIGURE 5.
Drop arm test.

Supraspinatus Test
The supraspinatus test result is positive for a tear in the supraspinatus tendon/muscle or neuropathy of the subsuprascapular nerve and is performed with the athlete's shoulder abducted 90 degrees with 0 rotation. The athlete then attempts to abduct the arm against resistance. At this point the shoulder is then medially rotated, angled forward at 30 degrees with the athlete's thumbs pointing toward the floor. An inability to perform this abducted maneuver or weakness represents a positive test result (Fig 7).[7]

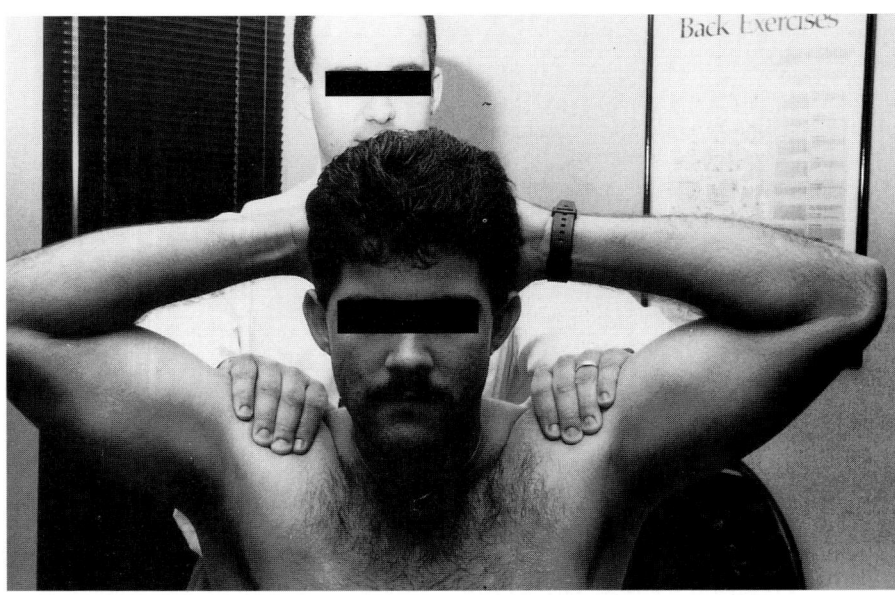

FIGURE 6.
Ludington's test.

Impingement Test

The impingement test result is positive for overuse injuries of the supraspinatus muscle biceps tendon and subdeltoid brusa and its extensions. This test is performed with the athlete's arm forcefully elevated through forward flexion and abduction. This procedure causes a jamming

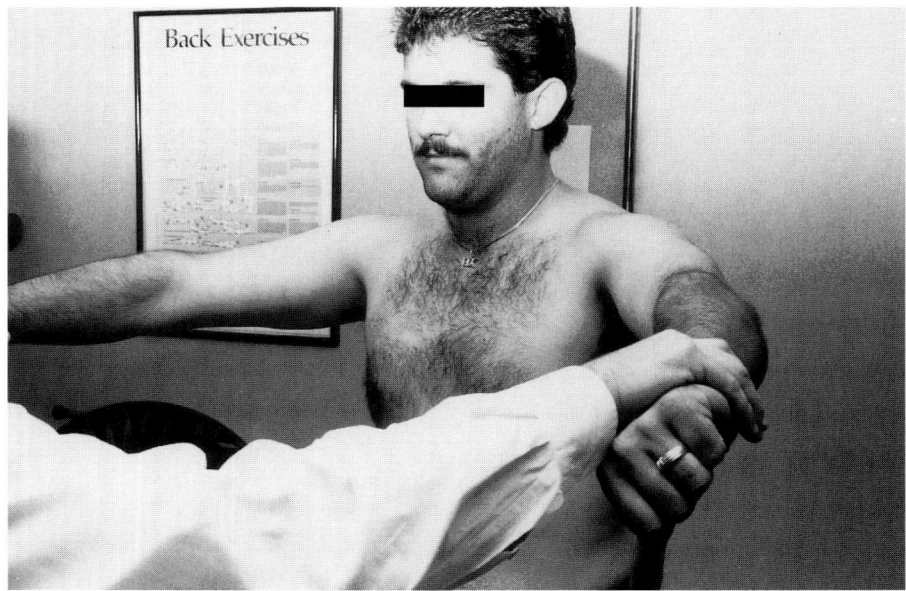

FIGURE 7.
Supraspinatus test.

of the greater tuberosity against the anteroinferior acromion surface. Pain on performing this maneuver indicates a positive test result.[7]

Hawkins-Kennedy Impingement Test
The Hawkins-Kennedy impingement test result is positive for supraspinatus tendinitis and is performed with the athlete standing and the examiner forward flexes the arm to 90 degrees, then forcefully internally rotates the shoulder. The supraspinatus tendon is forced against the anterior surface of the coracoacromial ligament, producing pain indicative of a positive test result.[7]

Gilchrest Sign
The Gilchrest sign test result is positive for bicipital tendinitis and is performed with the athlete standing while lifting a 2- to 3-kg weight overhead. The arm is then fully externally rotated and lowered to the side in the coronal plane. Pain located in the bicipital groove indicates a positive test result. An audible snap or pain may occur in the abducted position between 90 and 100 degrees.[7]

Lippman Test
The Lippman test result is positive for bicipital tendinitis and is performed with the athlete sitting or standing as the examiner holds the arm flexed to 90 degrees with one hand. The opposite hand palpates the biceps tendon 7 to 8 cm below the glenohumeral joint as the biceps tendon is moved from side to side within its groove. Sharp pain is indicative of a positive test result.[7]

Heuter's Sign
Heuter's sign is positive for biceps rupture and is performed by having the athlete flex the elbow as resistance is applied to the arm as it is pronated. The biceps tendon attempts to aid the brachialis muscle flex the elbow. Some supination will occur indicative of biceps tendon rupture.[7]

Pectoralis Major Contracture Test
A positive test result is indicative of a torn pectoralis major muscle and is performed with the athlete lying supine, clasping the hands together behind the head. The athlete then attempts to lower the arms, touching the examining table. If the athlete is unable to touch the table with his or her arms when they are lowered, a positive test result is indicated (Fig 8).[7]

Upper Limb Tension Test
This procedure tests the integrity of the median nerve and C-5 through C-7 nerve roots. It is performed with the athlete lying supine while the examiner abducts and laterally rotates the athlete's arm behind the acromial plane. When the shoulder girdle is pressed, the elbow is passively extended with the wrist in extension and the forearm in supination. A positive test result represents an aching or stretching sensation localized within the cubital fossa or the creation of tingling in the thumb and first three fingers. This represents tension of the dura mater within the cervical spine and tension of the median nerve (Fig 9).[7]

Tinel's Sign
Tinel's sign test result is positive for nerve root damage. The test is performed by having the examiner tap the scalene triangle over the area of

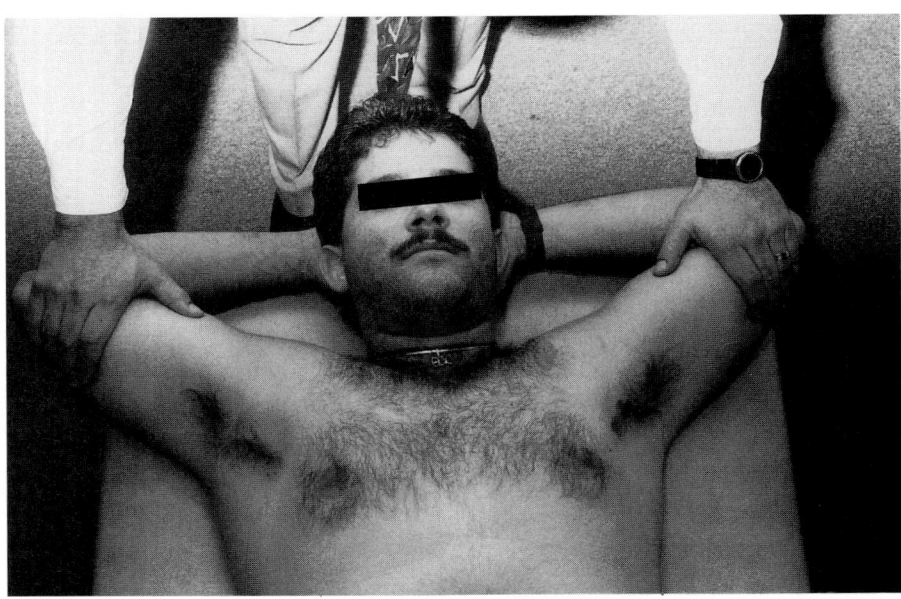

FIGURE 8.
Pectoralis major contracture test.

the brachial plexus just superior to the clavicle. The test is positive when a tingling sensation is created by this maneuver.[7]

Allen's Test
Allen's test result is positive for thoracic outlet syndrome and is performed with the patient's elbow flexed to 90 degrees as the shoulder is extended horizontally and laterally rotated. During this procedure the examiner palpates the radial pulse. While performing the maneuver, the patient rotates the head to the opposite side. Disappearance of the pulse during this procedure is indicative of a positive test result (Fig 10).[7]

Wright's Test or Maneuver
Wright's test result is positive for thoracic outlet syndrome and is performed with the athlete hyperabducting the arm overhead with the elbow and arm in the coronal plane. The test may also be performed by having the athlete take a breath and hold it or by having the athlete extend or rotate the head. A decrease in pulse is indicative of a positive test result.[7]

Adson's Maneuver
Adson's maneuver is positive for thoracic outlet syndrome and is performed by having the athlete rotate the head to the side being tested as the examiner palpates the radial pulse. The head is then extended as the examiner laterally rotates and extends the shoulder. Disappearance of the pulse as the athlete takes a deep breath and holds it represents a positive test result (Fig 11).[7]

Halstead's Maneuver
Halstead's maneuver is positive for thoracic outlet syndrome and is performed with the examiner applying a downward traction to the involved

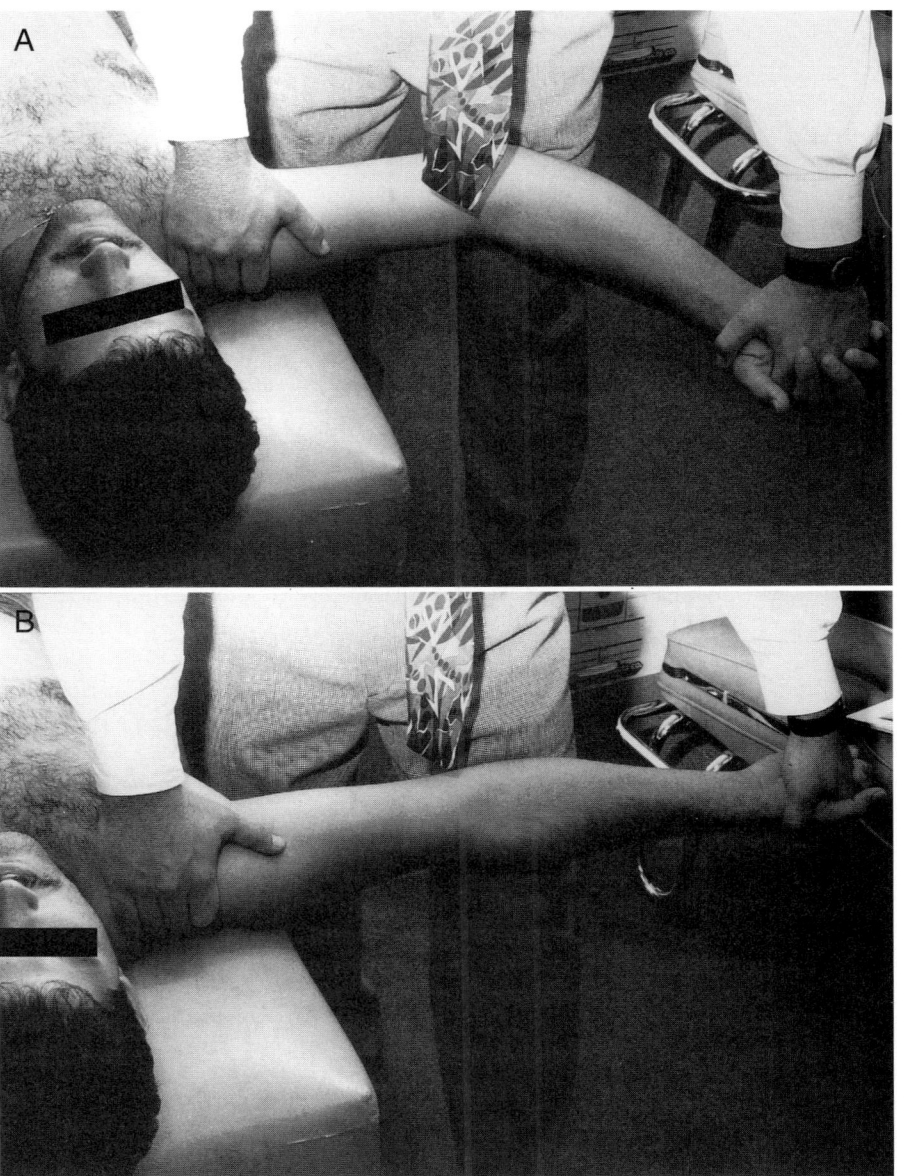

FIGURE 9.
Upper limb tension test.

extremity as the radial pulse is palpated. The athlete's neck is hyperextended with the head rotated to the opposite side. The absence of a radial pulse is indicative of a positive test result (Fig 12).[7]

Costoclavicular Test

The costoclavicular test result is positive for thoracic outlet syndrome and is performed by having the examiner draw the athlete's shoulder down and back while palpating the radial pulse. This simulates pain often ex-

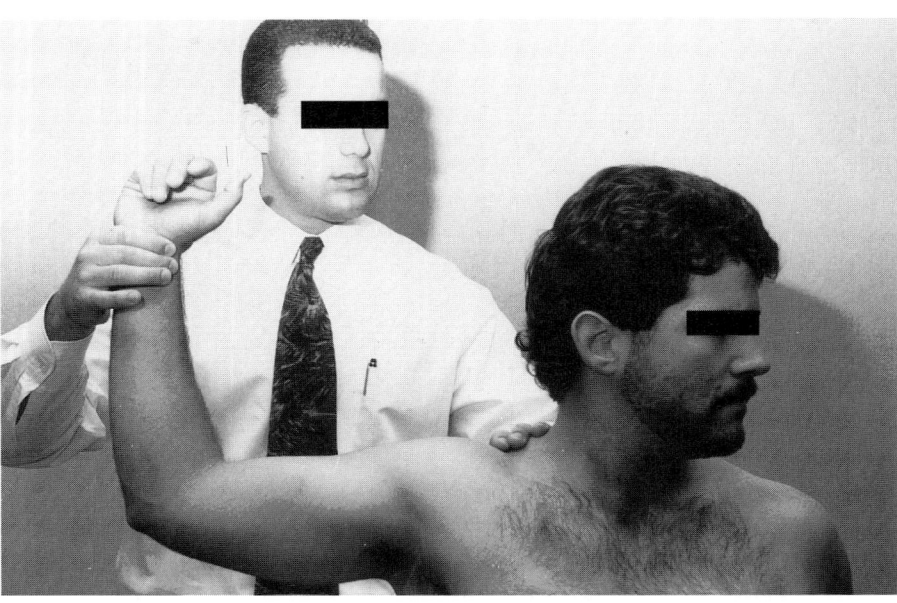

FIGURE 10.
Allen's maneuver.

perienced by athletes wearing backpacks. Absence of the radial pulse is indicative of a positive test result.[7]

Roos' Test
Roos' test result is positive for thoracic outlet syndrome and is performed by having the athlete stand while abducting the arms to 90 degrees with

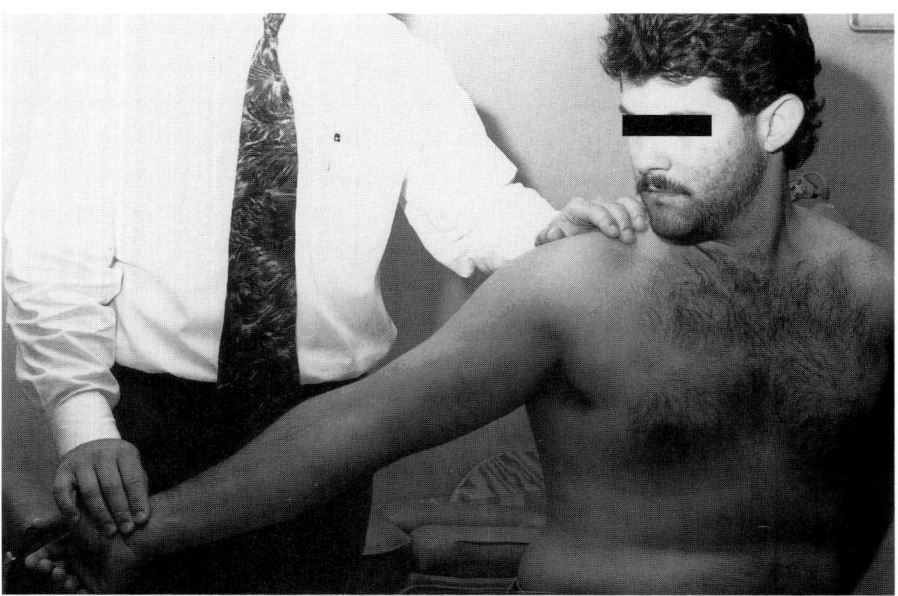

FIGURE 11.
Adson's maneuver.

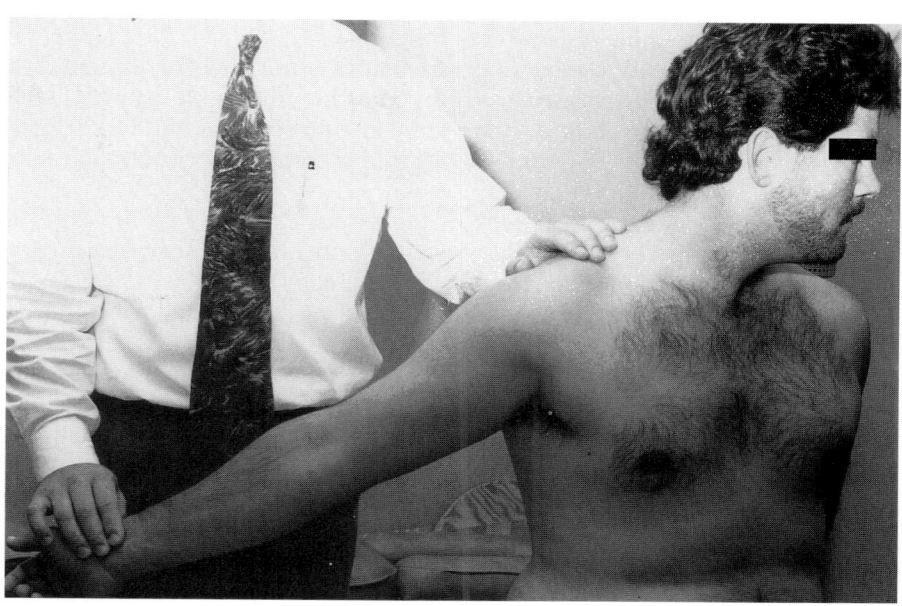

FIGURE 12.
Halstead's maneuver.

external rotation of the shoulder and the elbows flexed to 90 degrees. This position is maintained for a minimum of 3 minutes while the athlete continually opens and closes the hands slowly. An inability to maintain the arms in the starting position for a full 3 minutes while the patient complains of heaviness of the arm or numbness and tingling in the hand is indicative of a positive test result (Fig 13).[7]

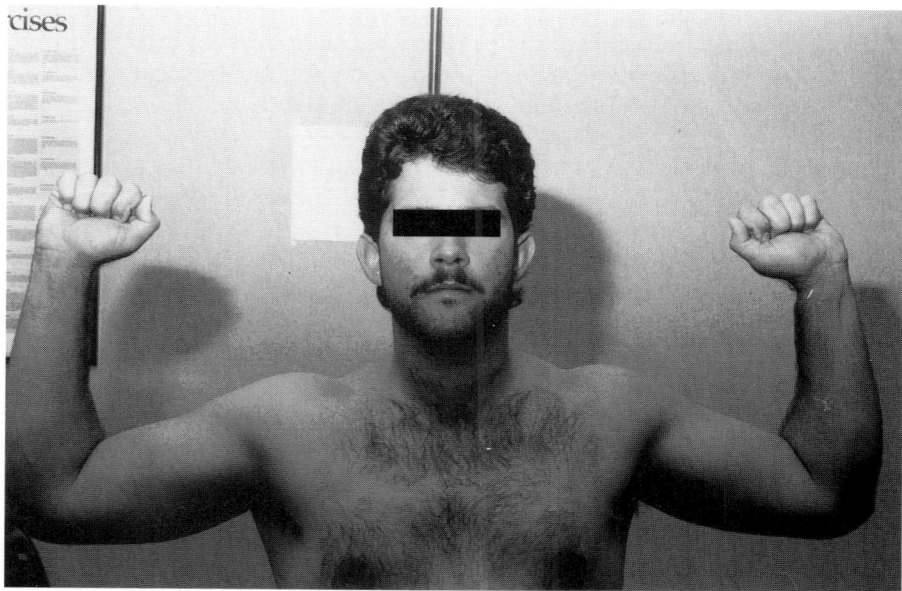

FIGURE 13.
Roos' test.

Provocative Elevation Test

The provocative elevation test result is positive for thoracic outlet syndrome and is performed by having the athlete elevate both arms above horizontal while rapidly opening and closing the hands 15 times. A positive test result is noted if the athlete complains of fatigue, cramping, or tingling.[7]

All reflexes are tested in the upper extremity to include the biceps, triceps, and brachioradalis routinely. In addition, the pectoralis major clavicular and sternoclavicular portions may be tested. These test the cervical nerve roots C-5 through T-1. The pectoralis major clavicular portion tests C-5 to C-6, where the sternocostal portion tests C-7 to C-8 and in some cases fibers from T-1. The biceps test C-5 to C-6 whereas the triceps test C-7 to C-8. The muscles of the upper extremity should also be tested to include biceps, triceps, deltoid, supraspinatus, infraspinatus, terres minor, terres major, subscapularis, trapezius, levator scapulae, pectoralis major, pectoralis minor, rhomboid major, and rhomboid minor. The strength and symmetry of each muscle group is tested via manual muscle testing. In addition, visualization and palpation of each muscle group should be performed by the examiner. Range of motion to include active, passive, and resisted should follow strength evaluation. Palpation of all bony landmarks should be a routine part of the physical examination. Bony structures palpated include the sternoclavicular joint, clavicle, acromioclavicular joint, humerus, coracoid process, scapula, and ribs.[8]

During the examination a number of symptoms often lead the examiner in establishing a diagnostic consideration. An arm hanging to the side may be indicative of shoulder dislocation, acromioclavicular joint separation, or fracture. Pain with burning or abnormal sensation may be indicative of brachial plexus lesions, shoulder dislocation, or fracture. Inability to abduct or decreased ability to move the arm with weakness of the associated shoulder muscles may be indicative of rotator cuff tear, biceps subluxation, dislocation, or fracture. Note that pain in the shoulder may be referred from the thoracic region, cervical region, or viscera. Tumors may also refer pain to the shoulder.

ACROMIOCLAVICULAR JOINT INJURIES

When injuries to any part of the body are assessed, understanding the mechanism of injury will aid in making a correct diagnosis. Injuries occurring to the acromioclavicular joint include separation, dislocation, sprains, and fractures. Injuries to the acromioclavicular joint can occur in many sports from horseback riding to tennis. Acromioclavicular dislocations typically occur when athletes land on the front of the shoulder, driving the acromion downward; sustain a blow from behind with the ipsilateral arm fixed on the ground, driving the clavicle forward and away from the acromion; or fall on an outstretched hand or elbow, creating a backward force on the acromion.[9]

Dislocations of the acromioclavicular joint according to a report published from Massachusetts General Hospital in Boston by E. F. Cave state that 12% of shoulder dislocations noted at the shoulder involve the acromioclavicular joint. As many as seven different types of dislocations have been described in the literature. Originally a three-level grading system was developed by Allman, which was later modified by Rockwood and Young. Type I sprains involve a partial disruption of acromioclavicular ligament and capsule. Laxity in the acromioclavicular joint is absent, and the examiner notes point tenderness over the joint. Type II sprains consist of a ruptured acromioclavicular ligament and capsule with incomplete injury to the coracoclavicular ligament, resulting in minimal acromioclavicular joint subluxation. Type III separations exhibit complete tearing of the acromioclavicular and coracoclavicular ligaments, possible deltoid-trapezius fascial injury, and dislocation of the acromioclavicular joint. Deformity is obvious, and the distal end of the clavicle is easy to palpate. A coracoclavicular interval increase of more than 25% indicates a type III separation. Type IV dislocations consist of a displaced clavicle that penetrates posteriorly into and through the trapezius muscle. The examiner can detect this condition by viewing the patient's shoulder from above. Type V dislocations are simply severe type II injuries with a greater coracoclavicular interval—100% to 300% more than an uninjured shoulder. Type VI injuries are rare, but whey they occur, the patient's clavicle is displaced inferior to the coracoid process. Rowe describes another acromioclavicular injury, type VII, in which a bifold or dislocation of the clavicle occurs with ruptures of the sternoclavicular and coracoclavicular ligaments (Fig 14).[9] Acromioclavicular joint separation or dislocation may appear cosmetically unacceptable to the athlete. Both surgical and nonsurgical approaches are used in the treatment of this disorder.

The injured athlete typically has severe pain localized over the acromioclavicular joint. Depending on the extent of structures damaged, ad-

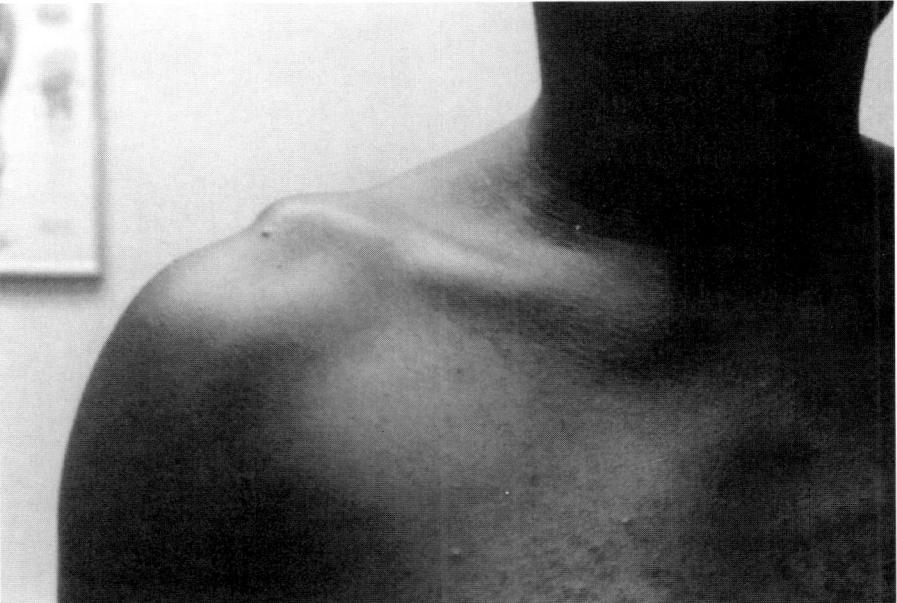

FIGURE 14.
Acromioclavicular joint with third-degree sprain. This athlete fell while riding a bicycle, landing on the lateral aspect of the shoulder.

ditional pain may be elicited along the clavicle and conoid process. Range of motion is typically decreased, especially in sprains greater than grade 1. Some elevation of the clavicle may be seen in second-degree sprains, but third-degree sprains make the deformity obvious. Edema typically is present in third-degree sprains but may be minimal to limited in first- and second-degree sprains.

RADIOGRAPHIC STUDIES

Radiographic studies should include the anteroposterior typically. Weights are not required for third-degree separations or dislocations, but they may be necessary in grade 1 or 2 sprains (Figs 15 and 16).

TREATMENT

Grade 1 injuries usually heal within a few days to several weeks, whereas grade 2 injuries require treatment for several weeks, typically 2 to 4. Grade 3 injuries treated conservatively may require treatment for several months or longer. Treatment can be surgical or nonsurgical, depending on the severity of the injury. First-degree sprains may be treated with ice and rest with pain-free range of motion as tolerated by the athlete. Rehabilitative exercises may be instituted, including range of motion, followed by the use of surgical tubing, progressing into isokinetic and free weight maneuvers. A second-degree sprain or separation is treated as before, but the lesion may take a longer period to recover. The athlete is often placed in a Kenny Howard sling advocated by some authors.[8] With a third-degree sprain treatment involves the use of a Kenny Howard sling for 6 to 8 weeks. Treatment of third-degree acromioclavicular separations should be

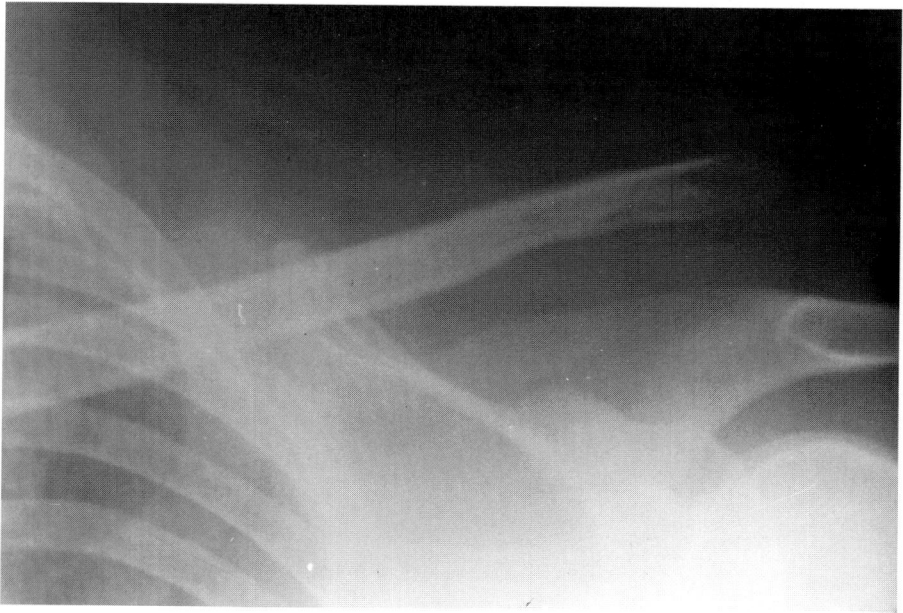

FIGURE 15.

Acromioclavicular joint separation. (Courtesy of Dr. Norman Kettner.)

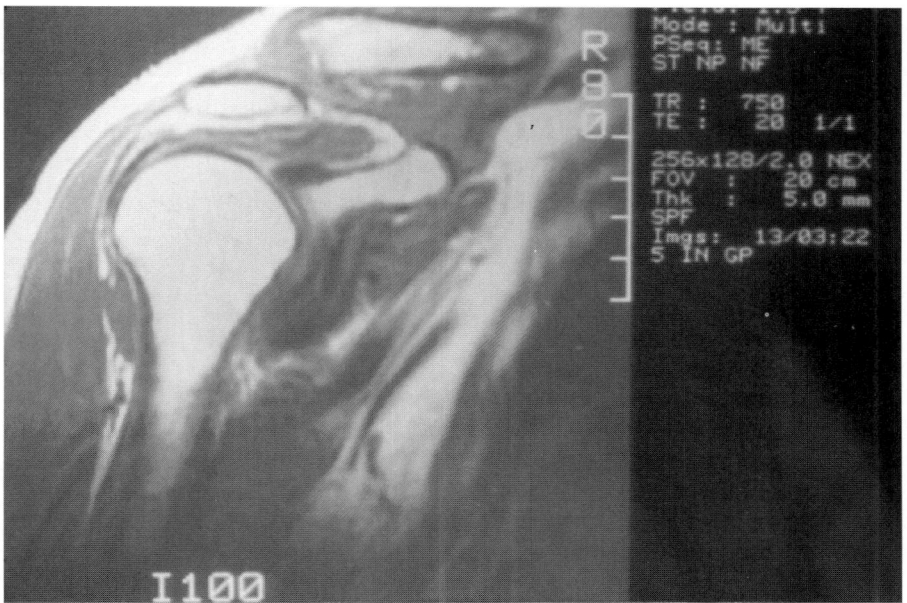

FIGURE 16.
MRI revealing acromioclavicular joint separation. (Courtesy of Dr. Norman Kettner.)

a joint decision by the athlete and physician. Not all third-degree sprains require surgery. This should depend on a number of factors, including level of competition by the athlete, dominant vs. nondominant shoulder, pain, and other complicating factors such as fracture, motivation, and willingness to undergo rehabilitation by the athlete. Bach et al.[9] indicate that the literature suggests that patients who are treated nonsurgically have equal if not greater strength than patients who undergo surgical treatment. Their review of nine studies revealed that the researchers who compared surgical and nonsurgical methods found no better results with surgery, with some suggesting that closed treatment was superior to surgical intervention.[9]

In a study of 29 male patients with complete acromioclavicular separations, MacDonald et al.[10] compared the results of 10 patients who had undergone surgical care with 10 who were treated nonsurgically. An initial 10 male patients were used as controls, and all were tested for comparison of strength between the dominant and nondominant limbs. The Kin-Com isokinetic dynamometer was used for muscle testing, whereas shoulder flexibility was tested using the Leighton Flexometer. Grip test was tested with a standard grip dynamometer. No significant differences were found between the nonsurgical and surgical groups in terms of strength and flexibility; however, the nonsurgical treated group was statistically superior to the surgical group in several areas. These included eccentric abduction at fast speeds, concentric external rotation at slow speeds, eccentric external rotation at fast speeds, eccentric abduction at slow speeds, and flexibility in external rotation. These findings suggested that nonsurgical treatment of a third-degree acromioclavicular separation was superior in restoring normal shoulder function in the first year after injury.[10] Conservative treatment should begin with range of motion in a pain-free state where pain-free range of motion is tolerated by the athlete. Surgical tubing exercises may follow as tolerated. Treatment using surgical tubing has been described by several authors. Christiansen[11] advocates four phases.

Phase 1 uses limited arc movement with a slow motion, slow pace, short range exercise. Phase 2 is a fast pace, short range to the point of fatigue. Phase 3 is a slow pace, full range exercise, and phase 4 is a fast pace, full range exercise. These exercises are to be done bilaterally, proceeding from minimal to maximal joint range of motion, always exercising caution and movement only into pain-free ranges of motion. Flexion, extension, abduction, adduction, horizontal abduction, and horizontal adduction with internal and external rotation are performed by the athlete.[11] Surgical tubing is available in various strengths, and the strength of the tubing used is determined by several factors: (1) the severity of the injury, (2) the stage of rehabilitation, (3) the size of the athlete, and (4) the overall strength of the athlete. Each exercise is performed for 1 minute. Roy and Irvine (personal communication) advocate full pain-free motion with a speed the athlete can tolerate, coupled with a pain-free range of motion, using each range of motion for 1 minute, again using the tubing bilaterally. Surgical tubing may also be used very similarly to weight lifting, prescribing for the athlete sets of repetitions ranging from three to five sets for each muscle group. The number of repetitions may range from a low of 10 to as many as 50, depending on the athlete's capabilities and the strength of the tubing used. Shoulder flexibility and maintenance of strength are crucial during the rehabilitation program. The athlete may progress from initial range of motion exercises, followed by tubing, and then into isotonic exercises with free weights or various machines. Exercises for the shoulder can include bench press, military press, deltoid raises (both lateral and forward), shrugs, curls, behind the neck presses, shoulder presses, and abduction and adduction exercises, as well as isolated exercises for the supraspinatus muscles. These include raises with the shoulder abducted, with the shoulder placed at 45 degrees, and the thumb down, internal and external rotation with the patient seated or supine. These may also be performed with the patient standing. During the latter stages of rehabilitation or in an athlete who wishes to further strengthen the shoulder, plyometrics may be introduced. Isometric exercises are typically recommended during the beginning stages of rehabilitation and may persist throughout the entire rehabilitative program.

ROTATOR CUFF INJURIES

Injuries to the rotator cuff are common in athletes using overhead motions and are more readily seen in pitchers, quarterbacks, tennis players, and swimmers. At the present time the exact mechanism of injuries to the rotator cuff is not fully understood. Angiographic studies have shown that the supraspinatus has a consistent avascular region near its tendinous insertion where tears to the tendon typically occur.[12] Hannaford[13] recognizes three common causes: sports-specific overuse (e.g., swimmer's shoulder); acute strains or tears, as experienced in contact sports; and coincidental degenerative lesions as seen in older patients. Most throwing injuries commonly seen during training are related to overuse of the rotator cuff. However, unrecognized instability, or silent subluxation, is becoming more apparent as our diagnostic ability and awareness improves.[14] The spectrum of rotator cuff disease begins with rotator cuff inflammation (stage 1), progresses to tendinitis (stage 2), and partial or full-thickness tears (stage 3).[15] Rotator cuff tendinitis or the pathology of rotator cuff tendinitis has been listed as:

I. Activity overuse
   A. Multiple repetitions
   B. Muscle tendon imbalances
      1. Strength
      2. Flexibility
   C. Glenohumeral instability (secondary impingement)
      1. Upward humeral migration
      2. Anterosuperior subluxation
II. Age
   A. Physiological
   B. Chronological
III. Heredity
   A. Mesenchymal syndrome (predisposition to tendinitis)
   B. Mechanical (primary impingement)
   C. Systemic factors (gout, estrogen, deficiency)[16]

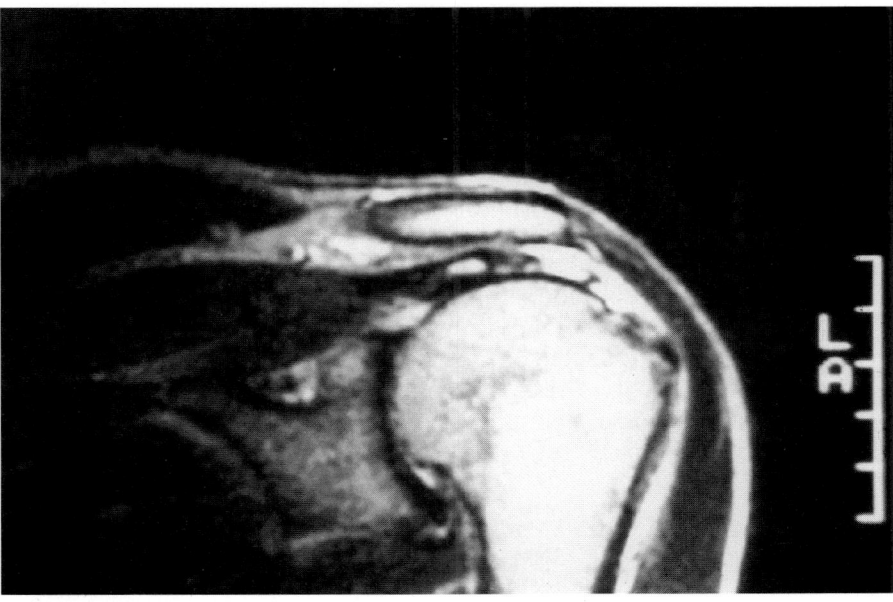

FIGURE 17.
T_1-weighted image showing tear of the supraspinatus tendon with accompanying exudate. (Courtesy of Dr. Norman Kettner.)

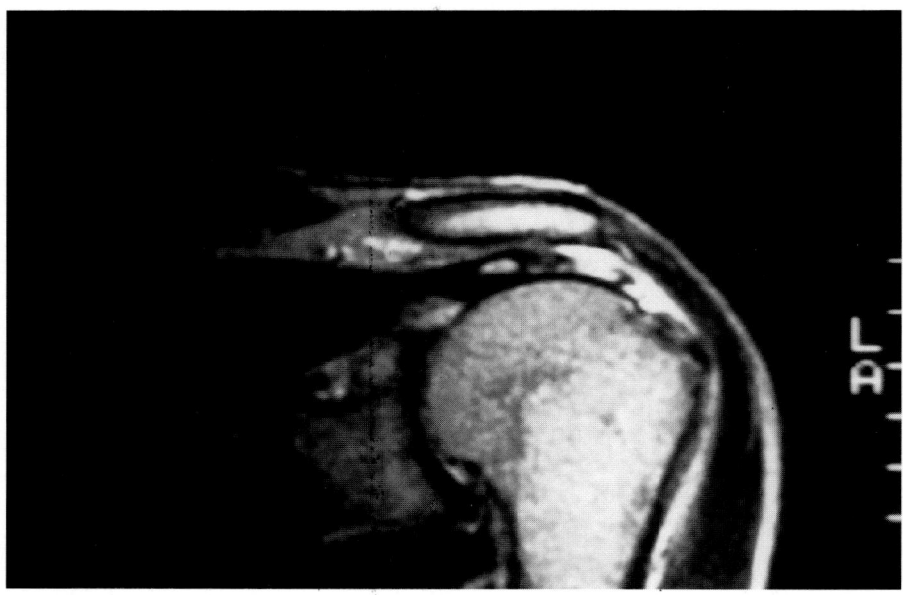

FIGURE 18.
T_2-weighted MR image showing the same tear as seen in Figure 17. (Courtesy of Dr. Norman Kettner.)

Rotator cuff disease is attributed to one of five modes of failure: primary compressive disease, secondary compressive disease, primary tensile overload, secondary tensile overload, and macrotraumatic injuries.[17] The athlete typically has pain but may also have early fatigue or loss of pitching control.[12] Pain is particularly present during performance of the activity. Complete tears of the supraspinatus will manifest with a positive arm drop test result and obvious muscle weakness. Athletes with a rotator cuff tear often have rest and night symptoms, whereas those with rotator cuff tendinitis develop pain with progressive shoulder activity.[14] Pain is felt in the superolateral aspect of the arm, sometimes with precise localization over the insertion of the affected muscle, and often with radiation around the lateral elbow and forearm.[13] Hannaford[13] grades swimmer's shoulder into four areas. In grade 1 the athlete experiences pain after activity only. In grade 2 pain is elicited with the onset of activity, then offset with activity (warming up), and recurs with association of activity. Grade 3 is constant pain with regional tenderness, which is often worse at night, whereas grade 4 is severe pain; tears may be present (Figs 17 and 18).

THROWING INJURIES

EXAMINATION

Evaluation of pain in the shoulder of the throwing athlete should include a careful history attempting to ascertain in which throwing phase the pain is reproduced. The presence of pain during the wind-up, early or late cocking, acceleration, or follow through may aid the examiner in determining what structure or structures have been traumatized. An anterior pop or clunk with certain motions may indicate a labral tear, whereas a burning-type pain noted after releasing the ball would be more indicative of rotator cuff tear.[18] In the early phase of cocking, the arm is abducted to 90 degrees and horizontally extended to 30 degrees, whereas late cocking involves external rotation of the shoulder and elbow flexion in the arm already abducted and extended. Both the infraspinatus and teres minor muscles provide external rotation. The subscapularis is seen to be most active during late cocking, whereas the supraspinatus activity also peaks during late cocking. Therefore, in either early or late cocking, these muscles are most likely to be injured.[19] During the acceleration phase the serratus anterior is most active during the cocking phase alone with the pectoralis major and latissimus dorsi. During the follow through phase, portions of the posterior deltoid, supraspinatus, teres minor, and infraspinatus are involved. In addition, the trapezius and rhomboids aid in decelerating scapular protraction, whereas the biceps works to decelerate elbow extension and forearm pronation.[19] Copeland[19] divides presenting symptoms into pain, clicking, dead arm, and night pain and ache.

Pain
During the evaluation of the athlete, the examiner must ascertain the phase in the throwing motion where pain is reproduced.

Clicking
The painful click may be most indicative of a possible torn intra-articular structure, particularly the glenoid labrum. Painless clicks are typically insignificant.

Dead Arm
During the acceleration phase of throwing, the athlete may complain of the arm becoming severely weak, dropping down by the side associated with pins and needles. Recovery may take anywhere from a few seconds to a few minutes. This is believed to be secondary to momentary subluxation of the glenohumeral joint and with compression of the brachial plexus.

Night Pain and Ache
Night pain and ache are most commonly associated with rotator cuff inflammation, with pain referred to the deltoid insertion. The athlete generally complains of an inability to sleep on the affected side and will wake up at night if he or she rolls on to the involved shoulder. Pain that prevents the athlete from falling asleep may be indicative of tendinitis.[19] Pain awakening the athlete at night necessitates a differential diagnosis of tumor and possibly metastatic disease (Fig 19).

With the number of injuries seen in overhead throwing motions, particularly pitching, concern has arisen as to how frequently the adolescent pitcher should throw. Adolescent pitchers who pitch frequently may place too great a demand on their rapidly growing shoulders, resulting in damage that may curtail and possibly end their playing careers.[20] Two helpful approaches according to Papas and Zawacki[20] are to limit the pitching frequency in games and to initiate total body conditioning programs that include developing or increasing flexibility, cardiopulmonary endurance, and lower extremity muscle strength and endurance.

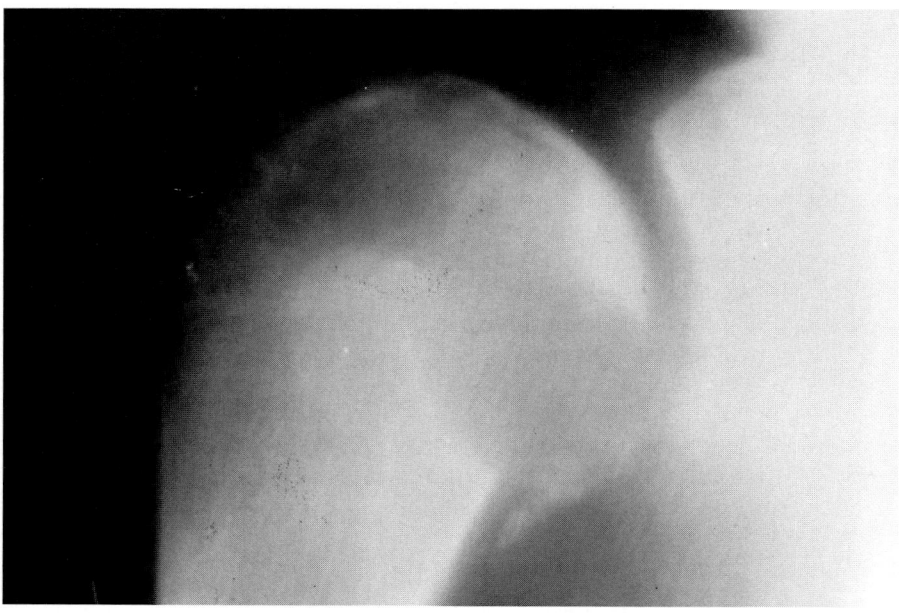

FIGURE 19.
Osteosarcoma. (Courtesy of Dr. Norman Kettner.)

BIOMECHANICS OF THROWING

Throwing a baseball with velocity and accuracy requires the thrower to generate kinetic energy. Using muscles in the lower extremity and torso, the energy can be generated and released through the throwing motion. After release of the ball, the retained energy must be dissipated. A failure in this mechanism to decrease energy may result in an injury to the shoulder.[21] During the wind-up phase, the athlete draws back on one leg, turning sideways, creating potential energy with the highest possible center of gravity. During subsequent stages, this center of gravity moves forward and lower. When the forward leg strikes the ground, the hips are then planted, allowing for turning and acceleration to occur in the upper half of the body. Acceleration then begins at the shoulder with external rotation and abduction and continues until ball release. The follow-through has potential for cumulative injury because it must dissipate the energy created. Rapid shoulder internal rotation and abduction must be reduced during the deceleration phase. These actions rely on the rotator cuff and shoulder adductors.[21] Proper biomechanics are essential, including those of the lower extremity during the overhand throw, in an attempt to reduce injuries to the shoulder. Injuries common in the athlete throwing overhead include tears of the glenoid labrum, overuse tendinitis, rotator cuff tears, and instability. During the overhead motion it appears that large shearing and compressive forces drive the humeral head anteriorly and posteriorly, creating trauma to the labrum, ultimately resulting in degenerative changes. These changes develop into frank tears or labral detachment as the shearing affect increases.[21] During shoulder abduction, the supraspinatus muscle and its tendon aid in depressing the humeral head. With continued use of the arm in the overhead position, fatigue may set in, ultimately leading to changes within the tendon and cuff.[21] As a result of continued degenerative changes, impingement syndrome may develop. Continued overload and secondary impingement may result in fiber failure and rotator cuff tears.[21] Tears may begin with partial disruption of the fibers, progressing with continued overuse into a complete tear. As changes to the glenoid labrum occur, followed by stretching of the inferior glenohumeral ligament, instability may ultimately develop.[21]

Jobe and Kvitne[22] classify anterior shoulder pain into one of four groups. Group 1 includes those patients with pure impingement and no instability who demonstrate a positive impingement sign and negative apprehension sign. Group 2 patients have primary instability due to chronic labral microtrauma with secondary impingement and will have a positive impingement sign experiencing pain but no apprehension. Group 3 patients consist of those with instability due to hyperelasticity, with subsequent impingement. These patients again will demonstrate a positive impingement sign and pain but no apprehension. Group 4 patients are those with pure instability (subluxation) without impingement demonstrating negative impingement but who will have pain with apprehension testing and relief of pain with the relocation test.[22]

Biomechanics

Overhead racket motion, such as that used when serving in tennis, may create the same shoulder stress as seen in throwing, causing rotator cuff injury, biceps tendon lesions, glenohumeral instability, and glenoid label tears.[27] The highly mobile shoulder joint is most susceptible to injury in the overhead use sports such as baseball, tennis, and swimming.[23] Sports-related shoulder injuries commonly occurring in the overhead-overuse are rotator cuff disease, glenohumeral instability, and acromioclavicular instability.[23] The rapid acceleration, deceleration, and rotational forces generated by the throwing motion impose adaptive changes and can cause injury to the shoulder.[24]

Throwing

The throwing motion has been broken down into five phases: windup, cocking (early and late), acceleration, deceleration, and follow-through. Windup begins with the thrower in a two-leg stance position and ends with the lead leg raised and the ball removed from the glove. The cocking stage follows and is divided into early and late phases. The cocking begins with removal of the ball from opposite the glove and ends with the shoulder at the point of maximum external rotation, approximately 180 degrees, and 100 degrees of abduction. Acceleration begins at the point of maximum shoulder external rotation and ends at ball release. These moves range from 180 to 90 degrees of external rotation at speeds of 7,000 degrees per second. Deceleration begins at ball release and ends at the completion of humeral rotation. The arm maintains an abducted position of about 100 degrees, and the shoulder internally rotates to about 0 degrees. This phase is recognized as the most violent phase of throwing and is marked by tremendous forces in compression, as well as force directed posteriorly and inferiorly.[17] Radiographs of the shoulder are typically normal unless an avulsion of the tendon is present.

OTHER CONSIDERATIONS

Other considerations should include surgery in the nonresponsive case. As with all surgeries, the criteria listed previously must be taken into consideration.

Neer's original theory of mechanical impingement suggested that the rotator cuff "impinges" against the rigid coracoacromial arch and was supported by the work of Bigliani and Morrison.[25] They describe three variations in the shape of the acromion: type 1, flat; type 2, curved; and type 3, hooked.[26] The size, shape, or slope of the acromion influences the amount of mechanical impingement, which, in turn, causes degenerative attritional changes within the rotator cuff in a critical area near the insertion of the supraspinatus tendon.[25]

Other causes of impingement of the rotator cuff include chronic microtrauma, vascular impairment, partial tears of the rotator cuff, and previous trauma. This condition is common in baseball pitchers, tennis players, and swimmers, particularly those performing the freestyle and butterfly.[8] The typical presenting symptom is that of pain, especially during the overhand pitch in baseball or overhand serve in tennis, as well as the butterfly stroke in swimming. Pain is localized over the posterolateral aspect of the shoulder at the junction of the supraspinatus muscle with its tendon. On some occasions the pain may not be as discrete and may be described more by the athlete as a diffuse pain. This condition is often accompanied by biceps tendinitis. Pain is typically elicited between 60 and 100 degrees of abduction. Failure to treat an early diagnosis of rotator cuff tendinitis may lead to rotator cuff rupture.[27] During examination, the supraspinatus can be checked for synchronous movement by having the patient stand with the arm in a neutral position at the side of the body and the humerus head internally rotated so the dorsum of the head faces the front of the body. The patient then abducts the arm very slowly for 20 to 25 degrees. If the movement is smooth, the supraspinatus is working normally. If the movement is not smooth (a racketlike or an erratic asynchronous movement), the supraspinatus needs to be synchronized. This is accomplished by having the patient do 3 sets of 10 repetitions abducting the arm 20 to 25 degrees very slowly for 4 days with no weight. Next have the patient do the same exercise with a 6-oz weight for 4 days. Finally, have the patient do the exercise with a 12-oz weight for 4 days.

TREATMENT

Initial treatment should consist of demobilization in a sling and ice. Early pain-free motion is a necessity, coupled with flexibility exercises and ultimately a strengthening program with isometric and isokinetic exercises. Early treatment consists of ice with limited range of motion within the athlete's tolerance. As pain and inflammation decrease, the athlete can begin resisted motions using surgical tubing, progressively advancing to isotonic rehabilitation. In the athlete unresponsive to conservative care, anti-inflammatory corticosteroid oral medication, as well as injections, may be beneficial. In the early stages the athlete should avoid any activity that produces pain. If corticosteroids are injected, it is advisable to abstain from any significant resistance exercises for 2 to 3 weeks because of the potential for corticosteroid-induced tendon atrophy.[29]

SHOULDER INSTABILITY

Anterior instability may be a result of repetitive stretching or acute trauma. This occurs typically in an anteroinferior direction. In up to 85% of such injuries, the labrum has been detached from the anteroinferior glenoid rim. It has been stated that the younger the athlete, the more likely dislocation is to recur. However, it does not recur as frequently in the nonathlete or if adequate immobilization and rehabilitation have taken place before the patient returns to sports.[3] Tearing of the labrum, with subluxation manifesting as clicking, has been identified in the anteroinferior glenoid in pitching and swimming. Posterior instability is classified as acute posterior dislocation, with or without a head impression fracture; chronic lock posterior dislocation; or recurrent posterior shoulder subluxation. The acute posterior dislocation and the posterior lock dislocation occur in sports from a fall on the elbow or outstretched hand when the arm is flexed forward, abducted, and internally rotated.[3] Shoulder instability may also be related to both rotator cuff and bicipital disorders. The patient with anterior subluxation is at risk for developing secondary impingement due to the architectural setup of the subacromial region.[1]

The overall incidence of shoulder dislocations is estimated to be 1% to 2%. Anterior instability is believed to account for 95% of the shoulder instability problems as a whole.[3] The instability is classified according to the cause (traumatic, atraumatic, overuse), timing (acute, recurrent, fixed), degree of instability (subluxation, dislocation), and direction of instability (anterior, posterior, multidirection).[30] Shoulder dislocation has been reported as high as 92%.[31] Research by Obrien has indicated that the inferior glenohumeral ligament is attached at two places at the shoulder joint, in front and in back of the glenoid cavity.[32] Originally the inferior glenohumeral ligament was thought to attach only in the front. Obrien states that this ligament is actually not a ligament but a thickening in the joint capsule and has both an anterior and posterior band with a thickened hammocklike structure connecting the two.[32] When the shoulder dislocates, typically in the anteroinferior direction, the humeral head moves through the foramen of Weitbrecht, moving between the superior and middle glenohumeral ligaments. A group of 20 weight lifters representing a total of 23 shoulders were examined for complaints of progressive instability. They were made to perform exercises with the upper extremity in the abducted, externally rotated position (the "at risk" position) because of pain.[33] In this study, 100% of the athletes experienced posterior shoulder pain while the shoulder was placed in this forced abduction and external rotation. Thirteen shoulders in 10 patients responded to conservative management, including aggressive rehabilitation and modification of technique to avoid the at risk position. The other 10 shoulders that did not respond to conservative treatment required surgical treatment to alleviate the symptoms. After treatment, all 20 athletes successfully returned to their previous weight lifting activities.[33]

Traumatic anterior glenohumeral dislocation may manifest with lesions such as avulsion of the anterior capsule and glenoid labrum from the glenoid rim (Bankart's lesion, compression fracture of the posterosuperior humeral head, Hill-Sachs lesion) and laxity of the joint capsule. Another common lesion is a lengthwise disruption of the rotator cuff at the interval between the subscapularis and supraspinatus tendon.[34] Orthopedic tests for instability were discussed earlier.

Standard radiographs of anteroposterior, internal and external rotation must be taken. In addition to the anteroposterior internal and external views, a modified axillary view and baby arm should be taken. Magnetic resonance imaging (MRI) may also be necessary and beneficial.

Autotraction, stress roentgenography of the shoulder, may be of use in the diagnosis of recurrent anterior subluxation and anteroinferior multidirectional instabilities.[35]

TREATMENT

For athletes sustaining anterior dislocation for the first time, treatment ranges from multiperiods of immobilization to the immediate implementation of conservative care. Others[30] recommended immediate surgery. In these athletes the recurrence rate is said to be 92%. Hovelius et al. performed a randomized study analyzing athlete's younger than 40 years with first-time documented anterior dislocations. The study compared athletes treated with 3 to 4 weeks of immobilization with those treated with early unrestricted motion using pain as the only inhibitor. They found an equal incidence of recurrence of one or more dislocations. The recurrence rates were stated to be 47%, 26%, and 13% for the three age groups less than 22 years, 23 to 29 years, and 30 to 40 years, respectively. A number of studies have shown that athlete's younger than 30 years have an increased rate of recurrence of anterior dislocation.[35-40]

It appears that the athlete greater than 40 years has a decreased chance of recurrence after the first incidence of shoulder dislocation.[30] After the dislocation, a sling is often used in the beginning stages, primarily until pain relief occurs.[30] Removal of the sling periodically, followed by range of motion within pain-free zones, should be implemented as soon as the athlete is able to tolerate movement. The ultimate objective is to return the athlete as quickly as possible to training and competition with the objective to strengthen and rehabilitate the shoulder in an attempt to reduce the possibilities of recurrence. The objective should include full range of motion and equal strength bilaterally. Once range of motion is improved in a pain-free state, the patient should begin gentle resisted exercises using surgical tubing. The strength of the tubing may vary depending on the size and ability of the athlete. Once the patient can comfortably handle tubing in all ranges of motion to include internal and external rotation, abduction, adduction, and forward and backward elevation, he or she may proceed to isotonic exercises. Return to training and competition will vary from athlete to athlete. Reasons for this may include motivation of the athlete, overall condition of the athlete before injury, severity of the injury, and the conservative program outlined by the treating physician and staff.

NEUROVASCULAR INJURIES

Injuries to the shoulder also include neurovascular disorders. The examination of the shoulder injury must include an evaluation of the neurovascular structures. The most commonly recognized neurovascular compression syndromes are axillary artery occlusion, effort thrombosis, quadrilateral space syndrome, and thoracic outlet syndrome.[41] Structures involved in these syndromes include entrapment of the axillary artery posterior to the pectoralis minor muscle, the first cervical rib, leading to venous thrombosis of the subclavian and axillary vein, and thoracic outlet syndrome, caused by either compression of the first rib, scalenus anticus muscle, or occlusion of the posterior humeral circumflex artery or axillary nerve in the quadrilateral space. Neurovascular symptoms may be vague, consisting of paresthesia, vascular insufficiency, and exertional fatigue.

The athlete with suspected axillary artery occlusion may have pain and tenderness over the pectoralis minor area, claudication, fatigue, diminished distal pulses, and cyanosis. Symptoms of effort thrombosis typically occur within 24 hours after repetitive, vigorous activities or blunt trauma. The symptoms consist of "dull, aching pain, numbness, and heaviness" of the upper arm and shoulder along with fatigue after activities involving the extremity.

The entire upper extremity may be swollen, the skin may be mottled and cold, and superficial veins may be prominent. Symptoms of quadrilateral space syndrome are generally poorly localized pain and paresthesia in the upper arm without associated trauma. Thoracic outlet symptoms may include venous engorgement, coolness, and paresthesia of the involved arm, and the patient may complain of arm weakness, heaviness, and fatigue.[41]

Specific orthopedic tests appropriate for several of these disorders has been discussed under the examination section. Some of the conditions require additional diagnostic work-ups, including vascular studies.

CERVICAL BURNERS

The cervical burner has been classified into a 1 through 3 system by Clancy[42]: Grade 1, resolved within 2 weeks; grade 2, delayed recovery up to 1 year; and grade 3, injuries greater than 1 year.

The injury is common in football whereby the athlete is struck on the helmet or delivers a blow head first with the helmet. Often traction on impact occurs between the cervical spine and the shoulder. Examination should consist of evaluation of the cervical spine and the integrity of the neurovascular structures of the upper extremity. Follow-up evaluation in those athletes whose symptoms persist is a must. In addition to overuse injuries resulting in neurovascular disorders, traumatic injuries may also produce the same entities. Another suspected cause of injury has been thought to occur secondary to traction when an athlete sustains a lateral flexion injury of the neck.[43] A study performed by Markey and DeBenedetto[43] on 32 players found a more common mechanism of injury resulting in the stinger syndrome, which is probably compression of the fixed brachial plexus between the shoulder pad and the superomedial scapula when the pad was pushed into the area of Erb's point, where the brachial plexus is most superficial.

TREATMENT

Both open and closed chain exercises have been recommended for shoulder rehabilitation. In this case we will discuss both open and closed chain exercises for neurovascular disorders.

Open vs. Closed Kinetic Chain

The concept of open vs. closed kinetic chain refers to viewing the body as a chain. Your limbs (legs and arms) serve as the opposite ends of the chain. If either set of limbs is involved in supporting your weight (e.g., a squatting exercise in which your legs are bearing the weight of your body or push-up in which your hands are partially shouldering the weight of your body), the physical endeavor is referred to as an example of a closed chain exercise. The end segment of the chain is closed (i.e., fixed.) On the other hand, if the end segment of the chain (your body) is not fixed (i.e., free, not supporting the weight of your body), the exercise is termed an open chain exercise. Closed chain exercises are much more functional and effective in facilitating the healing process than are open chain exercises.[45]

An open kinetic chain exercise refers to a combination of successively arranged joints in which the terminal segment can move freely, such as when a seated knee extension can be performed. During knee extension, motion at the knee joint occurs independently from motion at the hip and ankle joints. Motion at the glenohumeral joint occurs independently of motion at the elbow and wrist joints.[44] The closed kinetic chain occurs when neither the proximal nor distal segments can move. This creates a system where movement at one joint produces movement at all other joints in a predictable manner. Thus, in a true closed kinetic chain activity, movement never occurs in the extremities. Specifically, a closed kinetic chain exists when the terminal segment meets with some considerable external resistance that prohibits its free motion, such as when a squat is performed.[44] During closed chain exercises, motion at the glenohumeral joint is accompanied by motion at the scapulothoracic articulation (see Table 1).[45]

ADDITIONAL SHOULDER DISORDERS

OSTEOCHONDRITIS DISSECANS

Using a literature search over the past 60 years, Ishikawa et al.[46] found only four cases of osteochondritis dissecans involving the articular surface of the humeral head. They report a case of osteochondritis of the shoulder in a tennis player caused by trauma rather than overuse. When present, if the lesion is responsible for damage to the cartilaginous structures, the segment should be surgically removed.[46]

OSTEOLYSIS OF THE DISTAL CLAVICLE

Osteolysis of the distal clavicle was originally described as a sequela of acute trauma to the shoulder by Dupas et al. in 1936.[47] This condition may be seen after contusion of the shoulder, a clavicular fracture, or acromioclavicular joint dislocation. The condition has been seen in contact sports such as football, rugby, hockey, and judo, but most commonly it follows a fall or motor vehicle accident.

Approximately 100 cases of "stress"-induced osteolysis of the distal clavicle have now been reported.[47] In a group of weight lifters, seven cases of clavicular osteolysis were noted. There are cases of nontraumatic clavicular osteolysis.[48, 49] Cahill[49] believes that atraumatic osteolysis occurs primarily in young athletes who have a long history of training and performance, as well as in athletes who have an associated intense strength training program. If it is left untreated, the process of reduced bone strength and subchondral stress fractures continues. This can last for 12 to 18 months in traumatic cases and of an unknown period in nontraumatic cases, resulting in a 0.5- to 3-cm wide zone for varying radiolucency. If the sport is discontinued, the degenerative stage decreases gradually, and reparative changes take place over 4 to 6 months. The acromial end of the clavicle becomes smoother, but the joint space remains permanently wide.[48]

LEVATOR SCAPULA SYNDROME

The levator scapula inserts into the superior medial border of the scapula, but it originates from the transverse processes from C-1 through C-4. Spasm of this muscle will often result in severe pain in the cervical spine with decreased cervical range of motion, particularly in rotation and lateral flexion. Cervical extension may also be limited and painful. This condition has been observed in weight training while the athlete is performing incline presses with a straight bar, standing or seated presses either in front of or behind the neck, and latissimus pull-downs behind the head. This condition has been compared with tennis elbow in its causes, mechanisms, and treatment. In both conditions acute or chronic overload mechanisms are present.[50] Various soft tissue techniques, including active release technique, Nimmo, trigger point therapy, and proprioceptive neuromuscular facilitation, are used for treatment. Should this treatment fail, local injections may be beneficial, but caution should be taken to avoid pneumothorax.

INJURIES OF THE DISTAL CLAVICULAR PHYSIS IN CHILDREN

In a study of 10 adolescent males with distal clavicular physial injuries, 80% occurred on the right side. Nine of these were treated conservatively; one required surgical repair. Seven of the nine cases treated conservatively resulted in a deformity. No typical acromioclavicular dislocations occur in adults because the coracoclavicular ligaments remain intact.[51]

LATISSIMUS DORSI TENDINITIS

The latissimus muscle is a large flat triangular muscle extending primarily over the lumbar region and lower thoracic spine. Its tendon along with the tendon of the teres major unite at the lower borders near their humeral attachment. Tendinitis of the latissimus dorsi, although uncommon, has been reported because of overuse in throwing, with more than 100 cases reported.[52] Diagnosis is made via resisted arm depression, reproducing pain posterior to the shoulder and axillary regions.[52] Treatment is typically conservative, with the use of transverse friction massage as described by Cyriax, active release technique, and Nimmo, along with cessation of all activities producing the pain.

DISORDERS OF THE INFRASPINATUS MUSCLE

Motta and Carletti[53] report a case of a young female physical education teacher who, while falling from a chair, was caught and lifted by the shoulders just before hitting the floor. She suffered acute pain and felt a tearing sensation in the right scapular region. They[53] described the mechanism of injury as forced internal rotation and abduction of the shoulder. This injury resulted in complete rupture of the scapular insertion of the infraspinatus muscle. Treatment consisted of 2 weeks of rest, followed by physical therapy. One year follow-up resulted in no limitation of motion with only a feeling of heaviness after prolonged effort. Several cases of infraspinatus atrophy seen in volleyball players have been reported by Tengan et al.[54] In both cases, trauma did not exist. It is suspected that the atrophy was secondary to intense activity involving the shoulder joint. The authors[54] believed that the pathogenesis was related to traction of the distal branch of the suprascapular nerve during the act

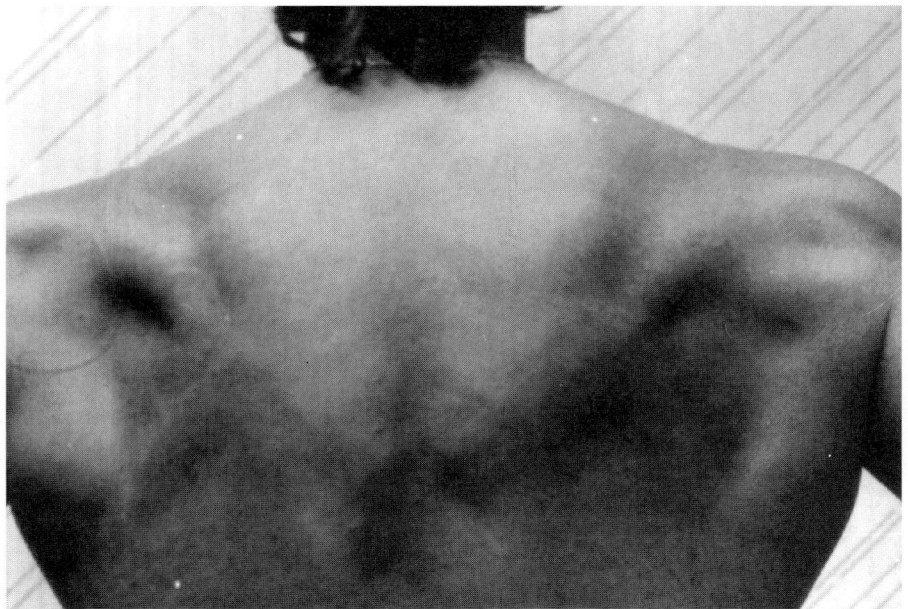

FIGURE 20.
Body builder displaying atrophy of the infraspinatus muscle on the left secondary to nerve damage caused by weight training.

of reception of the ball. One player ceased playing volleyball secondary to an ankle injury and within 1 year noticed decreased atrophy and weakness of the right shoulder. This weakness may lead to impingement. One player was treated conservatively; the second player continued playing with no signs of atrophy (Fig 20).

SHOULDER PAIN IN THE WHEELCHAIR ATHLETE

Athletes who are bound to wheelchairs seem to have an unusually high incident of shoulder pain and, in particular, rotator cuff tears.[55] It appears these injuries are secondary to the increased stress loads placed on the shoulder not only in weight bearing in the wheelchair athlete but the shoulder also serves as the primary mode of locomotion. All wheelchair athletes should be instructed in the proper mechanics of the shoulder and undergo appropriate strength training and flexibility with the intention of reducing the frequency of injuries sustained to the shoulder. Another study of shoulder pain in wheelchair athletes was conducted by Burnham et al.[56] They found shoulder rotator cuff impingement syndrome a common and disabling problem in the wheelchair athlete. Those athletes sustaining a rotator cuff impingement syndrome were weaker in adduction and external and internal rotation compared with the athletes without impingement syndrome. Conservative treatment should be the same as in any athlete with impingement syndrome.

SYNOVIOCHONDROMETAPLASIA

This condition is a benign atrophy characterized by synovial tissue undergoing metaplastic change to produce multiple foci of cartilaginous and osteocartilaginous nodules with an unknown cause. A case of synoviochondrometaplasia in a 41-year-old male tennis and softball player was reported by Leahy and Mock.[57] The patient was successfully treated with the use of myofascial active release technique and active exercise. After conservative care, complete range of motion without pain and almost total reduction of the chondrometaplasia was observed within 4½ months, with no recurrence of symptoms at 1 year.

FRACTURES

A number of fractures occur in and around the shoulder, including fractures of the humerus, clavicle, and scapula (Figs 21 to 23). Fractures of the acromion process of the scapula occur but are seen infrequently. The physician should be aware that fractures of the glenoid are often associated with dislocations of the glenohumeral joint.[58] Scapular border or body fractures are rare and represent approximately 1% of all skeletal injuries (most often associated with high-speed vehicular trauma[59]). Cain and Hamilton[59] report five scapular fractures caused by direct trauma in four football players between 1982 and 1988. All fractures responded to early active range of motion exercises and conservative care. One patient showed a delayed healing, which eventually healed with the aid of an electric bone stimulator.[59] Clavicular fractures are seen as a result of di-

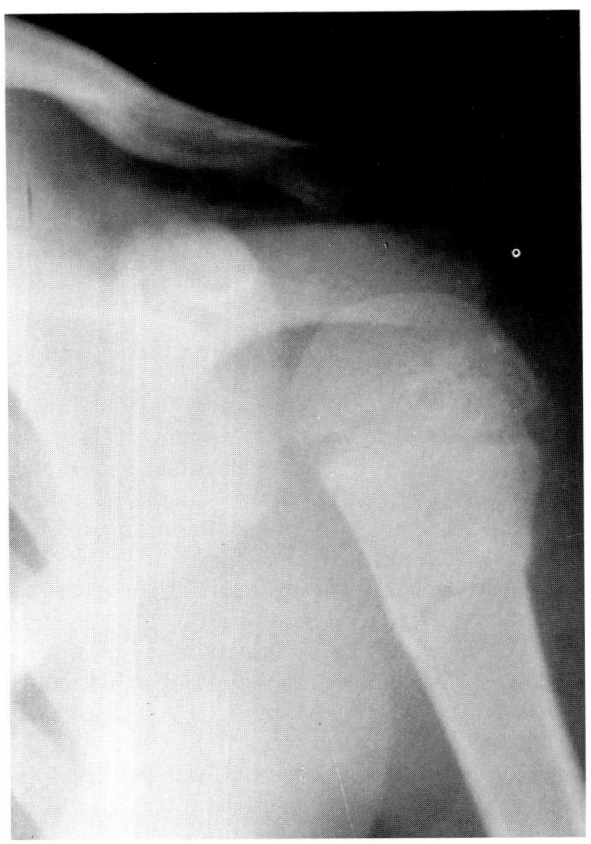

FIGURE 21.
Fracture of the proximal one third of the humerus. (Courtesy of Dr. Norman Kettner.)

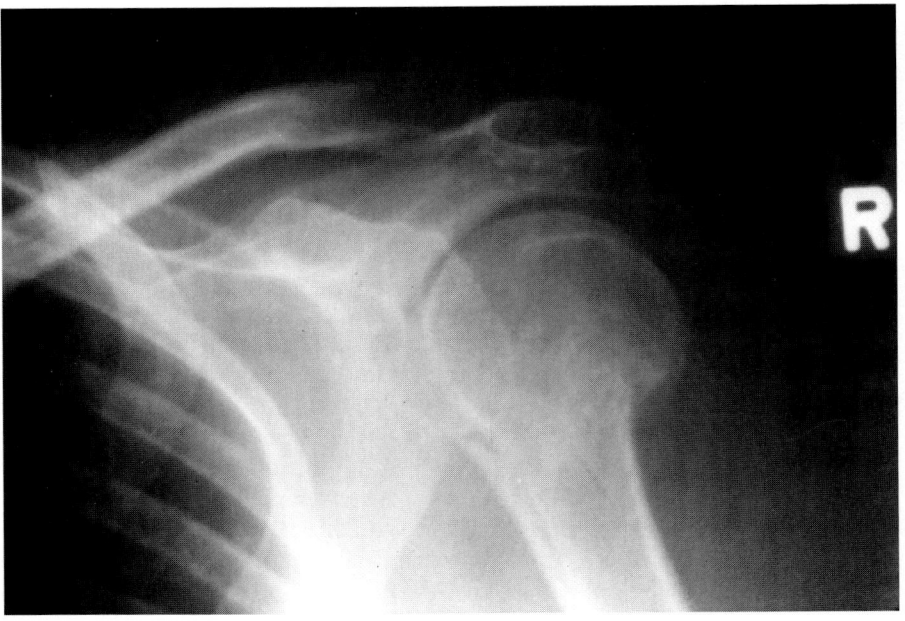

FIGURE 22.
Fracture of the surgical neck of the humerus. (Courtesy of Dr. Norman Kettner.)

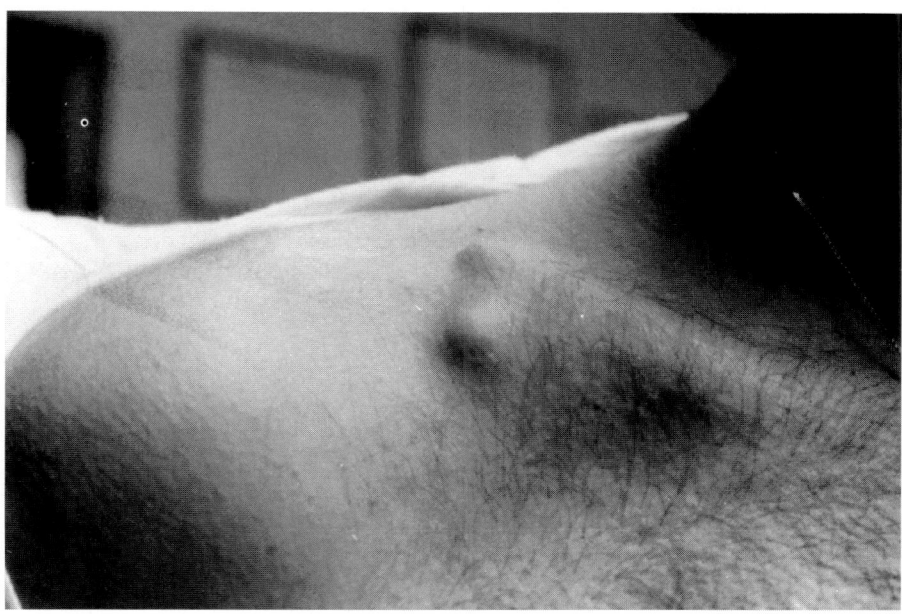

FIGURE 23.
Clavicular fracture occurring during a fall from a motorcycle while racing.

rect trauma and usually a result of the arm being outstretched or a result of a direct fall to the side of the shoulder (Fig 24). Fracture of the clavicle may occur in the clavicular region, as well as the medial and distal regions. The least common fractures are those to the inner or middle third, representing approximately 5% of all clavicular fractures. Fractures to the

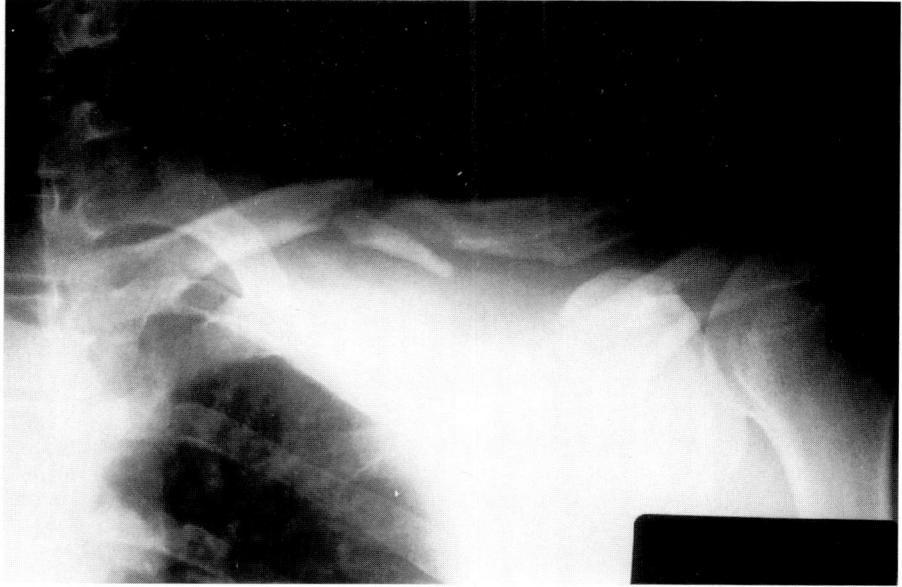

FIGURE 24.
Clavicular fracture. (Courtesy of Dr. Norman Kettner.)

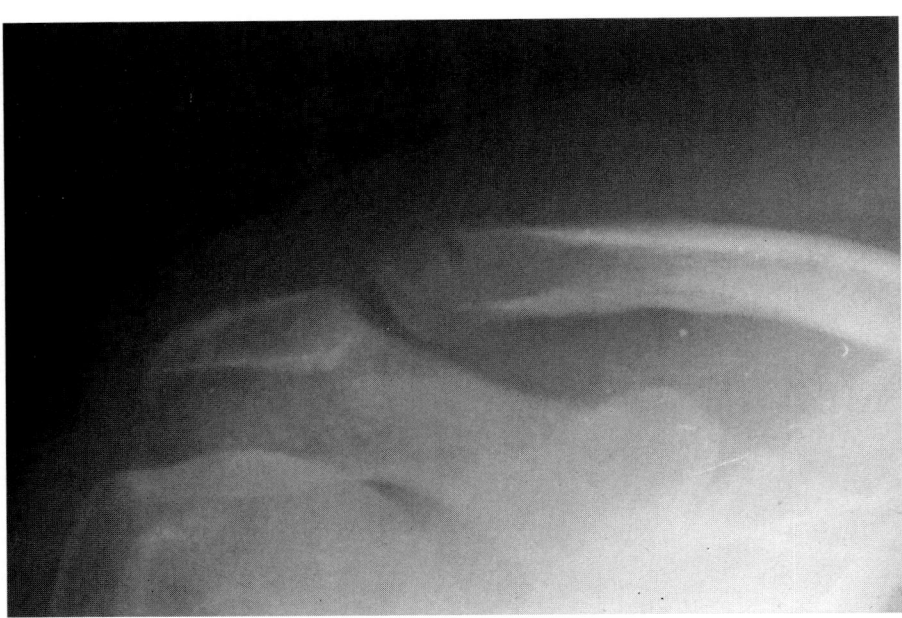

FIGURE 25.
Clavicular fracture of the distal aspect. (Courtesy of Dr. Norman Kettner.)

middle third of the clavicle comprise approximately 80%, with the remaining 15% occurring at the distal aspect (Fig 25).[60]

Salter-Harris fractures to the humerus should be ruled out in the adolescent athlete (Fig 26). The use of bone scans, computed tomography (CT) scans, and plain x-ray films may be beneficial in evaluating fractures.

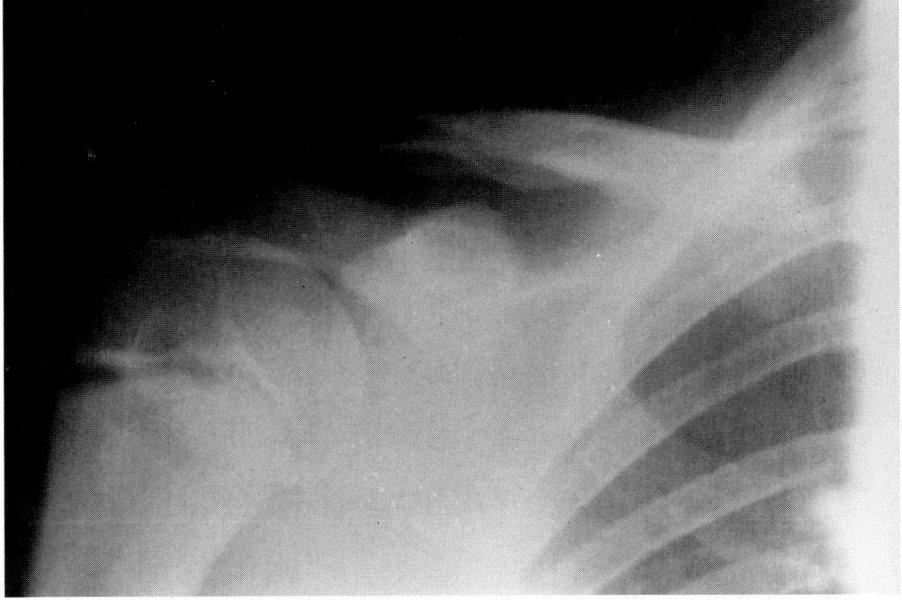

FIGURE 26.
Salter-Harris type I fracture. (Courtesy of Dr. Norman Kettner.)

Uhthoff and Sarkar developed an algorithm of the shoulder that appears to be beneficial in ascertaining a differential diagnosis and pain in the shoulder.[70]

CONSERVATIVE TREATMENT AND REHABILITATION CONSIDERATIONS

Soft tissue technique such as trigger point therapy as described by travel and active release technique is a beneficial means of treating soft tissue shoulder disorders. Isometric, isotonic, and isokinetic exercises may be employed as dictated. Active ranges of motion and assisted motion within pain tolerance should be initiated immediately. Ice and other modalities such as ultrasound, interferential current, heat, and muscle stimulation should be applied when appropriate. Resisted tubing exercises are an excellent means of rehabilitation for many injuries sustained to the shoulder.

- Phase I—A slow pace, short range exercise in which one gently, painlessly begins the exercise program.
- Phase II—A fast pace short range exercise to the point of fatigue.

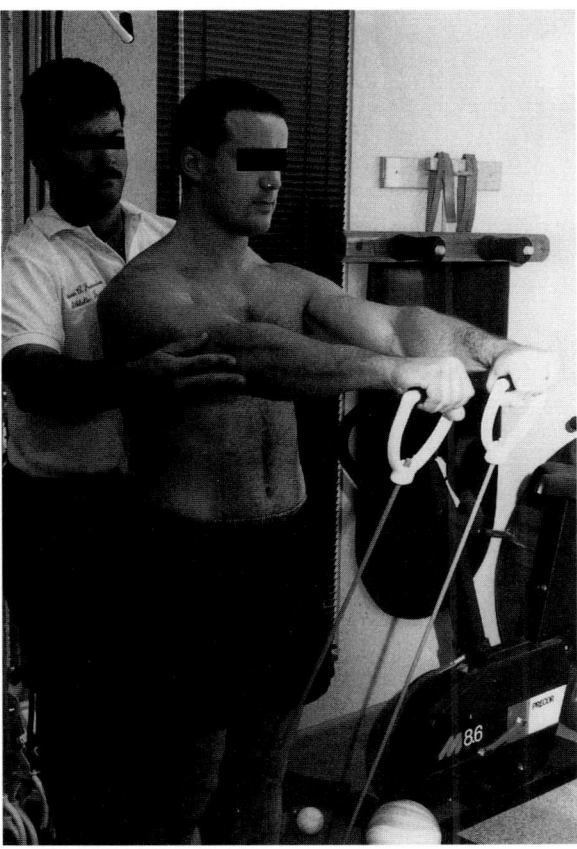

FIGURE 27.
Bilateral front deltoid raises using surgical tubing.

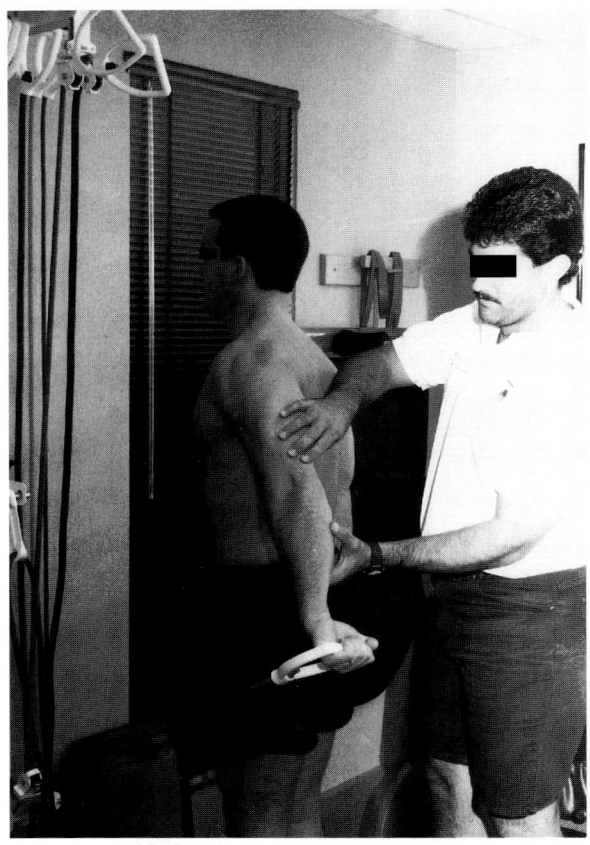

FIGURE 28.
Backward elevation using surgical tubing.

- Phase III—A slow pace, full range exercise in which one gently, painlessly increases one's abilities.
- Phase IV—A fast pace, full range exercise in which one fully reeducates muscle groups in their full functions (Figs 27 to 38).

Maintenance of cardiovascular fitness is a must during shoulder rehabilitation. Proprioception should be maintained, and exercises designed to enhance proprioception should be instituted as quickly as the athlete can tolerate. In the advanced stages of shoulder rehabilitation, the athlete can be introduced to isokinetics and plyometrics. The literature contains many references to rehabilitation of the shoulder. The reader is urged to consult this literature for specific rehabilitation and treatment schedules for particular shoulder disorders.

DIAGNOSTIC IMAGING

The initial diagnostic evaluation of injuries to the shoulder should include plain x-ray films. These should consist of anteroposterior internal and external rotation and baby arm. Suspected fractures of the clavicle

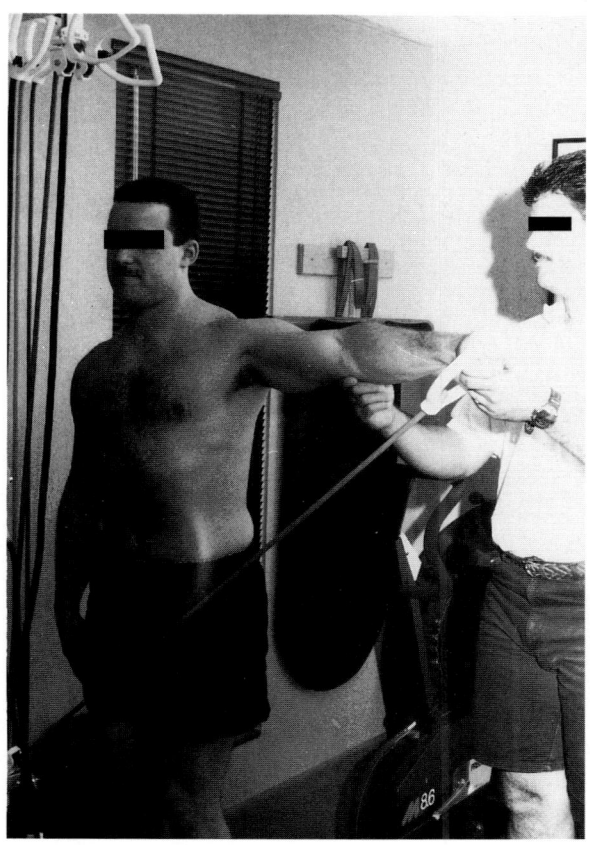

FIGURE 29.
Lateral deltoid raises during surgical tubing.

should include the posteroanterior clavicular and acromioclavicular. Additional views after trauma include the axillary and scapular Y or Neer views. For suspected Hill-Sachs deformities, the Rokous or West Point axillary view should be employed. An additional view known as the Stryker notch view may be useful in determining recurrent anterior dislocations. The anteroposterior view, particularly with internal rotation, seems important in the diagnosis of the unstable shoulder. The West Point axillary view is useful in identifying the presence of glenoid rim tears, whereas the Striker notch view aids in identifying the presence of Hill-Sachs lesions that may be absent on other radiographic views.[61]

Tomography may be helpful in the diagnosis of small neoplasms such as osteoid osteomas.[62]

Sonography is currently being used to detect tears in the tendon and abnormal motion patterns of the supraspinatus with arm rotation. This mode of diagnostic imaging continues to evolve, with a reported sensitivity and specificity of 91% detection of rotator cuff, according to Middleton et al.[62] High-resolution ultrasound using high-frequency, real-time transducers provides detailed images of small superficial structures, including the tendons, muscles, and subcutaneous tissues. These may be

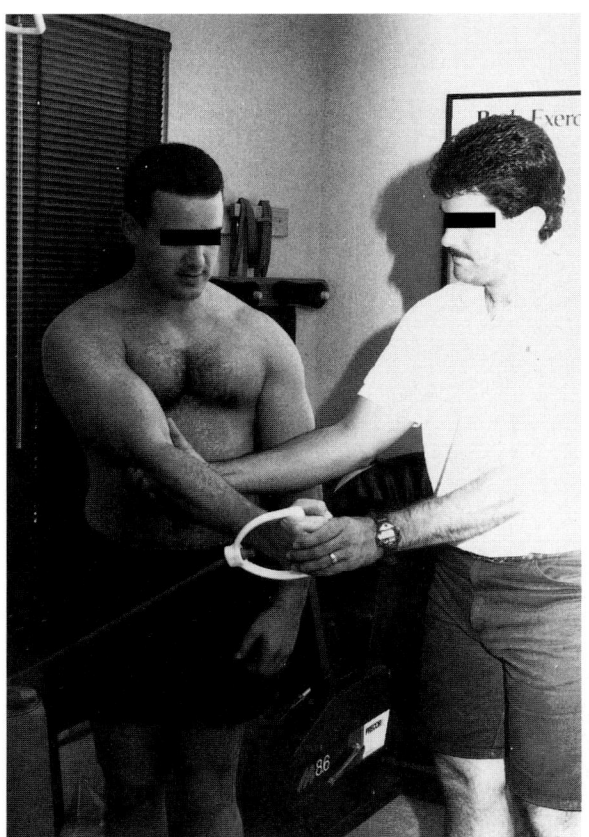

FIGURE 30.
Shoulder adduction using surgical tubing.

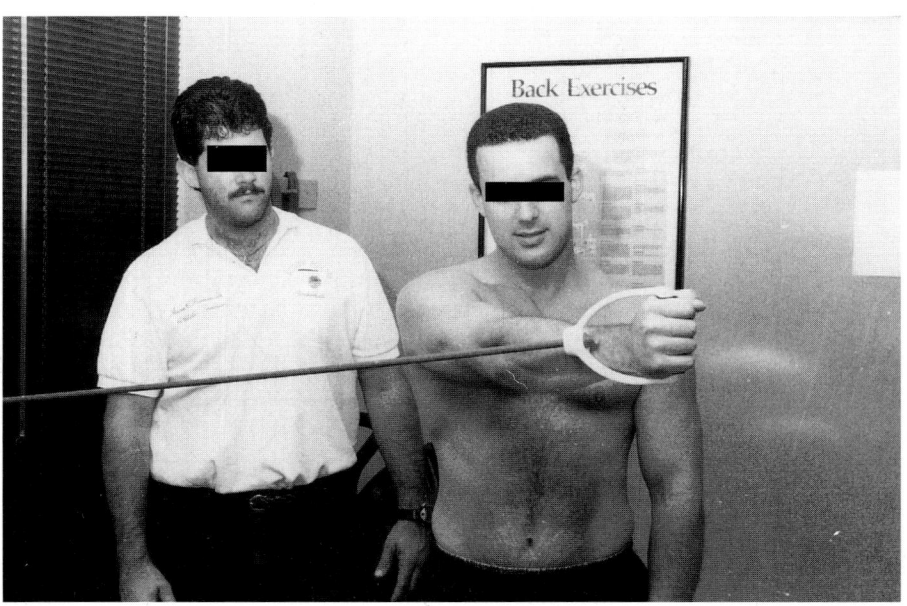

FIGURE 31.
Shoulder horizontal adduction using surgical tubing.

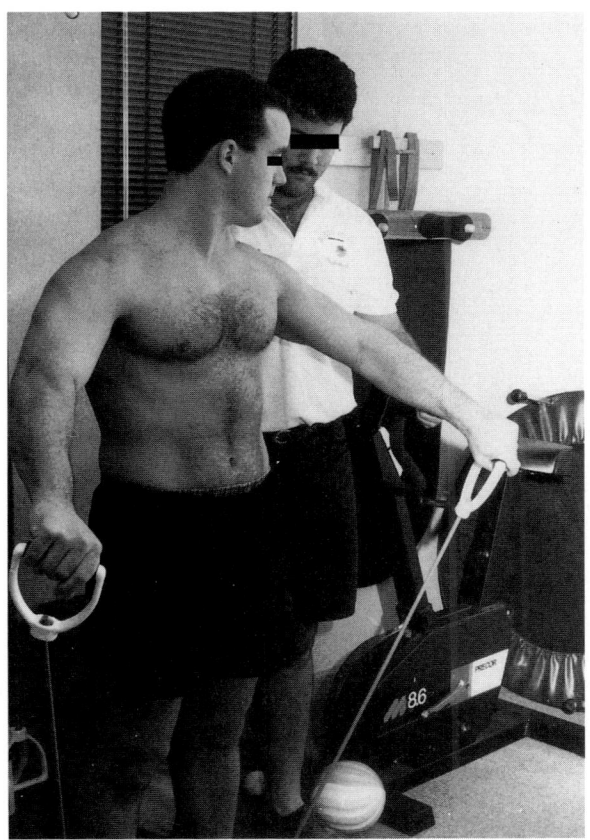

FIGURE 32.
Bilateral supraspinatus exercise using surgical tubing.

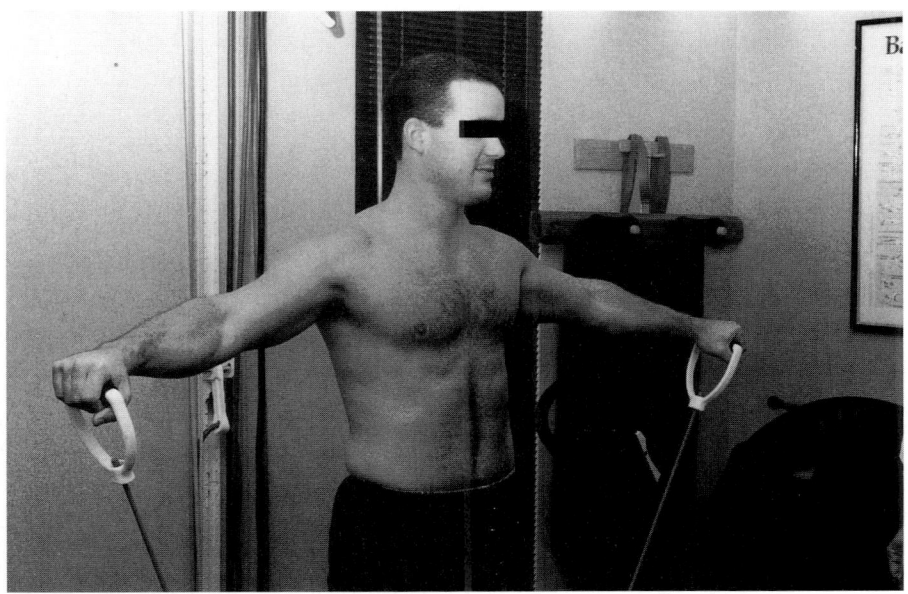

FIGURE 33.
Bilateral deltoid raises using surgical tubing.

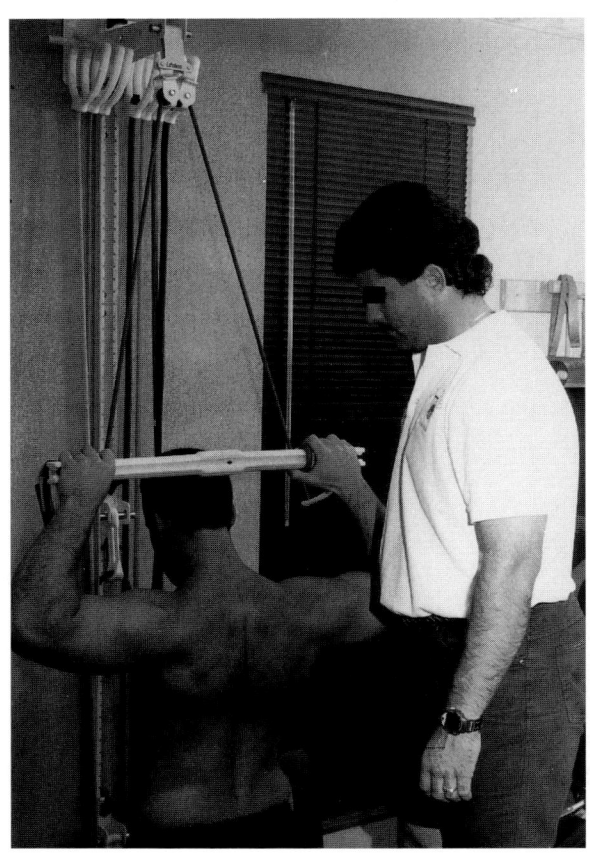

FIGURE 34.
Bilateral pull-downs for the latissimus dorsi, trapezius, and deltoids.

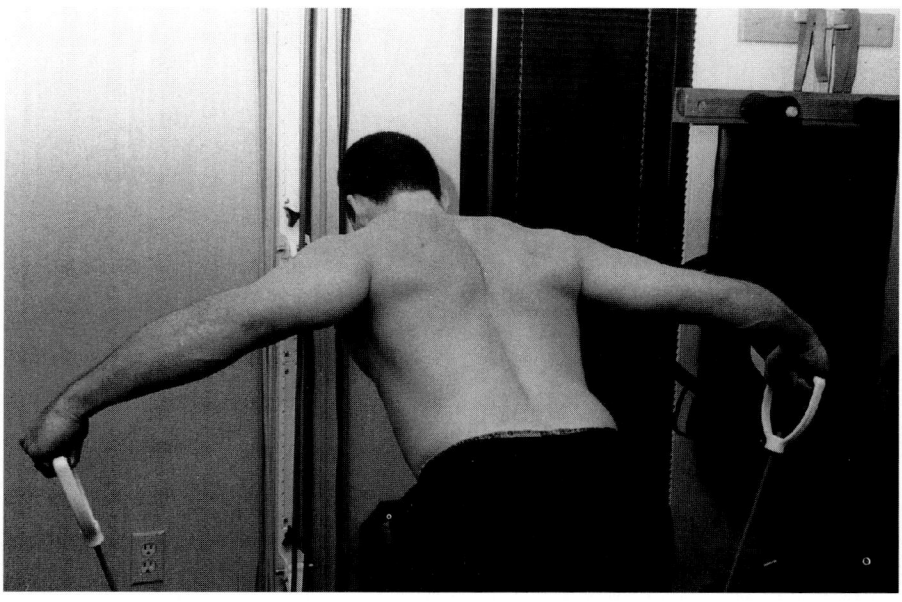

FIGURE 35.
Bilateral reverse flies working the rhomboids and posterior deltoids.

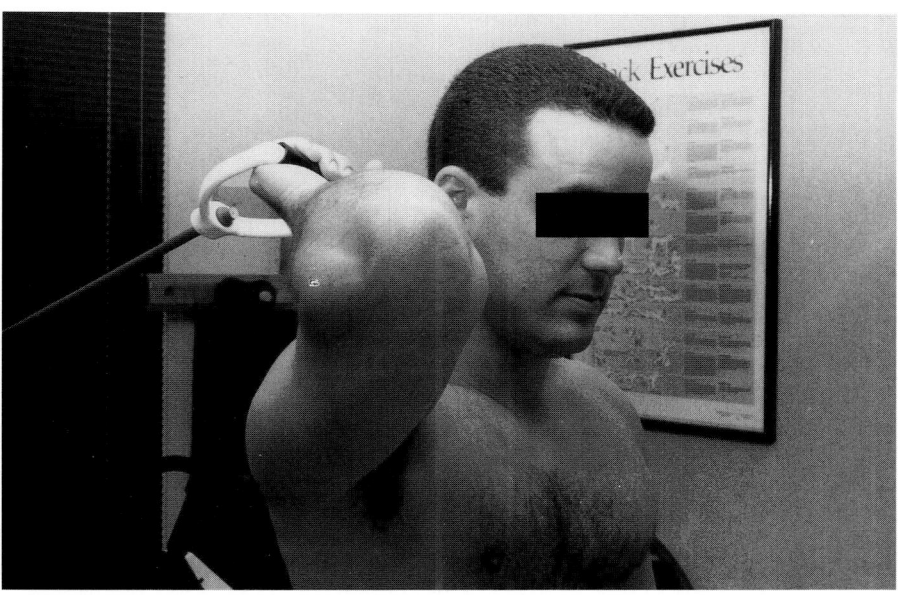

FIGURE 36.
Single arm triceps exercise.

assessed for disruption, masses, or fluid collections, as well as foreign bodies.[63]

Arthrography of the shoulder is used primarily in evaluating tears of the rotator cuff, adhesive capsulitis, and impingement syndrome. Double-contrast techniques, along with combined arthrography or arthrography and CT evaluation, appear to be more accurate.

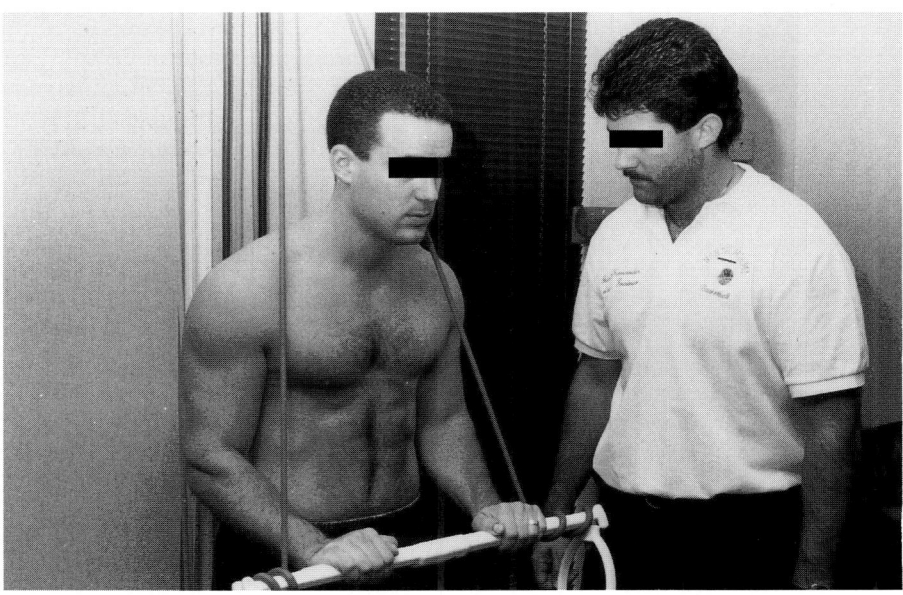

FIGURE 37.
Bilateral triceps push-downs.

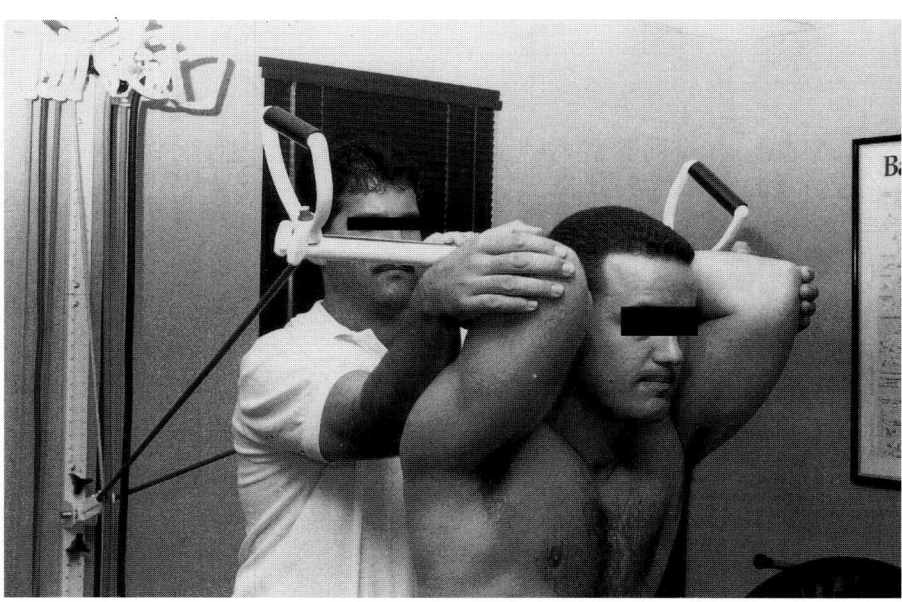

FIGURE 38.
Bilateral triceps exercise using Lifeline.

In recent years, MRI has been used quite extensively for evaluation of injuries to the shoulder. Tendon disease is best evaluated on long repetition times (TR), long echo times (TE) image acquisitions.[64] MRI is an effective means to evaluate the unstable glenohumeral joint, especially if the imaging takes place immediately after dislocation. This allows Bankhardt's lesions to be readily identified.[65] At the present time MRI is the investigation modality of choice for abnormalities associated with impingement syndrome, including compression of the subacromial bursa by bony spurs, capsule hypertrophy, or low-lying acromion.[66] Vellet et al.[67] state that present and future surgical and nonsurgical management of the shoulder will be shaped by MRI. When 21 patients with shoulder pain for more than 3 months were evaluated with ultrasonography and MRI, followed by CT arthrography, the results were compared with operative findings. MRI was found to be the most useful modality for the establishment of the cause of the pain in the shoulder due to disease of the rotator cuff, instability associated with abnormality of the glenoid labrum, subacromial impingement, stenosis of the coracoacromial arch, and osteoarthrosis of either the glenohumeral or the acromioclavicular joint. It must be noted that the accuracy of the MRI results was dependent on both the operator and the technique.[68]

A less often used diagnostic implement used is infrared thermography. Thermography has been shown to be sensitive for the detection of sympathetic maintained pain, primarily reflex sympathetic dystrophy, as well as some forms of headache.[69] It appears at this stage that the use of thermography is relatively minimal in the detection of injuries to the shoulder in athletes.

CT has been particularly useful in the detection of glenoid fractures and complex fractures.

CONCLUSION

This chapter covers only a very small portion of disorders affecting the shoulder, their diagnosis, conservative treatment, and imaging. With changing technologies geared toward expediting more accurate diagnoses and trends toward more conservative approaches to treatment and rehabilitation, future works will be necessary to adequately address these ever rapid changes. Conservative management of shoulder injuries, although a challenge, is both appropriate and effective when provided by a chiropractic doctor.

REFERENCES

1. DeLee JC, Drex D Jr: *Orthopaedic Sports Medicine Principles And Practice.* Philadelphia, WB Saunders, 1994, vol 2.
2. Lehman RC: *Clinics in Sports Medicine.* Philadelphia, WB Saunders, 1988, vol 71.
3. Nicholas JA, Hershman EB: *The Upper Extremity in Sports Medicine.* St Louis, Mosby, 1988.
4. Cailliet R: *Shoulder Pain,* ed 2. Philadelphia, FA Davis, 1988.
5. Williams PL, Warwick R, Dyson M, et al: *Gray's Anatomy,* ed 37. New York, Churchill Livingstone, 1989.
6. Danchik J, Karg M: *Conservative Management of Sports Injuries to the Shoulder.* Baltimore, Williams & Wilkins (in press), 1995.
7. Magee DJ: *Assessment.* Philadelphia, WB Saunders, 1992.
8. Roy S, Richard I: *Sports Medicine.* Englewood Cliffs, NJ, Prentice-Hall.
9. Bach BR Jr, VanFleet TA, Novak PJ: Acromioclavicular Injuries. *Phys Sports Med* 20:87–101, 1992.
10. MacDonald PB, Alexander MJ, Frejuk J, et al: Comprehensive functional analysis of shoulders following complete acromioclavicular separation. *Am J Sports Med* 16:475–480, 1988.
11. Christensen K: *Clinical Chiropractic Orthopedics.* Dubuque, Foot Levelers, Inc, 1984.
12. Noah J Jr, Giduman R: Rotator cuff injuries in the throwing athlete. *Orthop Rev* 17:1091–1096, 1988.
13. Hannaford P: Rotator cuff injuries of the shoulder. *Aust Fam Phys* 17:1091–1096, 1988.
14. Jobe FW, Bradley JP: Rotator cuff injuries in baseball. *Sports Med* 6:378–387, 1988.
15. Beach WR, Caspari RB: Arthroscopic management of rotator cuff disease *Orthopedics* 16:1007–1015, 1993.
16. Nirschl RP: Rotator cuff tendinitis, in *Basic Concepts of Pathoetiology,* pp 439–445.
17. Andrews JR, Meister K: Classification and treatment of rotator cuff injuries in the overhand athlete. *JOSPT* 18:413–421, 1993.
18. Savoie FH: Evaluation of the shoulder: Examination in throwing athletes. MSMA, 249–253.
19. Copeland S: Throwing injuries of the shoulder. *Br J Sports Med* 27:107–117, 1993;
20. Pappas AM, Zawacki RM: Baseball: Too much on a young pitcher's shoulders? Sports Med 27:107–117.
21. Abrams JS: Special shoulder problems in the throwing athlete: Pathology, diagnosis and nonoperative management. *Clin Sports Med* 10:839–861, 1991.
22. Jobe FW, Kvitne RS: Shoulder pain in the overhand or throwing athlete. The

relationship of anterior instability and rotator cuff impingement. *Orthop Rev* 18:963–975, 1989.
23. Greenan TJ, Zlatkin MB, Kalinka MK, et al: Posttraumatic changes in the posterior glenoid and labrum in a handball player. *Am J Sports Med* 21:153–156, 1993.
24. Andrews JR, Gidumal RH: Shoulder arthroscopy in the throwing athlete: Perspective and prognosis. *Clin Sports Med* 6:565–571, 1987.
25. Miniaci A, Fowler P: Impingement in the athlete. *Clin Sports Med* 12:91–110, 1993.
26. Bigliani LU, Morrison DS, April EW: The morphology of the acromion and rotator cuff: Importance. *Orthopedic Transactions* 10:228, 1986.
27. Ferguson AB: Shoulder impingement syndrome. A critical review. *Clin Orthop* 269:162–173, 1991.
28. Shrode LW: Treating shoulder impingement using the supraspinatus synchronization exercise. *J Manipulative Physiol Ther* 17:43–53, 1994.
29. Scheib J: Diagnosis and rehabilitation of the shoulder impingement syndrome in the overhand and throwing athlete. *Rheu Disease Clinics of North Am* 16:971–988, 1990.
30. Hawkins RJ, Mohtadi NGH: Controversy in anterior shoulder instability. *Clin Ortho Related Research* 272:152–161, 1991.
31. Rowe C: Prognosis in dislocations of the shoulder. *J Bone Joint Surg* 38:957, 1956.
32. Pacelli LC: Shoulder instability—a new approach. *Phys Sports Med* 18:103–106, 1990.
33. Gross ML, Brenner SL, Esformes I, et al: Anterior shoulder instability in weight lifters. *Am J Sports Med* 21:599–603, 1993.
34. Zarins B, McMahon MS, Rowe CR: Diagnosis and treatment of traumatic anterior instability of the shoulder. *Clin Orthop* 291:75–84, 1993.
35. Movelius L, Erickson GK, Fredin FH, et al: Recurrences after initial dislocations of the shoulder. *J Bone Joint Surg (Am)* 65A:343, 1983.
36. Henry JH, Genung JA: Natural history of glenohumeral dislocation. *Am J Sports Med* 10:135, 1982.
37. Kozar B, Relovsky E: Prognosis of primary dislocation of the shoulder. *Acta Orthop Scand* 40:216, 1969.
38. McLaughlin HL, Cavallaro WH: Primary anterior dislocation of the shoulder. *Am J Surg* 80:615, 1950.
39. McLaughlin HL, MacLellan DJ: Recurrent anterior dislocation of the shoulder. *J Trauma* 7:191, 1967.
40. Simonet WT, Cofield RH: Prognosis in anterior shoulder dislocation. *Am J Sports Med* 12:19, 1984.
41. Baker CL, Liu SH: Neurovascular injuries to the shoulder. *JOSPT* 18:360–364, 1993.
42. Silliman JF, Dean MT: Neurovascular injuries to the shoulder complex. *JOSPT* 18:442–448, 1993.
43. Markey KL, DiBenedetto M, Curl WW: Upper trunk brachial plexopathy. The stinger syndrome. *Am J Sports Med* 21:650–655, 1993.
44. Rivera JE: Open versus closed kinetic chain. *J Sport Rehabil* 3:154–167, 1994.
45. Gray G, Peterson JA, Bryant CX: Sense. *Fitness Manage* 4:31–33, 1992.
46. Ishikawa H, Yasuyuka V, Yonezawa T, et al: Osteochondritis dissecans of the shoulder in a tennis player. *Am J Sports Med* 15:547–550, 1988.
47. Matthews LS, Barry G, Simonson, MD, et al: Osteolysis of the distal clavicle in a female body builder. *Am J Sports Med* 21:150–152, 1993.
48. Scavebuys NM, Uverseb BJ: Nontraumatic clavicular osteolysis in weight lifters. *Am J Sports Med* 20:463–467, 1992.

49. Cahill R: A traumatic osteolysis of the distal clavicle. *Sports Med* 13:214–225, 1992.
50. Estwanik JJ: Levator scapulae syndrome. *Phys Sports Med* 17:57–68, 1989.
51. Havranek P: Injuries of distal clavicular physis in children. *J Pediatr Orthop* 9:213–215, 1989.
52. Fowler C, Potter GE: An uncommon shoulder injury. *Br J Sports Med* 24:125–126, 1990.
53. Motta F, Carletti T: Spontaneous rupture of the infraspinatus muscle. *Int Orthop* 14:351–353, 1990.
54. Tengan CH, Oliveira ASB, Kiymoto BH, et al: Isolated and painless infraspinatus atrophy in top-level volleyball players: Report of two cases and review of the literature. *Arq Neuropsiquiatr* 51:125–129, 1993.
55. Schaefer RS, Proffer DS: *Sports Medicine for Wheelchair Athletes.* 39:239–245, 1989.
56. Burnham RS, May L, Nelson E, et al: Shoulder pain in wheelchair athletes. *Am J Sports Med* 21:238–242, 1993.
57. Leahy PM, Mock LE: Synoviochondrometaplasia of the shoulder: A case report. *Chiropr Sports Med* 6:5–9, 1992.
58. Anderson T: Difficult sports-related shoulder fractures: *Clin Sports Med* 9:31–37, 1990.
59. Cain TE, Hamilton WP: Scapular fractures in professional football players. *Am J Sports Med* 20:363–365, 1992.
60. Henry J, Morley J: Clavicle fractures in bicyclists—a preventable injury? Case studies and recommendation. *Chiropr Sports Med* 4:42–45.
61. Engebretsen L, Craig CY: Radiologic features of shoulder instability. *Clin Ortho* 291:29–44, 1993.
62. Middleton, Kricun M: *Imaging of Sports Injuries.* Gaithersburg, Aspen, 1992.
63. Benson CB: Sonography of the musculoskeletal system. *Rheum Dis Clin North Am* 3:487–504, 1991.
64. Crues JV III, Fareed DO: Magnetic resonance imaging of shoulder impingement. 3:39–49, 1991.
65. Fischbach TJ, Seeger LL: Magnetic resonance imaging of glenohumeral instability. *Topics in MRI* 3:39–49, 1991.
66. Galloway H, Suh J, Everson L, Griffiths H: MRI and sports injuries. *Orthopedics* 15:249–256, 1991.
67. Vellet AD, Munk PI, Marks P: Imaging techniques of the shoulder: Present perspectives. *Clin Sports Med* 4:721–756, 1991.
68. Nelson MC, Leather GP, Mirschl RP, et al: Evaluation of the painful shoulder. *J Bone Joint Surg Am* 5:707–716, 1991.
69. Ben Eliyahu DJ: Infrared thermography in the diagnosis and management of sports injuries: A clinical study and literature review. *Chiropr Sports Med* 4:46–53, 1990.
70. Baumgartner K: An algorithm for shoulder pain caused by soft-tissue disorders. *DC Tracts* 3, 1991

The Many Faces of the Facets

Sharon A. Jaeger, D.C., D.A.C.B.R., F.I.C.C.
Secretary/Treasurer, Foundation on Chiropractic Education and Research; Board of Regents, Los Angeles College of Chiropractic, Whittier, California; Consulting Practice, Chatsworth, California; Private Practice, North Hollywood, California

Cynthia A. Baum, D.C., D.A.C.B.R.
Radiological Consulting Practice, Chatsworth, California; Postgraduate Faculty, Los Angeles College of Chiropractic, Whittier, California

Gary R. Lindquist, D.C., D.A.C.B.R.
Radiological Consulting Practice, Chatsworth, California; Postgraduate Faculty, Los Angeles College of Chiropractic, Whittier, California

PLANE FILM

Visualization of the facets on standard plane films in the cervical spine is best done on the lateral and oblique views. Boyleston's pillar views will better demonstrate the C-3 through C-7 facets and laminae on profile. The upper three or four thoracic vertebrae may also be visualized. The bilateral pillar view is taken with the patient supine or seated and the head hyperextended. The tube is angled caudally with a 25-degree tilt. The central ray should enter at the level of the thyroid cartilage. Unilateral pillar views are taken with the patient supine or seated with the head turned 45 degrees and slightly flexed. A 30- to 35-degree caudal tube tilt is used with the central ray entering at the thyroid cartilage (approximately C-4.) This can also be done with the patient prone if this position is more comfortable. A cephalic tube tilt is then employed. Both sides should be done for comparison. The degree of tube tilt should coincide with the amount of cervical lordosis.

The thoracic articular facets are best demonstrated on oblique projections. These may be taken either anteriorly (Oppenheimer's method)[1] or posteriorly (Fuch's method).[2] The anterior oblique views allow the facets closest to the film to be best delineated, whereas the posterior oblique views will visualize the facets furthest from the film. Again, whichever method is used, both sides should be done the same way. The patient is rotated approximately 20 degrees off true lateral (either anterior or posterior). In cases where the patient is hyperkyphotic, additional rotation may be necessary to visualize the upper- and lowermost facet levels.

The standard oblique views of the lumbar spine will in the majority of cases provide proper visualization of the facets. These may be performed either anteriorly or posteriorly. The opposite facets will be seen on the anterior oblique view. The facets on the same side will be depicted on posterior oblique views. The patient is rotated 45 degrees to the film. If the L-5 to S-1 facets are the prime area of interest or if this area is not imaged well on the standard view, obliquing the patient 30 degrees should rectify this.

The angle of the facets at the lumbosacral junction form an angle of 30 degrees whereas the L-1 to L-2 through the L-4 to L-5 facets form an angle of 45 degrees to the median coronal plane in most patients.[3]

IMAGING

Computed tomography (CT) can very accurately demonstrate inherent high contrast between bone and soft tissue[4] and is therefore probably the most sensitive method to evaluate the facet complexes.[5] The facets are directly imaged in the transaxial plane. When reconstruction methods can be employed, they can be presented in other planes such as coronal and sagittal. Various abnormalities of the facet joints, which can be identified by CT, include degenerative changes such as osteophyte formation, hypertrophy, joint space narrowing, and subchondral sclerosis. Erosions and cysts, vacuum formation (gas within the joints), synovial cysts, and periarticular calcifications are depicted. Subluxations related to retrolisthesis and spondylolisthesis and normal variations in size, shape, and ossification can be demonstrated. Spinal stenosis, primary bone neoplasm, metastatic disease, and inflammatory processes are well depicted. Three-dimensional CT imaging may provide more information and better perception of bone abnormalities than two-dimensional in spinal trauma.[5] Magnetic resonance imaging (MRI) is somewhat limited in evaluating the full spectrum of disease processes affecting the facets because the subchondral compact bone, the surrounding ligament structures, and any potential calcific formations all exhibit very dark images because their hydrogen is fixed in their molecular makeup. The facets and intervening joints can be seen in the sagittal plane but are best demonstrated in the transaxial plane. The normal articular capsule is difficult to distinguish on MR images.[4] Differentiation between spongy and cortical bone is best depicted on long time to repetition (TR)/short time to echo (TE) pulse sequences. The hyaline cartilage covering the facets (2–4 mm thick) is best imaged on gradient echo scans, where its increased signal stands out against the dark signal of underlying cortical bone. Synovial fluid accumulations within the joint display a bright signal on T_2-weighted images. The fatty marrow content within the medullary bone will exhibit a medium gray density on T_1-weighted images. MRI can also quantitatively image any hypertrophy of the facets leading to encroachment into the neural foramen. Short TR/short TE images are best for imaging the emerging nerve root surrounded by epineural fat within the radicular canal.[4]

ANATOMY

The apophyseal joints are encountered at each vertebral level from the upper cervical levels to the first sacral segment. All are true diarthrodial synovial joints. The articular processes arise from the caudal and cephalic aspects of the lamina-pedicle junctions on each side and constitute support structures for the articular facets or "zygapophyses." The superior (cephalic) facets generally face dorsally and are sometimes called "prezygapophyses"; the inferior (caudal) facets generally face ventrally and are called the "post(retro)zygapophyses."[6]

The articular surfaces of the facets are covered by hyaline cartilage, which measures 2 to 4 mm (in combined thickness). The cartilage may extend well beyond the limits of bony contact, particularly in the lower lumbar levels.

Joint space measures between 2 and 4 mm. It actually continues around on the posterior surface of the articular process in the lower lumbar spine. This smooth, rounded cartilage makes contact with the inside of the redundant capsule, aiding in stability from lateral thrust.

Loose ligamentous joint capsules (medially and laterally) enclose the joint. These are not attached to the articular margins but are reflected around and attach to the outer surfaces of the processes. These tend to be looser in the cervical spine than in the thoracic or lumbar region, allowing greater degree of motion. Anteromedially the capsule is thickened by the lateral attachment of the ligamentum flavum. The ligamentum flavum extends from the anteroinferior border of the lamina above to the upper posterior border of the lamina below.[5] The superior and inferior aspects of the capsule are synovial lined and contain fat. Two types of inclusions extend between the facets:

1. Fat-filled synovial folds (at superior and inferior poles of joint). These folds project between the articular surfaces 2 to 4 mm. These folds move freely in and out of the joint during movement.[7]
2. Meniscal-like rudimentary fibrous invaginations, which arise from dorsal and ventral portions of capsule.

These joint inclusions are thought to function as shock absorbers that allow for changing pressures within the joint. If they become incarcerated within a joint, the joint locks, reducing motion and producing pain.

NERVE SUPPLY

The loose capsule attached around the margins of the facets is supplied by medial branches of the dorsal rami of spinal nerves.[8] According to Wyke and Paris, the zygopophyseal joint is innervated from no less than three successive posterior primary rami (i.e., the nerve emerging at the level of the joint, plus the spinal nerve above and the spinal nerve below).[9] Articular nerves vary in number and course, and their areas of distribution overlap within joints. Articular nerves contain sensory and autonomic fibers.

Some of the sensory fibers form proprioceptive endings in the capsule and the ligaments, whereas others form pain endings. These are numerous in the joint capsules and ligaments. Studies have indicated that the fibrous capsule is highly sensitive,[10] whereas the synovial membrane is relatively insensitive.[11]

PLANE OF ORIENTATION

An important role of the posterior elements is the maintenance of spinal stability. The mobility between two adjacent vertebrae is determined primarily by the orientation of the planes of articulation. In the cervical spine, the orientation is more horizontal. This facilitates rotatory motion while allowing considerable flexion and extension and to a lesser degree lateral flexion. The facets in the thoracic spine are almost vertical; thus, these segments can flex and extend and rotate but allow only limited lateral bending. In the lumbar spine, the orientation of the articular facets changes from one level to the next. They allow flexion, extension, lateral bending, and minimal axial rotation. Sagittal orientation predominates in the upper lumbar region, rotating toward coronal predominance at the lumbosacral junction.

DEVELOPMENTAL VARIATIONS

The architecture of the facets is frequently different from what is described as "normal." In the cervical spine, a great deal of variation in re-

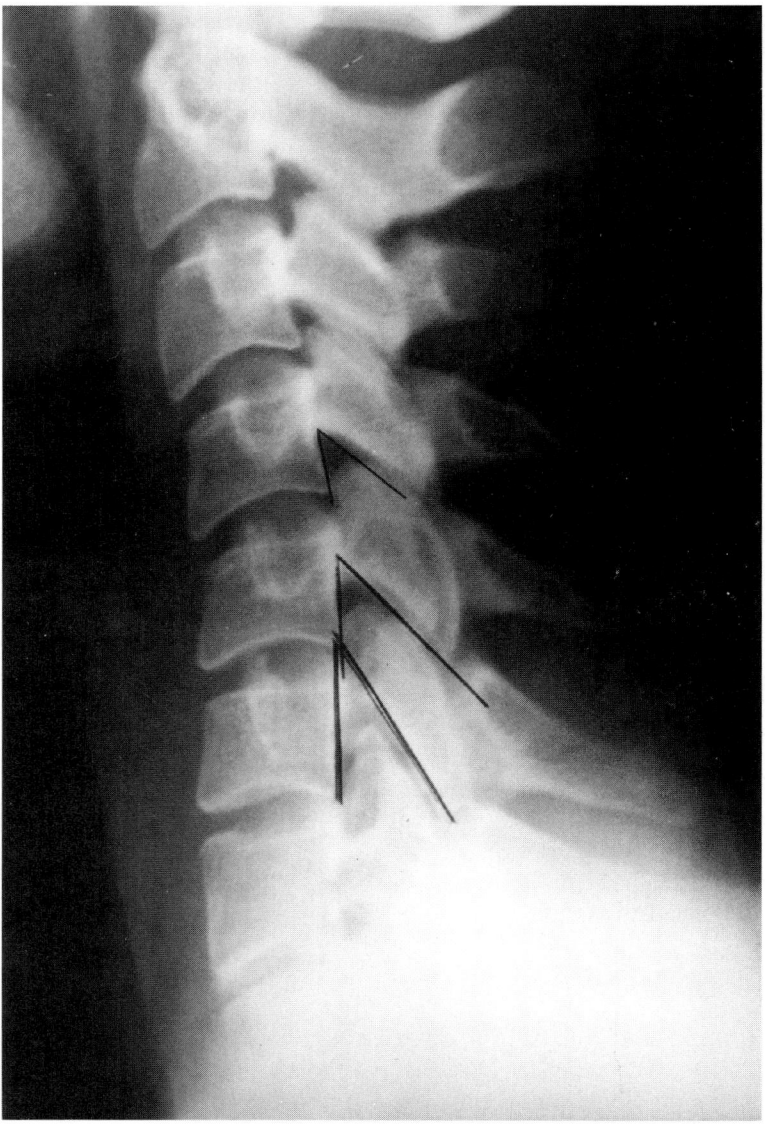

FIGURE 1.
Articular pillar angles (body facet angle). Normally this should not exceed 45 degrees.

gard to orientation is encountered at the C-2 to C-3 facet complex. They can appear fused on the lateral films. This is projectional in nature due to their obliquity. The C-3 through C-7 facets typically exhibit a body-facet angle of approximately 45 degrees. This angle is formed by lines drawn along the inferior facet surface to a vertical line along the posterior body margin (Fig 1). The height of the articular pillar usually does not exceed the height of the vertebral body. In addition, lines drawn along the plane of the superior and inferior facets should have a tendency to converge at some point posteriorly.

The cervical lordotic curve may be affected by developmental factors

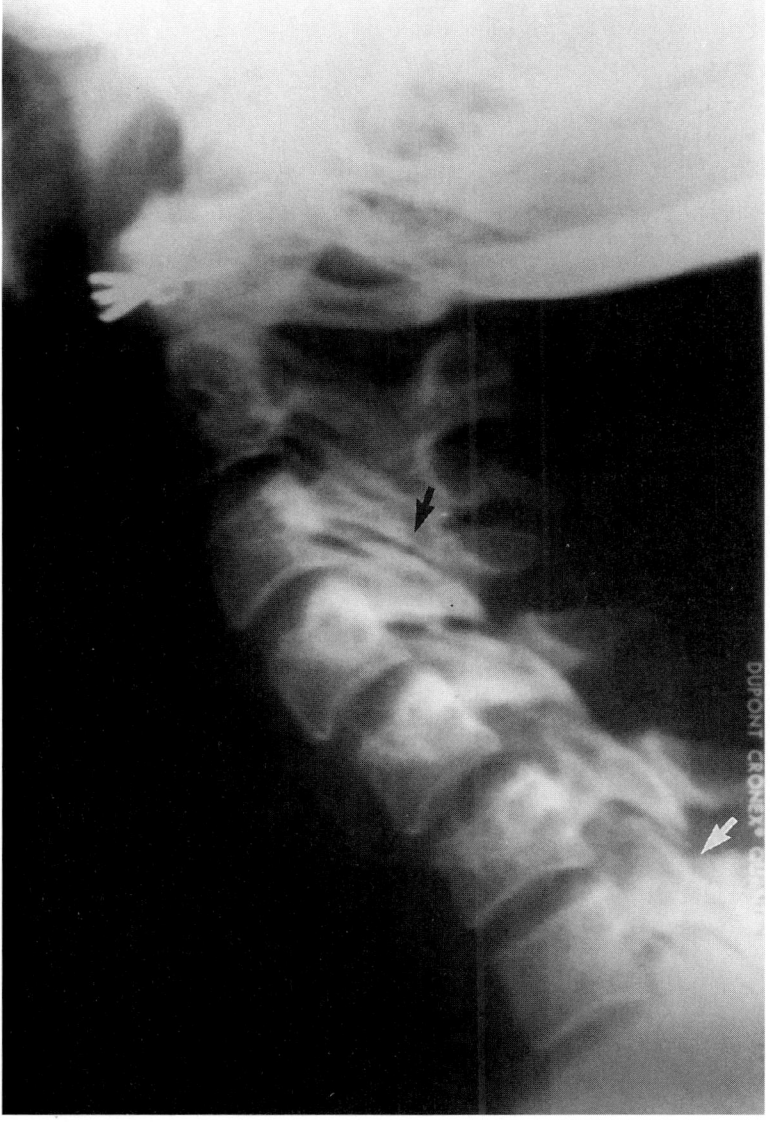

FIGURE 2.
There is a biphasic cervical curve created by the shape and angulation of the articular processes. The orientation of the upper facets is almost horizontal.

resulting in alordosis, hypolordosis, biphasic curve (Fig 2) or occasionally a kyphotic contour (reversed curve) (Fig 3). The following alterations may be encountered:

- Short pedicles or obliquely oriented pedicles that allow the articular pillars to overlay (lie lateral to) the posterior aspect of the body, as seen on lateral projections; usually generalized.
- Increased height of the articular pillar or developmentally short bodies (pillars are taller than the bodies); may be general or localized.

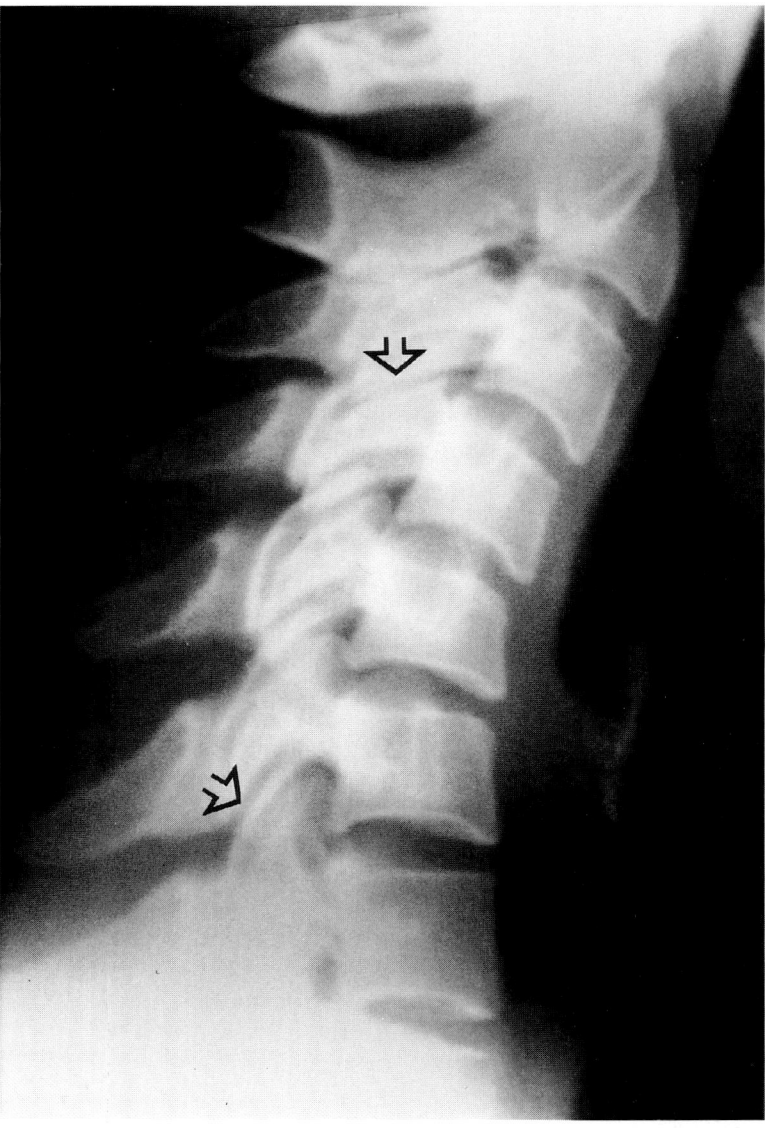

FIGURE 3.
Reversed cervical curve due to more horizontal orientation of the upper facets and vertical orientation of the lower facets.

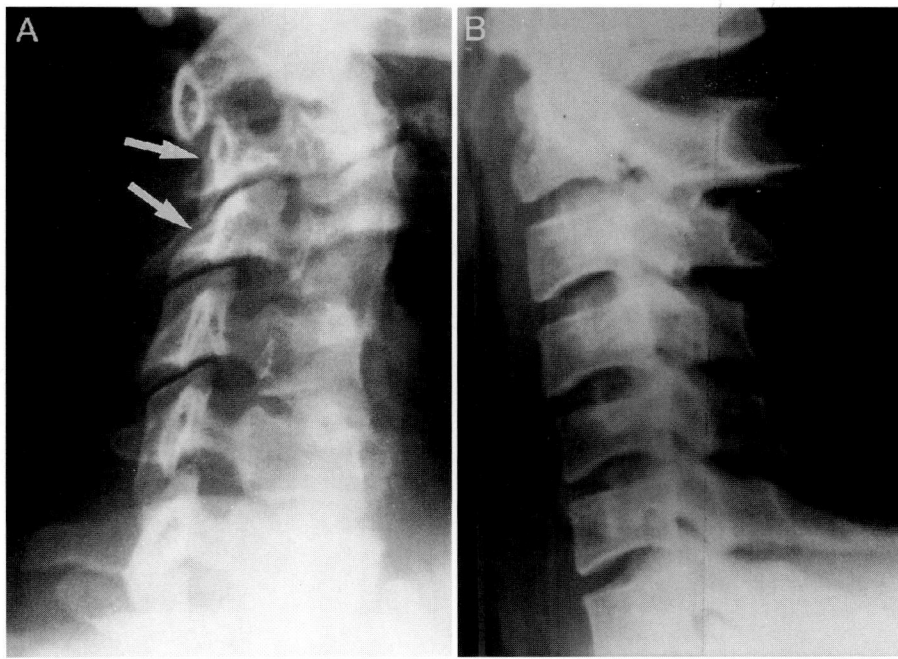

FIGURE 4.
A, hypoplastic C-3 and C-4 articular processes (*arrows*). **B,** the articular processes in this patient are hypoplastic. Note the large vertebral bodies compared with the small articular processes.

- Hypoplastic articular pillars or underdeveloped facets; usually generalized (Fig 4).
- Acute angulation of the body-facet angle (<45 degrees); localized or general (Fig 5).
- Facetal pillar planes, which are either *parallel* or posteriorly *divergent*; localized or general; may compensate with variable angulation at different levels.

FACET NOTCHING: GOUGE DEFECT

A gouge defect is a small notch seen along the posterior third of the superior articular facets in the lower cervical spine (Fig 6). It frequently occurs at C-7, less commonly at C-6. It suggests long-standing paradoxical motion between the lower cervical segments on attempted extension. For example, during cervical extension, C-7 paradoxically flexes while C-6 extends normally. The notch along the superior surface of the C-7 facet accommodates the C-6 inferior facet at the end of the range of motion. Some describe subchrondal reactive stress sclerosis below the notch.

In some patients, a small spurlike process projects superiorly from a point posterior to the notch. This acts as a bumper or stop to the normal posterior glide of the facet above the paradoxically flexing segment during extension motion.

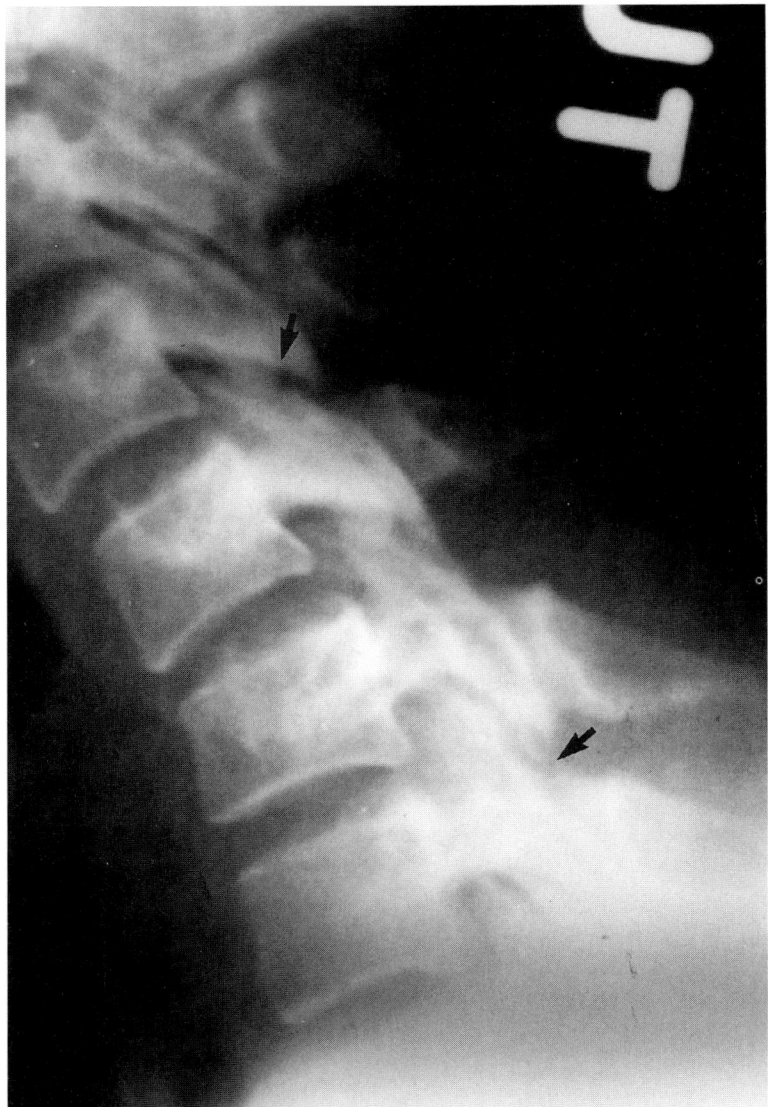

FIGURE 5.
Acute body facet angle *(upper arrow)*. Gouge defect *(lower arrow)*.

TROPISM

Tropism, defined as "turning" or "to turn" is a congenital anomaly. It is further defined as an asymmetry of 5 degrees or more in the horizontal plane of paired left and right facet joints that can occur at any spinal level (Figs 7 and 8). Tropism has been encountered in 21% to 37% of the population, most frequently at the lowest two lumbar levels. It is not uncommon at T-11 to L-1 (21%) and T-12 to L-1 (9%).[9]

Various controversial hypotheses have been described in the literature as to the clinical significance of tropism.

Goldthwait[12] and von Luckum[13] concluded that movements of asymmetrical articulations are irregular and may contribute to weakness in

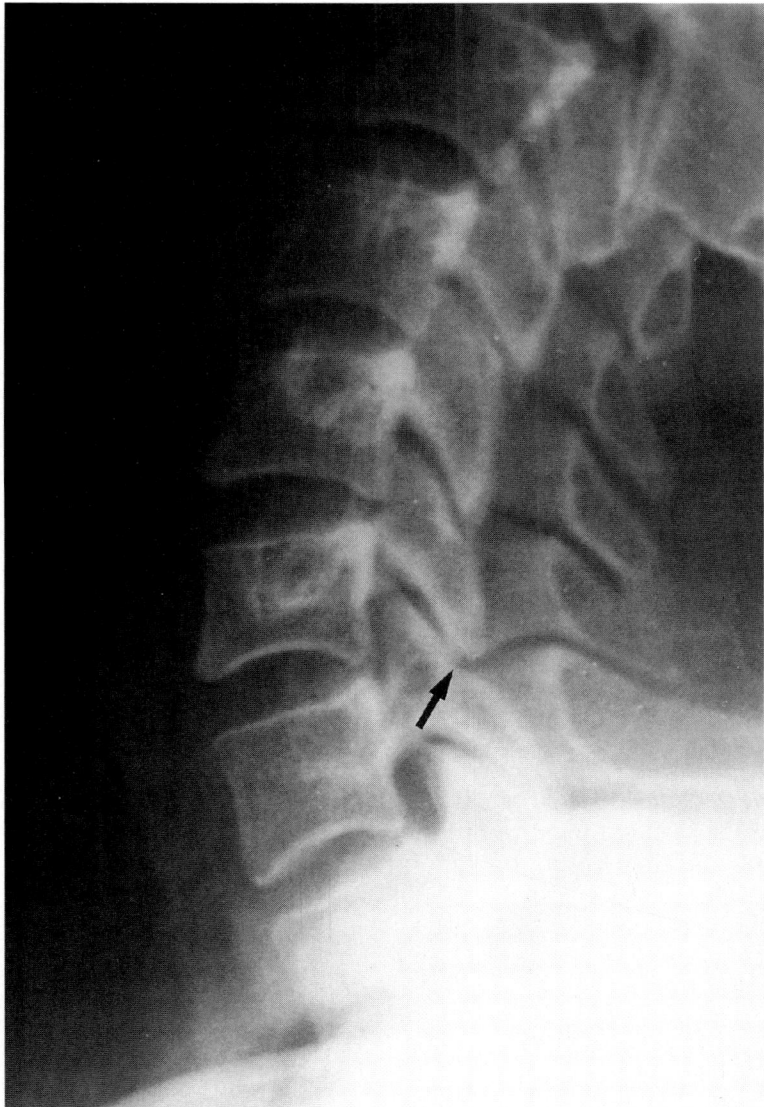

FIGURE 6.
Notched facet (arrow). The inferior articular process from the segment above fits nicely into the notch of the articular process below.

some parts of the mobile segment, particularly at the lumbosacral junction (mobile L-5 and immobile sacrum).

Putti[14] in 1927 was the first to comment on facetal tropism in the pathogenesis of low back pain and sciatica. He believed that it may alter the shape of the intervertebral foramen (IVF), reducing its capacity. The directional asymmetry may alter local spinal mechanics, resulting in premature osteoarthritis that could irritate the nerve trunk.

Ghormley[15] stated, "Articular tropism or asymmetry of the articular facets can lead to lumbar instability manifesting itself as joint rotation." This rotation occurs toward the side of the more oblique facet and can

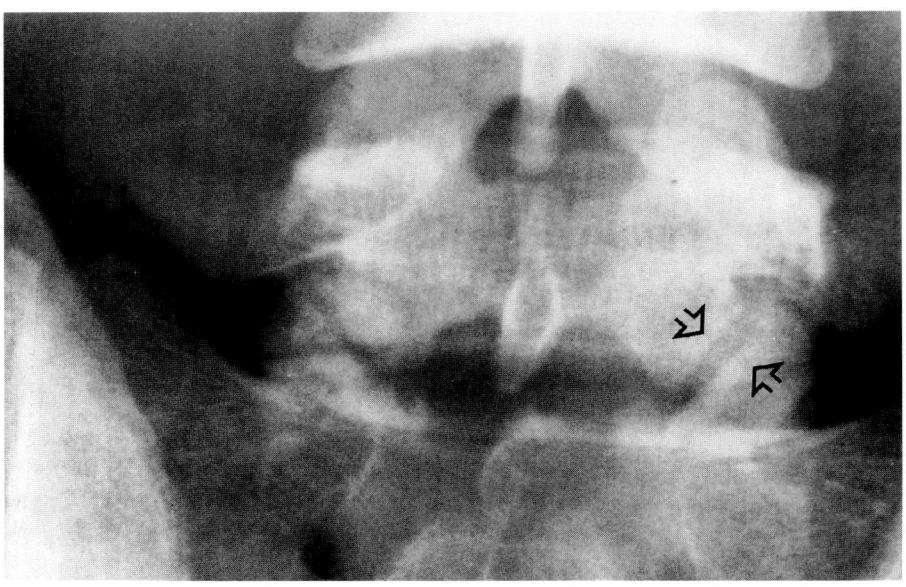

FIGURE 7.
Oblique orientation of the L-5 to S-1 facetal joints (arrows).

place additional stress on the annulus fibrosis of the intervertebral disk (IVD) and capsular ligaments of the apophyseal joints.

Ferguson[16] wrote that probably the worst type of facets mechanically were asymmetrical. In severe cases with one sagittal and one coronal, every movement must put undue strain on one or the other of these facets, because they do not operate in the same plane.

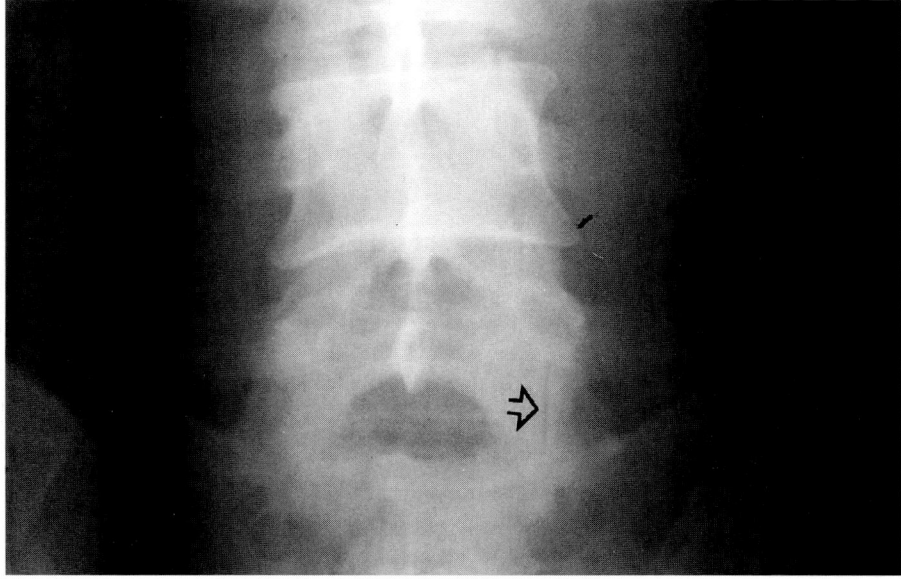

FIGURE 8.
Tropism. Sagittal facet (arrow), with coronal facet on opposite side.

Farfan and Sullivan[17] demonstrated a very high correlation of facet tropism with not only disk degeneration but with lateralization of nucleus pulposus and herniation as well. They proposed that these changes resulted from abnormal rotatory stress on the annulus. Protrusion will occur more often on the side of the more oblique joint surface.

Cyron and Hutton[18] reported that spines with asymmetrical facets produce instability, manifesting itself as rotation of the lumbar spine. This puts the ligaments of one facet joint under extra strain and greater interfacet forces in the more sagittally oriented facets at the lumbosacral junction. Sagittal facets are covered by significantly thinner hyaline cartilage, and the cross-sectional area is smaller than coronal facets.

Van Schaik et al.[19] found no correlation between asymmetry of the facet joints and the side of unilateral disk protrusion except in the case of gross asymmetry at the L-4 to L-5 level.

The Lobeck et al.[20] research focused on the association between the site of lumbar disk herniation and the orientation of the facets. Their results suggested that in patients with central herniations, the facet orientation was more symmetrical than with lateral herniations. Lateral herniations were found to be more likely on the side of the more coronal-facing facets. They argued that their results, like Farfan's, implicate torsional injuries in the cause of IVD failure at the L-5 to S-1 level.

The work of Gunzberg et al.[21] on axial rotation concluded that even though tropism has been described by many to be responsible for the development of abnormal rotations, nothing relating articular tropism to the amplitude of rotation has been found. He therefore concluded that no credence could be given to the view that torsion alone is responsible for disk damage or annular tears.

Vanharanta et al.[22] in 1993 did facet angle measurements on CT. Their data did not support the hypothesis that facet tropism is associated with degenerative lumbar disk disease or the production of clinical symptoms.

CONGENITAL BLOCKING

Failure of segmentation may involve the articular pillars unilaterally, bilaterally, or in concert with blocking of the bodies (Fig 9). Segmental laxity sometimes develops at the contiguous levels with the possibility of premature degenerative changes.

AGENESIS

Failure of formation of the facets is a relatively rare anomaly and seldom isolated. Various anomalies involving the posterior arch and bodies in the same location are often demonstrated. These findings should not be confused with a lytic lesion.

HYPOPLASIA OR HYPERPLASIA

Deficiencies of the articular facets are not uncommon (Fig 10). They can occur at any level but appear more frequently at the lumbosacral junction. Compensatory features are often present: hypoplasia at one level and hyperplasia at the contiguous levels (Figs 11 and 12). Local alterations in

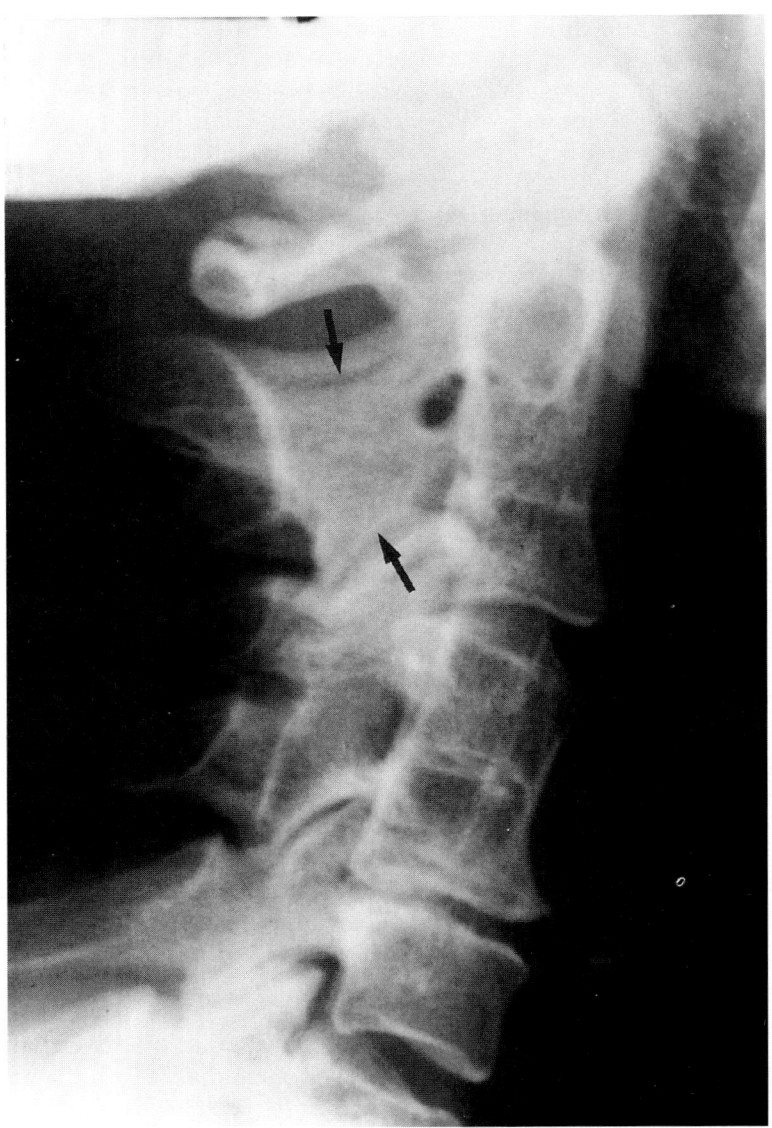

FIGURE 9.
Vertebral segments are blocked at C-2 through C-4 (*arrows*). The C-2 to C-3 facets are fused. The C-4 facets are hypoplastic.

biomechanics leading to stress sclerosis, pars impingement, and dysplastic forms of spondylolisthesis have resulted from these structural anomalies. Underdeveloped articular pillars are frequently the causative agent of cervical spondylolisthesis typically found at C-6.[23]

UNUNITED APOPHYSEAL GROWTH CENTERS: OSSICLES OF OPPENHEIMER

Secondary growth centers occur at the tips of both the superior and inferior articular processes (Fig 13). These usually ossify by age 25. The

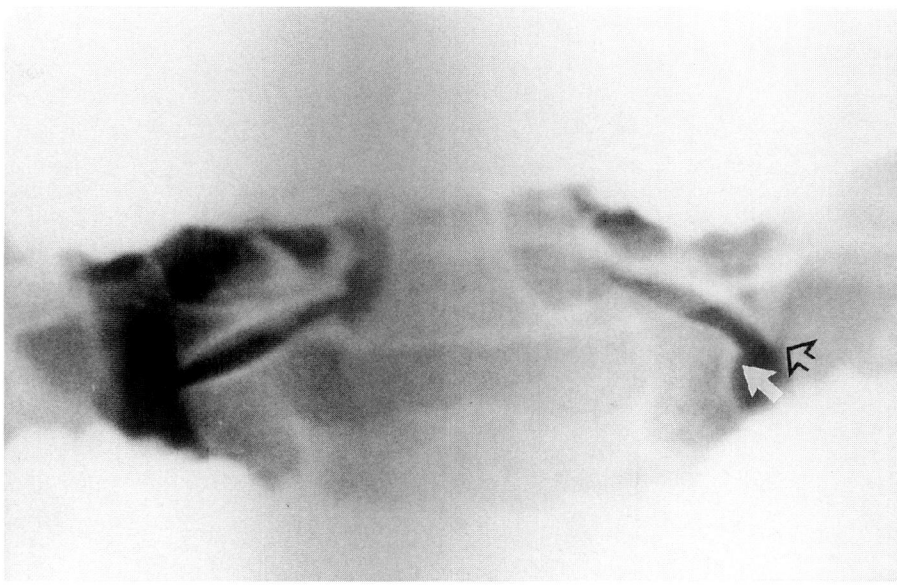

FIGURE 10.
Uneven development of the C-1 and C-2 facets (*arrows*). Note how the right C-1 apophysis overlaps the C-2 articular process. The lower facet is actually hypoplastic compared with the upper facet.

growth center may persist into adulthood as an accessory ossicle. Usually encountered in the lumbar region at the L-3 level, they are more common in males. The inferior articular processes are more commonly involved than the superior. These may be confused with a fracture, but an isolated fracture is very unlikely. If a fracture does occur, it would be the result of severe trauma of a rotary character. The fracture would most typically be accompanied by neural arch or body disruption. Marked pain and localized tenderness would accompany a traumatic fragment. They can be differentiated by their radiographic presentation. The ossicle is typically bulkier than the facets at the adjacent levels. The opposing contours of the bone are smooth, and the peripheral margins are somewhat rounded. Most sources agree that they are clinically insignificant. However, some claim that they may produce symptoms if they are large and mobile.

TRAUMA TO THE CERVICAL SPINE

LOCKED FACETS

One or both of the articular processes may be locked. Malgaigne described the differences between unilateral and bilateral interlocking thoroughly in 1855.[10] Interlocking is initiated by forward movement of the inferior articular facet of the upper vertebra over the superior articular facet of the underlying vertebra (Fig 14).

UNILATERAL FACET DISLOCATION: STABLE INJURY

The mechanism of injury is a combination of flexion, rotation, and distraction. On the side of dislocation the joint capsule and interspinous liga-

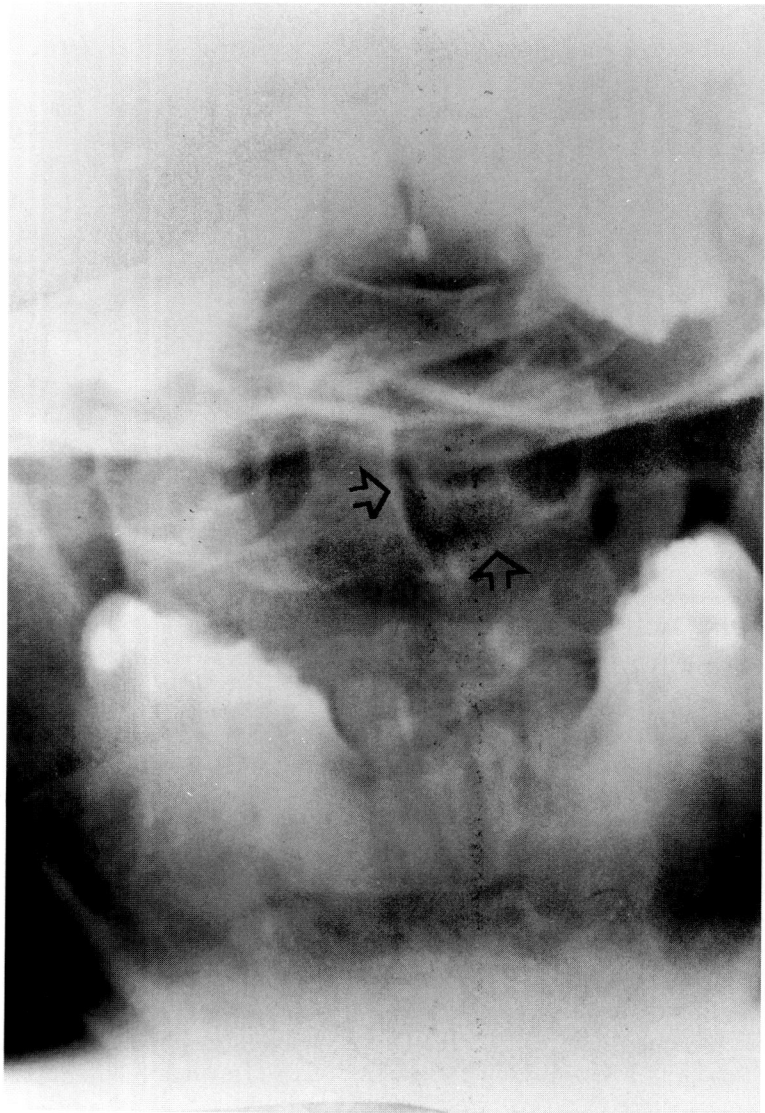

FIGURE 11.
Right angle atlas/axis (arrows).

ments must be torn to allow unilateral dislocation, whereas the posterior longitudinal ligament and annulus fibrosis may be only slightly damaged. On the opposite side, the ligaments of the zygapophyseal joint are usually torn. A fracture of the superior articular process is often present. Compression of the vertebral body directly below with possible lesions elsewhere in the cervical spine may be encountered.[10]

They are occasionally missed early on. Clinically they are well tolerated. An incorrect lateral view or vertebral rotation makes it difficult to interpret. After the muscle spasms and splinting have resolved, flexion and extension views will test for instability. Forward displacement of the

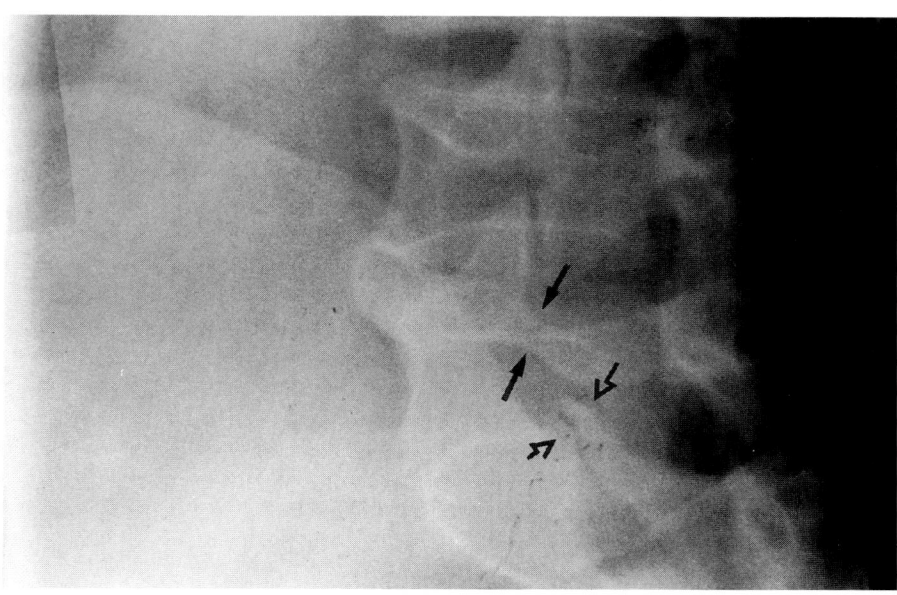

FIGURE 12.
Elongated pars interarticularis region at L-5 and hypoplastic L-5 to S-1 facets (open arrows).

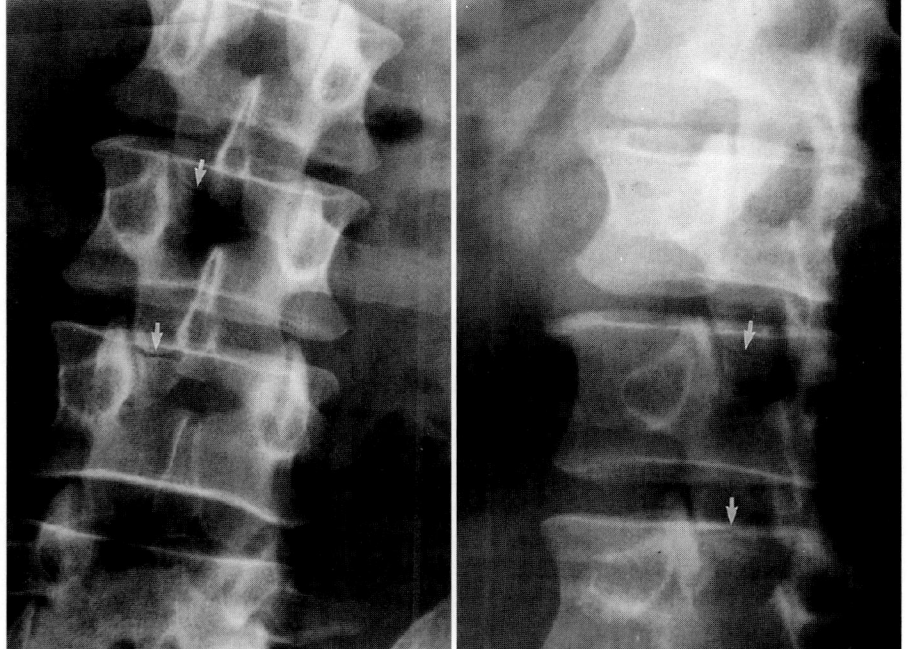

FIGURE 13.
A and B, ununited apophyses of the inferior articular processes of two contiguous segments. The margins are smooth, delineating it from fracture.

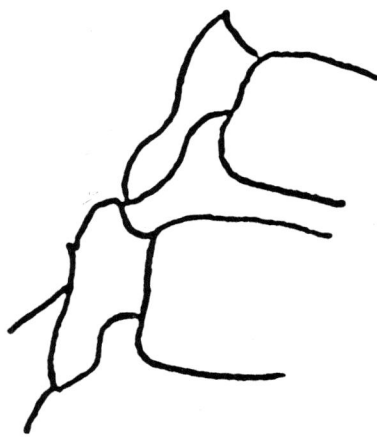

FIGURE 14.
Schematic of a locked facet.

body relative to the segment below will be present. The degree is 50% or less; 25% or less is probably a more accurate range. When visualized on the lateral view, the facetal joints will show greater obliquity from the level of injury above and remain in true profile below the level of injury (or vice versa). This may produce a bow tie or bat wing appearance (Fig 15) of the dislocated vertebra.

On the anteroposterior view, the spinous process is usually displaced to the side of the interlocking facets. Oblique or Boyleston views will illustrate the facet override to best advantage. The neural foramen on the side of injury is reduced and may be obscured by the rotated articular pillar. On CT, the superior articular process of the lower segment can be identified posterior to the inferior articular process of the upper segment. The nonarticular convex surfaces of the articular processes oppose each other, whereas the flat articular surfaces face in opposite directions. Normally the flat surfaces should be facing one another.

Neural involvement is rare. Cord injury occurs in only 30% of cases. If present, it may be isolated to a root. There may be transient motor weakness or paresis in all four limbs or limited to the upper extremity without sensory loss. Brown-Sèquard syndrome may be a residual. This involves unilateral motor paralysis and contralateral loss of pain and temperature sense.

There is a tendency for spontaneous stabilization of unilateral facet dislocation regardless of whether reduction is carried out or not. Healing leads to radiographically visible alterations. The damaged disk decreases in height with occasional ossification of the outer edge of the annulus fibrosis. This may ultimately connect the adjacent vertebral bodies. In time, osteoarthritis develops. Nearly always, the affected segments become immobile even in the interlocked state. Even though at times there is variable residual mobility, the risk of later progression of neurological symptoms is small in cases of unilateral locking without reduction.[10]

Moving?

I'd like to receive my ***Advances in Chiropractic*** without interruption.
Please note the following change of address, effective:

Name: _____

New Address: _____

_____

City: _____ State: _____ Zip: _____

Old Address: _____

_____

City: _____ State: _____ Zip: _____

Reservation Card

Yes, I would like my own copy of ***Advances in Chiropractic***. Please begin my subscription with the current edition according to the terms described below.* I understand that I will have 30 days to examine each annual edition. If satisfied, I will pay just $66.95 plus sales tax, postage and handling (price subject to change without notice).

Name: _____

Address: _____

City: _____ State: _____ Zip: _____

Method of Payment
○ Visa   ○ Mastercard   ○ AmEx   ○ Bill me   ○ Check (in US dollars, payable to Mosby, Inc.)

Card number: _____ Exp date: _____

Signature: _____

ls-0909

Your Advances Service Guarantee:

When you subscribe to *Advances*, we'll send you an advance notice of future volumes about two months before they publish. This automatic notice system is designed to take up as little of your time as possible. If you do not want *Advances*, the advance notice makes it quick and easy for you to let us know your decision, and you will always have at least 20 days to decide. If we don't hear from you, we'll send you the new volume as soon as it's available. And, of course, *Advances* is yours to examine free of charge for 30 days (postage, handling and applicable sales tax are added to each shipment.).

BUSINESS REPLY MAIL
FIRST CLASS MAIL   PERMIT No. 762   CHICAGO, IL

POSTAGE WILL BE PAID BY ADDRESSEE

Chris Hughes
Mosby-Year Book, Inc.
200 N. LaSalle Street
Suite 2600
Chicago, IL 60601-9981

NO POSTAGE
NECESSARY
IF MAILED
IN THE
UNITED STATES

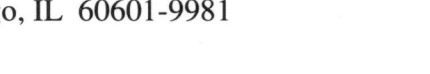

BUSINESS REPLY MAIL
FIRST CLASS MAIL   PERMIT No. 762   CHICAGO, IL

POSTAGE WILL BE PAID BY ADDRESSEE

Chris Hughes
Mosby-Year Book, Inc.
200 N. LaSalle Street
Suite 2600
Chicago, IL 60601-9981

NO POSTAGE
NECESSARY
IF MAILED
IN THE
UNITED STATES

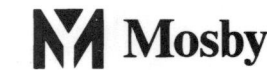

Dedicated to publishing excellence

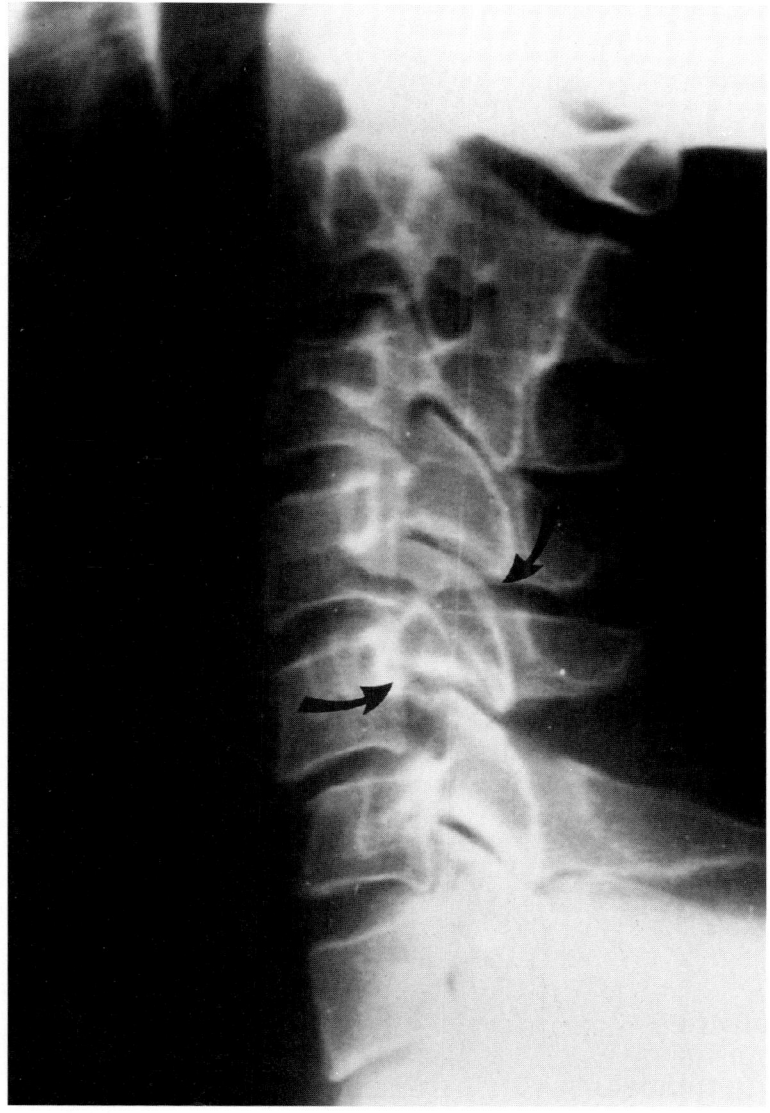

FIGURE 15.
The C-5 articular processes show a bow tie sign due to unilateral facet dislocation.

BILATERAL FACET DISLOCATION: UNSTABLE INJURY

The mechanism of injury is extreme flexion of the head and neck combined with distraction forces that cause disruption of interspinous-supraspinous ligaments, apophyseal joint capsule, posterior longitudinal ligaments, annulus fibrosis, and sometimes the anterior longitudinal ligament (Fig 16). C-4 through C-7 are usually involved. The body is displaced 50% or more relative to the segment below, allowing the inferior facets of the segment to lock in position anterior to the superior facets of the

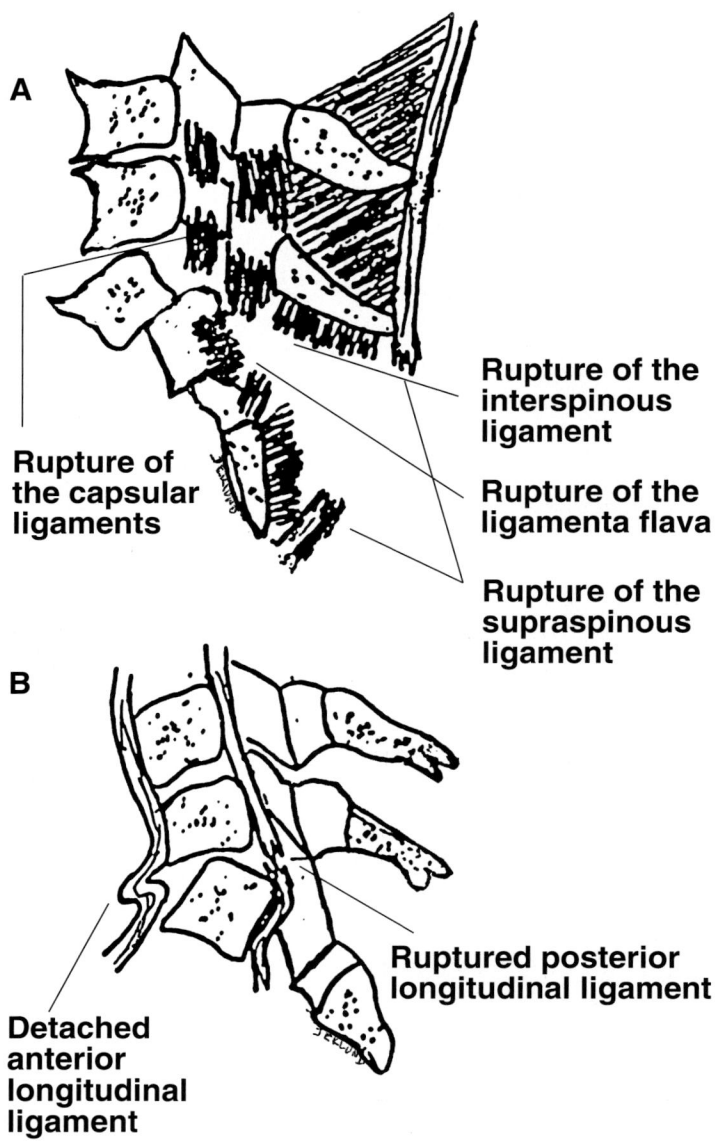

FIGURE 16.
A and B, schematics of ligamentous involvement associated with interlocking facets.

segment below. The spinous processes and laminae will flare (spread apart) because of the disruption of the ligamentum flava and the supraspinous and interspinous ligaments. The facets will come to lie within the neural foramen. Chip fractures often occur at the tips of the facets. Occasionally a fragment from the anterosuperior aspect of the vertebral body is torn off.[10] Neurological deficit is typically quite profound. The central spinal canal is mechanically compromised, and the cord injuries occur 85% of the time. Total motor and sensory loss below the level of injury is not uncommon. These injuries are primarily ligamentous. After reduction, stability is unlikely without surgical intervention such as wiring with fusion.

PERCHED FACETS

The inferior facet of the level above is perched atop the superior facet of the level below. The involved segment is flexed and displaced slightly anteriorly relative to the segment below. Angular reversal of the cervical lordotic curve is present with widening of the interspinous space. The disk space between these segments is wedged narrow anteriorly with greater posterior height (Fig 17).

On CT, the axial slices show the superior and inferior articular processes in different axial cuts. This creates the appearance of an unusually slender lateral mass without a joint space because the inferior articular facet of the level above sits atop the superior articular process of the level below.

DELAYED DISLOCATION

In cases of delayed dislocation, initial radiographs are normal, but some degree of subluxation becomes apparent on subsequent radiographs. These represent ligamentous disruptions either not recognized or not

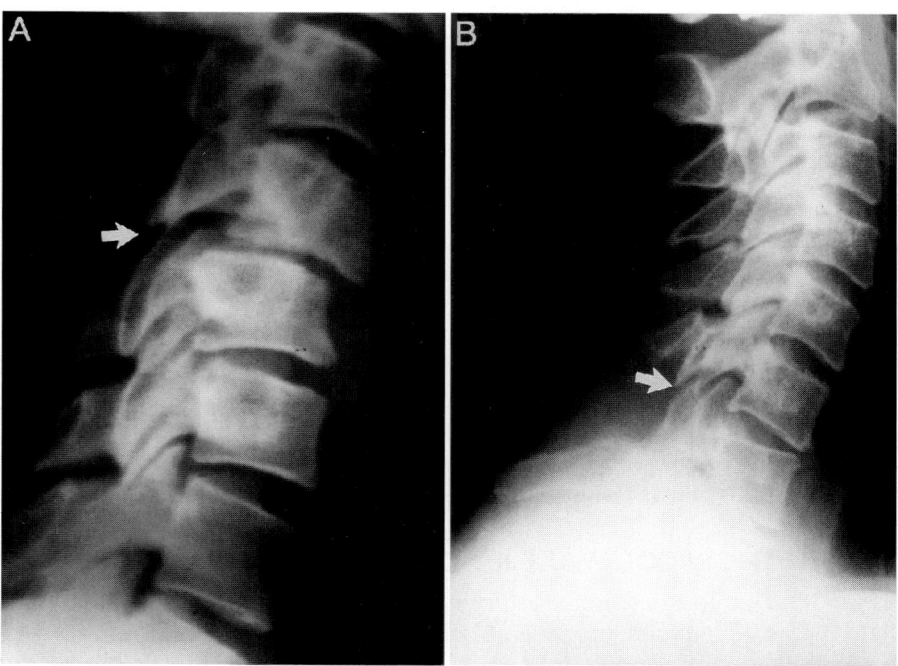

FIGURE 17.
A, perched facets in the cervical spine (*arrow*). Note how the C-3 facets lie at the superiormost aspect of the C-4 facets, creating a spondylolisthesis of C-3. This should not exceed 50% with perched facets. **B,** the C-7 segment is markedly flexed because of the perching of the C-6 facets on top of the C-7 facets (*arrow*). Note the widening of the interspinous space and narrow anterior disk height.

demonstrated on initial studies. Flexion and extension stress views will best illustrate these dysfunctions, but must be done carefully.

DISTRACTED FACETS

Hyperflexion and some hyperextension injuries may tear the joint capsules, resulting in widening of the facet joint. The joint space is abnormally wide on both plane film and CT, particularly on the latter. The widened space usually contains blood.

FACET FRACTURE

Combined severe compression and hyperextension forces can result in bilateral fractures. Unilateral facet fractures may result from sideways twist-type injuries (lateral bending with rotation). These are some of the most easily missed fractures to the cervical spine. Under optimal conditions, these may be detected on anteroposterior, lateral, and oblique films. Boyleston pillar views, however, are the view of choice. C-4 through C-7 are most frequently involved, with 40% of the cases occurring at C-6.

Avulsion of the fragment or fragments may result from ligamentous pull. Dislocation may or may not be manifested. Fractures vary in appearance. They may manifest as:

1. Vertical or horizontal line type.
2. Compression type (flattening or wedging of pillar), which is common.
3. Compression-distraction type; circular or elliptical lucencies within cancellous portion of pillar. These result from compression or crushing of the pillar with subsequent distraction of the fracture by opposing forces. This combination of forces is seen in cases of whiplash (pillar compression during hyperextension and distraction by hyperflexion).
4. Avulsion type.

TRAUMA TO THE THORACIC AND LUMBAR SPINE

Fractures of the first through the tenth thoracic vertebrae are generally stable because of the contiguous rib cage and ligament attachments. Although considerable violence is required to produce fractures and dislocations of the upper segments, the narrower spinal canal in this region allows less bone encroachment before neurological injury occurs.[24]

THORACOLUMBAR JUNCTION

Due to the configuration of the facet joint and the lack of supporting costal elements, considerably more motion is evidenced at this region. Acute hyperextension injuries may result in isolated fractures of the facets. These are rare though. The fracture line is characteristically obscure with little displacement.[25]

Fracture dislocations are commonly encountered at the thoracolumbar junction, primarily at T-12 to L-1. When they occur in the upper thoracic spine the T-4 through T-6 levels are most commonly involved. Facet joints are disrupted frequently with a fracture of the superior facet of the vertebral body below or a fracture through the lamina beneath the superior facet of the vertebra above the dislocation.[25] Locking or perching of the facets of the involved vertebrae with varying degrees of anterior displacement of the vertebral body above the dislocation will be present. The mechanism of injury is a combination of flexion, axial compression, and rotational shearing forces. These injuries are grossly unstable, and the majority involve neurological deficit.[26]

Less than 50% of anterior column compression suggests intact posterior structures. Again, CT will provide more accurate evaluation of the posterior elements and the middle column for 40% to 50% of anterior column compressions.

BURST FRACTURES

Burst fractures are also common at the thoracolumbar junction. They are distinguished from a simple compression fracture by loss of posterior body height with bony retropulsion into the neural canal and interpedicular widening. Posterior column injury may or may not be present. If the posterior column is intact, the fracture is considered to be stable. If there is interruption in the integrity of the posterior column, instability is suggested. Findings that may indicate probable posterior column injury include a kyphosis greater than 20 degrees, 50% or greater loss of anterior column height, and facet joint subluxation.[27]

Chance fractures are a flexion injury caused by an anteriorly placed fulcrum of motion, such as the lap belt. The classic injury is a horizontal fracture involving the vertebral body and posterior elements. Vertebral body height is typically maintained. Often a rotatory component contributes to the injury. Occasionally the spine will realign itself, resulting in minimal evidence of the significant underlying instability.[27] The incidence of facet joint subluxation is high, if not always present. Progressive deficits, widening of the disk, and kyphosis are not uncommon. These types of ligamentous injuries are very unstable and, if treated conservatively, must be monitored very carefully.

Some authors use the term "shingling" in reference to the normal anatomical overlay of one facet to its contiguous neighbor. Any disruption from this normal pattern might be referred to as "unshingling." Demonstration of facet unshingling and a naked facet are gross evidence of significant posterior element involvement and spinal instability. Plain films may establish more subtle radiographic evidence of capsular disruption. The findings include widening of the spinous processes on the anteroposterior films, subtle angulation on the lateral film, and facet unshingling on the oblique films (the inferior facet above riding high on the superior facet below).

CT sagittal reconstruction best demonstrates facet shingling and unshingling, posterior column distraction, and spreading of the facets. Axial (transverse) CT demonstrate the naked facet sign, with the inferior articular processes of the vertebra above lying naked without their companion superior articular processes of the vertebra below.[28] Figure 18 demon-

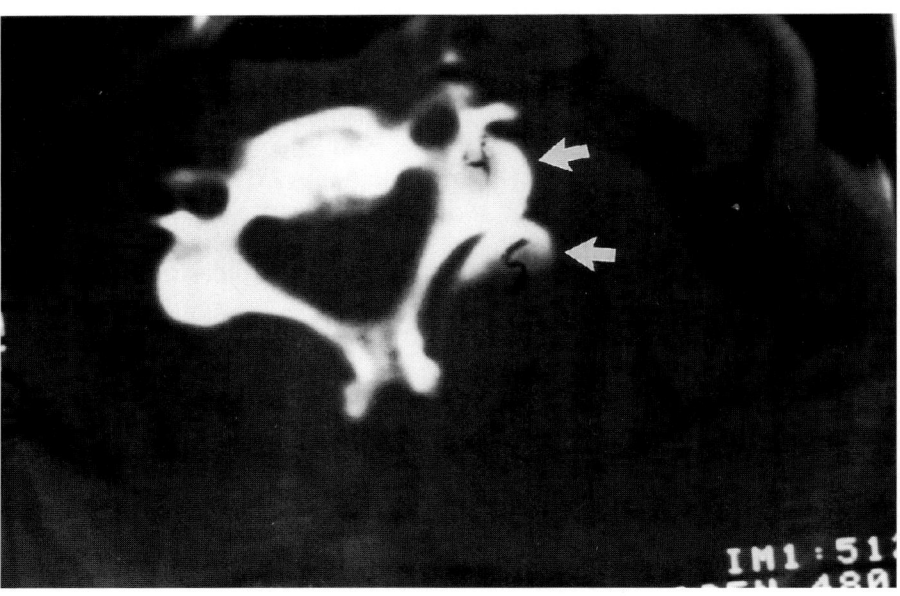

FIGURE 18.
C-4 to C-5 disrelationship, as evidenced by the rotation of the C-4 segment and the full visualization of the C-5 articular surface. "Naked facet" sign.

strates this in the cervical spine. The naked facet, which is a manifestation of a perched facet,[28] may be unilateral or bilateral and technically occur at almost any spinal level.

Lumbosacral dislocation, fracture-dislocation, and unilateral facet dislocation are rare.[28] The thick sagittally placed facets at the junction minimize the rotational components.[11, 29]

INFLAMMATORY SPONDYLOARTHROPATHY

Because the facetal articulations are synovial joints, they are susceptible to inflammatory synovitis or pannus. Such conditions include ankylosing spondylolitis, rheumatoid arthritis, juvenile rheumatoid arthritis, psoriatic arthritis, Reiter's arthritis, and enteropathic arthritis.

ANKYLOSING SPONDYLITIS AND ITS VARIANTS

The radiographic finding associated with ankylosing spondylolitis, psoriatic, Reiter's, and enteropathic arthritis are narrowed facetal joint spacing, ill-defined erosions of the articular surfaces, and subchondral reactive sclerosis. Marginal ankylosis, which may lead to complete fusion and/or firm adhesions or capsular ossification, may also result from the inflammatory process[30] and result in immobility. This is common in ankylosing spondylolitis and less common in Reiter's arthritis. Facetal involvement is very rare in psoriatic arthritis.

The combined effect of intra-articular osseous fusion and ligamentous capsular ossification creates on the frontal projection the "Railroad track sign." When combined with a third band composed of ossification of the supraspinous and interspinous ligament, the "trolley track sign" will be seen. These alterations can eventually extend throughout all three spinal regions. The articular pillars in the cervical column can fuse into a single pillar of bone from C-2 to C-3 through C-7 to T-1.

Due to the rigidity and associated vertebral body osteoporosis prevalent in ankylosing spondylolitis, fractures are not uncommon. Although they can occur at any level of the spinal column, they are particularly common in the lower cervical spine,[25] often related to the trivial trauma and usually the result of hyperextension forces. The fractures characteristically involve the posterior elements and an associated intervertebral disk space.

RHEUMATOID ARTHRITIS

Joint space narrowing and superficial erosions are common. Sclerosis is rare. Capsular ligamentous laxity can lead to instability, with resulting segmental subluxations. On motion stress, joint space widening and gapping will be demonstrated. The end result is usually fibrous ankylosis. Bony ankylosis can occur but is rare.

JUVENILE RHEUMATOID ARTHRITIS (JUVENILE CHRONIC ARTHRITIS)

Hypoplasia of the vertebral bodies and intervertebral disk spaces are demonstrated radiographically. The entire cervical articular pillar can be fused into a single block.

CRYSTAL DEPOSITION DISEASE

Calcium pyrophosphate dihydrate crystal deposition disease radiopaque crystals can be found in the articular cartilage, synovium, and ligamentous capsule of the facet complex. This can lead to narrowing and sclerosis of the joint, which may eventually result in bony ankylosis.

GOUT

Urate crystals may deposit in the facet joints.

OSTEOARTHRITIS (FACETAL ARTHROSIS)

Any level in the spine may be affected by osteoarthritis; however, the middle and lower cervical spine, upper and mid-thoracic spine, and the middle and lower lumbar spine are the predominate levels. Facets play a major role in resisting the stresses imposed on the vertebral segment. Nachemson concluded that the facets carry 18% of the total compressive load borne by the motion unit.[31] In pure flexion and lateral bending, the part played by the facets may be small. On extension, the resulting torsion and shear forces cause the facets to carry up to 40% of the total load applied to the vertebral segment.[31] Adams and Hutton[32] have shown that disk space narrowing can result in as much as 70% of the intervertebral load being transmitted across the facets. The excessive loads across the facet joints may result in the initiation of the degenerative process.[33,34]

The increase in load may also predispose the facets to injury.[35] In degeneration, the nucleus dehydrates and loses elasticity.[35] The annulus degenerates and loses torsional rigidity. The fulcrum of motion and torsional stresses are shifted posteriorly to the facets. Their normal gliding motion is now transformed to an abnormal rocking motion.

Repeated damage from injury to the posterior joints will lead to degeneration. Occasionally severe facet degeneration occurs without concomitant changes in the intervertebral disk.[36]

Posture also influences the arthritic process affecting the facets. These changes will more frequently be noted on the concave side of a scoliosis. Altered anteroposterior curves, such as cervical and lumbar hyperlordosis and a lumbar sway back posture, where stress points are again altered, often exhibit accelerated degenerative changes. Patients with a hyperkyphotic thoracic curve are also prone to alteration at the cervicothoracic junction.

Hypermobile segments adjacent to a hypomobile level, such as a blocked vertebra or transitional lumbosacral segment, are frequently affected.

The imaging choice to evaluate facetal arthrosis is CT.[37] A 1980 study demonstrated facet arthropathy on CT scans that was not evident on plain films. This supported the work of such people as Putti[14] and Rogoscino who believe that facet arthropathy was a cause of back pain. Modic et al.[29] have related that the "failed back" syndrome is because of undiagnosed facet disease. MRI is somewhat limited compared with CT. It is useful primarily in demonstrating hydrarthrosis of the facet joint in early degeneration and quantitatively documenting stenosis of the central canal, lateral recesses, and neural foramen.

FIVE SEQUENTIAL STAGES OF FACETAL DEGENERATION

The five sequential stages of facetal degeneration are synovitis, laxity of joint capsule, articular cartilage breakdown, subarticular erosions, and hyperostosis.

1. SYNOVITIS

Synovitis is composed of hyperemic and inflammatory cell infiltration. Resolution of CT and MRI is insufficient for full visualization. However, "hydrarthrosis" within the joint is seen as a bright signal on T_2-weighted MR images.

2. LAXITY OF JOINT CAPSULE

Exaggerated motion and gapping may be illustrated by motion studies.[23] Abnormal apophyseal motion is demonstrated on the static film as uneven widening of the joint space or excessive overall widening of the joint space. Excessive motion at the facets is evidenced as a faulty approximation of the facet surfaces, usually demonstrated as overriding of the facets where the superior facet extends down well below the lower margin of the inferior facet.[33]

3. ARTICULAR CARTILAGE BREAKDOWN

There are fibrillation and pitting (ulceration) of the articular cartilage. Partial or complete denudation of the cartilage surface will be viewed as diminished joint space (Fig 19).[5]

4. SUBARTICULAR BONE EROSION

Bone is exposed to synovial fluid, resulting in resorption.

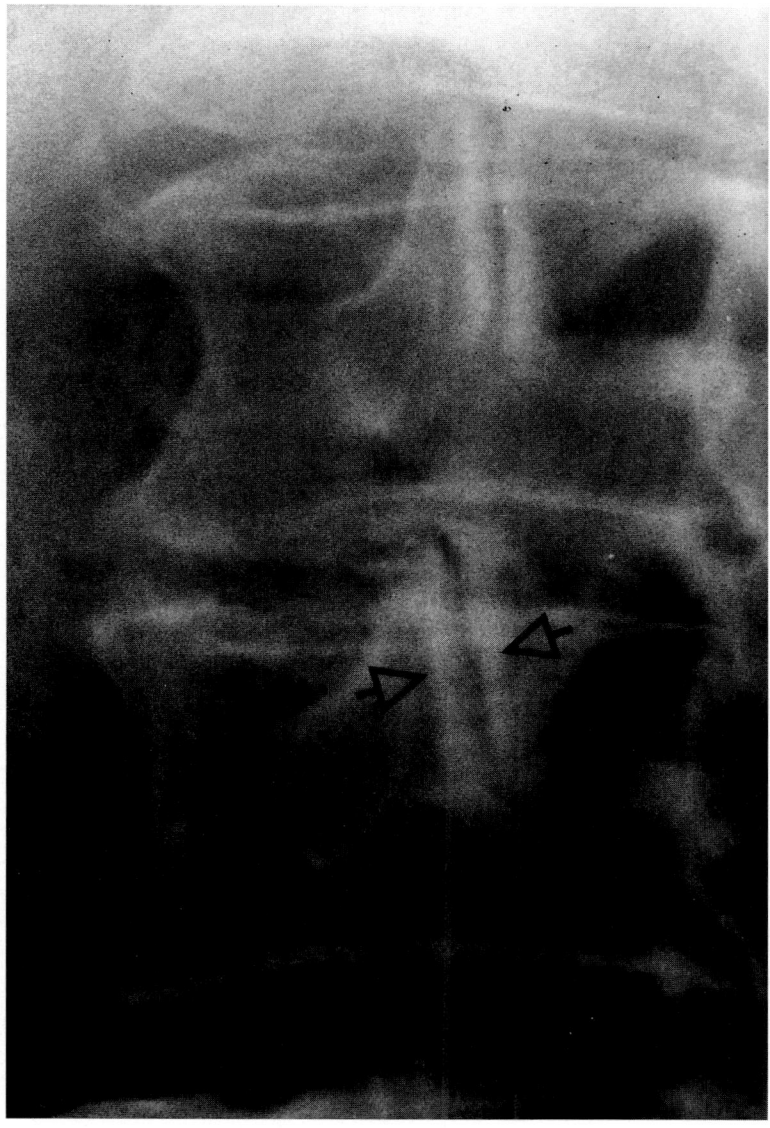

FIGURE 19.
Facetal arthrosis, which includes marginal sclerosis, narrowed spacing, spurring, and irregularity of the joint margins (arrows).

5. HYPEROSTOSIS

Hyperostosis refers to transformation of cancellous bone into compact bone (eburnation seen as reactive subchondral sclerosis) and the formation of marginal osteophytes (Fig 20) and hypertrophy of the facets (Fig 21). The latter is seen in long-standing disease.

Hypertrophy of facets, facet overriding, infolding or thickening of the ligamenta flava or of the lamina, and spur formation may affect the size of the central canal, lateral recess, and root canal. In 1922, Putti[14] described entrapment of an emerging nerve root in the subarticular gutter

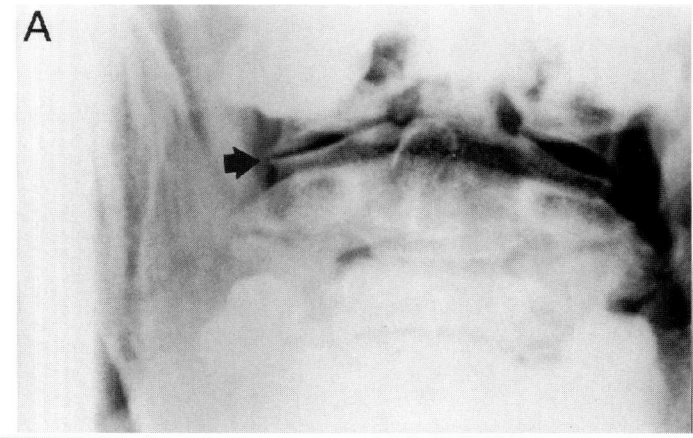

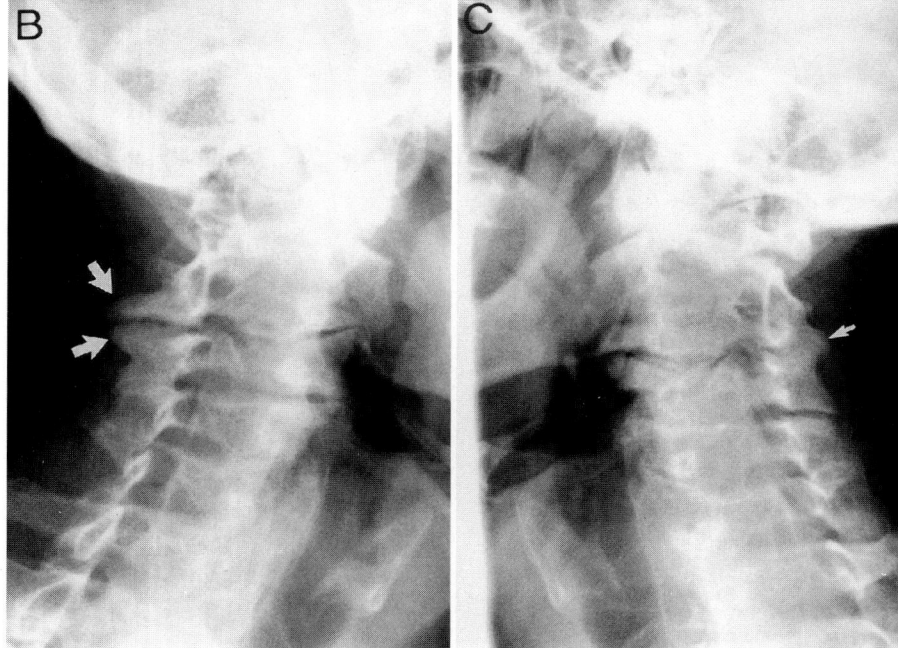

FIGURE 20.
A, arthrosis at the C-1 to C-2 facet joint *(arrow)*. Note the marginal spur and narrowed spacing compared with the opposite side. **B** and **C,** note spurs *(arrows),* which could create impingement on adjacent structures.

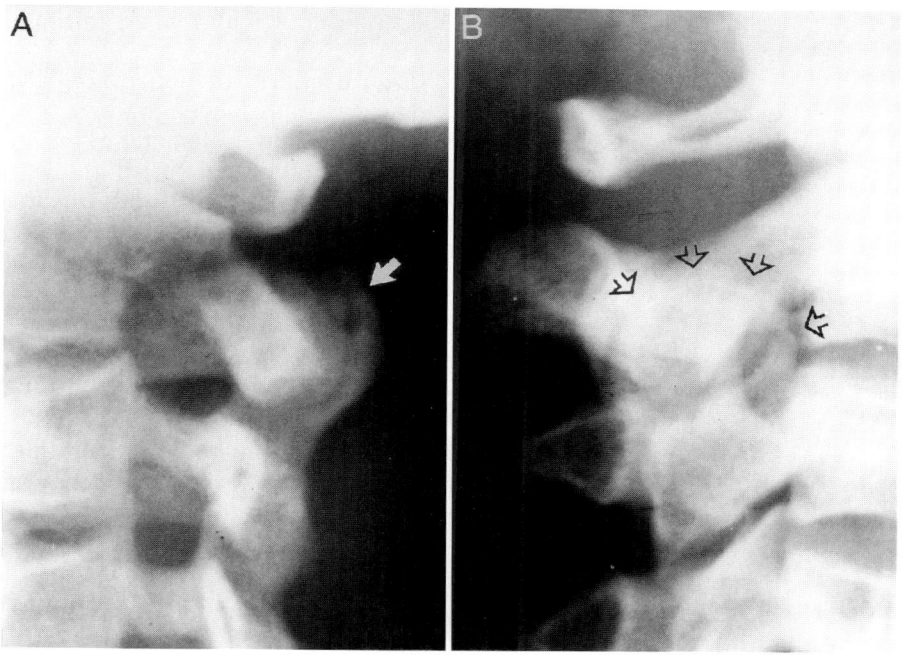

FIGURE 21.
A and **B,** markedly hypertrophied cervical facets. Note how the spurs are curved (*arrows*).

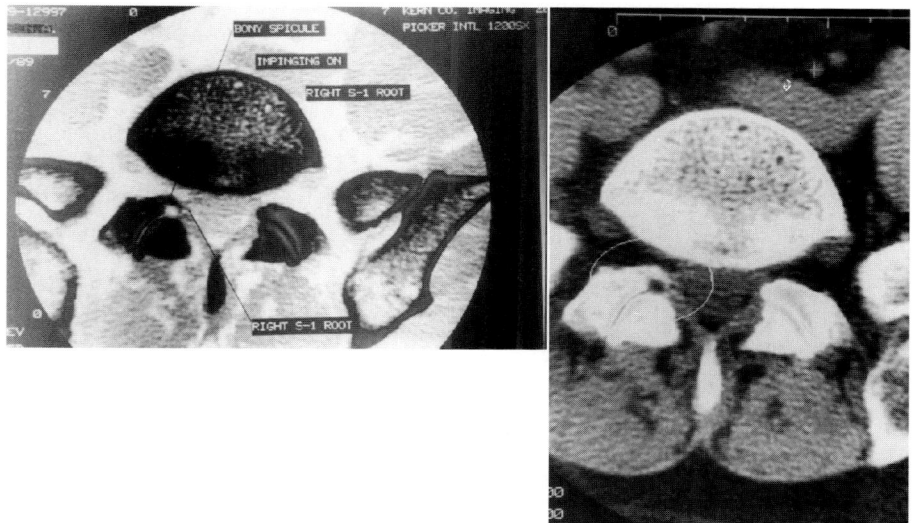

FIGURE 22.
A and **B,** bony spicule impinging on the right S-1 nerve root.

produced by overgrowth of the superior articular facet, particularly at the medial border (Fig 22).

The sagittal views on MRI are useful in demonstrating hypertrophy of the ligamentum flavum at the vertebral facets, grading the degree of foraminal stenosis, and measuring the sagittal diameter of the spinal cord. Images in the axial plane further facilitate the detailed analysis.[4]

Hyperostotic alterations can lead to mechanical impingement on the vertebral artery when spurring is pronounced off C-4 through C-7 due to the intimate relationship of the artery with the facet margins at these levels.

LESS COMMONLY MANIFESTED RADIOGRAPHIC FINDINGS
DEGENERATIVE OSSICLES

Small osteochondral fragments or ossicles may result from degenerative stresses. These may be introduced into joint or lay at the capsular margins.

SYNOVIAL HYPERPLASIA

Synovial villi, which are richly innervated and vascularized, have been reported between the articular surfaces. Pinching or crushing of these villi, which become hypertrophied in degenerative disease during motion, may be a source of pain.[38]

SEGMENTAL INSTABILITY

Segmental instability allows for subluxation, in other words, retrolisthesis (posterior displacement); anterolisthesis (spondylolisthesis forward displacement; Fig 23); and lateralisthesis (lateral offset).

VACUUM PHENOMENON

Vacuum phenomenon is a radiolucency seen within the joint space. It may indicate an abnormally lax joint capsule, uneven opposition of the joint surfaces, or possibly a normal joint under a distractive force due to position.[39]

DEGENERATIVE SYNOVIAL CYSTS
TARLOV CYST

Tarlov's cyst is most commonly found in the lower lumbar spine (L-4 to L-5). Synovial cysts arise from synovial outpouchings through points of weakened or destroyed capsular tissue.[5, 40–42] They may or may not have a detectable pedicle attached to a synovial sheath of joint capsule, which is filled with clear mucinous matter or gas.[5] The cyst will arise from the margin of the facet joint, usually medial to the ligamentum flavum, and extend into the central canal. They are round with the capsule of the cyst denser than the fluid filling. Not infrequently there may be calcification of the cyst wall, and occasionally it may contain lucent vacuum formation. The cyst is soft and may enlarge or collapse spontaneously. However, it does displace the epineural fat and can indent the thecal sac. MRI is valuable in making the diagnosis. CT is also helpful, especially if calcium is present.

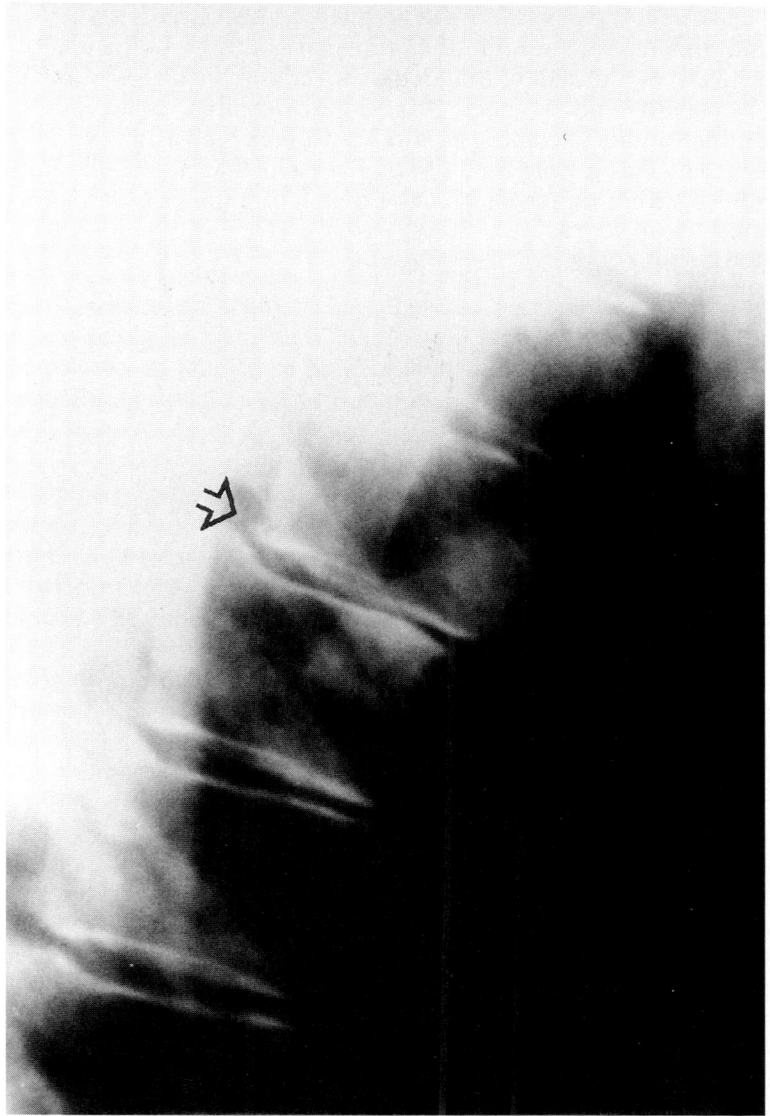

FIGURE 23.
Spondylolisthesis in the thoracic spine due to facet degeneration.

Ganglion cysts develop from mucinous degeneration of periarticular connective tissue. They contain a thick myxoid material. Both types of cysts share the common pathogenesis of being closely associated with degenerative joint disease that predisposed to their formation. It may be extremely difficult to distinguish between the two.

INTRA-ARTICULAR FUSION

Rarely in long-standing disease, fusion may take place. This, however, is usually limited to one motor unit. It has been argued in cases of degenerative facets, the menisci become entrapped between facets, resulting in a "catching-type pain." All the posterior joints contain small "meniscoid" structures that project into the joint space, similar to the alar folds of the knee, and are formed of tonguelike or semilunar fringes of the synovium.

Kos and Wolf[43] suggest that an "incarcerated" meniscoid may cause a sudden intervertebral joint block and that reposition of the meniscoid might be achieved by a passive movement that places the joint capsule under maximum tension, thereby distracting the opposed joint surfaces.

CHONDROMALACIA FACETAE

The histological changes seen with this condition resemble those of chondromalacia patellae, thus the name.[44] The speculated causes for this are variations of normal biomechanics due to trauma or genetic predisposition. Asymmetrical angulation may produce stresses sufficient to cause early articular cartilage injury.

DEGENERATIVE PSEUDOSPONDYLOLISTHESIS

This form of spondylolisthesis, which has an intact neural arch, was first described by Junghanns[45] in 1930. Approximately 4% of the mature population is affected, six times more frequently in females. It is almost never seen in patients less than age 40.

Some[46] describe the condition to be more common in patients who are diabetic, which may suggest a neuropathic cause (reported in 30%). L-4 on L-5 is the primary level of involvement, probably because L-4 is at the apex of the lordotic curve. The iliolumbar ligament attachments from L-4 to the iliac crest are not as strong and the facets are oriented more sagittally, allowing greater forward mobility.

Bony erosions, hypertrophy, and reactive remodeling of the articular processes result (Fig 24) in a more horizontal (transverse) orientation with an increased tendency toward forward slippage.[47] Transverse CT sections allow for a reliable, reproducible assessment of facet joint morphology. The amount of slippage is usually limited to 10% to 25% unless there is associated marked disk degeneration. The facetal remodeling and erosion caused by long-standing intersegmental instability[23] will result in an "obtuse-facet-pedicle angle" (Fig 25).

Degenerative changes of the superior articular processes are responsible for narrowing of the root canals (subarticular stenosis).[47] Forward displacement of the lamina may produce midline stenosis.[48] Narrowing may be slight and may not cause compression or may produce stenosis of varying severity.[47] The neurological effects of degenerative changes of the articular processes and spondylolisthesis are strictly related to the original dimensions of the vertebral canal. Degenerative spondylolisthesis in the cervical spine is typically in conjunction with hyperlordosis.

JOINT INSTABILITY

Facetal joint instability may appear soon after disk injury or the onset of disk degeneration.

Criteria to assess facet joint instability include abnormal gapping or widening of the joint space. Look for excessive widening of the joint space

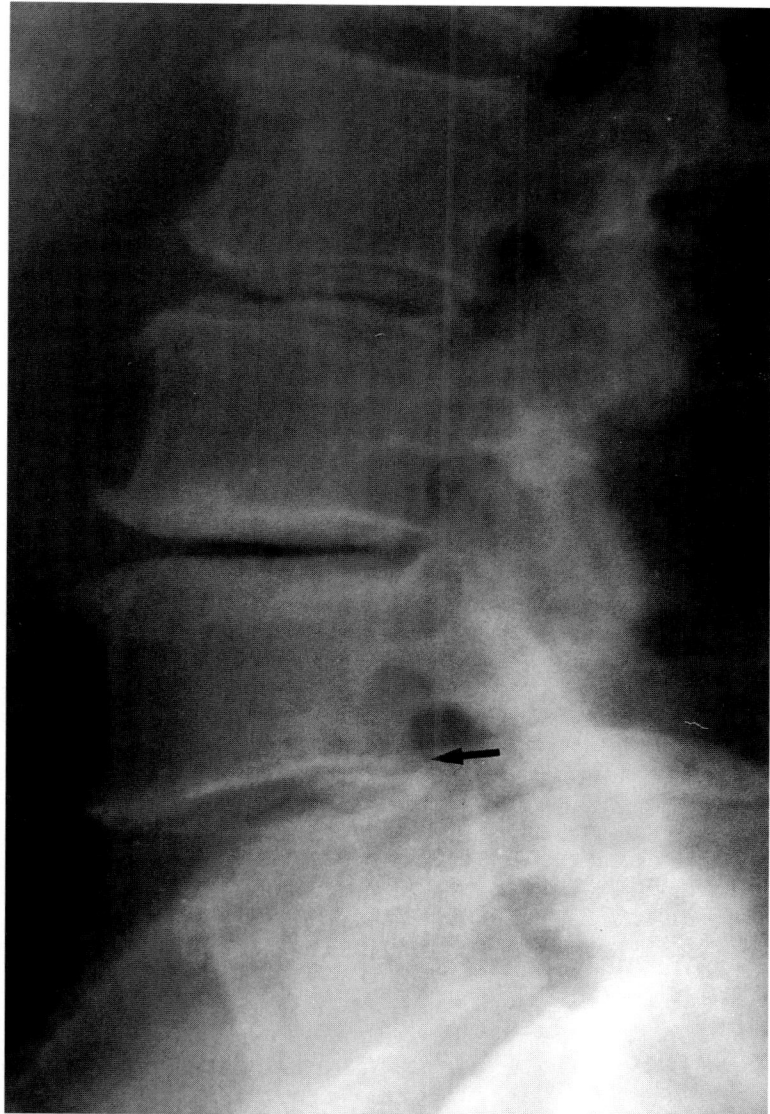

FIGURE 24.
Facetal degenerative changes in the lower lumbar spine have led to a grade 1 degenerative spondylolisthesis of L-4 (arrow).

in the cervical spine during flexion and extension motions. Excessive widening of the joint space of the lumbar spine is not as easily visualized as in the cervical spine.

According to Abel[33] abnormalities exist when

1. There is overall widening of the joint. The space is at least twice as wide as those of the adjacent levels.
2. One end of the joint is at least twice the width of the other end.
3. There is faulty facet opposition, such as imbrication, overriding, or telescoping.

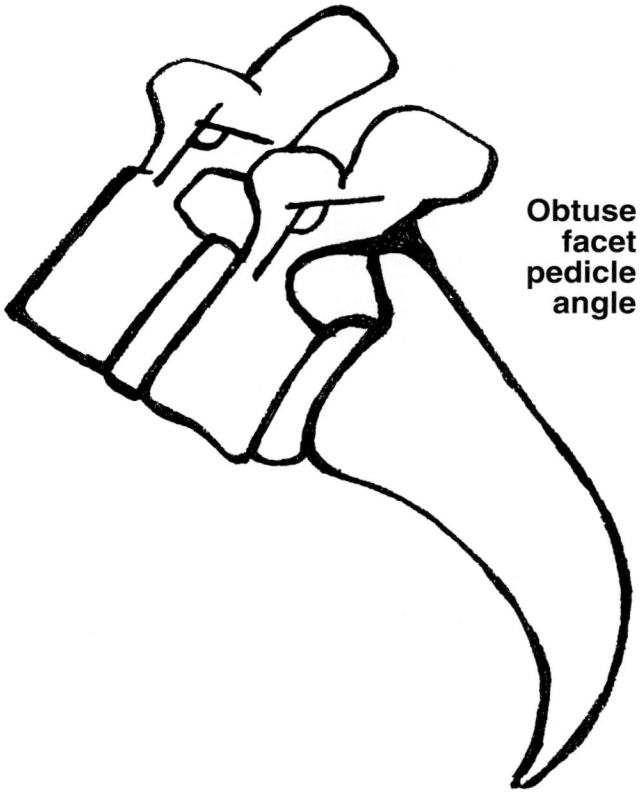

FIGURE 25.
Schematic of the obtuse facet pedicle angle.

FACETAL IMBRICATION (SHAKELIKE, OVERLAPPING, OR TELESCOPING)

When imbrication exists, there is disruption of the sliding approximation of the facets along their plane of orientation. The articular surfaces no longer register exactly opposite each other. This may allow a pulling stress to be placed on the capsule. It may manifest at any level but is usually described in the lower lumbar spine. Foraminal narrowing may result. In the lumbosacral spine, if there is postural extension of the region at the time of exposure, a false finding may be present because of the projection.

Imbrication is often encountered in patients with an increased sacral base angle, hyperlordosis, or sway back posture. A diminished sacral base angle and elongated articular processes may also be causative factors in this condition.

If imbrication is excessive, there can be a bony impingement between the tip of the articular process and the undersurface of the pedicle or transverse process of the level above (Fig 26). A fibrocartilage pad may develop at this point. Impingement can occur from above and below, resulting in "entrapment." Reactive eburnation or sclerosis can result at the

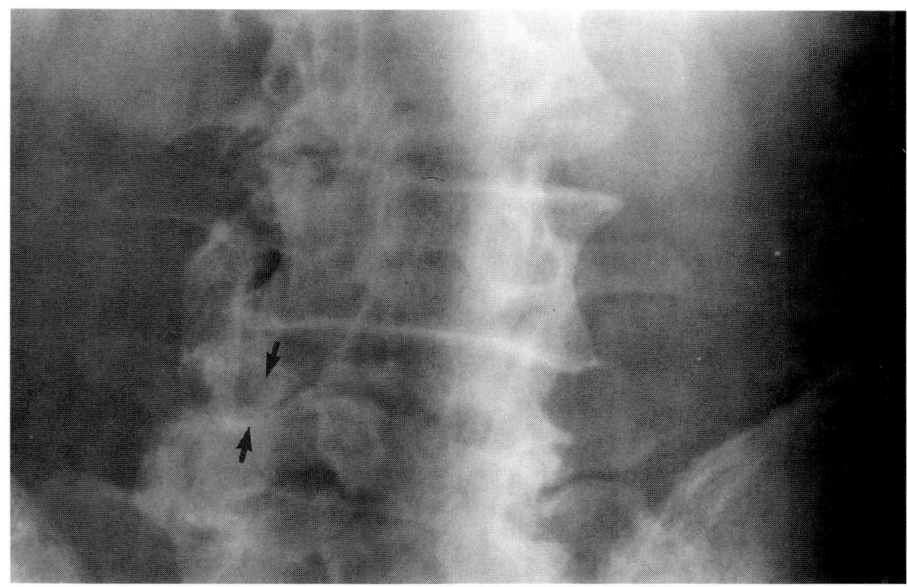

FIGURE 26.
Hyperplastic articular processes of L-4 to L-5 bilaterally (*arrows*). The articular processes of L-4 to L-5 are elongated, forming facetlamina joints bilaterally. The facets in the region are also degenerated, especially L-3 to L-4.

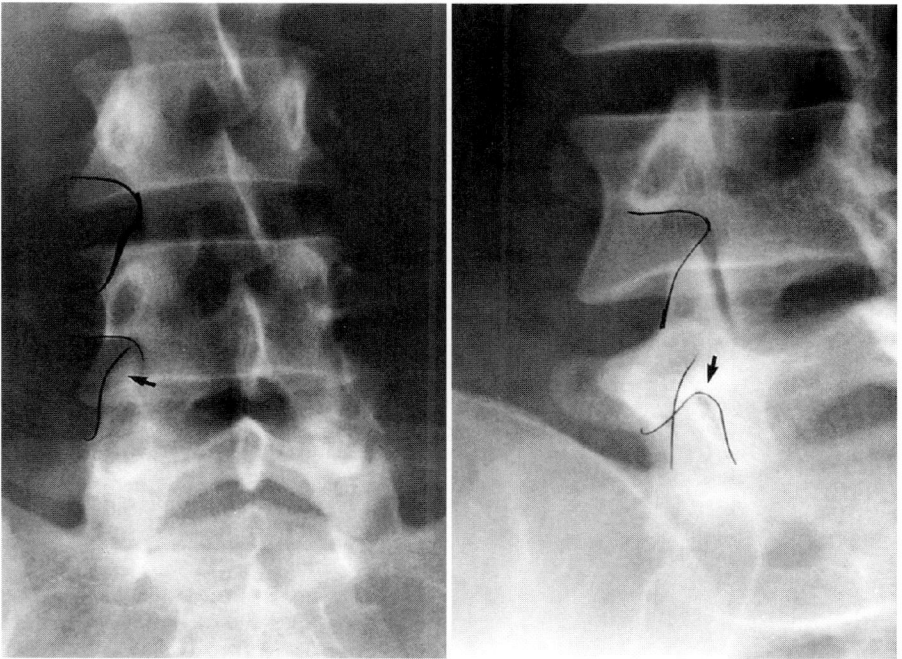

FIGURE 27.
A and **B,** Hadley's S curve (*arrows*). Note the failure of an S formation at the lower facet levels compared with the facets above.

point of impingement or entrapment to counteract local pressure stress. If stress continues, actual bony erosions develop at the site of pressure. Biomechanical parameters are identifiable on postural radiographs, which significantly correlate with the clinical syndrome of lumbar extension facet subluxations and herniation of the disk nucleus. Further, the entire lumbar posture is altered in these conditions either secondarily as in antalgia or primarily as a predisposing factor.[34] The postural complex in facet patients may include a shallow lumbosacral angle or flattened sacral base and yet a normal amount of lordosis from L-1 to L-5, causing a

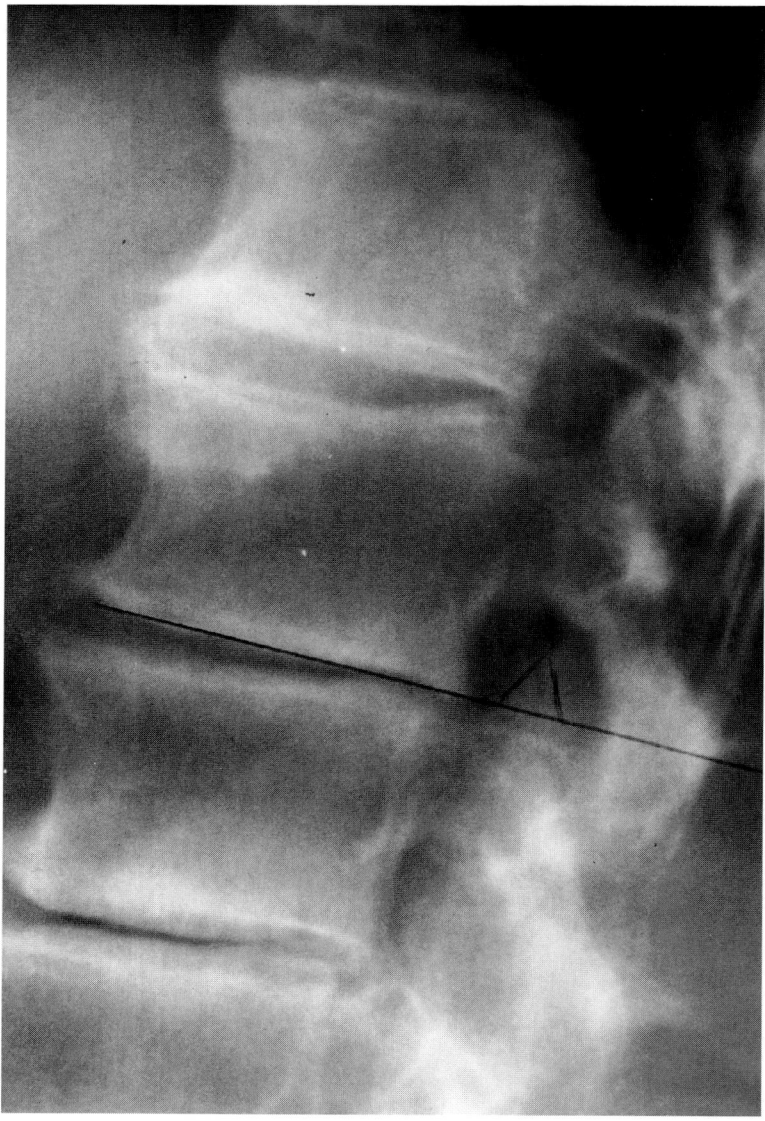

FIGURE 28.
MacNab's line intersects the superior articular facet of the level below, indicating facet imbrication.

posterior shift of the center of gravity in the sagittal plane. This increases the vertical facet load, predisposing it to an extension facet injury.[49]

SPINOGRAPHIC MEASUREMENTS RELATED TO THE FACETS
HADLEY'S S CURVE

Hadley's S curve is a line of mensuration forming an unbroken S curve drawn on anteroposterior or oblique lumbar views (Fig 27). The first line is drawn along the inferior aspect of the transverse process, continuing

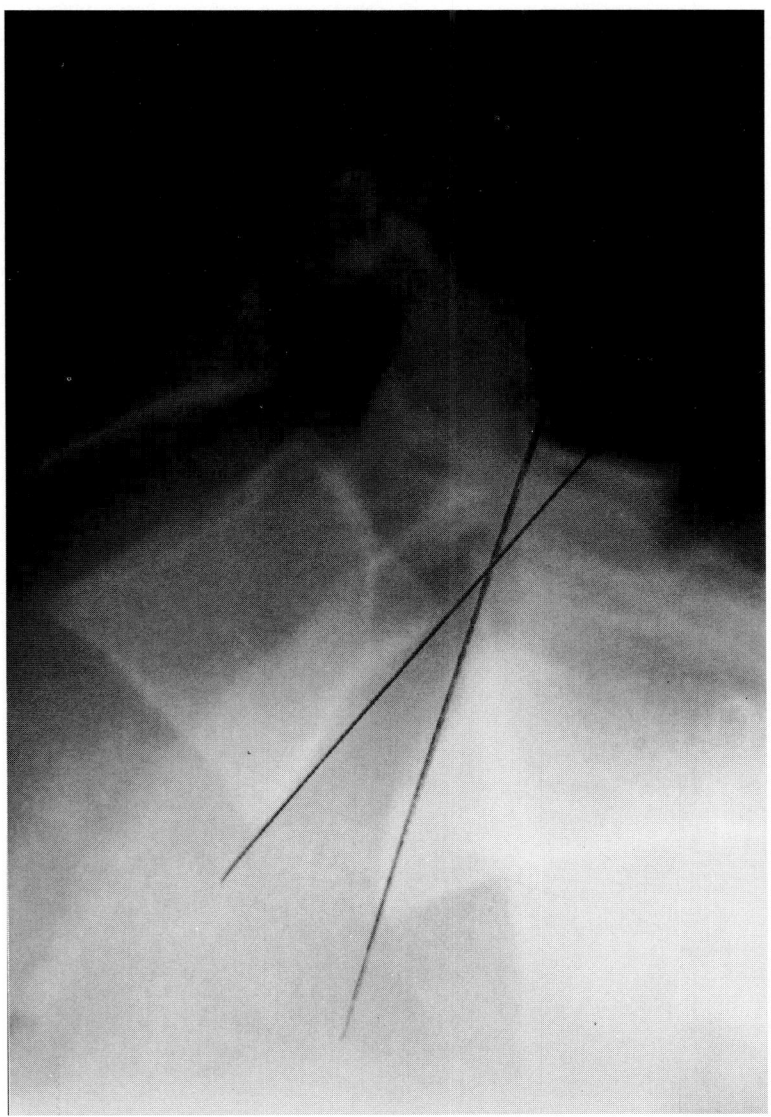

FIGURE 29.
Lumbar disk angle formed by intersecting lines along the inferior end plate of L-5 and superior surface of S-1.

along the lateral margin of the lamina. A second line is drawn upward along the lateral margin of the superior articular process of the segment below. The lines connect at the superior edge of the facet joint and should create a smooth curve. An abrupt disruption of the line suggests imbrication.[48]

MACNAB'S LINE (POSTERIOR JOINT BODY LINE)

Bony root entrapment syndromes are frequently associated with subluxations of the posterior facets.[48] This may be demonstrated on a lateral view

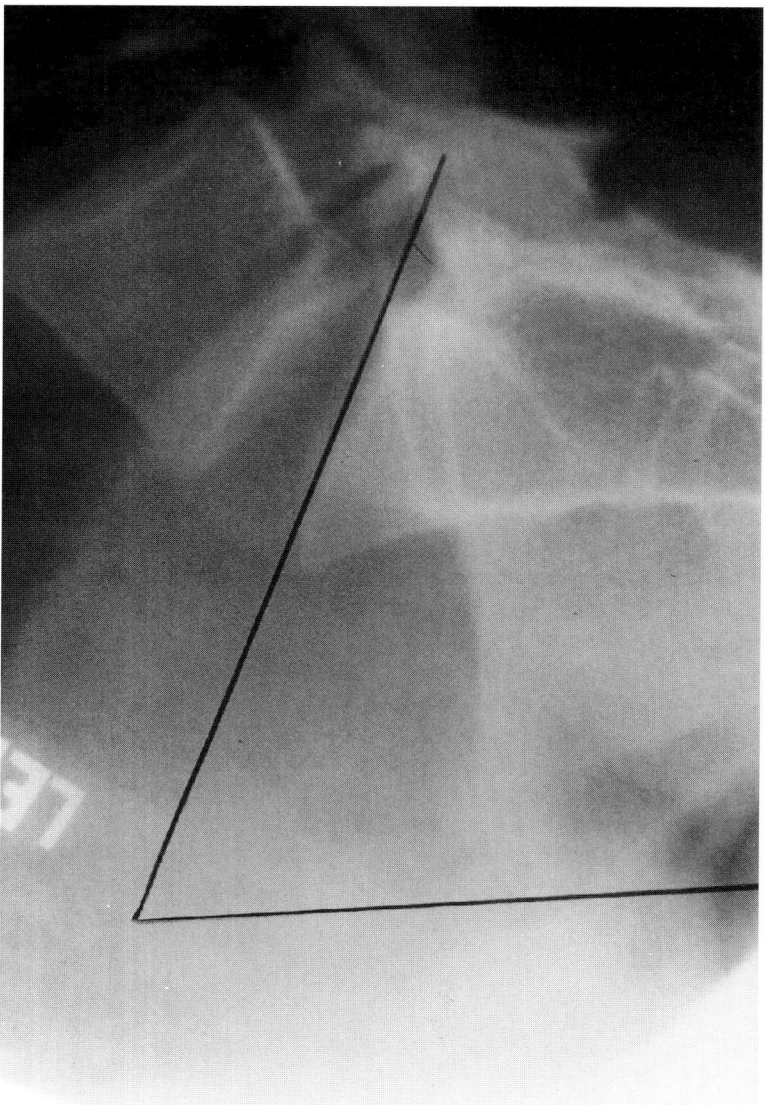

FIGURE 30.
Sacral base angle created by the angle formed by lines along the sacral promontory and one parallel to the floor.

of the lumbar spine. A line is drawn along the inferior end plate (caudal border) of the vertebra and extended posteriorly (Fig 28). Normally this should pass over the top of the superior articular facet of the segment below. If it cuts through the facet, it may indicate imbrication.[48]

LUMBOSACRAL DISK ANGLE

Lines are drawn along the inferior body surface of L-5 and the sacral base. Both lines are extended posteriorly until they intersect (Fig 29). They should intersect posterior to the facets. A measurement of greater than 15 degrees may be found in a hyperextension malposition and predisposes the facets to compression or impaction. A measurement of less than 11 degrees may be found in cases of acute facet inflammation and acute disk herniation.

SACRAL BASE ANGLE (FERGUSON'S SACRAL BASE ANGLE)

A line is drawn through the plane of the sacral base, and then a horizontal line is constructed (Fig 30). The angle formed has a wide range of 26 to 57 degrees. The measurement should be made on upright films. Variations in this angle may contribute to altered mechanical stresses on the facets.

WEIGHT BEARING: GRAVITATIONAL LINE OF L-3

A vertical line drawn from the center of the L-3 vertebral body should pass through the anterior one third of the sacral base. If this line passes anterior to the sacrum by more than 10 mm, an increase in shearing stresses in an anterior direction may be elicited between the lumbosacral facets. A posterior shift of weight bearing may indicate an increased load on the lumbosacral facets.

Often a combination of abnormal measurements and correlated clinical findings may allow for a diagnosis of facet syndrome to be made.

REFERENCES

1. Oppenheimer, A: The apophyseal intervertebral articulations roentgenologically considered. *Radiology* 30:724–740, 1938.
2. Fuchs AW: Thoracic vertebrae (part 2). *Radiogr Clin Photogr* 17:42–51, 1946.
3. Merrill V: *Atlas of Roentgenographic Positions and Standard Radiologic Procedures*, ed 4. St Louis, Mosby, 1994, vol 1, pp 255–256.
4. Grenier N, Kressel HY, Schiebler ML, et al: Normal and degenerative posterior spinal structures: MR imaging *Radiology* 165:517–525, 1987.
5. Wang AM, Wesolowski DP, Farah J: Evaluation of posterior spinal structures by computed tomography. *Spine* 2:439–465, 1988.
6. Hildebrandt RW: *Chiropractic Spinography: A Manual of Technology and Interpretation*. Des Plaines, Iowa, Hilmark, 1977, p 101.
7. Giles LGF, Taylor JR: Innervation of lumbar zygopophyseal joint synovial folds. *Acta Orthop Scand* 58:43–46, 1987.
8. Gardner E, Gray DJ, O'Rahilly R: *Anatomy. A Regional Study of Human Structure*, ed 4. Philadelphia, WB Saunders, 1975, p 534.
9. Giles LGF: *Anatomical Basis of Low Back Pain*. Baltimore, Williams & Wilkins, 1989, pp 60, 97.

10. Braakman R, Vinken PJ: Unilateral facet interlocking in the lower cervical spine. *J Bone Joint Surg (Br)* 49B:249–257, 1967.
11. Carl A, Blair B: Unilateral lumbosacral facet fracture-dislocation. *Spine* 16:218–221, 1991.
12. Goldthwait JE: The lumbo-sacral articulation. An explanation of many cases of "lumbago" "sciatica" and paraplegia. *Boston Med Surg J* 164:365, 1911.
13. von Luckum HL: The lumbosacral region. An anatomic study and some clinical observations. *JAMA* 82:1109, 1924.
14. Putti V: Lady Jones lecture on new conceptions in the pathogenesis of sciatic pain. Delivered at the Univ. of Liverpool on March 10, 1927. *Lancet* 2:53–60, 1927.
15. Ghormley RK: Low back pain with special reference to the articular facets with presentation of an operative procedure. *JAMA* 101:1773–1777, 1933.
16. Ferguson AB: The clinical and roentgenographic interpretation of lumbosacral anomalies. Presented at the Lake Keuka Medical Association, Lake Keuka, NY, July 14, 1933. *Radiology* 22:548–558, 1934.
17. Farfan HF, Sullivan JD: The relation of facet orientation to intervertebral disc failure. *Can J Surg* 10:179–185, 1967.
18. Cyron BM, Hutton WC: Articular tropism and stability of the lumbar spine. *Spine* 5:168–172, 1980.
19. Van Schaik JDJ, Verbiest H, Van Schack FDJ: The orientation and shape of the lower lumbar facet joints: A computed tomographic study of their variation in 100 patients with low back pain and a discussion of their possible clinical implications. in Post MJD (ed): *Computed Tomography of the Spine*, Baltimore, Williams & Wilkins, 1984, pp 495–505.
20. Lobeck D, Yong-Hing K, Cassidy D, et al: The relationship between facet orientation and lumbar disc herniation. The role of torsion to intervertebral disc failure. *Orthop Trans* 9:560, 1985.
21. Gunzberg R, Hutton W, Fraser R: Axial rotation of the lumbar spine and the effect of flexion. An *in vitro* and *in vivo* biomechanical study. *Spine* 16:22–28, 1991.
22. Vanharanta H, Floyd T, Ohnmeiss DD, et al: The relationship of facet tropism to degenerative disc disease. *Spine* 18:1000–1005, 1993.
23. Cox JM, Aspegren DD: Degenerative spondylolisthesis of C7 and L4 in same patient. *J Manipulative Physiol Ther* 11:195–203, 1988.
24. Bohlman HH, Freehafer A, Dejak J: The results of treatment of acute injuries of the upper thoracic spine with paralysis. *J Bone Joint Surg (Am)* 67A:360–369, 1985.
25. Rogers LF: *Radiology of Skeletal Trauma*. New York, Churchill Livingstone, 1982, p 332.
26. Juhl JH, Crummy AB: *Paul and Juhl's Essentials of Radiologic Imaging*, ed 6. Philadelphia, JB Lippincott, 1993.
27. Mann DC: Late-diagnosed post-injury spinal instability. *Spine* 7:189–202, 1993.
28. Kricun ME: *Imaging Modalities in Spinal Disorders*. Philadelphia, WB Saunders, 1988, pp 390, 446.
29. Modic MT, Masaryk TJ, Ross JS: *Magnetic Resonance Imaging of the Spine*, ed 2. St Louis, Mosby, 1994.
30. Eulderink F: Pathology of ankylosing spondylitis. *Spine* 4:507–528, 1990.
31. Tobias D, Ziv I, Maroudas A: Human facet cartilage: Swelling and some physicochemical characteristics as a function of age: 1. Swelling of human facet joint cartilage. *Spine* 17:694–700, 1992.
32. Adams MA, Hutton WC: The mechanical function of the lumbar apophyseal joints. *Spine* 8:327–330, 1983.

33. Abel MS: The unstable apophyseal joint: An early sign of lumbar disc disease. *Skeletal Radiol* 2:31–37, 1977.
34. Banks SD: The use of spinographic parameters in the differential diagnosis of lumbar facet and disc syndromes. *J Manipulative Physiol Ther* 6:113–116, 1983.
35. Shirazi-Adl A: Finite-element simulation of changes in the fluid content of human lumbar discs. Mechanical and clinical implications. *Spine* 17:206–212, 1992.
36. Fast A: Low back disorders: Conservative management. *Arch Phys Med Rehabil* 69:880–891, 1988.
37. Carrera GF, Haughton VM, Syvertsen A, et al: Computed tomography of the lumbar facet joints. *Radiology* 134:145–148, 1980.
38. Jeffries B: Facet steroid injections. *Spine* 2:409–417, 1988.
39. Peters RE: Facet syndrome. *Eur J Chiropr* 32:85–102, 1984.
40. Chen KTK: Synovial cyst of the spinal facet joint. *Arch Pathol Lab Med* 107:100–101, 1983.
41. Hemming LyH S, Daniels DL, Williams, AL, et al: Intraspinal synovial cyst: Natural history and diagnosis by CT. *Radiology* 145:375–376, 1982.
42. Pendleton B, Carl B, Pollay M: Spinal extradural benign synovial or ganglion cyst: Case report and review of the literature. *Neurosurgery* 13:322–326, 1983.
43. Kos J, Wolf J: Les ménisques intervertébraux et leur role possible dans les blocages vertébraux. *Annales de Medicine Physique* 15:203–217, 1972.
44. Warfield CA: Facet syndrome and the relief of low back pain. *Hosp Pract* 41–48, 1988.
45. Junghanns H, Schmorl G: *The Human Spine in Health and Disease*, ed 2. New York, Grune and Stratton, 1971.
46. Mink JH, Deutsch AL: *MRI of the Musculoskeletal System. A teaching file*. New York, Raven Press, 1990, pp 146–149.
47. Rauschning W: Pathoanatomy of lumbar disc degeneration and stenosis. *Acta Orthop Scand* 64(suppl 251):3–11, 1993.
48. MacNab I: The pathogenesis of spinal stenosis. *Spine* 1:369–381, 1987.
49. Banks SD: Spinographic assessment of treatment of spinal manipulative therapy. *J Manipulative Physiol Ther* 6:175–180, 1983.

SUGGESTED READINGS

Abumi K, Panjabi NM, Kramer KM, et al: Biomechanical evaluation of lumbar spinal stability after graded facetectomies. *Spine* 15:1142–1147, 1990.

Agur AMR, Lee MJ: *Grant's Atlas of Anatomy*, ed 9. Baltimore, Md, Williams and Wilkins, 1991.

Ahmed AM, Duncan MA, Burke DL: The effect of facet geometry on the axial torque-rotation response of lumbar motion segments. *Spine* 15:391–401, 1990.

Amevo B, Aprill C, Bogduk N: Abnormal instantaneous axes of rotation in patients with neck pain. *Spine* 17:748–756, 1992.

Aprill C, Bogduk N: The prevalence of cervical zygapophyseal joint pain. *Spine* 17:744–747, 1992.

Ayres CE: Further case studies of lumbosacral pathology with consideration of involvement of the intervertebral discs and the articular facets. *N Engl J Med* 213:716, 1935.

Bogduk N, Long DM: The anatomy of the so-called "articular nerves" and their relationship to facet denervation in the treatment of low-back pain. *J Neurosurg* 51:172–177, 1979.

Bogduk N, Marsland A: The cervical zygapophyseal joints as a source of neck pain. *Spine* 13:610–617, 1988.

Boger DC, Chandler RW, Pearce JG, et al: Unilateral facet dislocation at the lumbosacral junction. *J Bone Joint Surg (Am)* 65A:1174–1178, 1983.

Bullough PG, Boachie-Adjei O: *Atlas of Spinal Diseases.* New York, Gower Medical Publishing, 1988.

Burton AK, Tillotson KM: Is recurrent low back trouble associated with increased lumbar sagittal mobility? *J Biomed Eng* 11:245–248, 1989.

Calenoff L, Chessare JW, Rogers LF, et al: Multiple level spinal injuries: Importance of early recognition. *AJR* 130:665, 1978.

Carrera GF, Williams AL: Current concepts in evaluation of the lumbar facet joints. *Crit Rev Clin Imaging* 21:85–104, 1984.

Cotler JM, Herbison GJ, Nasuti JF, et al: Closed reduction of traumatic cervical spine dislocation using traction weights up to 140 pounds. *Spine* 18:386–390, 1993.

Cox JM, Shreener S: Chiropractic manipulation in low back pain and sciatica: Statistical data on the diagnosis, treatment and response of 576 consecutive cases. *J Manipulative Physiol Ther* 7:1–11, 1984.

Crock HV: Normal and pathological anatomy of the lumbar spinal nerve root canals. *J Bone Joint Surg (Br)* 63B:487–490, 1981.

Dall BH, Rowe DE: Degenerative spondylolisthesis. Its surgical management. *Spine* 10:668–672, 1985.

Das De S, McCreath SW: Lumbosacral fracture dislocations. *J Bone Joint Surg (Br)* 63B:58–60, 1981.

De Groot J, Chusid JG: *Correlative Neuroanatomy,* ed 21. Norwalk, Conn, Appleton & Lange, 1991.

Dosch J-C: *Trauma. Conventional Radiological Study in Spine Injury.* New York, Springer-Verlag New York, 1985.

Eisenstein SM, Parry CR: The lumbar facet arthrosis syndrome. Clinical presentation and articular surface changes. *J Bone Joint Surg (Br)* 69B:3–7, 1987.

Errico TJ: Techniques and management of cervical spine fractures. *Spine* 7:157–180, 1993.

Eyster EF, Scott WR: Lumbar synovial cysts: Report of eleven cases. *Neurosurgery* 24:112–115, 1989.

Farfan HF: Effects of torsion on the intervertebral joints. *Can J Surg* 12:336–341, 1969.

Finkelstein SD, Sayegh R, Watson P, et al: Juxta-facet cysts. Report of two cases and review of clinicopathologic features. *Spine* 18:779–782, 1993.

Gehwiler JA Jr, Osbourne RL Jr, Becker RF: *The Radiology of Vertebral Trauma.* Philadelphia, WB Saunders, 1980.

Giles LGF: Pathoanatomic studies and clinical significance of lumbosacral zygapophyseal (facet) joints. *J Manipulative Physiol Ther* 15:36–40, 1992.

Greenspan A: Orthopedic radiology. A practical approach. I. Trauma. Philadelphia, JB Lippincott, 1988, pp 8.2–8.7, 8.11–8.12, 8.21–8.24.

Grobler LJ, Robertson PA, Novotny JE, et al: Decompression for degenerative spondylolisthesis and spinal stenosis at L4-5. The effects on facet joint morphology. *Spine* 18:1475–1482, 1993.

Grobler LJ, Robertson PA, Novotny JE, et al: Etiology of spondylolisthesis. Assessment of the role played by lumbar facet joint morphology. *Spine* 18:80–89, 1993.

Gunzberg R, Sandhur A, Fraser RD: The value of computerized tomography in determining lumbar facet joint orientations. *J Spinal Disorders* 2:170–175, 1989.

Hadley LA: Apophyseal subluxation. *J Bone Joint Surg Am*18:428, 1936.

Hadley LA: Intervertebral joint subluxation, bony impingement and foraminal encroachment with nerve root change. *AJR* 65:377, 1951.

Hadley LA: *Anatomico-Roentgenographic Studies of the Spine.* Springfield, Ill, Charles C Thomas, 1981.

Haughton VM: MR Imaging of the spine. *Radiology* 166:297–301, 1988.

Helbig T, Lee CK: The lumbar facet syndrome. *Spine* 13:61–64, 1988.

Hickey RFJ, Tregonning GD: Denervation of spinal facet joints for treatment of chronic low back pain. *N Z Med J* Feb:96–99, 1977.

Hirsch C: Etiology and pathogenesis of low back pain. *Israel J Med Sci* 2:362–370, 1966.

Hirsch D, Ingelmark B, Miller M: The anatomical basis for low back pain. *Acta Orthop Scand* 33:1–17, 1963.

Holdsworth FW: Fractures, dislocations and fracture dislocations of the spine. *J Bone Joint Surg (Br)* 45B:6–20, 1963.

Howe JF, Loeser JD, Caluin WH: Mechanosensitivity of dorsal root ganglia and chronically injured axons: A physiological basis for the radicular pain of nerve root compression. *Pain* 3:25–41, 1977.

Jaeger SA, Pate DM: Case 14: facet syndrome. *Case Studies in Chiropractic Radiology*, Rockville, Md, Aspen, 1990, pp 87–94.

Kao CC, Winkler SS, Turner JH: Synovial cyst of spinal facet: Case report. *J Neurosurg* 41:372–376, 1974.

Keats TE: *Atlas of Normal Roentgen Variants that may Simulate Disease*, ed 4. Chicago, Mosby, 1988.

King AG: Functional anatomy of the lumbar spine. *Orthopedics* 6:1588–1590, 1983.

Leboeuf C, Kimber D, White K: Prevalence of spondylolisthesis, transitional anomalies and low intercrestal line in a chiropractic patient population. *J Manipulative Physiol Ther* 12:200–203, 1989.

Lewinnick GE, Warfield CA: Facet joint degeneration as a cause of low back pain. *Clin Orthop* 213:216–222, 1986.

Liang MH: Acute low back pain: Diagnosis and management of mechanical pain. *Primary Care* 15:827–847, 1988.

Lintner DM, Knight RQ, Cullen JP: The neurologic sequelae of cervical spine facet injuries. The role of canal diameter. *Spine* 18:725–729, 1993.

Lippitt AB: The facet joint and cervical spine's role in spine pain. Management with facet joint injections. *Spine* 9:746–750, 1984.

Lynch MC, Taylor JF: Facet joint injection for low back pain. *Bone Joint Surg (Br)* 68B:138–141, 1986.

MacNab I: *Backache*. Baltimore, Williams & Williams, 1977.

McClean ID: Ossicles of Oppenheimer. *Am Chiropractic Assoc J Chiropr* 22:6–56, 1988.

McRae JE: *Roentgenometrics in Chiropractic*. Toronto, Canadian Memorial Chiropractic College, 1983.

Moore KL: *Clinically Oriented Anatomy*, ed 3. Baltimore, Williams & Wilkins, 1992.

Murphy WA: The facet syndrome. *Radiology* 151:533, 1984.

Nicoll EA: Fractures of the dorso-lumbar spine. *J Bone Joint Surg Br* 31:376, 1949.

Penning L: Some aspects of plain radiography of the cervical spine in chronic myelopathy. *Neurology* 12:513–519, 1962.

Raymond J, Dumas JM: Intraarticular facet block—diagnostic test or therapeutic procedure. *Radiology* 151:333–336, 1984.

Resnick D, Niwayama G: *Diagnosis of Bone and Joint Disorders*, ed 2. Philadelphia, WB Saunders, 1988.

Roaf R: A study of the mechanics of spinal injuries. *J Bone Joint Surg (Br)* 42B:810–823, 1960.

Rorabeck CH, Roch MG, Hawkins RL, et al: Unilateral facet dislocation of the cervical spine. An analysis of the results in 26 patients. *Spine* 12:23–27, 1987.

Singer KP, Breidahl PD, Day RE: Variations in zygapophyseal joint orientation and level of transition at the thoracolumbar junction. Preliminary survey using computerized tomography. *Surg Radiol Anat* 10:291–295, 1988.

Smith WS, Kaufer H: Patterns and mechanisms of lumbar injuries associated with lap seat belts. *J Bone Joint Surg (Am)* 51A:239–254, 1990.

Swallow RA, Naylor E, Roebuck EJ, et al: *Clark's Positioning in Radiography*, ed 11.

Taylor JR, McCormick CC: The lumbar facet joint fat pads, their normal anatomy and their appearance when enlarged. *Neuroradiology* 33:38–42, 1991.

Taylor JR, Twomey LT: Age changes in lumbar zygapophyseal joints. Observations on structure and function. *Spine* 11:739–745, 1986.

Terrett ACJ, Vernon H: Manipulation and pain tolerance. A controlled study of the effect of spinal manipulation on paraspinal cutaneous pain tolerance levels. *Am J Phys Med* 63:217–225, 1984.

Torg JS, Pavlov H, Warren R, et al: The relationship of cervical canal narrowing ("stenosis") to permanent neurologic injury to the athlete: An epidemiologic surgery. Paper presented at the annual meeting of the American Academy of Orthopaedic Surgeons, New Orleans, Feb 8–13, 1990.

Tournade A, Patay Z, Krupa P, et al: A comparative study of anatomical, radiological and therapeutic features of the lumbar facet joints. *Neuroradiology* 34:257–261, 1992.

Weinstein J; Mechanisms of spinal pain. The dorsal root ganglion and its role as a mediator of low-back pain. *Spine* 11:999–1001, 1986.

White AA, Hirsch C: The significance of the vertebral posterior elements in the mechanics of the thoracic spine. *Clin Orthop* 81:2–14, 1971.

White AA, Panjabi MM: *Clinical Biomechanics of the Spine*, ed 2. Philadelphia, JB Lippincott, 1990.

Yagan R, AsimKhan M: Confusion of roentgenographic differential diagnosis of ankylosing hyperostosis (Forester's disease). *Spine* 4:561–575, 1990.

Yochum TR, Rowe LJ: *Essentials of Skeletal Radiology*. Baltimore, Williams & Wilkins 1987.

Ziv I, Maroudas C, Robin G, et al: Human facet cartilage: Swelling and some physicochemical characteristics as a function of age: 2. Age changes in some biophysical parameters of human facet joint cartilage. *Spine* 18:136–146, 1993.

Zoltan JD, Gilula LA, Murphy WA: Unilateral facet dislocation between the fifth lumbar and first sacral vertebra. *J Bone Joint Surg (Am)* 61A:767–769, 1979.

Chiropractic Today

Walter I. Wardwell, Ph.D.
Professor Emeritus of Sociology, University of Connecticut, Storrs, Connecticut

MEDIA ACCEPTANCE

There is no question that chiropractors today have obtained some acceptance, not only legally and by the public, but also professionally. As a result of resolution in 1991 of the Wilk et al.[1] antitrust suit, the most blatant antichiropractic activities of organized medicine have been curtailed, although its opposition can still be seen in presentations in the mass media (e.g., the *Wall Street Journal, Consumer Reports,* and the "20/20" television program by the American Broadcasting Company). Typically such releases acknowledge the scientific evidence that chiropractic and spinal manipulative therapy (SMT) benefit low back pain and other musculoskeletal conditions. But they go on to warn the public against chiropractors who treat serious spinal conditions or organic problems, and often they advise patients to see a physician first so as to avoid potential harm from chiropractic treatment or from delay in getting medical treatment. These are familiar antichiropractic arguments. The main difference now is that they acknowledge the potential benefits of chiropractic and SMT in ways not done 10 to 15 years ago. But because the negative comments seem to come as an afterthought and because they make the presentation seem more balanced, they may give it more credence.

LEGAL AND LEGISLATIVE ACCEPTANCE

In the legal, licensing, and scope-of-practice areas chiropractic status remains as varied as ever. The variability in legally authorized scopes of practice in different states, which Wilcher[2] documented in 1989, continues to confuse the public and third-party payers concerning what chiropractic is, what chiropractors do, and what they should be reimbursed for. Such inconsistency creates uncertainty for national health planners as to where chiropractors should fit into the health care system and gives organized medicine an opening wedge to oppose any chiropractic involvement.

So also does the debate over whether chiropractors practice general primary care or are simply portals of entry into the health care system. To combine these two things in the phrase "primary care portals of entry" only confuses the issue. This is not the place to debate the issue of primary care, but that term must be clearly defined and then used according to that definition. If primary care is defined to include all the services provided by family medical practitioners, chiropractors are not primary care providers even when they may be fully trained to identify and refer patients who have infectious diseases, need minor surgery, and so on. Chiropractors are, and always have been, portals of entry into the health care system because they see patients without referral from a physician. And like family physicians, they are competent to decide which patients they should refer to other health providers.

The shortage of medical primary care providers has motivated some chiropractors to try to define chiropractors as primary care providers to fill the gap. Nelson[3] presents excellent data and arguments showing that chiropractors are not and should not try to be primary care generalists—that they should be realists and call themselves what they actually are—"neuromusculoskeletal specialists." Chiropractors' academic and clinical training does not qualify them to be general practitioners, but it does qualify them to be back specialists, which is where the strongest evidence validating chiropractic is found. Nelson[3] argues that defining chiropractors as neuromusculoskeletal specialists offers the best chance of convincing organized medicine and third-party payers that chiropractic should be part of our health care system.

The argument that primary care should be chiropractors' goal has led to studies of chiropractors in rural areas lacking physicians, which is where chiropractors should be most likely to provide general primary care. A few chiropractors in such isolated rural areas do indeed see more of the conditions that patients would normally take to a physician, but they are an atypical minority of all chiropractors. In areas where choice of practitioner is possible, it has been well established that 85% to 95% of chiropractic patients are seen for neuromusculoskeletal problems. Callahan and Cianciulli[4] show that in the rural areas without physicians that they studied, the majority of respondents indicated that less than 10% of their patients are either referred in to them or referred out by them to other providers. Because this small percentage of cases referred out to physicians is the same percentage referred out by chiropractors in nonrural areas, the simple explanation may be that patients self-select whether to go to a physician or a chiropractor based on the illness they suffer, not whether it is more difficult to go to a physician, and that therefore they bring very few medical problems to chiropractors in both rural and nonrural areas. Hence, although chiropractors practice chiropractic primary care as back specialists, they do not provide medical primary care.

Although chiropractors are concerned that so few patients consult them for a wider array of complaints than they do, in actuality patient self-selection prevents chiropractors from treating conditions they might help but for which chiropractic has not yet been shown by solid research to be beneficial. Nelson[3] argues that the 3% to 5% of "visceral patients" that chiropractors treat require further research before medical authorities will take chiropractors' claims seriously. The recent proposal by Western States College of Chiropractic in Oregon to offer a new degree—doctor of chiropractic medicine (DCM)—could confuse the issue even further because it may widen the gap between traditional chiropractors and those who want to move in a more medical direction. The move to designate chiropractors as primary care practitioners could further alienate organized medicine, which is beginning to accept chiropractors as limited specialists.

Commissioning of chiropractors in the military was authorized by Congress in 1992 over strong medical opposition but has not yet been implemented, partly because of turmoil in the military over cutbacks necessitated by the end of the Cold War and also no doubt to the continued resistance of organized medicine. Congress has finally recognized the importance and prevalence of alternative medicines by appropriating several millions of dollars for their study to the National Institutes of Health (NIH), and several medical schools have introduced courses and research on alternative medicines. It is worth noting that chiropractic is sometimes included and sometimes excluded from lists of alternative medicines, which may indicate that chiropractic is no longer considered an alternative but has become established in our health care system. In any case, acceptance of chiropractic in the legal, scope of practice, and political areas has slowly improved over the past decade.

"Straight" states and "mixer" states still exist. Although model state licensing laws have been proposed, the political environment is so different in the different states that it is hard to see how uniformity can be obtained in the future. The straight/mixer division between the schools and the presence of ideologically competing associations in the states perpetuate these differences. Health planning decisions at the national level regarding chiropractors' competencies and scope of reimbursed practice could move the profession toward greater uniformity in scope of practice, but it is more probable that states' rights advocates will succeed in permitting the states to experiment with different health care plans and in authorizing chiropractors to practice in accordance with different state licensing laws.

The Federation of Straight Chiropractic Organizations (FSCO) has lost separate accreditation for its colleges, but the superstraight "s, p, and u" (specific, pure, and unadulterated) "philosophy" of chiropractic, which was derived from B.J. Palmer[5] and Stephenson,[6] continues to be taught (Strauss[7]), not only by the superstraight colleges but also by Life College and a majority of the practice builders. The word "philosophy" is put in quotation marks to indicate that it is not philosophy in the strict sense but is a mixture of scientific principles and B.J. Palmer's ideology. Not as well educated as his self-educated father, B.J. Palmer developed his "philosophy" primarily for political purposes, both to differentiate his school from competing schools and to gain separate examining boards and licensure for chiropractors. The fact that many other chiropractors accepted his use of the term "philosophy," rejected it, or developed one of their own does not justify perpetuating the error. There is no chiropractic philosophy different from that of medicine or of science in general. However, chiropractic operates from a somewhat different paradigm from that of medicine in that it emphasizes holistic healing, homeostasis, health maintenance, and illness prevention. James Winterstein,[8] president of the National College of Chiropractic, continues to use the term "philosophy" in presenting the chiropractic scientific paradigm as a list of 11 "principles."

ACCEPTANCE BY THE PUBLIC

Deyo and Tsui-Wu[9] analyzed data from the Second National Health and Nutrition Examination Survey, based on interviews between 1976 and 1980 with 10,404 U.S. adults older than 25 years. Fifty-nine percent of those with low back pain had consulted a general practitioner, 37% an orthopedist, 31% a chiropractor, and 14% an osteopath, some going to

TABLE 1.
Characteristics of Chiropractic Users and Nonusers in New Jersey*

	Nonusers† (%)	Users†‡ (%)	Total Sample§ (%)
Gender			
Male	42	38	41
Female	58	62	59
Education			
Less than high school	10	8	9
High school graduate	27	38	31
Some college	26	21	24
College graduate	24	23	24
Some graduate or professional school	3	2	2
Graduated from graduate or professional school	10	8	10
Ethnicity/race			
White (non-Hispanic)	69	73	71
African American	16	14	15
Hispanic	8	11	9
Asian	6	1	4
Other	1	1	1
Reported state of health			
Poor	2	3	2
Fair	10	16	12
Good	49	50	49
Excellent	39	31	37
Reported annual income			
No income (unemployed)	1	1	1
<$10,000	26	28	27
$10,001–$20,000	17	3	16
$20,001–$30,000	25	28	26
$30,001–$40,000	14	15	14
$40,001–$50,000	7	4	6
>$50,000	10	11	10

*From Sanchez JE: *J Manipulative Physiol Ther* 1991; 14:165–176. Used by permission.
†Four responses are missing; n = 449 (65% of total).
‡n = 240 (35% of total).
§N = 693.

more than one practitioner. Geographic distribution of those using a chiropractor was 45% in the West, 38% in the Midwest, and 30% in the South and Northeast. It was 14% for blacks and 39% for whites. It was 37% for those with a high school or college education, whereas for those with only an elementary school education it was 33%, due partly, no doubt, to the larger number of nonusing blacks with less education. Although chiropractic is still more popular in the West, it clearly is no longer used primarily by rural occupants, those less well educated, or those in lower occupational or income categories.[10]

The most thorough survey of the public's attitudes and reasons for using or not using chiropractors was reported by sociologist Sanchez (Table 1).[11] Telephone interviews with 693 randomly chosen New Jersey residents confirmed findings from other state surveys regarding satisfaction with treatment, attitudes among nonusers, and the demographic similarities between users and nonusers. Only 13% of nonusers held an unfavorable opinion of chiropractors, whereas other nonusers had not had a condition they thought chiropractors could help or were ignorant of the conditions that chiropractors treat. A *National Opinion Study* prepared for the American Chiropractic Association (ACA) by the Gallup Organization[12] produced results comparable to the state surveys.

Overall, about 40% of the U.S. population has visited a chiropractor at least once. Regular users probably comprise 8% to 10% of the total population, more in the West and Midwest than in the East and the South. It is estimated that about $6 billion is spent annually on chiropractors, with about 85% coming from third-party payers.

Acceptance of chiropractic in the sports world has been truly phenomenal, from local school teams to the International Olympics. Rehm[13] has documented the historically close relationship between chiropractic and professional baseball. Public advocacy of chiropractic by Joe Montana of the San Francisco Forty-Niners and by other world-class athletes has given chiropractic important public recognition.

Journals devoted to health and nutrition have often found common interest with chiropractors in advocating healthy diets, food supplements, and aerobic exercises. Public interviews on radio and television with chiropractors on general topics related to maintaining health have become common. Despite the negative comments in the *Wall Street Journal*, *Consumer Reports*, and the "20/20" television program, numerous favorable articles have appeared in newspapers and journals and on television. Overall, public acceptance and favorable media attention have increased greatly during the past decade.

PROFESSIONAL ACCEPTANCE

Professional acceptance of chiropractic and SMT has also increased considerably in the past decade. Although the National Academy of Manipulative (later Musculoskeletal) Medicine (NAAMM) has ceased to exist, it has been replaced by the American Back Society, which accepts chiropractors as full members and includes them in its programs. More chiropractors have published articles in medical journals, some coauthored with physicians. And more chiropractors have engaged in collaborative research with physicians. Terry Yochum became the first chiropractor to be appointed to a medical school faculty on the basis of his chiropractic credentials and publications.

Two medical school professors (Cherkin and MacCornack[14]) examined 457 patients with low back pain in the Puget Sound Group Health Cooperative, a well-known health maintenance organization (HMO). All patients were between 18 and 64 years old and chose whether to go to a family physician or a chiropractor. Although "chiropractic patients reported significantly more episodes of pain and had experienced pain for a longer period of time . . . the percentage of chiropractic patients 'very satisfied' with the care they received was triple that for patients of family physicians (66% vs. 22%)."[14] Chiropractic patients were about three times more satisfied with the information given them by their provider, twice as satisfied with the level of concern for them, and nearly three times as likely to perceive the provider as confident and comfortable in dealing with low back pain.

Professor Cherkin is also codirector of a 5-year $4,638,261 research grant from the National Center for Health Services Research to evaluate the effectiveness of care for low back pain patients. In addition, the U.S. Agency for Health Care Policy and Research awarded him $979,751 in 1993 for a 3-year study comparing chiropractic manipulation and McKenzie's physical therapy technique for low back pain in approximately 330 patients. In 1973 Congress appropriated $1.8 million for two research projects related to chiropractic: (1) a demonstration of how physicians and chiropractors can collaborate in treating spinal and low back conditions and (2) an interdisciplinary study of how chiropractic health care can be improved and expanded in rural areas.

In 1993 Manga et al.[15] from the University of Ottawa prepared an important report for the Province of Ontario, which found:

> On the evidence, particularly the most scientifically valid clinical studies, spinal manipulation applied by chiropractors is shown to be more effective than alternative treatments for LBP [low back pain]. Many medical therapies are of questionable validity or are clearly inadequate. . . . There would be highly significant cost savings if more management of LBP was transferred from physicians to chiropractors. . . . The major savings from chiropractic management come from fewer and lower costs of auxiliary services, much fewer hospitalizations, and a highly significant reduction in chronic problems and levels and duration of disability. . . . There is good empirical evidence that patients are very satisfied with chiropractic management of LBP and considerably less satisfied with physician management.*

They recommended:

> Chiropractic services should be fully insured under the Ontario Health Insurance Plan. . . . Chiropractic services should be fully integrated into the health care system. . . . Chiropractors should be employed by tertiary hospitals in Ontario. . . . Similar recommendations have

---

*From Manga P, et al: *The Effectiveness and Cost Effectiveness of Chiropractic Management of Low-Back Pain.* Toronto, Ontario Ministry of Health, 1993. Used by permission.

been made recently by government inquiries in Australia and Sweden, and following government funded research in the U.K. and other countries. Unnecessary or failed surgery is not only costly but also represents low quality care. The opportunity for consultation, second opinion and wider treatment options are significant advantages we foresee from this initiative which has been employed with success in a clinical research setting at the University Hospital, Saskatoon. Hospital privileges should be extended to all chiropractors for the purpose of treatment of their own patients who have been hospitalized for other reasons, and for access to diagnostic facilities relevant to their scope of practice and patients' needs. . . . Chiropractic education in Ontario should be in the multidisciplinary atmosphere of a university with appropriate public funding.*

A major research study in England was published in the *British Medical Journal* by Meade et al.[16] From a randomized comparison study of chiropractic and hospital outpatient treatment of 741 patients with low back pain of mechanical origin, they concluded that chiropractic treatment was more effective than hospital outpatient management, particularly for patients with chronic or severe back pain. "Chiropractic almost certainly confers worthwhile, long term benefit in comparison with hospital outpatient management. The benefit is seen mainly in those with chronic or severe pain. Introducing chiropractic into NHS (the National Health Service) should be considered."[16]

The study is all the more remarkable because 72% of the hospital outpatients received physical therapy manipulation using Maitland's[17] technique, whereas another 12% received the Cyriax[18] technique. The study therefore demonstrates the superiority of chiropractic technique according to an editorial in *Lancet*, "Chiropractors and Low Back Pain" (July 28, 1990), which noted that it took 15 years after the Cochrane Commission's recommendation for the Medical Research Council to authorize the clinical trial. The editorial concluded that although more studies are needed to confirm the results and to "dissect the causes, . . . chiropractic treatment should be taken seriously by conventional medicine, which means both doctors and physiotherapists. Physiotherapists need to . . . take on board the skills that chiropractors have developed so successfully." In 1994 chiropractors in England gained legal recognition and a plan to officially register them.

In 1994 the U.S. Agency for Health Care Policy and Research issued *Clinical Guideline Number 14: Acute Low Back Problems in Adults*, denigrating medical and surgical interventions, bed rest, corsets, and belts, but recommending spinal manipulation for most cases, along with moderate exercise and proper diet. It clearly gave chiropractic official endorsement by the U.S. government.

Chiropractors have been appointed to the professional staffs of about 100 hospitals and surgical centers in the United States. Although those hospitals have not been among the most prestigious, hospital appointment is an important symbolic achievement and is one of the results of victory in the Wilk[1] antitrust suit. In hospitals chiropractors coadmit with a physician or an osteopath, and in some hospitals they can order diagnostic tests, diets, and physical therapy in addition to providing SMT.

Manipulation under anesthesia (MUA) is an example of a collaborative procedure performed in a hospital in conjunction with a medical or osteopathic anesthesiologist on a patient who needs it. When chiropractors are members of hospital staffs, they are fellow practitioners of physicians, dentists, and podiatrists. When they become commissioned officers in the military, they will receive similar recognition. Although only a small percentage of chiropractors may enter the military or seek hospital staff privileges, for the big picture it is vitally important that some chiropractors achieve these advances.

At the clinical level, some chiropractic colleges have developed relationships with medical teaching hospitals permitting some chiropractic students to attend medical rounds. Relationships developed with medical students may continue into practice. Conclusive data are hard to obtain, but there is little doubt that referral by physicians to chiropractors is increasing, as it certainly should because full collaboration between chiropractors and physicians in diagnosis and treatment is the ultimate goal.

THIRD-PARTY REIMBURSEMENTS

The fee-for-service method of payment is disappearing from contemporary heath care in the United States. In an era of high costs, only the wealthy or the desperate will resort to it. It is ironic that just as chiropractors are winning their battles for recognition and against organized medicine, they must now battle on the economic front. Third-party repayment is dominated by medical thinking and medically oriented insurance functionaries, from the way diseases are categorized to the treatments provided and the terminology for them. Pressed to conserve funds, insurance companies resist paying more than they have to, and they often find that chiropractors are vulnerable targets. Not aware (until very recently) that they can save money by substituting conservative chiropractic treatment for aggressive and expensive drugging or surgery,[19, 20, 21] insurance companies often create problems for chiropractors by refusing to pay because of minor technicalities or by limiting the number or weeks of treatment they will pay for. They sometimes use unfair independent medical examinations (IMEs) to support their refusals.

Undoubtedly some chiropractors, like some physicians, have abused third-party payers by overtreating, overcharging, or even committing outright fraud. Chiropractors often view insurance scrutiny of them as a manifestation of antichiropractic bias. Even when other chiropractors perform the IMEs or serve as claims reviewers for insurance companies, there is suspicion that they have sold out their profession and turned traitor to their brethren. Insurance companies need to be educated concerning the cost savings that chiropractic provides, and chiropractors should discipline their wayward brethren.

MAJOR PROBLEMS IN THE 1990s

The biggest problem for chiropractic in the 1990s is reform of the health care system. Although President Clinton and First Lady Hillary Clinton are reported to be favorable toward chiropractors, their plan did not mention chiropractors (or podiatry or optometry), which all are presumed to continue in the future as they have in the past. The strong popular insistence on patient choice tends to reassure chiropractors, whereas the gatekeeper role in managed care plans causes them their greatest fear. Although chiropractors have mobilized their public and political supporters and seek to have chiropractic specifically named as an available health service, mere availability in the law is not sufficient if authorization by a physician is required to obtain it.

Existing managed health care systems offer various models for including chiropractic. Blue Cross/Blue Shield plans usually offer chiropractic services, sometimes in only the more expensive plans. Some HMOs provide chiropractic services without a physician gatekeeper and have found it to save on costs. Chiropractors hope to convince health planners that the cost savings from chiropractic will work in its favor. At this writing the outcome of health care reform remains in doubt. If chiropractic services are more cost effective, insurance companies should lead the way toward its greater use. However, the continuing ambiguous treatment of chiropractic in the mass media and in medically dominated federal agencies such as the U.S. Public Health Service and the Health Care Financing Agency (HCFA) shows that organized medicine's resistance persists and is still the most formidable obstacle to chiropractic's full acceptance. That is nothing new for chiropractors, who have become well accustomed to it during their century-long struggle to survive.

The second biggest problem facing chiropractic in the 1990s is the continuing ideological split between straights and mixers. Despite the use of different words (e.g., traditionalists vs. progressives), the problem persists, most obviously in the different associations at national and state levels. The ACA, as the largest national association, leads the profession in efforts to strengthen education, obtain favorable legislation, and support basic and clinical research. The International Chiropractors Association (ICA) continues to represent the traditional chiropractic position by focusing emphasis on the spinal subluxation complex, and it has become even more conservative since failure of the 1986 to 1988 merger attempt and loss of its moderate leadership to the ACA.

The FSCO has lost much of its clout now that its three schools must seek accreditation from the Council on Chiropractic Education (CCE), which insists that they teach a broader curriculum with more emphasis on diagnosis. It remains to be seen whether FSCO will continue on its current path or will ultimately merge with the ICA. To do so would strengthen the ICA but make it even more traditional than it is now. A straw in the wind may be the dropping of the word "straight" from Pennsylvania College of Straight Chiropractic. Worth noting is that there seems to be little difference between the ACA and the ICA over the question of whether chiropractors should treat organic conditions.

At the opposite pole from FSCO is a very small group that wants to limit chiropractic to musculoskeletal conditions and work more closely with physicians, if not completely under their direction. The National Association of Chiropractic Medicine (NACM) rejects all chiropractic "philosophy" and the use of chiropractic to treat any organic condition. It maintains that chiropractic's scope of practice should be limited to "functional biomechanics, gait, posture and rehabilitation of the locomotor systems with emphasis on the manipulative lesion, but to include physical medicine modalities for which scientific efficacy has been established."[22] It has affiliated with the new Orthopractic Manipulative Society of North America (OMSNA), which was begun in Canada in conjunction with medical associations and invites members of OMSNA to join. The NACM wants "to abandon the profession entirely and establish a new profession under the states' 'medical practice acts'."[22] Chiropractors would then become nearly indistinguishable from physical therapists, who are also eligible to become orthopractic manipulators and can now see patients without physician referral in about 30 states. Because the medical associations in Canada, Australia, and New Zealand, as well as the American Medical Association (AMA), support orthopractors, chiropractors view this development as yet another effort by organized medicine to "contain and then eliminate chiropractic," which was the goal the AMA set for itself in 1971.[23] Because some states have as many as four different chiropractic associations, each representing chiropractors of different ideological and political persuasions, that demonstrates the AMA's success in achieving that goal, which it set for itself in 1967 according to a memorandum of its Committee on Quackery: to encourage continued separation of the two national chiropractic associations.[23] However, it is worth noting that the AMA has not achieved its first two goals, which chiropractic successfully circumvented in the 1970s:

1. Doing everything within their power to see that chiropractic coverage under Title 18 of the Medicare law is not obtained.
2. Doing everything within their power to see that recognition or listing by the U.S. Office of Education of a chiropractic accrediting agency is not achieved.

Keeping chiropractic associations separate and contending with each other has served AMA's interests well, because it confuses health planners, legislators, and the public at large about what chiropractic is, does, and wants. It also gives third-party payers leverage for denying reimbursement for services that some chiropractors oppose. Although a fringe group, including many of the practice builders, still advocate chiropractic treatment for all possible pathological conditions, they are as extreme at one pole as the NACM, which opposes everything but a narrow musculoskeletal scope of practice, is at the other pole.

A third problem, fortunately one of decreasing importance, is variability in the curricula taught in different schools. CCE mandates academically sound training in the basic medical sciences taught by university-qualified instructors. The clinical courses, taught mainly by chiropractors, reveal greater variability due to differences in "philosophy" and ideology. But since spinal adjustments are the mainstay of chiropractic therapy, there is greater uniformity in the art of chiropractic. Colleges frequently hire faculty trained at other colleges, unlike in earlier periods when schools taught primarily the techniques of their founders. The colleges now permit outside technique teachers to visit and teach and often have student clubs devoted to particular manipulative techniques.

A fourth problem concerns research, which in the colleges is still hampered by shortages of funds, lack of a strong and continuing commitment by some administrators and the public at large, and a shortage of faculty competent to design and execute research projects that will attract funds from the Foundation for Chiropractic Education and Research (FCER), NIH, or private foundations. Too many chiropractors believe that because chiropractic works, the only research needed is that which proves, primarily to outsiders, that it works. Too few chiropractors understand that researchers must be objective, open minded, and question everything until objective evidence demonstrates otherwise. The profession will not attract significant research funds until it convinces fund-granting agencies that it supports truly objective research on chiropractic fundamentals and treatment outcomes.

A fifth problem still confronting the profession is the omnipresence of entrepreneurial practice builders who prey on the profession. Condemned as early as the 1954 ICA-sponsored report by Saunders Associates[24] as "glorified pep talks" and as "more inspirational than educational," their propounding of traditional "philosophy" and their Palmer-like appeals to save the world through chiropractic have been condemned as "that old-time religion." Also, their exhortations for lifetime wellness care may lead to the overtreatment that third-party payers do not consider "medically necessary" and will not pay for. Hence, to some degree the third-party payment system disciplines chiropractors tempted to overtreat.

Sixth, the colleges face several other serious problems. Financing remains uncertain because costs and pressures for improvement continually increase. Even the very best colleges have only small endowments. Because all the colleges depend mainly on tuition, only the best of them can be very selective about admissions. Even the best faculty often rely on outside income from practice or other sources, and all the colleges rely on the good will of manufacturers to donate much of the equipment needed for teaching and research.

Differences in orientation between the basic science and clinical faculties are more intense than in medical schools. Because the basic scientists have been educated in a medical environment, they sometimes retain an antichiropractic bias either because they reject the chiropractic "philosophy" still strong at some colleges or because they feel contempt for what they consider the less well-educated clinical chiropractors. At the 1989 meeting of the Association for the History of Chiropractic, one college administrator complained: "The clinical faculty is being 'eaten alive' by the students," whereas another said: "Not only the faculty but also the students are becoming demoralized." The earlier pattern where a basic science teacher almost automatically took chiropractic courses and qualified as a doctor of chiropractic, or where a qualified chiropractic student would also teach a basic science course has long since passed. Some of the hostility between the basic science and clinical faculties may decrease as more clinicians gain master's or doctoral degrees in a basic science and as more scientific evidence appears for chiropractic theory and its clinical success.

The mix of patients going to chiropractic clinics remains deficient in the range of ages and pathological conditions that a graduate will meet in practice. Too many college clinics still depend on student recruitment of patients. Recruitment from inner city neighborhoods helps, but the better solution is for students to have regular opportunities to join medical students on hospital rounds, where they will not only see a much wider variety of pathological conditions and learn about hospitals and medical procedures but will also rub shoulders with future medical consultants and potential collaborators in patient care. Thus far only the better chiropractic students in some of the better colleges have benefited from this important improvement in chiropractic education, but their numbers will increase as physicians learn that they and their students can also benefit from a chiropractic presence in their institutions. CCE should study this development and become a positive force in setting standards and goals for chiropractic education in medical hospitals.

CONCLUSION

Because it is certain that chiropractors will never accept the ancillary status of dependence on medical referral, nor is it likely that chiropractors will ever follow the path of osteopathy to become full medical practitioners, only two other possible courses of action remain open to them: to remain in their present ambiguous and unstable situation, which is not as marginal as it once was but is still not fully accepted by medical authorities, much of the public, and the public authorities that they influence; or to continue to move toward the medical pole by ceasing to reject most medical theories of illness and cure and demonstrating through scientific research the validity of chiropractic theories regarding neuromusculoskeletal mechanisms and the outcome benefits of chiropractic treatment compared with that of other practitioners. Chiropractic would then most likely become a limited medical profession similar to dentistry, podiatry, optometry, and psychology, all of which accept the major medical theories of disease but are limited in the parts of the body they treat and in the therapeutic modalities they can use.

Although some chiropractors refuse to acknowledge any limitations to chiropractic (and certainly all of its possible benefits have not yet been fully explored), there are obvious limitations in its legally authorized scope of practice and in what its colleges teach. If chiropractors claim to be primary care providers (beyond portals of entry), they clearly do not engage in the broad scope of practice available to physicians of family medicine, many of whose diagnostic tools and treatment modalities are denied to chiropractors. If chiropractors claim to be specialists, they are "back specialists," nearly all of whom give chiropractic adjustments to nearly all of their patients. In that respect they are much like dentists, podiatrists, optometrists, and psychologists, each of whom claims expertise in a particular part of the body but whose range of treatment is likewise severely limited.

Chiropractic could become accepted as a limited medical profession if current trends continue. Its schools offer excellent training in the basic medical sciences and in use of the latest high-tech diagnostic tests. Only a small minority of chiropractors still subscribe to Palmer's simplistic monocausal theory of illness and treatment. Chiropractors have obtained legal and legislative legitimacy as full participants in our health care system. Collaboration with physicians in diagnosis and treatment and in hospitals is increasing. What is still lacking is neurophysiological research relevant to the validity of chiropractic theories and research on outcomes documenting chiropractic benefits for additional types of illness, including organic and systemic ones. When that happens, the last remaining basis for organized medicine's resistance to chiropractic (except for economic competition) should disappear. In the terminology proposed by Australian sociologist Evan Willis,[25] chiropractic has already achieved "political-legal legitimation" based on "clinical legitimacy" (i.e., it "works"); what it still needs and seeks is "scientific legitimation," which organized medicine still hesitates to accord it.

REFERENCES

1. Wilk CA, et al vs. AMA, et al: Complaint 76C3777 filed Oct 12, 1976, in the US District Court for the Northern District of Illinois, Eastern Division.
2. Wilcher CC: National chiropractic standards. *Dynamic Chiropr* 7:40, 1989.
3. Nelson C: Chiropractic scope of practice. *J Manipulative Physiol Ther* 16:488–497, 1993.
4. Callahan D, Cianciulli A: *The Chiropractor as a Primary Health Care Provider in Rural Health Professional Shortage Areas of the U.S.: An Exploratory Analysis*, Arlington, Va, Foundation for Chiropractic Education and Research, 1994.
5. Palmer BJ: *The Science of Chiropractic: Its Principles and Philosophies.* Davenport, Iowa, Palmer School of Chiropractic, 1920.
6. Stephenson RW: *Chiropractic Textbook.* Davenport, Iowa, Palmer School of Chiropractic, 1927.
7. Strauss JB: *Chiropractic Philosophy.* Foundation for the Advancement of Chiropractic Education, 1991.
8. Winterstein J: Philosophy of chiropractic: A contemporary perspective. *J Chiropr* 31:28–36, 31:64–71, 1994.
9. Deyo RA, Tsui-Wu Y-J: Descriptive epidemiology of low back pain and its related medical care in the United States. *Spine* 12:264–268, 1987.
10. Wardwell WI: *Chiropractic: History and Evolution of A New Profession.* St Louis, Mosby, pp 229–241, 1992.
11. Sanchez JE: A look in the mirror: A critical and exploratory study of public perceptions of the chiropractic profession in New Jersey. *J Manipulative Physiol Ther* 14:165–176, 1991.
12. Gallup Organization: *National Opinion Study.* Paper prepared for the American Chiropractic Association, Princeton, NJ, 1991.
13. Rehm W: "Doc" Painter and the "Mighty" New York Yankees: Ruth, DiMaggio and Gehrig were his patients. *Chiropractic History* 12:10–11, 1992.
14. Cherkin DC, MacCornack FA: Patient evaluations of low back pain from family physicians and chiropractors. *West J Med* 150:351–355, 1989.
15. Manga P, et al: *The Effectiveness and Cost Effectiveness of Chiropractic Management of Low-Back Pain.* Toronto, Ontario Ministry of Health, 1993.
16. Meade TW, et al: Low back pain of mechanical origin: Randomised comparison of chiropractic and hospital outpatient treatment. *BMJ* 300:1431–1437, 1990.
17. Maitland GD: *Vertebral Manipulation.* London, Butterworth, 1984.
18. Cyriax JH: *Textbook of Orthopaedic Medicine: Treatment by Manipulation and Deep Massage,* ed 4. London, Cassell, 1975.

19. Wolk S: *An Analysis of Florida Workers Compensation Medical Claims for Back-Related Injuries.* Arlington, Va, Foundation for Chiropractic Education and Research, 1988.
20. Shifrin LG: *Mandated Health Insurance Coverage for Chiropractic Treatment: An Economic Assessment, with Implications for the Commonwealth of Virginia.* Richmond, Va, Virginia Chiropractic Association, 1992.
21. Stano M: Further analysis of health care costs for chiropractic and medical patients. *J Manipulative Physiol Ther* 17:442–446, 1994.
22. NACM seeks to create new profession: Orthopractors. *Dynamic Chiropr* 12(11):1, 42–43, 1994.
23. Trever W: *In the Public Interest.* Los Angeles, Scriptures Unlimited, 1972, pp 4, 123.
24. Saunders Associates: *The Chiropractic Profession.* New York, Public Relations Management Corporation, 1954.
25. Willis E: *Medical Dominance: The Division of Labor in Australian Health Care.* Sydney, Allen and Unwin, 1983.

Educational Issues in Chiropractic

Jennifer R. Jamison, Ph.D., M.B., B.Ch., Ed.D.
Professor of Diagnostic Sciences, School of Chiropractic and Osteopathy, Faculty of Biomedical and Health Sciences, Royal Melbourne Institute of Technology, Bundoora, Australia

The fundamental theme that largely guides contemporary issues in chiropractic remains the challenge to appropriately balance the sometimes conflicting exigencies of the art and science of health care. Chiropractic education is committed to preparing practitioners to practice within a health care system committed primarily to positivism, predictability, and classical determinism when the reality of patient care is embedded in relativity, uncertainty, unpredictability, and human freedom.[1] "In his commitment to action, his faith, his pragmatism, his subjectivism and his emphasis on indeterminancy, then, the practitioner is quite different from the scientist."[2] For the preparation of effective chiropractic practitioners, the dual aspects of clinical practice, the art and science of health care, need to be ingrained into the fabric of chiropractic education. Scientific validation sanctions the factual content of practice, and empathy empowers the healing process. Because "scientific norms concern knowledge and do not deal directly with practical outcomes" and "the goal of practice is healing,"[3] neither element can alone suffice. As Keating suggests, like the chiropractic art, "the primary purpose of chiropractic science is patient benefit."[4] Chiropractic practice and the knowledge base on which it rests is, like " 'medical knowledge' . . . the product of the dialectic between knowledge and practice/experience."[5] Retention of the humane aspects of clinical care while preparing chiropractors as practitioner-scientists[6] is a task that continues to demand the attention of chiropractic educators.

It is within the context of the paradigm disparities entrenched in the health care system and intrinsic to clinical practice that the educational ethos and best practice standards of chiropractic education are evolving. The chiropractic profession cognizant that "the study of our treatment—manipulation—no longer belongs exclusively to us,"[7] maintains that "the uniqueness of chiropractic is really not so much in its clinical methodologies per se—whether it be adjustments, manipulation or physiological therapeutics—but rather by its wholistic concerns for the total internal/external environment of the patient. . . ."[8] On the other hand, the chiropractic profession, concerned that it may lose "authority in the adjustive arts through lack of research,"[9] has encouraged the emergence of a "science-based" ethos in undergraduate chiropractic education. There is furthermore a discernible trend in chiropractic education toward the medical model,[10] even to the extent that Coulter estimates that as much as 70% of the current chiropractic curriculum in American colleges may be identical to medicine.[11] Because chiropractic education appears to be emulating medical education, it is important to appreciate that medical education is flawed. More than 10 years ago Clarke[12] identified an intrinsic defect in the management of medical education: "Medical education has evolved in parallel with changes in medical practice, and it has been molded by them . . . now we are approaching a situation in which medical education no longer can afford to tag along behind medical practice and social change." More recently medical education has been critically appraised, and changes are being implemented. Issues for contemporary medical education, identified by the Association of American Medical Colleges through the Project Panel on the General Professional Education of the Physician[13] include:

- A shift of emphasis in the curriculum so that the acquisition of values and attitudes that promote caring enjoy equal prominence to those concerned with the acquisition of clinical knowledge, the application of scientific methods in clinical practice and the skills of critical appraisal
- The placement of students in clinical setting most likely to meet their future practice needs
- Encouraging active and independent student learning
- The education of faculty to facilitate the implementation of appropriate changes.

Strategies for implementing change in medical education range from a system of peer and student evaluation of teaching and the curriculum through information integration by cross-disciplinary teaching and problem-based learning to improve assessment of clinical skills using objective structured clinical examinations (OSCEs).[14] The direction that postsecondary accrediting agencies recognized by the U.S. Secretary of Education and the Council of Postsecondary Accreditation, including the Liaison Committee on Medical Education, intend to follow is competency-based, outcome-assessed education.[15] Chiropractic shares the objectives of the greater academic community, and chiropractic colleges are actively pursuing excellence in education.[16] The American College, which has most specifically addressed the necessity for curricular changes, is perhaps Los Angeles College of Chiropractic. It is seeking to implement the recommendations of a situational analysis of their academic program, which advocates "adoption of a competency-based curriculum utilizing problem-centered educational methods to foster active student participation in their learning process, increased opportunities for independent learning, and development of skills in problem solving and critical thinking."[17] Other areas in which chiropractic education is demonstrating particular interest include achieving a more balanced evaluation of student performance by expanding the focus of assessment from traditionally accepted cognitive factors to include noncognitive factors deemed critical to chiropractic competence (Western States Chiropractic College)[18]; researching the correlation between patient satisfac-

TABLE 1.
Shift in Accreditation: New Look in Chiropractic Education

	Looking Back	**Looking Ahead**
Accreditation focus	Institutional compliance Program organization	Individual competence Program outcome
Assessment for	Conformity with tradition (course duration, content hours, staff qualifications, staff/student ratios)	Competence (appraisal of staff and student performance standards)
Approach	Quantitative	Qualitative
Measurement	Normative	Criterion referenced
Dominant paradigm	Mechanistic	Holistic

tion, a highly desirable outcome of chiropractic care, and academic variables (Palmer College of Chiropractic)[19]; and exploring student preferences for traditional vs. more innovative approaches (Canadian Memorial Chiropractic College).[20]

Reevaluation of chiropractic educational practices is not confined to America. In Australia an office of the Government's Department of Employment, Education and Training has funded research to identify the competencies required for acceptable chiropractic practice.[21] Once identified, the competencies are to be used as the objectives for chiropractic education in Australia and will constitute the desired outcome on which student assessment will be based. This Australian initiative is consistent with the shift of the Council of Chiropractic Education away from an approach that infers quality from institutional compliance with standards of program organization to one of outcomes assessment with the focus now on the performance of individuals (Table 1).[22]

Both the more global concept of outcomes assessment and the popular movement toward enhanced personal responsibility exemplify the drift toward increased individual accountability. In education this is clearly expressed not only in the trend toward competency-based student assessment[23] but also in the tendency toward independent student learning and staff appraisal. At the microteaching level such reforms include using problem solving in preference to rote memory learning, active rather than passive learning, and a student- rather than teacher-centered educational environment.[13] Contemporary changes in chiropractic education, like those in other areas of professional education,[24] are largely redefining education with an increased emphasis on the assumptions of the holistic paradigm.

GENERAL IMPLICATIONS OF PARADIGM ASSUMPTIONS ON TEACHING AND LEARNING

The assumptions underlying the mechanistic and holistic paradigm substantively modify the nature of the educational process. The mechanistic paradigm favors "objectification of knowing and of knowledge, additive and linear progress, quantification, right and wrong answers, mastery learning, and lack of consideration for context, meaning and personal purpose."[25] The educational repercussions of implementing this conceptual framework include (1) the use of behavioral objectives in developing a curriculum predicated on the belief that the dynamics of the whole can be understood in a piecemeal fashion; and (2) the generation of a controlled environment in which content sequencing and segmentation, the pace and focus of learning are teacher generated, and knowledge, perceived as incremental, is attained by the accumulation of sufficient data. Although understanding may be fragmented, skills, or ways of doing things, can be taught efficiently and effectively within a mechanistic paradigm. In contrast, "since holism understands human behaviour and growth as immanently active, meaning constructive, self-organizing, and self-regulating, there cannot be a sequentially organized, prescriptive approach to 'how to be holistic.' "[25] Successful learning is perceived to be transformative rather than additive, and understanding is achieved by investigating relationships rather than isolated pieces of knowledge. Learning is not limited to those experiences deliberately incorporated to convey particular concepts; it inevitably occurs in the absence of conscious effort merely by engaging in a shared activity.[26] Competence is achieved through experiential learning in realistic clinical situations. Attitudes evolve as learning and assessment focus on purposeful engagement in natural settings. The goals, teaching-learning relationships, and "classroom" environment envisaged by the mechanistic and holistic paradigms are different. Table 2 explores the communication between teacher and learner at the extreme poles of the mechanistic and holistic paradigms.

Because outcomes assessment implies evaluation of the educational product in the gestalt of a practice situation, the import of a holistic framework should not be underestimated. Neither should the contribution of the mechanistic paradigm be overlooked; the precision of manual skills requires structured repetition, and the development of a scientific mind-

TABLE 2.
Classroom Communication

	Mechanistic Paradigm	**Holistic Paradigm**
Goal of communication	Impose teacher's reality Teach right from wrong	Negotiate shared view Accommodate different perspectives
Aim	Convey information	Facilitate understanding
Knowledge	Propositional Universal	Propositional and tacit Personalized
Logic	Probability (normative)	Negative/positive feedback (self-renewal, self-transcendence)
Expectation	Add to student's knowledge	Enrich both participants
Learning experience	Additive	Transformation
Teaching model	Pedagogical	Andragogical

set demands the rigor of critical appraisal. The reductionist-holistic mix encountered in chiropractic education is consistent with contemporary trends in education. Although these paradigm anomalies may be acutely experienced by the theorist, the chiropractic educator is concerned with optimal student learning. However, "naming and giving language to non-reductionist values, beliefs, and principles of the teaching/learning process is an extremely difficult task since for so long most of the language we use in education has been associated with reductionism."[27]

COMPETENCY-BASED EDUCATION: A FORUM FOR PARADIGM INTERACTION

Competency-based education attempts to describe competencies in professional education according to essential knowledge, fundamental skills, and attitudes.[28] It draws from both the mechanistic and holistic paradigms in defining its desired outcomes (Table 3). Once defined, these competencies serve as a framework for determining curricular content.[29] Although bearing a strong resemblance to the rational models of curriculum development proposed by Tyler and Taba,[30] both of which emphasize outcome (objectives or competencies) and are prescriptive, competency-based education is context sensitive.[31] Learning in context substantially contributes to competent practice because the practitioner's knowledge is both propositional and tacit. Information is both overtly learned and covertly absorbed:

> There are generally two methods of learning: by replication of rules (you learn the rules and then apply them); or ostension (you learn to use the language through trial and error without formal rules). The knowledge that is built into the paradigm, both with respect to nature and to itself, is caught rather than taught. What is learned is not a formalized system of rules, but by exposure to a series of problem situations that the paradigm has confronted, the student comes to see situations as like each other (to see them within a certain gestalt).[32]

TABLE 3.
Dual Elements of a Competency-Based Education

	Mechanistic Paradigm	Holistic Paradigm
Educational ethos	Scientific appraisal	Empathic understanding
Process	Analysis	Synthesis
Desirable outcome	Acquisition of manual skills	Manual and interpersonal
Knowledge	Propositional	Propositional and tacit
Attitudes	Detached observer	Interactive carer
Content selection	Nomothetic clinical trials	Idiographic case study
	Statistical significance	Substantive significance
Data processing	Objective problem solving	Context-sensitive inquiring
Learning	Additive	Transformation
	Superficial	Deep
	Acquiring information	

Innovations emphasizing context sensitivity are "community-oriented" learning, which stresses content, and "problem-based" learning, which also focuses on the inquiry process.[33]

In competency-based education, "the curriculum is organized around the functions which the practitioner will be expected to perform."[34] The dominant function that the chiropractic practitioner is expected to perform is patient assessment and management. The teaching-learning strategy that best encompasses this ethos is the patient management problem. Patient management problems focus the content of the learning on realistic clinical situations and capture the process-based learning approach of problem solving. Patient management problems synthesize the well-recognized educational approaches of discovery learning and case studies. There are two fundamental postulates underlying this approach to learning. The first is that learning through problem solving is much more effective for creating in the student's mind a body of knowledge usable in the future than is traditional memory-based learning. The second is that the physician skills most important for patients are more closely linked to solving problems than recalling facts: "Learning through problem solving is much more effective for creating in the student's mind a body of knowledge usable in the future than is traditional memory-based learning."[35]

By increasing the focus on patient management problems, chiropractic colleges are effectively integrating disparate paradigms in their undergraduate curriculum.

PROBLEM SOLVING

Problem solving is the fundamental intellectual processing skill underlying both the science and the art of chiropractic clinical practice. The process itself is reductionist in that clinical reasoning traditionally condenses information through the processes of interpretation, hypothesis generation, and problem formulation. Nonetheless, understanding the strategies, values, and probabilities underlying problem solving may convert the student's learning task from one of memorizing opinions to one of reasoning and judgment[36]; it may transform the student from passive recipient to active participant.

The various stages of problem solving are well recognized.[37,38] The principal inquiry strategies used in clinical decision making are pattern recognition (intuition), systematic scanning (induction), and the exploration of provisional diagnoses (deduction).[39] Clinical memory of prevalent syndromes with strongly characteristic presentations may lead to immediate recognition, or intuitive, diagnosis. Pattern recognition, achieved through repetitive exposure, provides a global recognition strategy. Systematic scanning reasons from phenomena to theories in a circular process using hypotheses in a nonhierarchical sequence to establish familiarity with something previously discovered.[40] As possible explanations for the phenomena extend beyond the cognitive boundaries of the clinician, practitioners may limit their search area by adopting a hypotheticodeductive approach confined to familiar disease syndromes or well-established sign and symptom patterns. Hypotheticodeductive reasoning attempts to combine the creative acts of hypothesis or diagnostic idea generation with the logical structure of deductive inference. An "if-then" strategy applies. Problem solving in an inductive way is the most functional approach to clinical practice because it largely parallels the way in which patients present their problems. Diagnostic formulation in practice is more frequently based on hypotheticodeductive reasoning; alternately a tentative hypothesis may be formulated within seconds of the consultation using a form of pattern recognition.[41] Despite the inherently analytic and reductionist nature of problem solving, clinical decision making is, in practice, a multidirectional process in which analysis and synthesis and reductionism and holism play a part.

By comparing the data collected in the clinical situation with the information gleaned from critical appraisal of the literature, the chiropractic student can prepare for responsible practice in a health care system with a scientific ethos. Critical appraisal is a scientifically accepted approach to information evaluation. It involves implementation of problem solving skills according to a scientifically accepted framework. Clinically acceptable information, preferably conforming to a linear cause-effect relationship, is assessed according to universally defined and standardized criteria.[42] An information system, which values clinical information according to the manner in which the evidence on which it is based has been generated, is available.[43] Students are afforded an opportunity to perceive the strong interactions between cognitive processes and the structure of knowledge.[44]

PROBLEM-BASED LEARNING

When education aimed at critical thinking is concerned with developing a particular content and context rather than the abstract development of skills,[45, 46] problem-based learning is used. The reality of learning problem solving in clinical practice rather than attempting to acquire a content-free generic skill[47] constitutes the acquisition of an essential clinical competency in a contextually sensitive learning situation. Proponents of problem-based learning postulate that their approach takes cognizance of information processing principles. They emphasize that efficient knowledge acquisition and retrieval involves the activation of prior knowledge, encoding specificity, followed by knowledge elaboration.[48] In problem-based learning these processes are embedded in relevant problems. Encoding specificity implies that successful future retrieval of information is facilitated when retrieval cues that are to be reactivated are encoded under similar circumstances (i.e., the learning environment should strongly resemble the practice situation). Linking prior knowledge with information being acquired further enhances future accessibility, as does knowledge elaboration. Information is better understood, processed, and retrieved if it is elaborated on or manipulated during the learning process. Dynamic student interaction in a situation relevant to chiropractic practice is consequently beneficial. The paradigm paradox that arises from the use of a process such as problem solving, which adheres largely to analytic and reductionist principles, in contextually sensitive learning situations is that subject boundaries are diminished. Problem-based learning employs an integrated code; it values a weak frame.[49] The selection of appropriate problems facilitates the acquisition of a core of relevant knowledge and lays down new knowledge in a clinically accessible rather than discipline-dictated format. In reality chiropractic practice is not discipline based. In practice, regardless of whether a course is constructed along innovative or traditional lines, as students progress the use of patient management problems can serve to convert a discipline-based perspective to an integrated frame and can replace segmented with integrated reasoning.[50] When the presenting problem is reduced to its component parts, the process of problem solving fails to recognize discipline-determined boundaries, and problem-based learning becomes a synthesizing activity. By linking the interactive nature of discovery learning with the context sensitivity of the case study, problem-based learning fulfills many of the criteria of learning within the holistic paradigm.

Although the competency-based nature of professional education requires a standardized level of practice, neither a discipline-based nor teacher-centered educational style is predicated. A curriculum that emphasizes problem solving is less likely to rely heavily on a teacher-centered style, which values didactic instruction and fosters unthinking and noncritical acceptance of material.[51] A problem-based curriculum encourages active student involvement by shifting the responsibility from teaching to learning. At the very least, problem-based learning encourages student control over the pace of learning. It is furthermore of substantive significance to heed the observation that adult learners appear to select teaching/learning formats that offer opportunities for self-pacing, problem solving, and frequent feedback.[52] In view of the variety of strategies available for teaching, such considerations should be borne in mind when teaching options are selected for chiropractic courses.

TEACHING STRATEGIES

Adequate preparation for the gestalt of apprenticeship in the clinic requires a diversity of skills, some of which are best acquired through a repetitious mechanistic approach, others of which are best perceived holistically. The manual skills of chiropractic care are learned through reduction of each technique to its component parts. The nuances of clinical management are better perceived through experiential learning.[53] The linear reductionist's world view, expressed in Tyler's orderly objectives-based curriculum, or Skinner's behavioral model, which assumes the determinism of systematic reinforcement, stimulus control, linear sequencing, and the generation of cumulative change, is well suited to the manual aspects of patient assessment and treatment. Successful patient involvement, however, is more effectively acquired through consideration of the patient's total life world.[54] Despite its focus on context, competency-based learning all too often reverts to lists of specific tasks, neglecting higher level competencies, and to analysis of desirable practitioner attributes in isolation from routine practice requirements. Problem-based learning directly addresses this issue intrinsically linking context sensitivity with student learning.

Like community-based education, in which the venue defines the scope of problem selection, patient management problems, by being less abstract and focusing on more concrete practice problems, offer a more realistic learning experience. Patient management problems provide a forum for acquiring both the inquiry skills and contextual sensitivity to deliver a form of problem-based learning tailored to achieving competence in chiropractic practice. "Patient management problems," rather than constituting a particular teaching strategy, provide a flexible approach that uses a variety of teaching strategies (Table 4). The core concept of patient management problems in no way restricts the teaching formats that can be employed. "Many different strategies can be used to teach problem solving. These may include the use of simulated patients, case presentations, computer-aided course work, small group assignments and independent study sessions."[55]

Although the patient may provide the most beneficial experiential learning opportunity, use of a diversity of alternate approaches can ensure that all chiropractic students share a common curriculum and that each student entering the clinical situation has had an equivalent opportunity to attain a critical level of proficiency. Simulated or standardized patients provide a relatively nonstressful, safe learning format for acquiring competence at collecting data and interacting with patients. Simulated patients provide a milieu conducive to refining skills in history taking, physical examination, counseling, and patient education. Actors, instructors, and students can be trained to simulate cases. Simulated patients can also provide helpful student feedback. Although clinicians may be better qualified to comment on the logical sequencing of data collection, lay patients are more sensitive to the learner's communication skills and are excellent judges of certain examination maneuvers, particularly those involving palpation. The interactive videodisk patient-simulation model provides an additional option.[56] Students leaving an

TABLE 4.
Patient Management Problem: The Ethos—A Problem-Solving Inquiry Process in a Chiropractic Clinical Context Resulting in Problem-Based Learning

Learning stimulus
   Chiropractic clinical problem
Form of learning trigger
   Written: Manual, computer
   Model: Auditory, palpatory, visual
   Patient: Simulated, standardized, real
Student evaluation
   Written: manual (essay, short answer, multiple choice
    questions); electronic (computerized, interactive)
   Observed: Checklists
   Charts: Examiner, patient
   Verbal: *Vive voce* (oral)
   Mixed: Objective structured/sequential clinical examination

interactive videodisk patient-simulation session feel as if they have interacted with an actual person!

Learning options supported by sophisticated technology are becoming increasingly popular. Computer-based instruction, recognized as useful in spinal anatomy, can be developed for a variety of areas in the chiropractic program.[57] A variety of computer-based instructional systems are available. They range from the most simple text-based question and answer systems, through tutorial systems following a structured course outline and hypertext for studying topics in varying depths, to the more intellectually demanding option of problem-based learning and more technically progressive systems using interactive multimedia.[58] Multimedia systems in which traditional computing functions are combined with a range of possibilities for recording and using sound, video, and still images provide a gestalt experience for the learner. The use of interactive multimedia is furthermore not necessarily geographically confined. So advanced is contemporary educational technology that it is feasible for students on one side of the globe to clarify, in real time, a concept with a lecturer teaching on the other. The technology is available for the development of a global chiropractic campus. Time changes aside, chiropractic students could in practice share and simultaneously attend on their home campuses the lecture of a chiropractic expert. Students in the United States, Canada, Australia, England, and South Africa could ask the lecturer questions, with the resulting answers being discussed in front of a participating global chiropractic student audience. Telephone conferencing in which participants could be linked by sound has been superseded by video conferencing in which distant sites could be linked by both audio and visual signals. Interactive television is another alternative in which video and audio signals are transmitted from the teaching site; students on different campuses can see and hear the lecturer, but only audio signals are received from the student sites. Already available and used by chiropractic colleges are the older, cheaper systems of information dispersal such as audiotapes, videotapes, electronic mail, and Compact Disc ROMs. The technology is available for chiropractic education to be undertaken in a distance education mode.

Access, economic considerations, flexibility, and more effective use of personal time all are compelling reasons to consider the potential for teaching of chiropractic by distance education.[59] Certain aspects of chiropractic competence do, however, demand individual student-instructor interaction that goes beyond group visual and verbal communication. The acquisition of psychomotor skills is one such example. The importance of critical feedback, not merely the intrinsic feedback received during the performance of a psychomotor task, requires that adequate learning of psychomotor skills is undertaken within a situation in which there is dynamic, preferably one-on-one, teacher-learner interaction. Students deprived of such dynamic, experiential interaction may fail to modify poor technique with practice, achieving consistency rather than competence.[60] Provided students are ensured of opportunities to acquire the practical skills characteristic of chiropractic practitioners, there is no reason to preclude a mixed mode option for chiropractic education. On the contrary, advances in educational technology coupled with the conceptual change of the teacher from lecturer to learning facilitator would suggest this is a logical progression. In the development of those aspects of the program that are to be undertaken by distance education, however, it is essential to design programs that promote and support independent learning skills.

LEARNING PREFERENCES

Active student participation in education breaks the shackles of education within a mechanistic paradigm and encourages implementation of a holistic approach. With the waning of the behaviorist school, learning outcomes that depend to a greater extent on the student's intentions, interpretations, and active knowledge construction assume substantive significance.[61] Instead of external control with the student the passive recipient, as predicated by the mechanistic paradigm, the holistic paradigm encourages personal involvement by the student (Table 5). In place of atomistic information processing in which factual content is absorbed and compartmentalized, deep-level information processing emerges, and the

TABLE 5.
Teaching and Learning in the Chiropractic Curriculum

	Behaviorist Pedagogy of the Mechanistic Paradigm	**Andragogy of the Holistic Paradigm**
Teacher	Information fountainhead	Facilitator
Teaching process	Teacher centered	Student centered
	Prescriptive	Negotiable
Teaching assumptions	Cause-effect model (student responds to external stimuli)	Self-organizing model (interaction of external plus internal stimuli)
Teaching style	Didactic	Facilitation
Teaching climate	Formal	Informal
	Competitive	Collaborative
	Judgmental	Supportive
Communication	Unidirectional	Interaction
Tasks for providing information	Isolated skill training	Professional behavior training
	Task Analysis	
	Handouts	Problem-based scenarios
		Interaction
View of the learner	Submissive	Participatory
	Passive recipient	Active negotiator
	Detached	Involved
Valued learning style	Dependent	Self-directed
Learning	Unidirectional	Bidirectional
	Directed/assigned	Experiential
	Passive	Active
	Fact based	Concept based
	Superficial	Deep

semantic content of subject matter is considered and related to previously acquired cognitive structures. Application of the principles of motivational theory would also appear well suited to enhancing learning in chiropractic programs cognizant of the assumptions of the holistic paradigm.[62] "The inherently active, self-regulating organism is the pivotal cornerstone of the shift from reductionist or stimulus-response explanations of learning to the assimilative or response-stimulus explanation fundamental to dialectical theories—and the holistic paradigm."[63]

The standardization required by professional registration boards limits the freedom of chiropractic students to personally generate curricular learning goals. It is nonetheless efficient to encourage students to personally identify problems relevant to their future professional life because independent learning skills appear to be fostered when learning issues are student rather than faculty generated.[64] Learner-generated goals evoke enhanced motivation and commitment. Despite the context sensitivity of professional education somewhat precluding a student-centered curriculum, active student participation need not be hindered. Student-centered programs, whether or not they incorporate an opportunity for working toward learner-generated goals, take the learning preferences of their students into consideration when modes of instruction are determined.

In combination, problem-based learning and self-directed (learner-centered) learning are regarded as interventions providing the wisest available strategy for managing courses regarded as excessively long and detailed, lacking in critical thinking, or demonstrating continuing obsolescence and inflexibility to social change.[65] Although students in problem-based learning curricula do appear to acquire behaviors that reflect self-directed learning,[66] the use of a problem-based framework does not automatically confer a learner-centered approach.[67] The inclusion of student-generated learning issues needs to be actively pursued and included in the program. An alternate approach to problem-based learning that uses a similar problem-solving process but may be inherently more sensitive to student issues is inquiry-based learning.[68] Inclusion of opportunities for inquiry-based learning may enhance the opportunities for self-direction in competency-based programs. Student involvement in self-assessment has also been found to sharpen skills required for successful continuing self-education and independent learning.[69, 70]

Self-direction in professional courses requires that the student is proficient in identifying learning needs, converting these to learning goals, selecting learning strategies, and monitoring personal progress.[71] "An essential component of clinical competence [which] is the ability to identify the limits of one's knowledge and skills and to organize resources to learn more."[72] Self-direction in education is a fundamental assumption of the andragogical or adult learning model and contrasts sharply with pedagogical constructs.[73] Although all chiropractic students are adults, not all have a preference for independent learning. A diversity of cognitive styles have been described,[74-76] and application of certain of these to chiropractic education has been considered.[77] Although learning and information processing may be most efficient when the cognitive processing style and the dominant instructional style match, it is essential that all students maximize their proficiency at independent learning. Self-directed learning is a prerequisite to the continuing education lifestyle required of chiropractic practitioners. Because all students do not share a preference or equivalent capacity for self-directed learning, faculty may find it helpful to identify which students most need assistance with the development of independent learning skills. An inventory for determining the student's learning preferences has been developed[78] and may be used by the teacher as a guide to the amount of guidance a student requires at a particular stage of the program. Chiropractic students in later years of their course have been found to have a greater preference for independent study than those in earlier years.[79] Opportunities for independent learning and self-pacing are available. One such option is the portable patient problem pack. Canadian Memorial Chiropractic College uses these "card form" standardized patient packs to augment and enhance clinical learning.[80] Self-study is complemented by the choice of group discussion.

ASSESSMENT OPTIONS

Changes in assessment may be anticipated to accompany modifications in teaching and learning. Traditionally assessment has been normative. Normative assessment, influenced by the apparent precision and objectivity of mathematical symbols, ranks students rather than providing information on the competence of any individual candidate. Assessment of student learning in this framework focuses on detecting deficiencies, not on evaluating accomplishments. Norm-referenced assessment epitomizes the mechanistic paradigm's assumption that reality can be adequately represented through an abstract mathematical symbol system. Reliance on propositional knowledge as predicated by the mechanistic paradigm has furthermore almost certainly contributed to a situation in which medical students are "trained to use biological reductionistic action models, producing a 'culture of practice' in which clinicians consider only narrow technical hypotheses and generally do not care to see the connection of these disease stages to the lives of their patients."[81] In this model "detached concern"[82] rather than empathic involvement is regarded as desirable behavior.

In contrast, holistic assessment is concerned with real life processes, and accomplishments are documented. Criterion-referenced assessment, based on examinations that specifically ascertain the acquisition of knowledge, values, and skills, is increasingly supplanting the more traditional norm-referenced option. The goal of assessment has changed from a desire to rank students to one that provides information on whether the student has achieved competence. Accompanying the swing toward criterion-referenced assessment is an increased emphasis on continuous rather than terminal assessment. Continuous student evaluation can be formal or informal, formative or summative. Methods may range from direct patient examination to simulated-patient observation, from oral examinations to computer simulations, from logbooks to objective structured clinical examinations. Current trends in chiropractic education, like that of other health professionals,[83, 84] suggest an increased emphasis on continuous and criterion-referenced assessment. Terminal and norm-referenced assessment is more consistent with a mechanistic paradigm, continuous and criterion-referenced evaluation with a holistic approach (Table 6). The OSCE[85] (or Observed Sequential Competency Examination[86]) is an examination innovation that draws from both paradigms and matches the notion of competency assessment. It captures both the dispassionate nature and formal configuration of traditional assessment while globally assessing examinees performing a variety of clinically relevant tasks. The OSCE employs the construct of criterion-referenced assessment in the context of problem-based evaluation. This combination ensures that the OSCE provides a useful examination format for the measurement of specific performance.[87] It creates a forum wherein clinical proficiency may be analyzed in a standardized, controlled environment. It furnishes a format in which both content and process can be probed and factual knowledge, cognitive, interpersonal and manual skills can be examined. It has been suggested that "the OSCE has emerged as the state-of-the-art method for testing clinical skills."[88] Seminal work on the development of OSCEs was published by Harden and Gleeson.[89] As chiropractic colleges increasingly require competency examinations for graduation, the use of OSCEs patterned after problem-based approaches are likely to increase.[90]

The OSCE, rather than constituting a particular testing method, provides a flexible approach that uses a diversity of assessment methods. A variety of standardized clinical stations are created. A series of independent stations are designed. Examinees rotate through these stations. Each station requires the completion of a single task. The task at any one station may focus on history taking, physical examination, diagnostic decision making, special investigations, and therapeutic decision making. Different triggers and evaluation formats are used. The clinical scenario may be triggered by a simulated patient, a slide, a lifeform model, or an auscultatory sound. The most expensive stations are those that feature real or, more usually, simulated patients. A useful evaluation of clinical proficiency can be achieved by requiring examinees to perform a variety of clinical tasks at a series of "stations."[91]

By going beyond the evaluation of theoretical competence and providing an assessment format wherein practical tasks can be performed and from which potential clinical proficiency can be extrapolated, OSCEs provide a more realistic assessment format on which to predict a particular student's clinical performance. The OSCE format also facilitates standard-

TABLE 6.
Assessment Options

	Mechanistic Paradigm	**Holistic Paradigm**
Meaningful measurement	Statistically significant (mathematical terms)	Substantive significance (proficiency terms)
Objective	Quantify outcome	Recognize quality performance
	Relative standard	Acceptable standard
	Normative	Criterion referenced

ization of skills assessment.[92] Observers rate the student's interpersonal skills, attitude, empathy, and manual skills. In certain cases nonphysicians, trained to play the role of patients, can also be trained as observers and serve as models on which to assess clinical skills.[93] Such simulated-patient observers provide a unique insight into patients' perceptions of the patient-practitioner encounter.[94] It has been suggested that such simulated patient-based assessments are better able to detect individual examinees performing at marginal levels than more traditional examination formats.[95] The cost of the overall examination can be significantly reduced through the use of nonclinician raters. One study achieved a rater cost saving of some 70% by replacing physicians by nonphysicians.[96] Investigations to further improve standardization of simulated patients are under way.[97, 98]

The ultimate standardized format currently available is the interactive videodisk patient-simulation.[56] Standardization of each examinee's performance at different stations is also being undertaken. Rating forms specifically prepared for each station list the items or actions deemed necessary to cover the essentials of the clinical task. Rating possibilities vary from dichotomous to multiple-point scales. "Highly structured rating forms help raise the OSCE's level of standardization and objectivity over that of other examination methods that include the observation of clinical tasks."[99] A similar observation may be made about checklists. Although both are acceptable assessment formats, interrater agreement is greater for checklists than rating forms.

In contrast to the observer station, clinical situations can be created using models, sounds, and pen-and-pencil scenarios. Curricular content or clinical competencies such as the interpretation of laboratory results, the recognition of sounds, or the detection of palpable abnormalities can be assessed by multiple choice or short answer questions. The simulation of initial medical problem-solving (SIMP) layout, which consists of short case histories, followed by the question "What would you do as a physician in this situation?"[100] provides a particularly helpful context into which visual, auditory, and palpatory triggers can be introduced.[101] This contemporary variant of the traditional problem-based essay has been designed to better simulate the clinical reality of patient care while retaining the benefits traditionally associated with essay questions. Essay questions are generally considered to provide an opportunity for in-depth assessment of both the students' knowledge and their ability to integrate information in a clinically relevant fashion. Providing a more global insight into student knowledge, essays are particularly helpful for assessing the ability of the examinee to formulate and defend a course of action. They create an opportunity for students to display logical clinical decision making and, in the absence of cuing, to take cognizance of the nodal points of clinical decision making.[102] Essays provide an opportunity to explore deep learning. Consistent with assessment in an examination system that has traditionally been dominated by the mechanistic paradigm, guidelines are available for enhancing the objectivity of essay marking.[103]

When student feedback is gathered, the objective nature of assessment can be maintained and the overall cost at OSCE stations curtailed through the use of multiple choice and short answer questions. When examinees are required to record a diagnosis, however, it has been found that free-response forms yield a more accurate measure of the student's clinical skills.[97] Reflecting on the discrepancies detected between cued- and free-response formats, the authors[97] suggest that the cued formats tended to overestimate the student's diagnostic skills. The desirability of using short answer rather than multiple choice assessment is tempered, however, because it appears, from at least one reputable study, that essay "scores fail to capture a sizable unique aspect of competence over and above multiple-choice questions."[104] Although multiple choice questions are criticized as being largely confined to testing recall and evaluating superficial learning, some researchers[105] believe that careful construction of multiple choice questions can enable objective assessment of clinical judgment. Multiple choice questions are routinely used to probe the diagnostic decision-making skills of final year chiropractic students using a fixed-response OSCE.[106]

STAFF APPRAISAL

Evaluation of staff performance, increasingly an integral component of academic life, is one aspect of quality management.[107] The increased emphasis on faculty appraisal implies not only that the performance of staff is actively scrutinized but also that staff are assisted to enhance their professional competence.[108] Faculty development is emerging as a strategy to address diverse dilemmas, including the excessive length of undergraduate training, which is partially attributed to ineffective educational techniques.[109] The role of faculty is changing. The mandatory competencies of faculty extend beyond those of a good clinician to incorporate demonstration of proficiency as an academic. The perception that staff serve as fountainheads of knowledge is being supplanted by the expectation that they perform as information resource facilitators. It has been suggested that chiropractic clinical educators, in addition to good patient management skills, need "talents in motivation, critical thinking, interprofessional relations, group dynamics and a multitude of patient evaluation and care areas."[110]

In a study of family medicine faculty (tenured and nontenured) and medical staff in other areas, differences were identified in the competencies that each group considered essential.[111] Nonfamily medicine faculty regarded all aspects of research as essential, whereas tenured family medicine faculty, although acknowledging the importance of research, were clearly less research oriented. Nontenured family medicine faculty regarded teaching as more important and were the only group who considered the task of counseling learners with a view to facilitating students' development of self-evaluation skills as essential. It may be surmised that chiropractic educators could identify with family medicine staff. Certainly a recent survey of medical centers[112] identified a dilemma experienced by chiropractic educators. This survey found that clinician-educators have little free time to engage in research or written scholarship because of their patient care commitments. Jacobs[112] in this study identified scholarship as the cornerstone on which guidelines for promotion of clinician-educators could be developed. He[112] suggested that scholarship include

1. The Scholarship of Application, i.e., building bridges between theory and practice, applying knowledge to consequential problems
2. The Scholarship of Teaching, i.e., communicating knowledge, inspiring trainees, transforming the difficult-to-understand to the easy-to-assimilate
3. The Scholarship of Integration, i.e., creative synthesis or analysis, looking for connections across disciplines, bringing new insights to bear on original research, "horizontal" scholarship
4. The Scholarship of Discovery, i.e., the elucidation of new knowledge, research in its traditional sense, "vertical" scholarship

Whatever guidelines chiropractic colleges choose to adopt, faculty appraisal carries with it the requirement that opportunities are provided for professional development. General options used in medical education range from self-assessment inventories such as that devised for evaluation of clinical teaching techniques,[113] through experiential workshops on teaching,[114] to faculty "journal" clubs designed to help staff acquire specific skills such as critical appraisal of the literature.[115] In chiropractic education in Australia personal performance contracts and action plans are used.

In Australia, chiropractic staff are subject to the same terms and conditions of employment of other university staff. These chiropractic educators have the requirement of staff development linked to their industrial award.[116] Professional development review is a condition of employment. Although the original intention of staff appraisal was that it form the basis for individualized staff development, both academic promotion and unsatisfactory performance have become inextricably linked to faculty evaluation. Although the nuances of distinguishing between these two notions has become an issue between Australian academics and university management, these changes have resulted in government funds being allocated to staff development.

EDUCATION IN THE INTERSTICES OF PARADIGMS

Chiropractic education and its outcome are influenced by the assumptions underlying both the mechanistic and holistic paradigms. Socialization as a chiropractor occurs overtly through curriculum content and covertly through the processes used in teaching and learning. Technique drills suggest unidirectional reinforcement, but the preparation of chiropractors as self-directed lifelong learners presupposes interaction. Much of the content and certain of the teaching learning processes suggest an educational approach consistent with the mechanistic paradigm, yet the global educational experience is compatible largely with the ethos and nuances of holism. Models that avoid the extremes of paradigm purity have been framed in the interstices of the mechanistic and holistic paradigms. Two such models, both of which have virtue for chiropractic education, are constructivism and critical multiplism. These options deserve consideration by chiropractic educators and other professionals working in the interstices of paradigms.

The constructs of holism and constructivism are cognitively distinct yet clearly removed from the mechanistic perspective. In contrast to holism, which brings into focus feeling and intuition, constructivism places more emphasis on cognitive processes by describing learning in terms of the building of knowledge through transformation and self-regulation.[28]

> Constructivists posit that learning is a process whereby new meanings are created (constructed) by the learner within the context of her or his current knowledge. The new meanings that are constructed by the learner are products of transformations that occur between the new experiences to be learned and all other previous and current learning experiences (i.e., one's spiral of knowledge) . . . . These transformations are self-regulatory, in that our own "spiral" delimits what we will or will not learn, given all that we currently know, our developmental readiness, and so forth. To the constructivist learning is not simply the taking in of new information as it exists externally (in adult minds, in the curriculum or text), it is the natural, continuous construction and reconstruction of new, richer, and more complex and connected meanings by the learner. . . . Holistic education tends to de-emphasize developmental limitations and emphasize more the role of affect, intuition, and sociopolitical forces in learning. Further, holists stress the role of interest, self-concept, connectedness, trust, and expectations in learning, factors that are overlooked by cognitive learning theorists.[28]

Neither holists nor constructivists believe that learning is best achieved piecemeal or by means of task analysis, but constructivists recognize that learning often proceeds from whole to part to whole. This belief is practiced in chiropractic education. After an initial phase of searching for new experiences, shaping new questions, and independent browsing, a second reductionist phase is entered in which precision is valued and details are determined. The subsequent phase of generalization recreates a gestalt that incorporates both detail and interrelationships. Both holists and constructivists emphasize the current knowledge and personal experience of the learner as a vital predictor of future learning; holists emphasize emotional involvement or personal interest as a substantive determinant of learning. In contrast to a mechanistic model in which the learner is often perceived to be a passive recipient of information, constructivists view the learner as an active participant in an ongoing learning process. In contrast to a mechanistic model of unidirectional reinforcement, constructivists envisage interactive self-regulation. At the very least, "the healing relationship is best conceived as a form of dialogue."[117]

The inadequacy of a stance confined to either empirical-analytical cause-effect determinism or the discovery of meaning through interpretation of person-environmental interactions raises the issue of dialectical multiplism.

> Critical multiplism is a strategy in which quantitative and qualitative methods are reconciled within a third world view and model of scientific inquiry. "Multiplism" is a strategy in which multiple perspec-

tives are used to define research goals: to choose research questions, methods and analyses; and to interpret research results. "Critical" refers to the critical, thoughtful selection of multiple procedures.[118]

A program embracing critical multiplism as a strategy for conceptualization in the interstices of paradigms would contemplate multiple options and select particular strategies based on a discourse on the strengths and limitations of each option given a particular context. Critical multiplism provides an apt description of the current state of chiropractic education. In this instance, critical multiplism may be construed as the pragmatic response of chiropractic educationalists and researchers to the paradigm anomalies experienced by the chiropractic profession. This mode of information processing selectively brings the mechanistic paradigm's analytic, deductive reasoning approach, its reduction of complex issues, and its abstraction of ideal forms to a world where reality is more holistically conceived through the social creation of knowledge through intuition, observation, and rhetoric. Critical multiplism creates the possibility for incorporating both objectifying and expressive-interpretive approaches.[119] It allows for the acquisition of task-oriented skills while providing the openness of exposure to practice. It uses the reductionist approach to solving problems in an environment in which student attitudes are shaped and changed by role modeling and mentoring.[120] Where clinical exposure is not possible:

> Learning from narratives, although not a perfect solution to bridging the gap between general stereotypes and completely idiosyncratic notions of persons, is a way of recognizing shared cultural beliefs, values and experiences while respecting them as diverse individuals . . . narratives can assist . . . in learning about clients' everyday experiences, priorities, needs and goals.[121]

In addition to profoundly influencing teaching/learning formats, critical multiplism facilitates contemplation of revolutionary assessment possibilities to the extent that practitioners may "be able to hold each other accountable not only for specific procedures but also for delivering care, as perceived by the client."[122] Critical multiplism values precision, predictability, and control, but it also recognizes the language of possibility with its inherent uncertainty and ceaseless becoming.

A diversity of experiences are required to produce practitioners who are skilled in both manual intervention and interpersonal relationships, who have a conceptual understanding and tacit experience of reductionism and holism, and who are themselves lifelong self-directed learners.

CONCLUSION

It appears that in the area of research, "the most important task is the establishment of a legitimate holistic paradigm."[123] In the area of practice, it is the provision of responsive health care,[124] and in the area of education it is acquisition of the knowledge and skills to practice in the interstices of paradigms. Constructivism and critical multiplism are two eclectic models that draw from both paradigms and provide a framework within which chiropractic education can pursue its committment to outcomes assessment. With outcomes assessment as the ultimate goal, chiropractic educators are progressively introducing competency-based education and reflectively selecting from an array of traditional and innovative teaching/learning strategies.

REFERENCES

1. Pretorius PJ: A foundation for physiology. *Med Hypotheses* 31:121–130, 1990.
2. Freidson E: *Profession of Medicine*. New York, Harper & Row, 1970, p 169.
3. Greer AL: The two cultures of biomedicine: Can there be consensus? *JAMA* 258:2739, 1987.
4. Keating JC: Scientific epistemology and the status of chiropractic: We are what we do. *Eur J Chiropr* 41:81–88, 1993.
5. Young AA: Mode of production of medical knowledge. *Med Anthropol* 2:107, 1978.
6. Keating JC: The chiropractic practitioner scientist: An old idea revisited. *Am J Chiropr Med* 1:17–23, 1988.
7. Vernon H: Toward a clinical philosophy within the discipline of chiropractic. *J Chiropr Assoc* 34:187–188, 1990.
8. Hildebrandt RW: The scope of chiropractic as a clinical science and art: An introductory review of concepts. *J Manipulative Physiol Ther* 1:17, 1978.
9. Keating JC: Which philosophy of chiropractic? *J Manipulative Physiol Ther* 11:325–327, 1988.
10. Wiese G: A review and comparison of medical and chiropractic education. *J Chiropr Educ* 4:127–139, 1993.
11. Coulter ID: Is chiropractic primary health care? *J Can Chiropr Assoc* 36:96–101, 1992.
12. Clarke R: Undergraduate medical education: Prognosis and priorities. *Med J Aust* 1:389–391, 1979.
13. Report of the Project Panel on the General Professional Education of the Physician: Physicians of the twenty-first century. *J Med Educ* 59(suppl 2):5–27, 1984.
14. ACME-TRI Report: Educating medical students. *Acad Med* 68(suppl 6):S11–S46, 1993.
15. Kassebaum DG: The measurement of outcomes in assessment of educational program effectiveness. *Acad Med* 65:293–296, 1990.
16. Proceedings of the Second Congress of Chiropractic Educators: Excellence in chiropractic education. *J Chiropr Educ* 4:45–73, 1992.
17. Adams AH, Miller JA, Miller G: The development and implementation of an innovative curriculum in chiropractic education: The LACC experience. *J Chiropr Educ* 4:122–127, 1991.
18. Harris JA: Non-cognitive evaluations for chiropractic education. *J Chiropr Educ* 7:3–17, 1993.
19. Goff PJ: Use of selected elements of patient perception of care in the evaluation of clinical training. *J Chiropr Educ* 5:115–132, 1992.
20. Gatterman MI: Teaching-learning options for the study of chiropractic principles: A case study. *J Chiropr Educ* 6:93–104, 1992.
21. Kleynhans AM: *Competency-Based Professional Standards for Chiropractic*. Mornington, Victoria, Australia, Australasian Council on Chiropractic and Osteopathic Education (in press).
22. Wiese G, Peterson D: An overview of chiropractic educational institutions, 1986 to the present. *J Chiropr Educ* 4:104–113, 1990.

23. Council on Chiropractic Education: Standards for chiropractic institutions—clinical competency document. West Des Moines, Iowa, Council on Chiropractic Education, 1991.
24. Griffey DC: The future of graduate study in teacher preparation in physical education. *Quest* 39:174–178, 1987.
25. Heshusius L: The newtowian mechanistic paradigm, special education, and contours of alternatives: An overview. *J Learn Disabil* 22:403–415, 1989.
26. Greene M: Philosophy and teaching, in Wittrock MC (ed): *Handbook of Research on Teaching*. New York, Macmillan, 1986, p 485.
27. Poplin MS: Holistic/constructivist principles of the teaching/learning process: Implications for the field for learning disabilities. *J Learn Disabil* 21:401–416, 1988.
28. Gonczi A, Hager P, Oliver L: Establishing competency-based standards in the professions. Canberra, Australia, Australian Government Publishing Service, 1990, pp 23–26.
29. Kleynhans AM: Curriculum content II—methods of monitoring to ensure competency. *J Chiropr Educ* 5:59–63, 1991.
30. Print M: Curriculum development and design. Sydney, Allen & Unwin, 1987, pp 21–27.
31. Kleynhans AM: The establishment of competency-based professional standards for chiropractors. *Aust Chiropr Assoc* 22:98–104, 1992.
32. Coulter ID: The defense of Thomas Kuhn (and chiropractic). *J Manipulative Physiol Ther* 15:392–401, 1992.
33. Friedman CP, De Bliek R, Greer DS, et al: Charting the winds of change: Evaluating innovative medical curricula. *Acad Med* January:8–14, 1990.
34. Beenhakker JC: Determinant in physiotherapy education. *Med Teacher* 9:161–166, 1987.
35. Jonas S: Foreword, in Barrows HS, Tamblyn RM (eds): *Problem-based Learning: An Approach to Medical Education*. New York, Springer-Verlag, 1980, p viii.
36. Balla J, Cox K: How to teach clinical decision making, in Cox K, Ewan CE (eds): *The Medical Teacher*. New York, Churchill Livingstone, 1988, pp 115–120.
37. Barrows HS, Tamblyn RM: *Problem-based Learning: An Approach to Medical Education*. New York, Springer-Verlag, 1980, pp 2, 37–56, 149–150.
38. Joorabchi B: Medical information processing skills: Guideposts to clinical assessment. *Med Teach* 11:331–337, 1989.
39. Cox K: How to teach clinical reasoning, in Cox K, Ewan CE (eds): *The Medical Teacher*. New York, Churchill Livingstone, 1988, pp 102–107.
40. Ridderikhoff J: Medical problem solving: An exploration of strategies. *Med Educ* 25:196–207, 1991.
41. Pietroni P: Alternative medicine: Methinks the doctor protests too much and incidentally befuddles the debate. *J Med Ethics* 18:23–25, 1992.
42. Sackett DL, Haynes RB, Tugwell P: *Clinical Epidemiology*. Boston, Little, Brown, 1988, p 298.
43. Canadian Task Force: The periodic health examination. *Can Med Assoc J* 121:1193–1254, 1979.
44. Glaser R: Education and thinking: The role of knowledge. *Am Psychol* 39:93–104, 1984.
45. Hostetler K: Community and neutrality in critical thought: A nonobjectivist view on the conduct and teaching of critical thinking. *Educ Theory* 41:1–12, 1991.
46. Russell IJ, Hendricson WD, Harris GD, et al: A comparison of two methods for facilitating clinical data integration by medical students. *Acad Med* 65:333–340, 1990.

47. Sternberg RJ: Intelligence, wisdom, and creativity: Three is better than one. *Educ Psychol* 21:175–190, 1986.
48. Schmidt HG: The rationale behind problem-based learning. *J Med Educ* 17:11–16, 1983.
49. Bernstein B: Class, codes and control. London, Routledge & Kegan Paul, 1971, vol 1, pp 202–230.
50. Jamison JR: Curriculum development in diagnosis for contemporary chiropractic practice. *J Aust Chiropr Assoc* 14:147–152, 1984.
51. Neame RLB: Problem-based medical education: The Newcastle approach, in Schmidt HG, Lipkin M, de Vries MW, et al (eds): *New Directions for Medical Education*. New York, Springer Verlag New York, 1989, pp 112–146.
52. Berman J, Bergen MR, Skeff KM: Feasibility of incorporating alternative teaching methods into clinical clerkships. *Teach Learn Med* 2:98–103, 1990.
53. Jamison JR: Dietary assessment—experiential learning in nutritional intervention for chiropractic students. *J Aust Chiropr Assoc* 18:63–66, 1988.
54. Jamison JR: *Health Promotion for Chiropractic Practice*. Baltimore, Md, Aspen, 1991.
55. Good CJ: The McMaster problem based learning method: An analysis and its relevance to chiropractic education. *J Chiropr Educ* 6:85–91, 1992.
56. Harless WG, Duncan RC, Zier MA, et al: A field test of the TIME patient simulation model. *Acad Med* 65:327–333, 1990.
57. Cramer G, Darby S: Computer based instruction. *J Chiropr Educ* 3:10, 1989.
58. Fysh PN: Development and implementation of multi-media computer based learning systems. *J Chiropr Educ* 5:15–20, 1991.
59. Kleynhans AM: Implications of distance education for chiropractic. *J Chiropr Educ* 6:55–67, 1992.
60. Good CJ: Aspects of learning issues relevant to the chiropractic adjustment. *J Chiropr Educ* 7:59–67, 1993.
61. Leino-Kilpi H: Learning to care—a qualitative prespective of student evaluation. *J Nurs Educ* 28:61–66, 1989.
62. Kleynhans AM: Motivation and learning. *J Chiropr Educ* 5:147–152, 1992.
63. Reid K: Reflections on the pragmatics of a paradigm shift. *J Learn Disabil* 21:417–420, 1988.
64. Blumberg P, Michael JA, Zeitz H: Roles of student generated learning issues in problem-based learning. *Teach Learn Med* 2:149–154, 1990.
65. Pallie W, Carr DH: The McMaster medical education philosophy in theory, practice and historical perspective. *Med Teach* 9:59–71, 1987.
66. Blumberg P, Michael JA: Development of self-directed learning behaviors in a partially teacher-directed problem-based learning curriculum. *Teach Learn Med* 4:3–8, 1992.
67. Blumberg P, Michael JA, Zeitz H: Roles of student-generated learning issues in problem-based learning. *Teach Learn Med* 2:149–154, 1990.
68. Feletti G: Inquiry based and problem based learning: How similar are these approaches to nursing and medical education? *Higher Educ Res Dev* 12:143–156, 1993.
69. Rezler AG: Self-assessment in problem-based groups. *Med Teach* 11:151–155, 1989.
70. Calhoun JG, Haken JDT, Woolliscroft JO: Medical students' development of self- and peer assessment skills: A longitudinal study. *Teach Learn Med* 2:25–29, 1990.
71. Hammond M, Collins R: Self-directed learning to educate medical educators: I. How do we use self-directed learning? *Med Teach* 9:253–260, 1987.
72. Wilkerson L, Armstrong E, Lesky L: Faculty development for ambulatory teaching. *J Gen Intern Med* 5(suppl):S44–S53, 1990.

73. Knowles M: *Self-Directed Learning*. Chicago, Follett, 1975.
74. Merrit SL: Learning styles: Theory and use as a basis for instruction. *Rev Res Nurs Educ* 2:1–31, 1989.
75. Partridge R: Learning styles: A review of selected models. *J Nurs Educ* 22:243–248, 1983.
76. Kolb DA, Rubin IM, McIntyre JM: *Organizational Psychology: an Experiential Approach*. Englewood Cliffs, NJ, Prentice Hall, 1971.
77. Olsen E, Nyiendo J, Jones R: An introduction to Myers-Briggs type indicator (MBTI) theory with applications for chiropractic educators. *J Chiropr Educ* 5:123–131, 1992.
78. Rezler AG: Learning preference inventory. *Med Teach* 5:107–109, 1983.
79. Jamison JR: Motivational factors in continuing self-education. *Eur J Chiropr* 39:27–32, 1991.
80. Mrozek JP: Problem solving facilitation in chiropractic education using the portable patient problem pack (P4). *J Chiropr Educ* 6:105–110, 1992.
81. De Vries MW, Berg RL, Lipkin M: On the use and abuse of medicine: A conclusion, in De Vries MW, Berg RL, Lipkin M (eds): *The Use and Abuse of Medicine*. New York, Praeger, 1982, p 274.
82. Pfifferling J-H: Medicalization and physician socialization. In De Vries MW, Berg RL, Lipkin M (eds): *The Use and Abuse of Medicine*. New York, Praeger, 1982, p 190.
83. Maudsley RF: Effective in-training evaluation. *Med Teach* 11:285–290, 1989.
84. Turnbull JM: What is . . . normative versus criterion-referenced assessment. *Med Teach* 11:145–151, 1989.
85. Harden RM: Twelve tips for organizing an objective structured clinical examination (OSCE). *Med Teach* 12:259–264, 1990.
86. Sandefur R: Use of problem-based learning methods in the chiropractic college classroom. *J Chiropr Educ* 4:81–83, 1990.
87. Cater JI, Forsyth JS, Frost GJ: The use of structured clinical examination as an audit of teaching and student performance. *Med Teach* 13:253–257, 1991.
88. Reznick R, Smee S, Rothman A, et al: An objective structured clinical examination for the licentiate: Report of the pilot project of the Medical Council of Canada. *Acad Med* 67:487–494, 1992.
89. Harden RM, Gleeson FA: ANSAME Medical Education Booklet No 8: Assessment of medical competence using an objective structured clinical examination (OSCE). *Med Educ* 13:39, 1979.
90. Sandefur R: Use of problem-based learning methods in the chiropractic college classroom. *J Chiropr Educ* 4:81–83, 1990.
91. Peden NR, Cairncross RG, Harden RM, et al: Assessment of clinical competence in therapeutics: The use of the objective structured clinical examination. *Med Teach* 7:217–223, 1985.
92. Bouhuijs PAJ, Van der Vleuten CP, Van Luyk SJ: The OSCE as a part of a systematic skills training approach. *Med Teach* 9:183–191, 1987.
93. Van der Vleuter CPM, Swanson DB: Assessment of clinical skills with standardized patients: State of the art. *Teach Learn Med* 2:58–76, 1990.
94. Vu NV, Marcy ML, Verhulst SJ, et al: Generalizability of standardized patients' satisfaction ratings of their clinical encounter with fourth-year medical students. *Acad Med* 65:S29–S30, 1990.
95. Stillman PL, Regan MB, Swanson DB, et al: An assessment of the clinical skills of fourth-year students at four New England medical schools. *Acad Med* 65:320–326, 1990.
96. Stillman PL, Regan MB, Haley HA, et al: Validity studies using standardized-

patient examinations: Standardized patient potpourri. *Acad Med* 67:S57–S59, 1992.

97. Stillman PL, Regan MB, Haley HL, et al: A comparison of free-response and cued-response diagnosis scores in an evaluation of clinical competence utilizing standardized patients. *Acad Med* 65:S27–S28, 1990.
98. Abrahamowicz M, Tamblyn RM, Ransay JO, et al: Detecting and correcting for rater-induced difference in standardized patient tests of clinical competence. *Acad Med* 65(suppl 9):S25–S26, 1990.
99. Kachur EK, Green S, Dennis C: Written comments on objective structured clinical examination rating forms: An exploratory study. *Teach Learn Med* 2:225–231, 1990.
100. DeGraaff E: Simulation of initial medical problem-solving: A test for the assessment of medical problem solving. *Med Teach* 10:49–55, 1988.
101. Jamison JR: Clinical competence: The use of simulators/models in diagnosis of visceral conditions. *J Manipulative Physiol Ther* 12:10–14, 1989.
102. Jamison JR: Diagnostic decision making. In Lawrence D (ed): *Seminars in Chiropractic*. Baltimore, Williams & Wilkins, 1991, vol 2, pp 12–13.
103. Bandaranayake R: Can I really grade essays fairly? *Med J Aust* 1:595–597, 1978.
104. Day SC, Norcini JJ, Diserens D, et al: The validity of an essay test of clinical judgement. *Acad Med* 65(suppl 9):S39–S40, 1990.
105. Van Susteren TJ, Cohen EB, Simpson DE: Alternate-choice test items: Implications for measuring clinical judgment. *Teach Learn Med* 3:33–37, 1991.
106. Jamison JR: The fixed response OSCE: A useful adjunct for assessing competence in diagnostic decision making. *J Manipulative Physiol Ther* 15:261–266, 1992.
107. Piper DW: Quality management in universities. Canberra, Australia, Australian Government Publishing Service, 1993.
108. Miller GA: Faculty performance appraisal: The process is as important as the product. *J Chiropr Educ* 6:119–125, 1993.
109. Seddon TDS: Medical education's black mark institutionalized abuse. *ANZAME Bull* 21:3–11, 1994.
110. Mootz RD, Cohen PA: Chiropractic clinical teaching. *J Manipulative Physiol Ther* 15:471–476, 1992.
111. Stritter FT, Bland CJ, Youngblood PL: Determining essential faculty competencies. *Teach Learn Med* 3:232–238, 1991.
112. Jacobs MB: Faculty status for clinician-educators: Guidelines for evaluation and promotion. *Acad Med* 68:126–128, 1993.
113. Farquhar LJ, Holdman H: Preferred styles of clinical teaching: measuring physician control over students in patient care encounters. *Med Teach* 4:104–109, 1982.
114. Tiberius R, Silver I, Fleming S, et al: Teaching physicians about teaching: An experiential workshop. *Med Teach* 12:23–31, 1990.
115. Moyer VA: Learning critical appraisal skills at the faculty level: Methods and benefits. *Teach Learn Med* 4:115–117, 1992.
116. Lublin JR: Staff development, staff assessment and industrial awards. *Higher Educ Res Dev* 11:73–83, 1992.
117. Zaner RM: Medicine and dialogue. *J Med Philos* 15:303–325, 1990.
118. Coward DD: Critical multiplism: A research strategy for nursing science. *Image J Nurs Scholarship* 22:163–167, 1990.
119. Lieberman PB: "Objective" methods and "subjective" experiences. *Schizophr Bull* 15:267–275, 1989.
120. Kobert L, Folan M: Coming of age in rethinking the philosophies behind holism and nursing process. *Nurs Health Care* 11:308–312, 1991.

121. Stevens PE, Hall JM, Meleis A: Narratives as a basis for culturally relevant holistic care: Ethnicity and everyday experiences of women clerical workers. *Holistic Nurse Pract* 6(3):49–58, 1992.
122. Lang NM, Krejci JW: Standards and holism: A reframing. *Holistic Nurse Pract* 5(3):14–21, 1991.
123. Caplan RL: Chiropractic in the United States and the changing health care environment: A view from outside the profession. *J Manipulative Physiol Ther* 14:46–50, 1991.
124. Jamison JR: Chiropractic holism: Interactively becoming in a reductionist health care system. *Chiropr J Aust* 23:98–105, 1993.

Chiropractic Technique: An Overview

Thomas F. Bergmann, D.C., F.I.C.C.
Professor, Department of Chiropractic Methods, Faculty Clinician, Center for Clinical Studies, Northwestern College of Chiropractic, Bloomington, Minnesota

In spite of the fact that manipulation has been described clinically since the days of Hippocrates, there is a dearth of information about the scientific foundations of the indications for and the effects of manipulation in any form.[1] Chiropractic care generally and spinal manipulative therapy specifically continue to grow in popularity and acceptance despite the controversies that exist in clinical practice and the lack of appropriate validation. Though there are a few published clinical trials investigating the use of manipulation for back pain, as well as empiric literature and anecdotal information claiming its usage for other problems, the chiropractic profession has yet to experimentally substantiate the clinical value of any uniquely chiropractic method of health care.[2] Although manipulative therapy has been used for centuries and still occupies small niches in medical, osteopathic, and physical therapy practices, the chiropractic profession has done the most to promote its use in the treatment of neuromusculoskeletal dysfunction.[3] The chiropractic profession has remained dedicated to the use of manipulative therapy and, specifically, the adjustment as a form of clinical intervention.

The clinical practice of manipulative therapy should be based on experimentation and testing. It is important to identify and eliminate ineffective treatment procedures and inaccurate diagnostic procedures while preserving those tests and treatment procedures that provide clinical benefits compared with costs and risks. The focus must be on such principal issues as the identification of parameters, relation to known information, and published research. It is not certain what really does help patients, or what is worse, what is useless, and what may even be harmful.

Before any therapy can be employed, physicians must first ascertain if there is a clinical basis for their specific form of treatment. The chiropractor considering manual or adjustive therapy must first establish if conditions exist that support this form of treatment. Painful conditions affecting the locomotor system are very common disorders and tend to originate from the joint systems and contiguous structures.

A working knowledge of the causes of joint pain and dysfunction, as well as clinical patterns, should allow the practitioner to develop a logical and confident approach to the treatment of the individual patient. However, treatment patterns tend to vary based on the training and philosophy of the practitioner rather than the specific clinical picture displayed by the patient. This process forces the patient to fit the doctor's treatment rather than fitting treatment to the specific needs of the patient (Table 1).

Manual therapy has been proposed as a treatment for a wide variety of conditions, but it is most commonly associated with disorders that have their origins from mechanical alterations of the articulations that make up the locomotor system. The identification of the common functional components of the dysfunctional joint lesion is therefore critical to the management of conditions affecting the neuromusculoskeletal system. This has, however, contributed to the misconception that all manipulative disorders have the same pathological basis. Although many disorders that are purported to be effectively treated with chiropractic manipulative procedures display joint and somatic functional alterations, a myriad of pathological processes are capable of inducing dysfunction of the locomotor system. When joint dysfunction is perceived as the sole cause of the disorder being considered for treatment, adjustive therapy may stand alone. However, when dysfunction is secondary to other disorders, therapy directed to treat the source of the problem should be provided or made available to the patient. The neuromusculoskeletal system remains the most clinically overlooked system in the body though it comprises over half of the body's mass. Although chiropractic health care does place a focus on the evaluation and treatment of neuromusculoskeletal disorders, the multiple potential etiologies of ill health and the complex nature of health maintenance are not disregarded.

It has long been a basic premise of chiropractic that a relationship exists between dysfunction of the nervous system and disease. It is also fundamental that some aberration within the spinal column produces the neurological dysfunction. To bring about this disturbance, a force of some kind must be applied to the vertebra or supporting structures. If the force

TABLE 1.
Treatment Patterns Tend to Vary Based on Type of Practitioner

My Treatment Is:	Therefore, 90% of My Patients Have:
1. Disk surgery	1. Disk disease
2. Exercise	2. Weakness, stiffness
3. Muscle relaxants	3. Muscle spasm
4. Pain medication	4. Pain
5. Nonsteroidal anti-inflammatory agents	5. Inflammation
6. Manipulation	6. Joint dysfunction
a. Activator technique	a. Leg length inequality, isolation tests
b. Applied kinesiology	b. Muscle tests, therapy localization
c. Sacral occipital technique	c. Arm fossa test, heel tension, dollar sign
d. Gonstead technique	d. Radiographic measures, temperature changes
e. Diversified technique	e. Fixations, misalignments

is of a severe nature or allowed to continue over time, the effect on the vertebral motion segment will likely be joint dysfunction. One of the proposals for a better understanding of locomotor dysfunction is an attempt to view joint pain not as a strictly local problem but as a disorder that involves the motor system in general, both the osteoarticular and nervous components.[4] The use of manipulative therapy emphasizes the restoration of free movement between articular surfaces but also affects the contiguous soft tissues.

An important function for the spine is permitting movement in and through the body's three planes. The spinal motion segment, composed of two vertebrae and the continguous soft tissues, is the smallest component capable of performing the characteristic functions of the spine. Normal movement of the spinal articulations occurs in the sagittal (flexion/extension), transverse (axial rotation), and coronal (lateral flexion) planes (Fig 1). It is essential to understand and correlate the pathomechanics of the spine with clinical manifestations to develop rational and effective treatment.

Joint evaluation, therefore, becomes the focal point of the patient examination. It is the chiropractic spinal examination that sets apart chiropractic from other areas of the healing arts.[5] The role of the chiropractic spinal examination is to accurately and objectively detect and monitor joint dysfunction by noninvasive procedures. There is, however, no con-

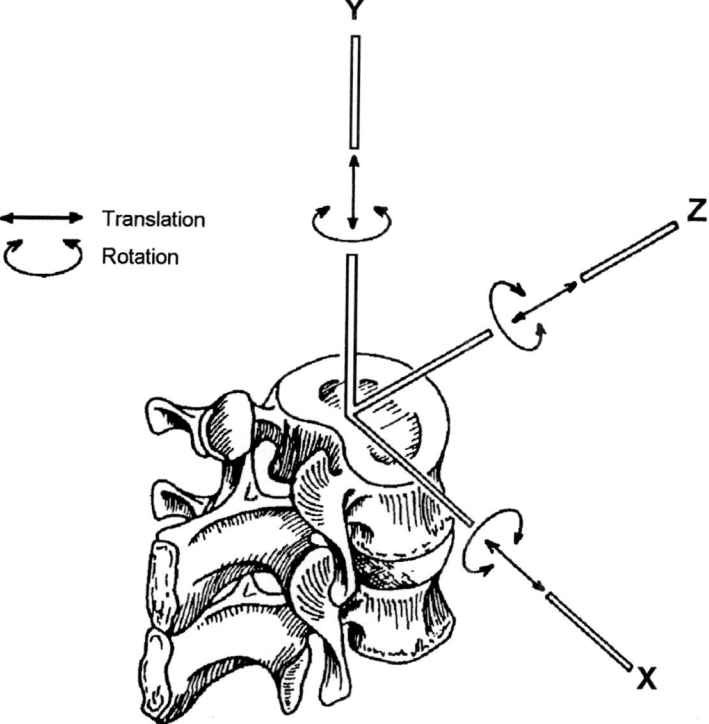

FIGURE 1.
The three-dimensional coordinate system demonstrating the possible rotational and translational movements around or along three axes, respectively.

sensus at this time on the most valid, objective, and efficient means of detecting joint dysfunction. Because the human body and specifically the neuromusculoskeletal system is so complex, it would seem most appropriate to employ a system that combines clinical indicators to decide on those joints in greatest need of intervention. Clinical experience suggests that doctors frequently employ an informal system of combining clinical indicators to make this decision.[6] Structural evaluation of the neuromusculoskeletal system should then be viewed in terms of a multidimensional index of segmental abnormality.[6,7]

The methods used in the joint assessment process are the same as those in other aspects of evaluation, that is, observation, palpation, percussion, and auscultation. By far, palpation is emphasized most. By using the acronym PARTS, the five diagnostic criteria for spinal dysfunction are identified as[5]:

> *P*—pain/tenderness. The perception of pain and tenderness may be evaluated in terms of location, quality, and intensity. The patient's description and location are obtained through history, and the location and intensity of tenderness are identified through palpation of osseous and soft tissues. Changes in pain intensity can be objectified using visual analog scales, algometers, and pain questionnaires.
>
> *A*—asymmetry/alignment. Asymmetrical qualities on a sectional or segmental level are noted. This would include observation of posture and gait, as well as palpation for misalignment of joint structures. X-ray evaluation may also be used to evaluate joint derangements.
>
> *R*—range of motion abnormality. Changes in active, passive, and accessory joint motions are noted. These changes may be an increase or a decrease in mobility. Abnormalities of motion can be identified through motion palpation procedures and through the use of functional radiographs.
>
> *T*—tissue tone, texture, temperature abnormality. Changes in the characteristics of contiguous and associated soft tissues, including skin, fascia, muscle, and ligament, are noted. These changes are identified through the procedures of observation, palpation, instrumentation, and tests for length and strength.
>
> *S*—special tests. Those testing procedures that are specific to a technique system are performed. In addition, visceral relationships, as well as other testing procedures deemed necessary from data previously obtained, are considered.

The evaluation process must be an ongoing procedure, because no matter how thorough, the initial examination cannot be expected to provide all of the answers. A treatment trial should be instituted with its effects assessed to determine whether it should be continued or a different plan devised. The detection of joint dysfunction is not an exact science, as any of the examination procedures used to detect joint dysfunction may produce false positives, false negatives, and equivocal results. Furthermore, very little has been done in the area of validity assessment. Nearly all examination procedures used in the detection of joint dysfunction have not been subjected to validity testing.

FORMS OF MANUAL THERAPY

The most specialized and significant therapy employed by the doctor of chiropractic involves the adjustment of the articulations of the human body. Sandoz[8,9] defines the chiropractic adjustment as a passive manual maneuver during which the three-joint complex is suddenly carried beyond the normal physiological range of movement without exceeding the boundaries of anatomical integrity. Various forms of manipulation exist affecting different aspects of joint function.

The common factor in all of these methods is the application of external forces to the body for the purpose of affecting the flexibility and comfort of the spine and its contiguous tissues.[10] Lewit[11] identifies that another common feature of most methods is they act reflexively, that is, they act on sensor receptors—usually in the region where the pain is felt, or even better, where it originates—to produce a reflex response. Pain is mainly a warning against harmful functioning, and it is disturbance of function that is the most common cause of pain originating in the locomotor system. Movement restriction (blockage) at the segmental level and disturbed motor patterns at the central level may serve as examples.[11] The form of therapy used must vary according to the structures on which it is to act. The most adequate treatment of joint or spinal segment movement restriction is manipulation; the most adequate treatment of disturbed motor patterns is remedial exercise.[11] However, regardless of the form of therapy used, it is always difficult to determine whether any improvement in a patient's condition results from the treatment offered.[12]

Although manipulation is a term broadly used to define the therapeutic application of a manual force, chiropractors emphasize the application of specific adjustive techniques. Chiropractic technique should not be confused with chiropractic therapy or treatment, which includes the application of all the primary and ancillary procedures appropriate in the management of a patient with a given health disorder. These procedures are limited by individual statutory practice acts but may include such procedures as joint mobilization, therapeutic muscle stretching, soft tissue manipulation, sustained and intermittent traction, meridian therapy, physical therapy modalities, application of heat or cold, dietary and nutritional counseling, therapeutic and rehabilitative exercises, and biofeedback and stress management.[13] It is necessary to understand that a wide variety of methods exist, so the assumption that all forms of manual therapy are equivalent must be avoided.[14] Some factors that influence the selection of manipulative procedures have been identified (Table 2).[15]

Unfortunately, even with its identification with manipulative procedures, the chiropractic profession has not developed a common professional definition and classification scheme. The profession has made recent laudable attempts to address this inconsistency but still faces significant variation. A classification scheme has been suggested and published[16] but has not been put through any consensus process for professional acceptance. At issue is whether adjustments should be defined by therapeutic intention or defined and classified by physical characteristics. The basis for distinguishing and classifying adjustive procedures should incorporate its measurable characteristics and not be based solely

TABLE 2.
Factors That Influence the Selection of Manipulative Procedures*

Age of patient
Acuteness or chronicity of the problem
General physical condition of the patient
Clinician's size and ability
Effectiveness of previous and/or present therapy

*Adapted from Greenman P: *Principle of Manual Medicine.* Baltimore, Williams & Wilkins, 1989, p 46.

on therapeutic intention.[13] The central physical feature distinguishing chiropractic adjustments from other manual procedures is the delivery of a precisely gauged adjustive thrust of controlled velocity, depth, and direction.[8] Although amplitude and velocity of the adjustive thrust may vary, often it is a relatively high-velocity, low-amplitude force.

Through a consensus process, Gatterman[17] defines manual therapy, manipulation, mobilization, and adjustment (Table 3).

A widely used form of chiropractic adjustment is characterized by a specific high-velocity and short-amplitude thrust. This type of adjustive thrust is characterized by a transmission of force using a combination of muscular power and body weight of the practitioner. The force is delivered with controlled speed, depth, and magnitude through a specific contact on a particular structure such as the transverse or spinous process of a vertebra.[18]

TABLE 3.
Manual Therapy Terminology*

Manual therapy
  Procedures by which the hands directly contact the body to treat the articulations and/or soft tissues.
Mobilization
  Movement applied singularly or repetitively within or at the physiological range of joint motion, without imparting a thrust or impulse, with the goal of restoring joint mobility.
Manipulation
  A manual procedure that involves a directed thrust to move a joint past the physiological range of motion, without exceeding the anatomical limit.
Adjustment
  Any chiropractic therapeutic procedure that uses controlled force, leverage, direction, amplitude, and velocity directed at specific joints or anatomical regions; chriopractors commonly use such procedures to influence joint and neurophysiological function.

*Adapted from Gatterman MI: *J Manipulative Physiol Ther* 17:302–309, 1994.

Haldeman[19] implies that though there are a large variety of techniques within the entire field of spinal manipulation, each has different therapeutic goals, and each is administered according to different biomechanical or physiological principles; the most commonly used manipulative technique is the short-lever, high-velocity adjustment. He characterizes this technique as a quick, small-amplitude, high-velocity thrust delivered to one of the small vertebral processes (specific short-lever contact) in a specific direction.

Although technique applications may be highly variable, the underlying principles are fairly constant. Hoag et al.[20] state that a major subdivision of osteopathic manipulative therapy involves technique directed mainly to osseous structures and designed to restore normal joint mobility and weight distribution. They describe the procedures used as positioning the patient in such a way that the force to be applied will cause motion between the affected segments and not be dissipated by the elasticity or mobility of other spinal or appendicular structures. After tension is taken up in muscles and ligaments from above and below the site to be mobilized, a force is delivered, usually to the upper of two segments, in a direction most likely to restore normal motion or apposition. They add that frequently the procedure is accompanied by a cracking sound, which is regarded by patients and, unfortunately, by some physicians as the indication of proper osteopathic treatment. They further describe the thrust movement as rapid (high velocity) and of short distance (low amplitude) and carefully calibrated according to the age and condition of the patient and the nature of the skeletal disorder.

Greenman[15] also writes that the high-velocity, low-amplitude thrust technique is one of the oldest and most widely used forms of manual medicine and remains one of the most frequently used forms of manual medicine. He states that such thrusts are usually applied as precisely as possible to a single joint level and for specific joint motion loss. He believes that the high-velocity, low-amplitude thrust appears to be much more effective in subacute and chronic conditions than in acute somatic dysfunction, though he offers no support for these statements. Cremata et al.[21] describe the Gonstead-type adjustment as a high-velocity, low-amplitude thrust applied to short-lever arms such as a spinous process or transverse process. These authors believe that specificity is critical in the contacts taken, as well as in the line of correction used, but offer no evidence or rationale as to why such specificity is important or whether it is achievable.

Adjustive contacts are usually established in close proximity to the joint being treated, and the thrust is delivered within the limits of anatomical integrity. Adjustive therapy is commonly associated with an audible articular crack, but the presence or absence of joint cracking should not be the test for determining whether or not an adjustment has been performed.

Properly applied adjustments are usually painless, though some minimal discomfort may be experienced by the patient who has long-standing dysfunction with some degree of periarticular soft tissue contracture. Adjustive procedures that induce increased pain should be considered only if directed toward reducing joint dysfunction or subluxation. Adjustments should never be forced in a situation where pain, hesitancy, or protective resistance is encountered.[13]

The chiropractic profession has emphasized specific short-lever procedures, theorizing that these procedures would be more precise in correcting local subluxation/dysfunction without inducing stress or possible injury to adjacent articulations. This may be especially pertinent in circumstances where there is adjacent joint instability. However, by applying principles of joint localization, long-lever procedures become more precise, and the assumption that short-lever adjustments are inherently more specific than long-lever adjustments may not always apply.

Until a professional standard of care is established, each practitioner must use reasonable and conservative clinical judgment in the management of subluxation and dysfunction. The decision to treat must be weighed against the presence or absence of pain and the degree of noted structural or functional deviation. Minor structural or functional alteration in the absence of a painful manifestation may not warrant adjustive therapy.

ADJUSTIVE MECHANICS[22]

The science of chiropractic is now beginning to investigate the art of chiropractic. Especially important in the performance of adjustive techniques is an awareness of spinal and extremity joint architecture, facet plane orientations, and arthrokinematics. When subluxation and dysfunction are identified, the chiropractor must be able to effectively induce joint separation and corrective joint movements without producing joint compression, injury, or distraction at undesired segmental levels. Most adjustive techniques are directed at producing joint distraction either along the articular plane or at right angles (perpendicular) to the articular plane. This cannot be efficiently and effectively accomplished without an understanding of how joints are configured and how they move.[22]

To illustrate this point, consider the application of prone adjustive techniques in the treatment of thoracic flexion and extension dysfunction. In the thoracic spine the articular surfaces are relatively flat. The superior articular processes underlie the inferior articular processes at an angle of approximately 60 degrees from the horizontal plane toward the coronal plane. During segmental flexion in the thoracic spine, the posterior joint surfaces separate and glide apart along their joint surfaces. During extension the posterior joint surfaces approximate and gap at their superior margins at the end range of motion. When performing prone thoracic adjustments, the doctor typically develops adjustive vectors that either approximate the disk plane or the facet planes. The thrust, which parallels the disk plane, is perpendicular to the spine and facet facings and will likely induce approximation of the facets in the joint below the contacted vertebrae and perpendicular gapping in the joint superior to the contacted vertebrae. In contrast, a thrust delivered cephalically along facet planes should induce longitudinal distraction in the facet joint inferior to the point of contact and gliding approximation in the joint superior to the point of contact. Therefore, thrusts that parallel the disk plane induce movements approximating extension in the joint below the contact and perpendicular gapping above. Thrusts directed cephalically along the facet plane induce movements that approximate flexion in the joint below the contact and extension above. These deductions would not have been possible without knowledge of joint anatomy and arthrokinematics (Fig 2).

Each grouping of adjustments has its own mechanical characteristics dependent on adjustive contacts, patient positioning, doctor positioning, and adjustive vectors. Efficient and effective selections cannot be made without an understanding of each adjustment's unique physical attributes.[22]

ADJUSTIVE LOCALIZATION

Adjustive localization refers to the preadjustive procedures designed to localize adjustive forces and joint distraction. They involve the application of physiological and unphysiological positions, the removal of articular "slack," and the development of appropriate patient positions, contact points, and adjustive vectors. These factors are critical to the development of appropriate preadjustive tension and adjustive efficiency. Attention to these components is intended to improve adjustive specificity and to further minimize the distractive tension on adjacent joints.[22]

PATIENT POSITIONING

Appropriate preadjustive joint tension and localization are critically dependent on patient placement and leverage. Localization of adjustive forces may be enhanced by using patient placement to position a joint at a point of distractive vulnerability. Locking adjacent joints and positioning the joint to be adjusted at the apex of curves established during patient positioning enhance this process and adjustive specificity. Joint localization and joint distraction may be further enhanced if forces are used to either assist or oppose the adjustive thrust. Assisting or opposing forces may be generated either during the adjustive setup or during the adjustive thrust. Assisted and resisted patient positions refer to the principles

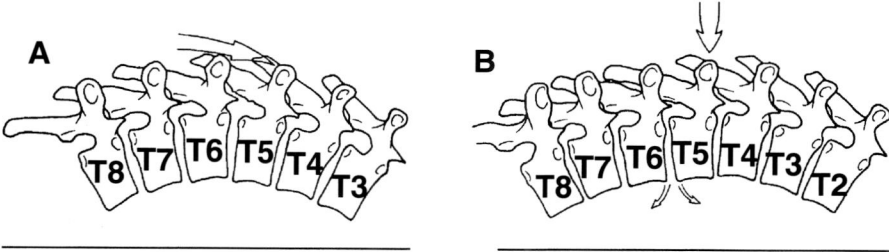

FIGURE 2.
Graphic depiction of the effects of a thrust vector in line with the facet plane (**A**) and the disk plane (**B**). With the facet plane thrust applied to T-5 transverse processes there will likely be translation and approximation of the facet joints above (T-4 to T-5) and separation and cavitation of the facet joints below (T-5 to T-6). With the disk plane thrust applied to T-5 transverse processes there will likely be approximation and translation of the facet joints below (T-5 to T-6) and separation and cavitation of the facet joints above (T-4 to T-5).

involved during the adjustive setup and development of preadjustive tension, not to the generation of assisted or resisted thrusts.[22]

ASSISTED AND RESISTED POSITIONING

The notion of applying assisted and opposing forces during the performance of manipulation was first described relative to thoracic manipulation by the French orthopedist Robert Maigne.[23] In the chiropractic profession, Sandoz[8] was the first to describe similar terms. Sandoz proposed using the terms assisted and resisted to describe patient positions that either assist or resist adjustive thrusts. Recently, Good[24] has presented examples of these concepts in relation to diversified technique. As originally described, assisted and resisted methods were applied only to side posture lumbar adjustments and those procedures involving a single primary thrust.[8] Both methods are employed to improve the localization of preadjustive tension. Their application is based on the mechanical principle that the point of maximal tension will be developed at the point of opposing counterrotation. Assisted and resisted methods are distinguished from each other by the positioning of vertebral segments relative to the adjustive thrust. In both circumstances the trunk and vertebral segments superior to the adjustive contact are prestressed in the direction of desired joint movement. In the assisted method the contact is established on the superior vertebral segment and movement of the trunk and the thrust are directed together. Assisted procedures are designed to induce preadjustive tension and positions that assist the adjustive thrust. Resisted procedures employ patient positions in which the segments superior to the adjustive contact are stabilized or moved in a direction opposing the adjustive thrust. In the resisted method the contact is established on the lower vertebral segment, and the direction of trunk movement and adjustive thrust are in opposing directions. Sandoz[8] has suggested that resisted positions bring maximal tension to the articulation superior to the established contact (e.g., contact at the L-3 mammillary, inducing tension at the L-2 to L-3 motion segment), and assisted positions bring maximal tension to the articulation inferior to the established contact (e.g., L-2 spinous contact, inducing tension at the L-2 to L-3 motion segment). In the assisted method the point of countertension is inferior to the point of contact because the segments below are stabilized or rotated in a direction opposite the adjustive thrust. In the resisted approach the site of countertension is superior to the point of contact because the segments above are stabilized or rotated in a direction opposite the adjustive thrust. Therefore, either method can theoretically be used to induce cavitation and motion within the same articulation. Although the movement generated is the same, the points of contact and the line of drive are different. With the assisted method the contact is established on the superior vertebrae of the dysfunctional motion segment, and in the resisted method it is established on the inferior vertebrae. The thrust is oriented in the direction of restriction when the assisted method is used and against the direction of restriction when the resisted method is used. Assisted and resisted methods have been most frequently discussed relative to the development of rotational tension of the spine, but the same methods and principles may be applied to treat dysfunction in lateral flexion or flexion and extension.

EFFECTS OF ADJUSTIVE THERAPY

Though various forms of manual therapy exist affecting different aspects of musculoskeletal function, most will result in passive movement of joint surfaces with the purpose of restoring normal articular relationship and function, as well as reestablishing neurological integrity and influencing physiological processes. The nature and extent of individual joint motion are determined by the joint structure and specifically by the shape and direction of the joint surfaces. No two opposing joint surfaces are perfectly matched, nor are they perfectly geometric. Because of the incongruence between joint surfaces, some joint space and "play" must be present to allow free movement. This joint play is an accessory movement of the joint that is essential for normal functioning of the joint.[13]

The joint capsule must allow this play for full movement of the joint to occur. The joint demonstrates joint play in the neutral or close-packed position, which is then followed by an active range of motion under the control of the musculature. A small degree of passive movement then occurs, followed by an elastic barrier of resistance called end-feel or end-play. A loss of either joint play or end-feel can result in a restriction of motion, pain, or both. Active movements can be influenced through exercise, and passive movement can be influenced with traction and mobilization; however, joint play and end-feel movements are affected only when the joint is taken beyond the elastic barrier, creating a sudden yielding of the joint and typically a cracking noise. This sudden separation of a joint that produces the cracking sound is termed "cavitation." Movement of the joint beyond the paraphysiological space would take the joint beyond its limit of anatomical integrity, causing joint trauma or abnormality (Fig 3).

Paris proposed a mechanism for intervertebral joint dysfunction that began with an episode of rotational or compressive trauma to the three-joint complex, which then leads to posterior joint strain and a stress to the annular fibers.[25] This causes a minor facet subluxation characterized by synovitis and pain. This process stimulates sustained segmental hypertonicity of muscle, which itself becomes ischemic and painful through altered muscle metabolism. The muscle contraction results in a splinting of the posterior joint that maintains the subluxation and perpetuates the posterior joint strain.

The changes that occur in the posterior joints are the same as those characteristics of any synovial joint. They consist first of synovitis, which may then proceed to the formation of a synovial fold that projects into the joint between the articular surfaces. These changes lead to fibrosis. The three-joint complex then becomes dysfunctional. With continued stress or further trauma, progressive changes will be seen.[26]

When joint dysfunction occurs, particularly in a vertebral motion segment, reflex changes may also occur in the same spinal segment. The effects may be evident in dermatomes, myotomes, and/or sclerotomes. The term "segmental facilitation" has been used to describe this phenom-

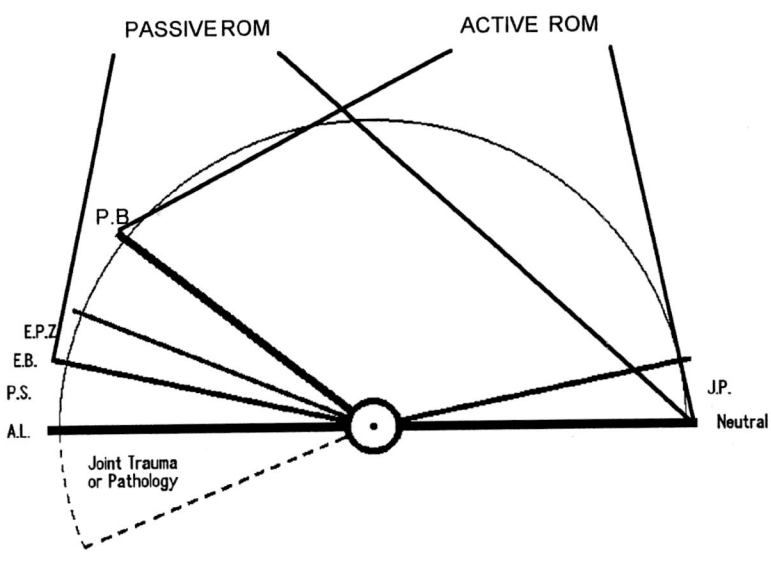

FIGURE 3.
Joint motions. Joint play occurs in the neutral position, followed by the active and passive ranges of motion. The passive range of motion goes beyond the active range of motion, engaging the elastic barrier in the end play (feel) zone. After cavitation, the paraphysiological space extends the passive range of motion. JP = joint play; PB = physiological barrier; EPZ = end play zone; EB = elastic barrier; PS = paraphysiological space; AL = anatomic limit.

enon.[27] Lewit[11] described an experiment where 10 patients were examined for cervical spine joint dysfunction before abdominal surgery. They were reexamined while they were under anesthesia. The joint restrictions continued to be evident and, in fact, more easily recognizable with the patients under the anesthesia. Furthermore, a significant factor in musculoskeletal function is the musculature and its nervous control. Each individual will have a postural personality that is an expression of the individual's muscular patterns and posture. A frequent cause of joint dysfunction would therefore be faulty movement patterns due to muscular imbalance and postural overstrain.[11]

Manual therapy, with its emphasis on joint movement, has become increasingly important for the treatment of pain and dysfunction of the neuromusculoskeletal system. The rationale used to explain the success of manual therapy has changed radically in recent years. Current biological research shows the value of movement in maintaining the health and strength of collagenous, muscular, and bony tissues while emphasizing the need for joint movement and relatively high levels of activity throughout the life cycle. The musculoskeletal system thrives on stress and movement and reacts adversely to prolonged rest or immobilization.[28] A number of clinical trials have also demonstrated effective results for manipulation in treating spinal pain compared with a control group, medical care, physical therapy, or combination thereof.[29-44]

The goals of manipulation include a combination of mechanical, soft tissue, neurological, and psychological effects. These divisions are academic, however, and are used only for ease in understanding. It is not to imply that the effects of manipulation can occur singularly or in isolation. It would be absurd to think that one could make a mechanical effect without affecting the soft tissues or joint receptors.

MECHANICAL EFFECTS

The mechanical effects of an adjustment include changes in joint alignment and motion, as well as spinal curvature dynamics. Generally, then, the mechanical effects will be on derangements or disorders of the somatic structures of the body that have altered joint function resulting from acute injury, repetitive use injury, faulty posture or coordination, aging, congenital or developmental defects, or other primary disease states.[13]

Studies done by Roston et al.[45] and Unsworth et al.[46] demonstrate that as tension is applied, causing a separation of the joint, there is a point where the joint surfaces jump apart that coincides with a cracking noise. Once the tension is removed from the joint, the surfaces approximate themselves once again but at a distance slightly more apart. A correlation of these studies with intervertebral joint adjustment is seen in Figure 4.[47]

As the elastic barrier is passed, the articular surfaces separate suddenly, a cracking noise can be heard, and a radiolucent space appears within the joint space. The explanation of the radiolucent space rests with the fact that there is normally a small negative pressure present in a synovial joint. Its purpose is to maintain the cartilage surfaces in apposition and help to maintain the stability of the joint. Separation of the joint surfaces beyond the elastic barrier creates a drop in the interarticular pressure, and gas is suddenly liberated from the synovial fluid to form a bubble in the joint space. The bubble bursts almost immediately with an audible crack. Analysis of the gas produced by synovial fluid cavitation was shown to consist of more than 80% carbon dioxide.[46]

Herzog[48] at the University of Calgary is studying changes in mechanics when a thrusting force is applied to a specific area. The forces exerted by a chiropractor in the deliverance of a high-velocity, low-amplitude thrust have been measured in the sacroiliac articulation, the thoracic spine, and the cervical spine. In the study of the thoracic spine it was found that cavitation may not be solely related to peak force in all cases but may depend on other mechanical factors such as speed of applied force or the impulse applied during a manipulative thrust.

A synovial joint may also become dysfunctional through entrapment or extrapment of a synovial fold or fibroadipose meniscoid.[49] These project from the inner surface of the superior and inferior capsules, serving a protective function for the joint. When joint movement occurs, the meniscoids cover exposed articular surfaces.[50] A common clinical manifestation described by patients is bending forward in flexion with an acute inability to straighten up because of pain. Although the pathology of this acute locked back remains unknown, a theoretical explanation is meniscoid extrapment.[50,51] The application of an adjustive thrust will separate the articular surfaces and may release the entrapped or extrapped synovial fold.[52]

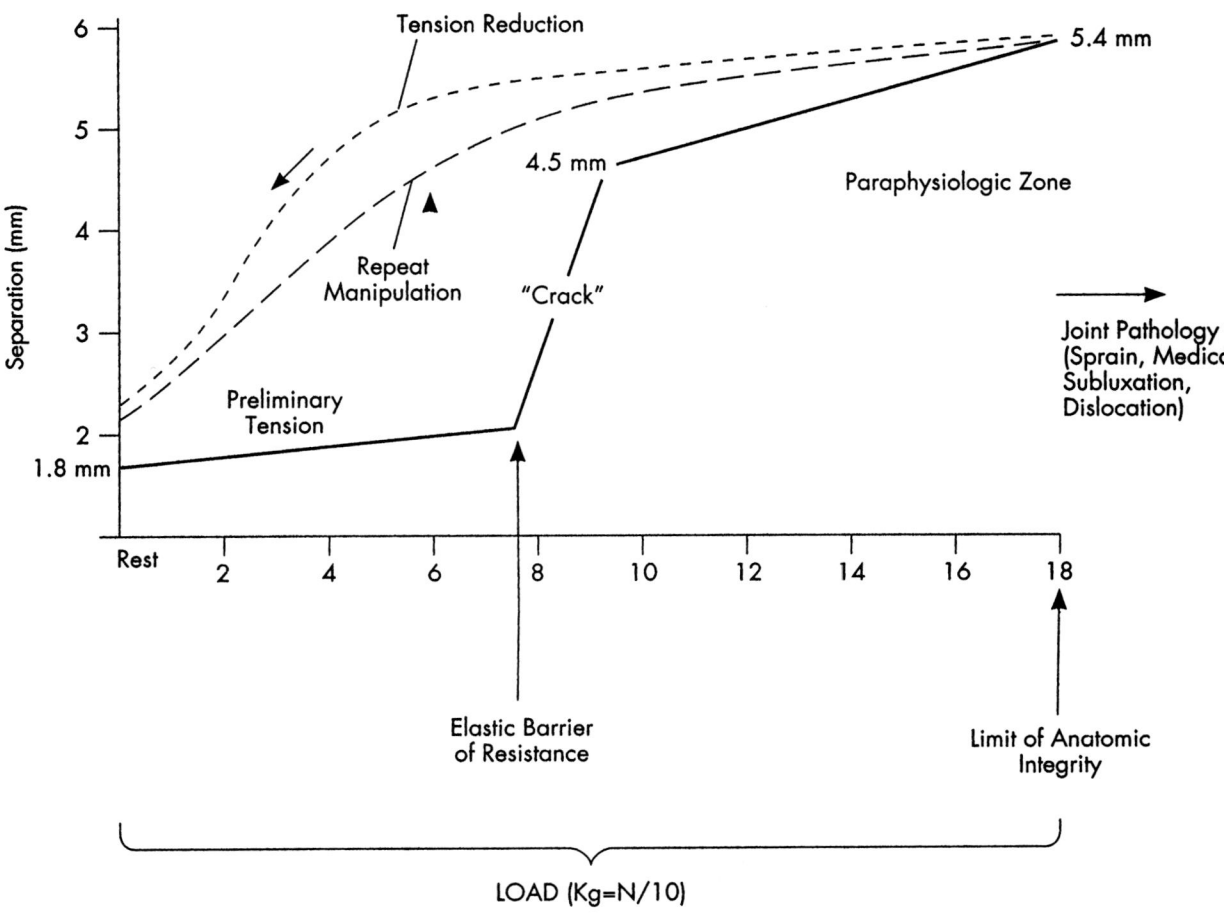

FIGURE 4.
Graph representing the effects of joint separation and cavitation: as the joint tension increases with joint surface separation, a quick and dramatic separation occurs and a cracking noise is produced; the resting joint spacing is increased, but further joint separation results in no further cavitation response. (Adapted from Sandoz R: *Ann Swiss Chiropr Assoc* 4:47, 1969.)

SOFT TISSUE EFFECTS

Soft tissue effects include changing the tone and strength of supporting musculature and influencing the dynamics of supportive capsuloligamentous connective tissue (viscoelastic properties of collagen). Connective tissue elements lose their extensibility when their related joints are immobilized.[53] With immobilization, water is released from the proteoglycan molecule, allowing connective tissue fibers to contact one another, encouraging abnormal cross linking, and resulting in a loss of extensibility.[54] It is hypothesized that manipulation can break the cross linking and any intra-articular capsular fiber fatty adhesions, thereby providing free motion and allowing water inhibition. Furthermore, action of the adjustment can stretch segmental muscles, stimulating spindle reflexes that may decrease the state of hypertonicity.[55]

NEUROLOGICAL EFFECTS

Neurological effects include reducing pain, influencing spinal and peripheral nerve conduction, thereby altering motor and sensory function, and influencing autonomic nervous system regulation. Wyke[56] identified that manipulative procedures may stimulate the mechanoreceptors associated with synovial joints and thereby affect joint pain. He has identified four types of receptors. The first three, types I, II, and III, are corpuscular mechanoreceptors, which detect static position of the joint, acceleration and deceleration of the joint, direction of movement, and overdisplacement of the joint. The fourth receptor, type IV, is a network of free nerve endings that have nociceptive capabilities. Type IV receptors are usually inactive under normal conditions; however, if noxious mechanical or chemical stimulation occurs or if type I to III receptors are not able to function, type IV receptors become active and pain results. If manipulative therapy can restore normal function to the joint, allowing types I to III receptors to function, type IV pain receptors should be inhibited, thereby decreasing the patient's pain. The structures most sensitive to noxious stimulation are the periosteum and joint capsule.

There are many controversies in the application of manipulative therapy. Of significance is the role of pain in deciding when or if to manipulate. Mitchell[57] states that if one treats the part where the patient experiences the pain, one will be treating the wrong part of the body most of the time. He goes on to quote Osler with "pain is a liar." Mitchell bases this idea on the concept that in the musculoskeletal system, pain almost always develops and persists in the structures stressed the most by the adaptation to the dysfunction. The opposite idea is extolled by Lewit,[11] who states that if manipulative treatment is successful, it will usually produce immediate relief of pain. He adds that by far the most frequent cause of pain is disturbed function. This may concern passive mobility (joints), active movement patterns, or body statics. Manipulative treatment is directed to movement restriction of joints or motion segments of the spinal column. Pain in the locomotor system is therefore looked on as a warning sign of harmful functioning that should be corrected in time before it causes permanent damage. Lewit[11] also emphasizes that undiagnosed impairment of motor function is the most frequent type of pain without a specific diagnosis, and treatment of the pain as such, without a thorough clinical understanding of the functioning of the locomotor system, is courting failure.

In addition, current research provides evidence that the spinal adjustment decreases pain, increases range of motion, increases pain tolerance in the skin and deeper muscle structures, raises β-endorphin levels in the blood plasma, and has an impact on the nerve pathways between the soma and viscera that regulate general health.[58-66]

PSYCHOLOGICAL EFFECTS

The psychological effect of the lying on of hands cannot be denied or overlooked. Paris[67] states that with the addition of a skilled evaluation involving palpation for soft tissue changes and altered joint mechanics, the patient becomes convinced of the interest, concern, and manual skills of the clinician. If at the conclusion of the examination manipulation is performed, resulting in an audible pop or snap, the placebo factor will be undeniably high. It is no wonder that some patients report total relief within 1 or 2 seconds of manipulation, far too short a time for any genuine benefit to be appreciated. The astute clinician accepts and reinforces this report, recognizing that the patient is in need of all possible assistance.

The chiropractic profession has a long empirical history of noting positive responses to treatment for a variety of neuromusculoskeletal disorders and pain syndromes. It is these conditions that have historically been the major reason for which chiropractors are consulted.[68, 69] Furthermore, chiropractic patients have repeatedly expressed satisfaction with the quality and effectiveness of chiropractic care. In comparative studies for the treatment of back pain, patients consistently rate chiropractic care as being superior to medical care.[70-72]

TEACHING OF CHIROPRACTIC TECHNIQUE

Curricula at accredited chiropractic colleges are designed to ensure that certain information is imparted to the student body. As such the colleges teach a comprehensive program that incorporates elements of basic science and clinical science while also providing a clinical experience.

Though the curriculum is standardized to assure the public that the graduates have been provided a competent education, each college does not necessarily teach its students the same chiropractic manipulative techniques. Although all forms of chiropractic technique have many elements in common, there can be substantial differences and disparities in their approaches and nomenclature. Furthermore, a plethora of technique procedures are available to the profession in the form of postgraduate seminars, many of which are not under the influence of any regulatory body or accrediting procedure necessary to ensure an adequate scholastic level. A number of these "system" techniques are identified in Table 4.

The majority of chiropractic technique systems were started by chiropractors who noticed a regularity in their results and began to ask why those results occurred. This was largely a bootstrapping effort, where the impetus to gain and disseminate new knowledge was primarily self-driven.[73] The apparent fallacy to many of these system approaches is that the evaluative procedure linked to the manipulative procedure is often singular, very simplistic, and untested. Relying on a single evaluative tool for the sole application of a therapeutic intervention is not sound clinical practice.

A challenge for the future is to classify and place all chiropractic techniques into a framework that allows the determination as to whether any of them has a basis in fact. The profession can then begin to eliminate unacceptable procedures. Studies designed to compare effectiveness of the many forms of chiropractic technique systems have not been done. It must therefore be emphasized that no technique system or evaluative procedure has been demonstrated to be more or less effective than any other for any condition. Studies comparing the effectiveness and efficiency of

TABLE 4.
Various Forms of Chiropractic Technique

Technique	Developer	Technique	Developer
Access Seminars	Weigant, Bloomenthal	Howard System	Howard
Activator Technique	Fuhr (Lee)	Keck Method of Analysis	Keck
Alternative Chiropractic Adjustments	Wiehe	King Tetrahedron Concept	King
		Lemond Brain Stem Technique	Lemond
Applied Chiropractic Distortion Analysis	Kotheimer	Logan Basic Technique	Logan, Coggins Bartlett
Applied Kinesiology	Goodheart, Walters, Schmitt, Thie	Master Energy Dynamics	
		Mawhinney Scoliosis Technique	Mawhinney
		McTimody Technique	McTimody
Applied Spinal Biomechanical Engineering	Aragona	Mears Technique	Mears
		Meric Technique System	Cleveland, Palmer, Loban, Forster, Riley
Aquarian Age Healing	Hurley		
Arnholz Muscle Adjusting	Arnholtz		
Atlas Orthogonality Techinque	Sweat	Micromanipulation	Young
Atlas Specific	Wernsing	Motion Palpation	Gillet, Faye
Bandy Seminars	Bandy	Muscle Palpation	Spano
Bio Kinesiology	Barton	Muscle Response Testing	Lepore, Fishman, Grinims
BioEnergetic Synchronization Technique (BEST)	Morter	Musculoskeletal Synchronization and Stabilization Technique	Krippenbrock
Bioenergetics	Broeringmeyer Stoffels, Borham, Broeringmeyer		
Biomagnetic Technique		Nerve Signal Interference	Craton

Continued.

TABLE 4 (cont.).
Various Forms of Chiropractic Technique

Technique	Developer	Technique	Developer
Blair Upper Cervical Technique	Blair	Network Chiropractic	Epstein
Bloodless Surgery	Lorenz, Failor, DeJarnette	Neuro Emotional Technique	Walker
		Neuro Organizational Technique	Ferrari
Body Integration	Espy	NeuroLymphactic Reflex Technique	Chapman
Buxton Technical Course of Painless Chiropractic	Buxton	NeuroVascular Reflex Technique	Bennett
		Olesky 21st Century Technique	Olesky
Chiro Plus Kinesiology	Dowty	Ortman Technique	Ortman
Chiroenergetics	Kimmel	Perianal Postural Reflex Technique	
Chirometry	Quigly	Pettibon Spinal Biomechanics Technique	Pettibon
Chiropractic Concept	Prill		
Chiropractic Manipulative Reflex Technique (CMRT)	DeJarnette	Pierce-Stillwagon Technique	Pierce, Stillwagon
		Polarity Technique	Sinclaire
Chiropractic Neuro-Biochemical Analysis		Posture Imbalance Patterns	Morrheim
		Pure Chiropractic Technique	Reaver, Pierce
Chiropractic Spinal Biophysics	Harrison	Reaver's Fifth Cervical Key	Nimmo
CHOK-E System		Receptor Tonus Technique	Riddler
Clinical Kinesiology	Beardall	Riddler Reflex Technique	DeJarnette
Collins Method of Painless Adjusting	Collins	Sacro-occipital Technique	Rees
		Soft Tissue Orthopedics	Ford
Concept Therapy	Fleet, Dill	Somatosynthesis	Spears
Cranial Technique	DeJarnette, Denton Goodheart	Spears Painless System	Nemiroff
		Specific Majors	Ward
Craniopathy	Cottam	Spinal Stress (Stressology)	Rosquist
Directional Nonforce Technique -DNFT	Van Rumpt, Johns	Spinal Touch Technique	Forster, Riley
Distraction Technique	Cox, Markey, Leander	Spondylotherapy	

Diversified Technique	Beatty, Bonyun, Carver, Crawford, DeGiacomo, Frank, Grecco, Logan, LeBeau, Metzinger, Reinert, States, Stonebrink, Stierwalt	Thompson Terminal Point Technique	Thompson, Stucky, Mitchell
		Tiezen Technique	Tiezen
		Toftness Technique	Toftness
		Top Notch Visceral Techniques	Portelli, Marcellino
		Tortipelvis/Torticolis	Barge
		Total Body Modification	Frank
Endonasal Technique	Gibbons, Lake, Broeringmeyer	Touch for Health	Thie
		Truscott Technique	Truscott
Extremity Technique	Burns, Grecco, Christenson, Gertler, Hearon, Malley, Schawn	Ungerank Specific Low Force Chiropractic Technique	Ungerank
		Upper Cervical Technique—HIO, Toggle	Palmer, Duff, Grostic, Kale, Life, NUCCA
Focoalizer Spinal Recoil Stimulus Reflex Effector Technique	George	Variable Force Technique	Leighton
Freeman Chiropractic Procedure	Freeman	Von Fox Combination Technique	Von Fox
Fundamental Chiropractic	Ashton	Zindler Reflex Technique	Zindler
Global Energetic Matrix	Babinet		
Gonstead Technique	Gonstead		
Herring Cervical Technique	Herring		
Holographic Diagnosis and Treatment	Franks, Gleason		

Chiropractic Technique: An Overview **431**

technique systems are long overdue. Serious investigation into some of these systems is under way, but more needs to be done. It is the responsibility of the developers and followers of a specific technique to establish efficacy, not through anecdotes and testimonials but through properly documented case reports leading to clinical trials.

Practitioners of manipulative therapy need to continue to develop skills and knowledge, not only in the area of therapeutics but also in recognizing potential patients at risk. Studies to collect the facts should serve to quell fears in the minds of practitioners and disarm the opponents of manipulative therapy who aim to denigrate by alarming the public with information that is distorted and overstated and implanting in the public mind a fear of a genuinely safe and effective form of health care.[74] Even in light of the fact that the disastrous complication of permanent neurological damage is indeed so rare an event, the term "acceptable risk" is suitable when applied to manipulative therapies.[75]

SUMMARY

This chapter attempts to provide clarification to various aspects of chiropractic technique, including the definition of some terms, identification of a rationale for the use of chiropractic technique, criteria for application, and the role that chiropractic technique may play in the treatment of dysfunctional changes in the neuromusculoskeletal system.

ACKNOWLEDGMENT

Acknowledgment is given to David Peterson, Western States Chiropractic College, for his insights and contributions to the science of manipulation incorporated in this chapter.

REFERENCES

1. Bergmann TF: Various forms of chiropractic technique. *Chiropr Technique* 5:53–55, 1993.
2. Keating JC: Traditional barriers to standards of knowledge production in chiropractic. *Chiropr Technique* 2:78–85, 1990.
3. Bergmann TF: Short lever, specific contact articular chiropractic technique. *J Manipulative Physiol Ther* 15:591–595, 1992.
4. Janda V: Pain in the locomotor system—a broad approach, in Grieve G (ed): *Modern Manual Therapy*, New York, Churchill Livingstone, 1994, pp 148–151.
5. Bergmann T: The chiropractic spinal examination, in Ferezy JS: *The Chiropractic Neurological Examination*, Gaithersburg, Md, Aspen Publications, 1992, pp 97–110.
6. Keating JC, Bergmann TF, Jacobs GE, et al: Interexaminer reliability of eight evaluative dimensions of lumbar segmental dysfunction. *J Manipulative Physiol Ther* 13:463, 1990.
7. Faucret B, Mao W, Nakagawa T, et al: Determination of bony subluxations by clinical, neurological, and chiropractic procedures. *J Manipulative Physiol Ther* 3:165–176, 1980.
8. Sandoz R: Some physical mechanisms and affects of spinal adjustments. *Ann Swiss Chiropr Assoc* 6:91, 1976.

9. Sandoz R: Some reflex phenomena associated with spinal derangements and adjustments. *Ann Swiss Chiropr Assoc* 7:45, 1981.
10. Triano JJ: Studies on the biomechanical effect of a spinal adjustment. *J Manipulative Physiol Ther* 1992; 15:71–75.
11. Lewit K: *Manipulative Therapy in Rehabilitation of the Motor System.* New York, Butterworths, 1985.
12. Nachemson A: A critical look at the treatment for low back pain. *Scand J Rehabil Med* 11:143–147, 1979.
13. Bergmann TB, Peterson DH, Lawrence DJ: *Chiropractic Technique.* New York, Churchill Livingstone, 1993, pp 127–128.
14. Haldeman S: Spinal manipulative therapy and sports medicine. *Clin Sports Med* 5(2):277–293, 1986.
15. Greenman P: *Principles of Manual Medicine.* Baltimore, Williams & Wilkins, 1989, p 46.
16. Bartol KM: A model for the categorization of chiropractic treatment procedures. *J Chiropr Technique* 3:78–80, 1991.
17. Gatterman MI: Development of chiropractic nomenclature through consensus. *J Manipulative Physiol Ther* 17:302–309, 1994.
18. Grice AS: Biomechanical approach to cervical and dorsal adjusting. In Haldeman S (ed): *Modern Developments in the Principles and Practice of Chiropractic.* New York, Appleton-Century-Croft, 1980.
19. Haldeman S: Spinal manipulative therapy: A status report. *Clin Orthop* 179:62–70, 1983.
20. Hoag JM, Cole WV, Bradford SG: *Osteopathic Medicine.* New York, McGraw-Hill, 1969.
21. Cremata EE, Plaugher G, Cox WA: Technique system application: The Gonstead approach. *Chiropr Technique* 3:19–25, 1991.
22. Peterson DH: Principles of adjustive technique. In Bergmann TB, Peterson DH, Lawrence DJ (ed): *Chiropractic Technique.* New York, Churchill Livingstone, 1993.
23. Maigne R: *Orthopedic Medicine,* ed 3. Springfield, Ill, Charles C Thomas, 1979.
24. Good C: An analysis of diversified (lege artis) type adjustments upon the assisted-resisted model of intervertebral motion unit prestress. *Chiropr Technique* 4:117–123, 1992.
25. Paris SV: in, Kirkaldy-Willis WH (ed): *Managing Low Back Pain,* ed 3. New York, Churchill Livingstone, 1993, p 106.
26. Kirkaldy-Willis WH, Burton CV: *Managing Low Back Pain,* ed 3. New York, Churchill Livingstone, 1993, pp 105–119.
27. Korr IM: Proprioceptors and somatic dysfunction. *J Am Osteopath Assoc* 74:638, 1975.
28. Twomey LT: A rationale for the treatment of back pain and joint pain by manual therapy. *Phys Ther* 72:885–892.
29. Meade TW, Dyers S, Browne W, et al: Low back pain of mechanical origin: randomized comparison of chiropractic and hospital outpatient treatment. *BMJ* 300:1431–1437, 1990.
30. Arkuszewski Z: The efficacy of manual treatment in low back pain: A clinical trial. *Manual Med* 2:68–71, 1986.
31. Coxhead CE, Inskip H, Meade TW, et al: Multicentre trial of physiotherapy in the management of sciatic symptoms. *Lancet* 1:1065–1068, 1981.
32. Coyer AB, Curwin I: Low back pain treated by manipulation. *BMJ* 1:705–707, 1955.
33. Edwards BC: Low back pain and pain resulting from lumbar spine conditions: A comparison of treatment results. *Aust J Physiol* 15:104–110, 1969.

34. Evans DP, Burke MS, Lloyd KN, et al: Lumbar spinal manipulation on trial: 1. Clinical assessment. *Rheum Rehabil* 17:46–53, 1978.
35. Farrell JP, Twomey LT: Acute low back pain: Comparison of two conservative treatment approaches. *Med J Aust* 1:160–164, 1982.
36. Godfrey CM, Morgan PP, Schatzker J: A randomized trial of manipulation for low back pain in a medical setting. *Spine* 9:301–304, 1984.
37. Hadler NM, Curtis P, Gillings DB, et al: A benefit of spinal manipulation as adjunctive therapy for acute low back pain: A stratified controlled trial. *Spine* 12:703–706, 1987.
38. Hoehler FK, Tobis JS, Beurger AA: Spinal manipulation for low back pain. *JAMA* 245:1835–1838, 1981.
39. Matthews JA, Mills SB, Jenkins VM, et al: Back pain and sciatica: Controlled trials of manipulation, traction, sclerosant, and epidural injections. *Br J Rheum* 26:416–423, 1987.
40. Nwuga VC: Relative therapeutic efficacy of vertebral manipulation and conventional treatment in back pain management. *Am J Phys Med* 61:273–278, 1982.
41. Ongley MJ, Klein RG, Dorman TA, et al: A new approach to the treatment of chronic low back pain. *Lancet* 2:143–146, 1987.
42. Rasmussen GG: Manipulation in the treatment of low back pain—a randomized clinical trial. *Manuelle Med* 1:8–10, 1979.
43. Sims-Williams H, Jayson M, Young S, et al: Controlled trial of mobilization and manipulation for patients with low back pain in general practice. *BMJ* 2:1338–1340, 1978.
44. Waagen GN, Haldeman S, Cook G, et al: Short term trial of chiropractic adjustments for the relief of chronic low back pain. *Manipulative Med* 2:63–67, 1986.
45. Roston JB, Wheeler Haines RW: Cracking in the metacarpophalangeal joint. *J Anat* 81:165, 1947.
46. Unsworth A, Dowson D, Wright V: Cracking joints, a bioengineering study of cavitation in the metacarpophalangeal joint. *Ann Rheum Dis* 30:348, 1971.
47. Sandoz R: The significance of the manipulative crack and other articular noises. *Ann Swiss Chiropr Assoc* 4:47, 1969.
48. Herzog W: Biomechanical studies of spinal manipulative therapy. *J Can Chiropr Assoc* 35:156–164, 1991.
49. Giles LGF: Lumbosacral and cervicozygoapophyseal joint inclusions. *Manual Med* 2:89, 1986.
50. Bogduk N, Twomey LT: *Clinical Anatomy of the Lumbar Spine*, ed 2. New York, Churchill Livingstone, 1991, pp 33–34.
51. Bogduk N, Engel R: The menisci of the lumbar zygapophyseal joints. A review of their anatomy and clinical significance. *Spine* 9:454–460, 1984.
52. Bogduk N, Jull G: The theoretical pathology of acute locked back: A basis for manipulative therapy. *Manual Med* 1:78–82, 1985.
53. Akeson WH, Amiel D, Woo S: Immobility effects of synovial joints: The pathomechanics of joint contracture. *Biorheology* 17:95, 1980.
54. Akeson WH, Amiel D, Mechanic GL, et al: Collagen cross linking alterations in joint contractures: Changes in reducible cross links in periarticular connective tissue collagen after 9 weeks of immobilization. *Connect Tissue Res* 5:5, 1977.
55. Burger AA: Experimental neuromuscular models of spinal manual techniques. *Manual Med* 1:10, 1983.
56. Wyke BD: Articular neurology and manipulative therapy. In Glasgow EF, Twomey LT, Schull ER, et al (eds): *Aspects of Manipulative Therapy*. New York, Churchill Livingstone, 1985.

57. Mitchell FL: Elements of muscle energy technique. In Basmajin JV, Nyberg R (eds): *Rational Manual Therapies*. Baltimore, Williams & Wilkins, 1993, pp 318–319.
58. Terrett ACJ, Vernon H: Manipulation and pain tolerance. *Am J Phys Med* 63:217–225, 1984.
59. Cassidy JD, Quon J, LaFrance L, et al: The effect of manipulation on pain and range of motion in the cervical spine. Presented at North American Spine Society, Quebec, June 1989.
60. Vernon HT, Dhami MSI, Howley TP, et al: Spinal manipulation and beta-endorphin: A controlled study of the effect of a spinal manipulation on plasma beta-endorphin levels in normal males. *J Manipulative Physiol Ther* 9:115–123, 1986.
61. Vernon HT: Pressure pain threshold evaluation of the effect of spinal manipulation on chronic neck pain: A single case study. *J Can Chiropr Assoc* 32:191–194, 1988.
62. Hood RP: Blood pressure results in 75 abnormal cases. *Digest Chiropr Econ* 16:36–38, 1974.
63. Tran TA, Kirby JD: The effectiveness of upper cervical adjustment upon the normal physiology of the heart. *Am Chiropractic Assoc J Chiropr* XIS:58–62, 1977.
64. Sato A, Swenson RS: Sympathetic nervous system response to mechanical stress of the spinal column in rats. *J Manipulative Physiol Ther* 7:141–147, 1984.
65. Briggs L, Boone WR: Effects of a chiropractic adjustment on changes in pupillary diameter: A model for evaluating somatovisceral response. *J Manipulative Physiol Ther* 11:181–189, 1988.
66. Dhami MSI, Coyle BA, Menke JM, et al: Evidence for sympathetic neuron stimulation by cervicospinal manipulation. In *Proceedings of the First Annual Conference on Research and Education of Specific Consortium for Chiropractic Research*, Sacramento, Calif, California Chiropractic Association, 1986, pp A51–A55.
67. Paris SV: Spinal manipulative therapy. *Clin Orthop* 179:55–61, 1983.
68. Nyiendo J, Haldeman S: A prospective study of 2,000 patients attending a chiropractic college teaching clinic. *Med Care* 25:516, 1987.
69. Shekelle PG, Brook RH: A community-based study of the use of chiropractic services. *Am J Public Health* 81:439, 1991.
70. Cherkin DC, MacCornack FA: Health care delivery, patient evaluations of low back pain care from family physicians and chiropractors. *Zoes J Med* 150:351, 1989.
71. Cherkin DC, MacCornack FA, Berg AO: The management of low back pain—a comparison of the beliefs and behaviors of family physicians and chiropractors. *West J Med* 149:475, 1988.
72. Cherkin DC: Patient satisfaction as an outcome measure. *Chiropr Technique* 2:138–142, 1990.
73. Lawrence DJ: General overview of the chiropractic profession. In Bergmann TB, Peterson DH, Lawrence DJ: *Chiropractic Technique: Principles and Procedures*. New York, Churchill Livingstone, 1993, p 6.
74. Terrett AGJ: Vascular accidents from cervical spine manipulation: Report on 107 cases. *J Aust Chiropr Assoc* 17:15–24, 1987.
75. Ferezy JS: Neural ischemia and cervical manipulation: An acceptable risk. *Am Chiropractic Assoc J Chiropr* 22:61–63, 1988.

Contemporary Approach to Understanding Chiropractic Technique

Robert Cooperstein, M.A., D.C.
Associate Professor, Palmer College of Chiropractic West, San Jose, California

Chiropractors today, as in the past, tend to affiliate themselves with certain named *technique systems*, or *proprietary techniques*. How this has come about, in what ways it may be changing, and in response to what driving forces are the subjects of this chapter.

CHIROPRACTIC AS ART, SCIENCE, AND PHILOSOPHY—BUT ESPECIALLY ART

Although it is often stated that chiropractic is an art, a science, and a philosophy,[1,2] the science and the philosophy would be of little interest if the art of chiropractic, *clinical chiropractic technique*, were not so effective. The evidence in support of this contention was most recently and comprehensively evaluated by economist Pran Manga[3] in a review funded by the Ontario Ministry of Health. The profession has bred a sizable and enthusiastic following of exceedingly loyal patients[4] and an equally enthusiastic hoard of enemies and rivals consumed by fear and loathing. Neither the loyalty nor the hatred devolve primarily from people's attitudes about the science or philosophy of chiropractic, the superstructures that are erected above the real, material practice of clinical chiropractic. What energizes advocates and detractors alike, the phenomenon that ushers the profession toward its centennial celebration alive and well, is that chiropractic might very well be the most effective treatment for somatogenic pain.

Two tracks in empirical research have converged to put a favorable spotlight on chiropractic treatment. On the one hand, there have been randomized clinical trials (RCTs) of manipulation and subsequent meta-analysis of these trials[5] that clearly indicate manipulation of the spine to be more effective than other treatments, including the treatment of no treatment. A recent Rand report, following an extensive review of the literature, lists many of these RCTs.[6] On the other hand, there have been so-called *pragmatic studies*, most recently the Meade study, where patients are randomly assigned to either "medical" or "chiropractic" treatment.[7] These studies tend to support the relative superiority, both clinically and economically, of chiropractic treatment. The RCTs of manipulation and the chiropractic vs. medicine pragmatic studies intersect at the interpretive point where chiropractic, uniquely among the professions that practice manual medicine, specializes in manipulation.[8]

CHIROPRACTIC TECHNIQUE QUA TECHNIQUE

The practice of science involves knowledge that has been attained through specialized methods of fact finding, research, and interpretation. These methods establish ways of thinking and understanding that distinguish their practitioners from the quotidian mental habits and limited knowledge base of the average citizen. The ensemble of such methods warrants the descriptive term "technique" in the sense of a body of technical and conceptual procedures by which the knowledge accrues and the science advances. Any particular scientific profession—economics, psychology, physics, chiropractic, and all the rest—consists in the tooled knowledge,[9] the *technique*, that establish its unique professional identity. Chiropractic science, or technique in the expanded sense of the term, is thus a kind of tooled knowledge that has focused historically on "the relationship between structure (primarily the spine) and function (primarily the nervous system) of the human body that leads to the restoration and preservation of health."[10]

Unlike professions in which the toolbox is primarily or even exclusively conceptual (e.g., economics), chiropractic technique employs a very significant psychomotor component as well. This means it has something in common with the "technique" of a dancer or martial artist: an appreciable component of chiropractic technique has to do with the perfection of a series of physical maneuvers. This fact partially explains the great diversity in proprietary chiropractic techniques, each distinguished from the others by both its unique physical style and what may be called the *artistic conception* from which it derives its animus. Nevertheless, chiropractic technique is more than the sum of its named technique systems and very much more than the collection of psychomotor skills with which it is occasionally equated. More amazing than the mind-numbing gaggle of separate technique systems[11] is the mind-boggling success of the chiropractic profession to keep it all under one technique hat. How do so many strange bedfellows get along so well? Probably because no matter how substantively different and even inconsistent the techniques may be, the great majority of them seem equally at home among just a few sweeping phrases and organizing principles: Subluxation, Nerve Interference, the Adjustment, and the relationship of structure and function.

It may seem odd at first to emphasize the moderating, harmonizing role of the chiropractic technique umbrella, given how often we are reminded that "chiropractors have been waging war against themselves for 90 odd years,"[12] and that "the chiropractic technic wars go on, with 'new' technics coming and going as frequently as woman's fashions."[13] The conventional wisdom at play here fails to appreciate that "technic wars" are not entirely unlike Pepsi vs. Coke confrontations, where both beverage companies have a common long-term interest in promoting cola vs. flavored teas, no matter the short-term struggle over market share. Likewise, the chiropractic wars are very often largely over infrastructure: scope of practice, terminology, case management, billing practices, relations with allied health professionals, and college curricula.

These *ideological confrontations* stand apart from and may even conceal essential agreement over the basics: chiropractic treats the spine, usually with manipulation, which helps the nerves, which promotes health. Two chiropractors who could kill one another over the vaccination issue might be in perfect accord on subluxation detection and correction, whereas another pair of doctors at odds over manipulative vs. soft tissue techniques might be willing to live and let live, provided they share the ultimate goal of reducing "nerve interference."[14] Of course, this would not stop either one from claiming his or her own methods would be a better way to achieve the desired end!

PROLIFERATION OF CHIROPRACTIC TECHNIQUE SYSTEMS

Granted a certain degree of technique congruity at the highest level of abstraction, chiropractic has always enjoyed a somewhat startling variety of different implementations (Table 1) of that universal technique.[15-17] Almost from the beginning chiropractic fragmented into a series of competitive, often mutually exclusive techniques,[18] each claiming to be largely self-sufficient for addressing either the totality or an expansive range of human ailments.[11]

A similar situation prevails in the field of martial arts. Although all practitioners share a certain kinship as martial artists, none of them would think of incorporating, say, a karate move into a jujitsu routine. When it comes to the martial arts (read: one of the proprietary chiropractic tech-

TABLE 1.
Partial Listing of Proprietary Techniques

Activator Methods	Logan Basic
Applied Kinesiology	Mears
Applied Spinal Biomechanical Engineering	Meric
	Motion Palpation
Atlas Orthagonality	Network
Atlas Specific/HIO	Neuro Organization
Bioenergetic Synchronization	Nimmo Receptor Tonus
Blair Upper Cervical	Nucca
Chiropractic Biophysics	Ortmann
Concept Therapy	Pettibon Spinal Biomechanics
Cox Flexion-Distraction	Pierce-Stillwagon
Craniopathy	Sacro-Occipital
Directional Non-force	Stressology
Diversified	Thompson
Endonasal	Toftness
Gonstead	Total Body Modification
	Truscott

niques), purity is everything, and allegiance to the sensei (technique innovator) is automatic. Although one supposes that chiropractors on the average tend to be less rigid than martial artists, they remain arguably closer to the rigidity of the latter than to the flexibility one would expect in an integrated approach to patient care.

Although medicine in its entirety is not divided up in an analogous fashion into proprietary technique systems, a similar phenomenon does exist within at least one of its specialties: psychiatry. The Freudian, Jungian, Reichian, gestalt, and other psychoanalytic techniques constitute complete systems, offering up very different diagnostic and treatment approaches to the same range of psychoneurotic conditions. Psychiatrists are not exactly thrilled with this internal technique war but are no more able than chiropractors to escape the consequences of highly imperfect knowledge, one of the primary causes of technique proliferation, discussed later on.

WHY THERE ARE SO MANY TECHNIQUE SYSTEMS

The bewildering array of mutually exclusive chiropractic techniques, each claiming to be the legitimate pretender to the medical throne, requires some explanation. Although much of this spectacle is of little redeeming value, it remains entirely possible that where back care languishes for lack of imagination, even chaos has its advantages. It is easy to point an accusatory finger at the custodians of proprietary technique—yes, they confuse the public, make insupportable claims, and ignore standard scientific method—but these same technique mavens, past and present, are the ones who have reduced to practice much of what will evolve into the more responsible generic technique just over the horizon. The technique spectacle, past and present, deserves no less than a healthy admixture of constructive and destructive criticism.

DEVELOPMENT AT THE MARGIN

Chiropractic today displays just the sort of methodological diversity that one would expect of a discipline that developed on the fringes of the organized health care profession. It is always at the margins of society that freedom of experimentation commingles with reckless adventurism, that lack of regulation breeds simultaneously bold innovation and abject quackery. The phenomenon is not unlike the explosion of new life forms that is seen when existing species rush in to exploit a new biological niche that suddenly opens up after a geological catastrophe or other rapid and major environmental change.

Human society can hopefully exercise more restraint than natural selection, which, although ensuring survival of the fittest, undoubtedly discards many promising biological innovations that are unfortunately coupled to environmentally unsuccessful strategies, what amount to failed genetic experiments. It would be unfortunate if under the guise of bringing order to the house of technique the chiropractic profession were to throw out the kernels of analytic truth and clinical utility that surely reside in some of its most dirty bathwater. This fear is acknowledged in both the chiropractic and medical settings when every measure to standardize the delivery of health care evokes the same refrain: "Cookbook health care will stifle research and innovation."[19] Of course, it is equally true that continued technique chaos will risk excluding chiropractic from national health care and worsen its position in a managed care environment.

LACK OF MARKET PENETRATION

Revolutionaries without a revolution always do the same thing. When their messianic zeal to transform society stumbles in the face of the predictable establishment backlash, their movement fragments into an assortment of political sects that have no option left except to transform each other (e.g., the American "New Left" around 1975). Rage against the status quo transmutes into multilateral civil war, which flares up from time to time in direct proportion to the magnitude of the lost opportunities. Chiropractic, which has always behaved like and regarded itself as something of a movement, cannot escape the internal consequences of long-term marginalization.

Although chiropractic is the nation's third largest primary health care profession, with 50,000 practitioners in North America alone, only 1 in 20 Americans obtains chiropractic treatment in any one year.[15] Given that the point prevalence of low back pain alone is 5% to 30% and that 80% of all people suffer from low back pain at some time in their lives,[3, 20, 21] it does not appear that chiropractors have been able to take their case effectively to the public. No doubt medical and media chiro-bashing have compounded the problem. For an entire century chiropractic has struggled to become a mass movement but has been unable to attract suitable numbers of adherents (patients). Although failed movements go away and victorious movements immediately close ranks, the frustrations of partial success sow disunity and foster internecine struggle. Such is the situation of chiropractic today, as it has always been.

THE ECONOMIC ADVANTAGE OF RETAINING SEVERAL TECHNIQUES

Consumers are presented with a bewildering array of choices in the health care market: medicine, chiropractic, acupuncture, nutritional supplements, biofeedback, and so forth.[22] Health care providers, just like the vendors of other sorts of goods and services, are subject to market forces that drive them to strive for product diversification and the establishment of brand names.

To some extent consumer choice is governed by pure geography, the amount of space occupied on the shelf by given brands, say, of health care professions. Assume the simplest competitive case imaginable: that consumers are constrained to choose between medical and chiropractic care. Let us suppose that the choice is purely dichotomous, that the public is indifferent between the two, and that both chiropractic and medicine wind up with half of the market. Now, have some chiropractors segment themselves into a number of well-defined, mutually exclusive techniques: technique 1, technique 2, and technique 3. Classic microeconomic theory predicts that the market share for chiropractic as a whole will probably increase relative to medicine, because the consumers' choice is no longer purely dichotomous, medicine vs. chiropractic, but multilateral: medicine vs. chiro-technique 1 vs. chiro-technique 2 vs. chiro-technique 3 (Fig 1).[23]

Although proprietary chiropractic techniques are not literally brands on the shelf, consumer choice is still governed partially by such *psychogeographic* considerations.[24] The chiropractic alternative to medicine occupies a larger psychic space in the consumer's mind to the extent it is divided into several technique systems. Of course, there is no net benefit to any existing individual chiropractic producer when a new brand of technique is invented, because his or her market share may decline even if chiropractic as a whole were to increase its share relative to medicine. As for the newcomer, he or she is bound to observe Boulding's *principle of minimum differentiation*: "Make your product as like the existing products as you can without destroying the differences."[25]

Technique proliferation may reach a point where the variety of techniques itself becomes confusing, especially if some of the brands are of very questionable quality. In such a case, each new product introduction risks engendering what economists call a "negative externality," a kind of backlash effect. The public may eventually develop a preference for health care services sold in a more stable and coherent market. We all know how hard medicine has worked to be that preferred market but not without some deep misgivings about sacrificing market share to a suite of more exciting "unconventional" therapies.[22]

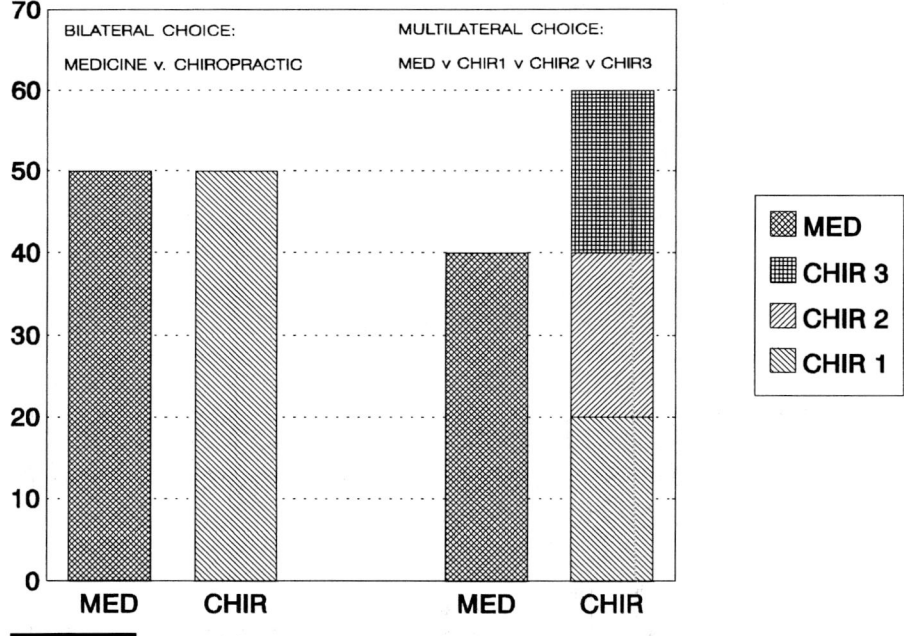

FIGURE 1.
Chiropractic and medicine: market segmentation.

THE CHIROPRACTOR AS A GENERALIST

The chiropractor who wishes to distinguish himself or herself from another—and there are always purely commercial reasons to do so—must do so on the basis of the particular type of technique used rather than conditions or types of patients treated. This accrues to the simple fact that most chiropractors claim to be generalists treating a great variety of diseases, even though most patients have musculoskeletal complaints.[15] By comparison, the majority of medical doctors are specialists, distinguishing themselves from one another by the organ systems addressed and the range of patients and diseases treated.

MERCANTILE BENT OF THE FOUNDERS

There is no need to harp on the fact that both of the Palmers, especially the son, were very susceptible to purely commercial considerations and were not adverse to lurid, sensationalist advertising claims for the advantages of chiropractic care.[26] Chiropractors certainly possess no monopoly on the possession of a certain human frailty by which entrepreneurial interests occasionally displace scientific and clinical concerns off to the side. The question is not so much why overtly philistine technique vendors have been so numerous, but *why they have gone so unchecked and even unopposed* until fairly recently.

LACK OF KNOWLEDGE

Although *actual data* and *substantive research* should constitute the best potential check on technique hyperbole, there have been many phenomena germane to chiropractic procedures that have so far defied explanation and resisted investigation. Throughout most of its history, chiropractic, not unlike other "soft sciences," has endured wild speculation concerning its basic phenomena. It has witnessed a plethora of hypotheses governing the nature of the chiropractic subluxation and the mechanism of the chiropractic adjustment. Such speculation is not only necessary but desirable, insofar as future knowledge takes root in the theoretical constructs of the present.

Although it is never true that "one opinion is as good as another," until fairly recently the research community was simply not up to the task of counteracting the endless unfolding of the technique spectacle. In a word, the technique innovators on the medicine ball circuit flourished because they *could*. Competition has been fierce.

Everyone knows about the lack of funding for research and how long it took to develop the quantity and quality of human resources required to get research done in chiropractic (the current status of which is arguably the best in any field of manual medicine). Apart from the lack of a research-based moderating influence, chiropractic has suffered from the presence of endemic, intraprofessional obstacles to developing a chiropractic science. Keating[27,28] discusses three intraprofessional barriers to the emergence of chiropractic science: a theosophic, fundamentalist belief in innate intelligence; a rationalist bent toward deducing chiropractic methods from the "immutable laws of biology"; and the empiricist "belief that private, uncontrolled clinical experience is sufficient to support, legitimize, and guide the art and science."

Although the fairly recent explosion of data has narrowed down the field of legitimate conjecture considerably, not everyone has noticed. As a teacher in a chiropractic college, I have observed that a significant minority of students, confronted with a research study that invalidates some cherished chiropractic procedure, are likely to respond, "Oh, those crazy researchers, there they go again." Such remarks are also common in the letters section of our journals and other trade publications. On the other hand, Robert Jansen's large-scale survey on chiropractors' attitudes toward practice standards and the organizations developing them showed surprising support for research; for example, only 8% agreed with the statement that "chiropractic methods do not need to be validated."[8]

THE QUEST FOR "NERVE INTERFERENCE"

Because chiropractors have always hung their hat on the hook of "nerve interference," it should be noted that the consequences of a hypothetical subclinical neuropathy, occurring at the histological level, may be extraordinarily difficult to detect.[29] No one has any problem in diagnosing severe nerve damage, because there are obvious neurological deficits: anesthesia, muscle weakness, altered deep tendon reflexes, and so forth. In the absence of so-called hard neurologicals, chiropractors have claimed to detect neuropathy by the presence of pain, tenderness, altered galvanic skin response, surface skin temperature asymmetry, peculiar electromagnetic radiations, "reflexes" of different kinds, and so on.

Because few of these have been particularly convincing, a perennial market has been created for the proclamation of new and increasingly outlandish indicators, which has greatly enriched the technique spectacle. If anything over the years has represented something of a chiropractic golden fleece, it would be the heroic effort to demonstrate "nerve interference," that is, mild or even subclinical neuropathy, that would supposedly accompany minor articular misalignment and altered motion characteristics.

THE ALLURE OF BRAND NAME TECHNIQUES[30]

Chiropractic science has developed to the point that like other maturing sciences, it has been able to cast off the tiresome arrogance of the neophyte, having assumed instead a firm grasp on its limitations. Although this exercise in humility has been necessary and desirable, it has inadvertently rendered chiropractors and chiropractic students increasingly vulnerable to the exploitation of the technique hawkers. They offer us what a disabused appraisal of the state of the arts cannot: absolute conviction in the value of the technique for sale, including the smoke and mirrors of its ideological accounterment.

The simple truth is that those technique evangelists who incessantly denounce "The Subluxation" and deify "The Adjustment" can gather up quite a bit of monomaniacal steam and, like Ahab in pursuit of the whale, be seen as invested with undauntable purpose. They can skillfully link their particular bag of metaphysical and psychomotor tools with a whole set of purely extraneous, unrelated values: loyalty to chiropractic, staunch opposition to medical expropriation, quality service to patients, and above all, the daily accomplishment of miracles.

Scientifically based chiropractors do not rant and rave about "The Subluxation" and "The Adjustment." Good science by its very nature automatically desanctifies the standard totems. However, deconsecrating religious symbols has its price, especially if no secular model of equal interest is constructed. It is unrealistic to expect chiropractors to become as excited about "research" as they were about "subluxation" and "adjustment." Likewise, it is more difficult to promote generic technique than brand name techniques, which bear the stamp of the guru and the cross of religious conviction. The most sought-after item on today's seminar circuit is the promised relief from the anxiety of negative research findings. This mandates to the colleges and the journals the task of reconciling clinical chiropractic with clinical uncertainty, which entails directly confronting the anachronistic barking of the technique evangelists.

THE GLASS HOUSE EFFECT

No hard and fast line separates what is known from what is not known, not even science from myth. Rather, there is a continuum that defines the fabric of reality, stretching from abject nonsense to proven fact. Where an individual practitioner situates himself or herself on this very elastic fabric is to some degree a question of taste. In a science where so much remains "investigational," traditionalist chiropractors seek comfort in the science of myth, whereas more contemporary practitioners seem more at home in the myth of science.[31]

Ideally speaking, the chiropractic profession would weed from its garden those methods that stretch credibility to the point of incredulity, but there is a fundamental problem in doing so: only the thinnest of margins separate officially endorsed "mainstream" chiropractic methods from those out of the mainstream. These latter earn a variety of epithets, anything from "unorthodox" to "experimental" to "quackery," depending on the nay-sayer's degree of charity and sometimes professional rivalry. Admittedly, it may seem odd that Doctor X gets his listings from aura analysis and adjusts the spine with forces not in excess of 1 oz, but where is the evidence that Doctor Y, a motion palpator, possesses superior diagnostic acumen or gets better clinical outcomes? To apply an old adage, those who live in glass houses shouldn't throw stones.

I attend meetings of a chiropractic grouping that is routinely approached by the various states that seek an opinion on what defines a legitimate chiropractic technique, what is mainstream compared with what is fringe. Up to now, this group has been unwilling to render such positions and only partially because of the legal exposure attached to taking positions that could cause material harm to individual technique innovators and organizations. Individuals within this grouping are uneasy that the same logic that drives a particular state to reject some techniques will one day point the finger at their own favored techniques. It is not clear whether they should be defending practice rights for all but the most obviously eccentric "doctors," or enjoining the nascent profession-wide attack on quackery. One sees a similar kind of dilemma (although over political, not scientific issues) when an organization such as the American Civil Liberties Union defends the rights of neo-Nazis to hurl ugly epithets at holocaust survivors.

THE SPECTACLE OF PSEUDOSCIENTIFIC TECHNIQUE

The generally perceived need for more research in chiropractic seems to have become important at about the time the profession was becoming more nationally accepted by the mid-1970s. In the absence of hard data, this need was at first filled by two groups of allied practitioners.

First, there were technique innovator/vendor types who promoted *chiropractic scientism*, primarily in the form of abstract spinal models and abstruse adjusting formulas. These developed mostly as a full-spine application of the formularized upper cervical work that began in the 1930s. (Economist Hayek[9] used the term "scientism" to refer to the inappropriate attempt to emulate the methods of mathematical physics in an inappropriate field.) The innovator/vendor types overreacted to the well-nigh absence of research in chiropractic by claiming for themselves a level of precision and of certainty that would be considered unattainable in the hard sciences, even with their more extensive financial and human resources.

Second, there arose *marketing experts* who intuitively understood that pseudoscience would soon become the most contemporary and effective means of product differentiation on the chiropractic technique circuit. In their hands, the uncertainty with which chiropractors routinely deal has led to a genre of "research" that may as well be called the *plausibility study*: "Since this study described a neuroma associated with a glandular problem, then it may be true that subluxation can account for problems x, y, and z."

Keating,[28] writing of such plausibility studies, states that "rationalism involves the belief that methods of clinical practice that are logically derived, or potentially derivable, from knowledge of the basic sciences are therefore 'scientifically valid' (and implicitly effective and safe)." These largely one-sided reviews of the literature tend to select studies hypothetically in support of chiropractic theories and ignore contrasting evidence. The cited articles are often unrelated to the points being made.

If the scientismists capitalize on the spectacle of technique, the marketeers exploit the technique of spectacle. That is why they often wind up on the same program at association meetings and on the seminar circuit. The techniques elaborated by the scientismists and the plausibility studies amassed by the marketeers, rather than replacing the more traditional proprietary techniques, stood side by side in a now-enlarged technique pageant.

There is no point in condemning those who put forth the facade of research to fill the research vacuum, no matter how crass their motives or how much violence was done to accepted standards of scientific work. These individuals served the historical role of irreversibly formulating a new agenda for chiropractic: in the future, it would have to prove and not merely posit its clinical utility and, what's more, demonstrate that its methodology in concept and practice was consistent with normal science. If the scientismists made mistakes, so be it. If someone had not made these mistakes, thrown down the research gauntlet to the colleges and the journals, it is highly unlikely that the bona fide research milieu would have taken the strides that now usher the profession toward rational technique.

By the mid-1980s less ambitious but more careful researchers were painstakingly gathering data on the types of patients and conditions seen by chiropractors and performing small-scale but often effective studies on the reliability of chiropractic diagnostic procedures. This type of research is less dramatic than that of the model crunchers and armchair speculators, but is a harbinger of better times to come.

CHIROPRACTIC TECHNIQUE AND THE COLLEGES

Given the awesome diversity of techniques practiced in the field, it is not immediately obvious how the chiropractic colleges should decide on a technique curriculum. The difficulty in establishing defensible criteria by which fringe and mainstream techniques could be distinguished becomes exceedingly problematic in the chiropractic colleges, where the decision to teach a given technique is invariably interpreted by some students as a decision not to teach some other technique. As Lawrence[32] points out, "The grass is always greener on the other side"—at the other chiropractic colleges, at the weekend technique seminar that rolls into town, during the lunchtime technique club meetings, at the offices of local field doctors, and so on.

A lack of up-to-date, comprehensive textbooks has compounded the problem. Nothing defines the scope of a subject better than a textbook, even a poor book. There have always been works that could be construed as textbooks of chiropractic, but they were limited in one way or another. Many have limited themselves to discussion of the particular technique system espoused, some were simple technique manuals or seminar notes, others were de facto treatises on philosophy, and still others were little more than pictorial albums of moves. This situation has changed rapidly, with a recent explosion of chiropractic textbooks (Table 2).

Chiropractic colleges must first decide whether they want to teach named techniques in their purity, devise an eclectic program of generic technique, or compromise on the issue in some way. Most seem to have settled on this last option, featuring a core curriculum of generic technique that is supplemented by electives and college-sponsored continuing education programs featuring named techniques.

A generic technique core curriculum solves several problems:

1. It avoids inculcating the absurd notion that a patient with a given problem could be successfully treated by any number of mutually exclusive and very clinically different technique methods.
2. It deals honestly with the time limitations common to all the colleges by emphasizing elements that different technique systems have in common.

TABLE 2.
Recently Published Comprehensive Chiropractic Textbooks

Title	Author	Yr
Clinical Biomechanics: Musculoskeletal Actions and Reactions, ed 2	Schafer RC	1987
Chiropractic Management of Spine-Related Disorders	Gatterman MI	1990
Fundamentals of Chiropractic Diagnosis and Management	Lawrence DJ (ed)	1991
Principles and Practice of Chiropractic, ed 2	Haldeman S (ed)	1992
Textbook of Clinical Chiropractic: A Specific Biomechanical Approach	Plaugher G (ed)	1993
Chiropractic Technique	Bergmann T, Peterson DH, Lawrence DJ	1994
Chiropractic Therapy: Diagnosis and Treatment	Eder M, Tilsher H	1990

3. It keeps the college at least formally independent from the crass commercialism of the technique vendors and the sensationalism of the snake oil circuit.
4. It is harmonious with the contemporary emphasis on practice guidelines and standards of care, which is strictly incompatible with the anarchy and autonomy that rules in the land of proprietary techniques.

TAXONOMY OF CHIROPRACTIC TECHNIQUE

The quantity of stand-alone chiropractic techniques out there boggles the mind, and one must be thankful that some individuals and organizations have had the temerity to attempt cataloging the mass.[15, 16, 33, 34] It is now necessary to go one step further by producing a Linnaean-type classification of chiropractic techniques, hopefully allowing reduction categorization according to a few key organizing principles. Given this task is well beyond my current scope, it might be helpful to list and briefly describe a few of the relevant parameters, emphasizing issues that have become bones of contention.

The profession currently entertains a variety of debates that are not herein discussed because they involve technique only indirectly. These issues include the appropriate scope of practice, the chiropractor as primary care provider, and the effect of chiropractic care on visceral conditions.[35, 36]

Some of the distinctions in the discussions that follow transect some of the others, creating in effect a multidimensional matrix of technique characterizations. The term "subluxation" is used not in its medical dictionary sense but to signify (for the sake of convenience) the spinal pathologic condition that the majority of chiropractors profess to treat. Although in some cases representative examples are given that conform mostly to the categorizations, it should be remembered that no shoe ever fits perfectly.

SEGMENTALISM VS. POSTURALISM

Given that few individual chiropractors reside entirely within one of these two extreme positions, for the purposes of discussion we will characterize them as mutually exclusive methodological positions. The *segmentalist* believes that cranial-spinal-pelvic entities occur at specific motion segments consisting of two bones, be they vertebrae, the skull, any of the pelvic bones, or combinations thereof. The subluxation in the specific motion segment may result in postural distortions such as scoliosis in the frontal plane and loss or exaggeration of the two kyphotic and two lordotic curves in the sagittal plane. These postural distortions are seen as *compensatory* consequences of specific motion segment subluxations and not as the problems in and of themselves. Examples of segmentalism include the Gonstead[37, 38] and Diversified Techniques.[39, 40]

The *posturalist* (Montgomery uses the term "structuralist" to refer to a similar position[18]) sees postural distortion as the subluxation in and of itself and offers up a language of listings that describes the linear and angular relationship of entire regions of the cranial-spinal-pelvic articulations. A given motion segment may exhibit more signs and symptoms of dysfunction than another, but this is the consequence rather than the cause of the primary postural distortion. The posturalist claims that the spine subluxates as groupings of adjacent vertebrae and is to be adjusted accordingly, with relatively nonspecific contacts. Examples of posturalism include the Chiropractic Biophysics Technique,[41] Spinal Biomechanics,[42] and Logan Basic Technique.[43]

MISALIGNMENT VS. FIXATION

Although it has been traditional for chiropractors to emphasize the static positional relationships of vertebrae, the last 15 years have witnessed a heightened and perhaps even dominant interest in the function of vertebral motion segments.[44, 45] When it comes to describing the spinal entity under treatment, chiropractic traditionalists continue to favor the word "subluxation" in the sense of bony misalignment, whereas the motion palpators tend to use the word "dysfunction." It is likely that very few chiropractors situate themselves at either the "crooked bone" or "sticky joint" extremes and that most of them can be located somewhere on a continuum where both sets of considerations are taken into account.

Those who continue to emphasize vertebral misalignment can trace their lineage in virtually every detail straight back to the founder himself, DD Palmer. Bones misalign, partially occlude the intervertebral foramen, produce nerve interference, and eventually cause disease.[1, 10, 46]

Regarding the motion palpators, in its purity their main methodological position is that if all segments of the spine and pelvis are free to move in all their anatomically allowable ranges of motion, the neuromuscular control mechanism will achieve that organization that maximizes the efficiency of body function. At the limit, the disregard for positional relationships is so extreme that it vanishes: even what appears to be a hyperextended segment should be adjusted toward greater extension, if examination shows that to be a direction in which movement is limited.[46]

Arguably the most extensively tested of the chiropractic diagnostic procedures, motion palpation has not been shown to have the reproducibility one would expect of a procedure so dominant at the chiropractic college level. Indeed, "fixation" resembles some kind of spinal "ether": virtually everyone is quite certain it is there, but no one can really touch it. Triano[47] reflects that "several efforts have been made to critically examine interrater reliability with very troubling results." (One wonders how many negative studies were never published.)

STRUCTURE VS. FUNCTION

Until fairly recently the majority of chiropractors took it for granted that chiropractic clinical intervention fundamentally addressed the structure of the body, because the body's structure supposedly determined its function, unlike architecture where "form follows function." In this way chiropractic doctors would treat the structural "cause of dis-ease," whereas the competition, the medical profession, would treat only its symptoms, expressed as disturbance of function.

The fundamental problem that has come up is that in the majority of cases, the anatomical cause of the back pain, the actual pain generator, is unknown.[48, 49] Therefore, it would be very difficult to say whether the pain is related to structural or functional problems. It has become clear that there is very poor correspondence of imaging results, including degenerative changes, and patient symptoms.[21, 50, 51] The question raised is what are we to say about back pain for which no specific pathoanatomical lesion can be demonstrated objectively? Do we continue to say that surely there must be some structural lesion, even though we just can't seem to find it? Or do we relegate all of these cases to a gigantic garbage can, a default option called "dysfunction" or maybe "functional disturbance"? In other words, *are we to believe in structure or function?*

Clouding the issue is the fact that about the only *outcome measures* that are holding up are essentially functional in character, especially pain reduction and patient subjective satisfaction. Of course it is one thing to validate functional outcome assessment and quite another to opine that the patient's lesion is functional in character. Worse yet would be to suppose that "functional" treatment of muscles and soft tissues is preferred to spinal manipulation. These are perfect non sequiturs. How sad it would be if the chiropractic profession, after one century of defending osseous spinal manipulation, were to become so seduced by the admitted utility of functional outcome measures that it actually forgot what it was that produced the outcomes being measured!

ANATOMICOPHYSIOLOGICAL VS. REFLEX TECHNIQUES

What is at issue here is the basic conception of how the body works. Some techniques are essentially physiological in that the examination and treatment measures are applied in keeping with the standard anatomicophysiological description of body function. Such technique systems understand that much remains to be learned but do not invent largely data-free, previously nondescribed, and wildly imaginative alternative physiologies to fill in the voids in the meantime.

By "reflex technique" we denote technique systems in which observations, palpatory contacts, or other maneuvers relevant to a given part of the body or organ system can provide information or achieve distant effects at other points—muscles, organs, joints—even in cases where no known anatomical or physiological connection can be demonstrated. (Of course, there are many contexts in which the term "reflex" is used in the usual way: deep tendon reflex, somatovisceral reflex, pathological reflex, etc.) Each of the following reflex techniques finds adherents in chiropractic today: iridology, auricular therapy, occipital fiber palpation, organ-muscle relationships, and neurovascular points. Examples of reflex technique include Sacro-Occipital Technique[52] and Applied Kinesiology.[53]

FORCEFUL VS. LIGHT-FORCE (AND EVEN NON-FORCE) TECHNIQUES

Although chiropractors, both in their own and in the public mind, have always been chiefly identified with the high-velocity, low-amplitude (HVLA) thrust, there has always been a strong undercurrent of light-force and even purported non-force[54] technique systems. Expanded interest in soft tissue rehabilitation in recent years has perhaps increased interest in light-force methods.

Although "light-force" technique is sometimes regarded as synonymous with "reflex" technique, this is not entirely accurate. Logan, for example, considered the mode of correction of his light contact to be purely mechanical, in opposition to some of his critics at the time who opined that the basic contact exerted its effects through a neurological reflex. The latter presumed an influence on ganglion impar, where the two pelvic sympathetic trunks converge anterior to the coccyx.

Another common misconception is to suppose that light-force and soft-tissue oriented practitioners have somehow abandoned the traditional concept that vertebral misalignment results in nerve interference and altered body function. Nimmo[14] and his contemporary followers[55] have suggested that bones subluxate largely because muscles pull them into misalignment. Take care of the muscles, by direct digital pressure on trigger points, and the spine will take care of itself. Nimmo[14] looked with some derision on such chiropractors as Bennett[56] and osteopaths such as Chapman (whose work is described by Chaitow[57]) who were contemporaneously developing systems of organ therapy based on somatic reflex points—neurovascular or neurolymphatic points, respectively.

In a way, despite his apparent disdain for the direct manipulative thrust, Nimmo is a perfectly traditionalist chiropractor, because his therapeutic goal is to reduce nerve interference using the muscles more than the bones as egress into the system. This illustrates the lack of distinction of osseous from soft tissue techniques at the level of the neurological sequelae that have been postulated. Examples of light-force techniques include activator,[58] Logan Basic,[43] and Nimmo's Receptor Tonus.[14]

CHARACTERIZATION OF TECHNIQUE PROCEDURES

Bartol[17, 59] engaged in a concerted effort to categorize specific treatment procedures but not named techniques per se (Fig 2). Procedures are classified as either manual or nonmanual. If manual, they are further classified as either articular or nonarticular. If articular, they are then classified as specific, nonspecific, mechanically assisted, or mechanical, and finally, as HV-HA, HV-LA, LV-HA, or LV-LA (where H is high, L is low, V is velocity, and A is amplitude).

Good[60] went further in a kinematic direction, attempting to categorize the *mechanisms* of manual, articular procedures as a function of the doctor's setup and manner of thrusting.

Kaminski et al. developed an algorithm (Fig 3) by which the status of a chiropractic procedure may be evaluated and classified according to the following schema: provisional acceptance, full acceptance, or unsubstantiated.[61, 62]

PRACTICE PARAMETERS

The National Board of Chiropractic Examiners (NBCE) recently produced a comprehensive study entitled *Job Analysis of Chiropractic*,[15] in which there were 5,000 respondents to a survey instrument on the practice characteristics of chiropractic today. They were asked to indicate "the primary technique approach" used in their practices, where the possible choices were full spine, upper cervical, or other. The majority (93.3%) said they used primarily a full spine approach (Fig 4).

The NBCE survey also asked the respondents to check off those "adjustive techniques" among a supplied list of 20 that they had used during the last 2 years. Only four techniques—Diversified, Gonstead, Cox's, and Activator—were used by a majority of practitioners. The average practitioner reported using 5.7 of the techniques in his or her practice. It is interesting that 5 of the top 10 techniques would be classified as primarily soft tissue or reflex. Diversified, which probably comes closer to being generic (in the sense of eclectic) than any other of the listed techniques, is by far the most practiced technique system (Fig 5).

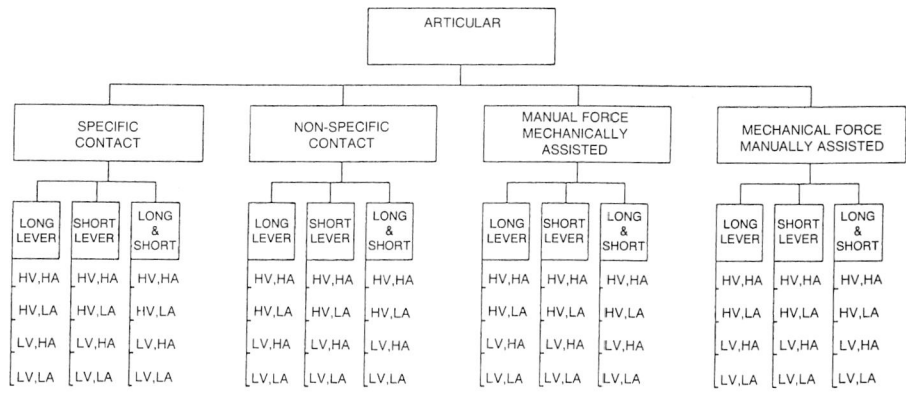

FIGURE 2.

Bartol's technique procedure algorithm. (From Bartol KM: *Chiropractic Technique* 4:8, 1992. Used by permission.)

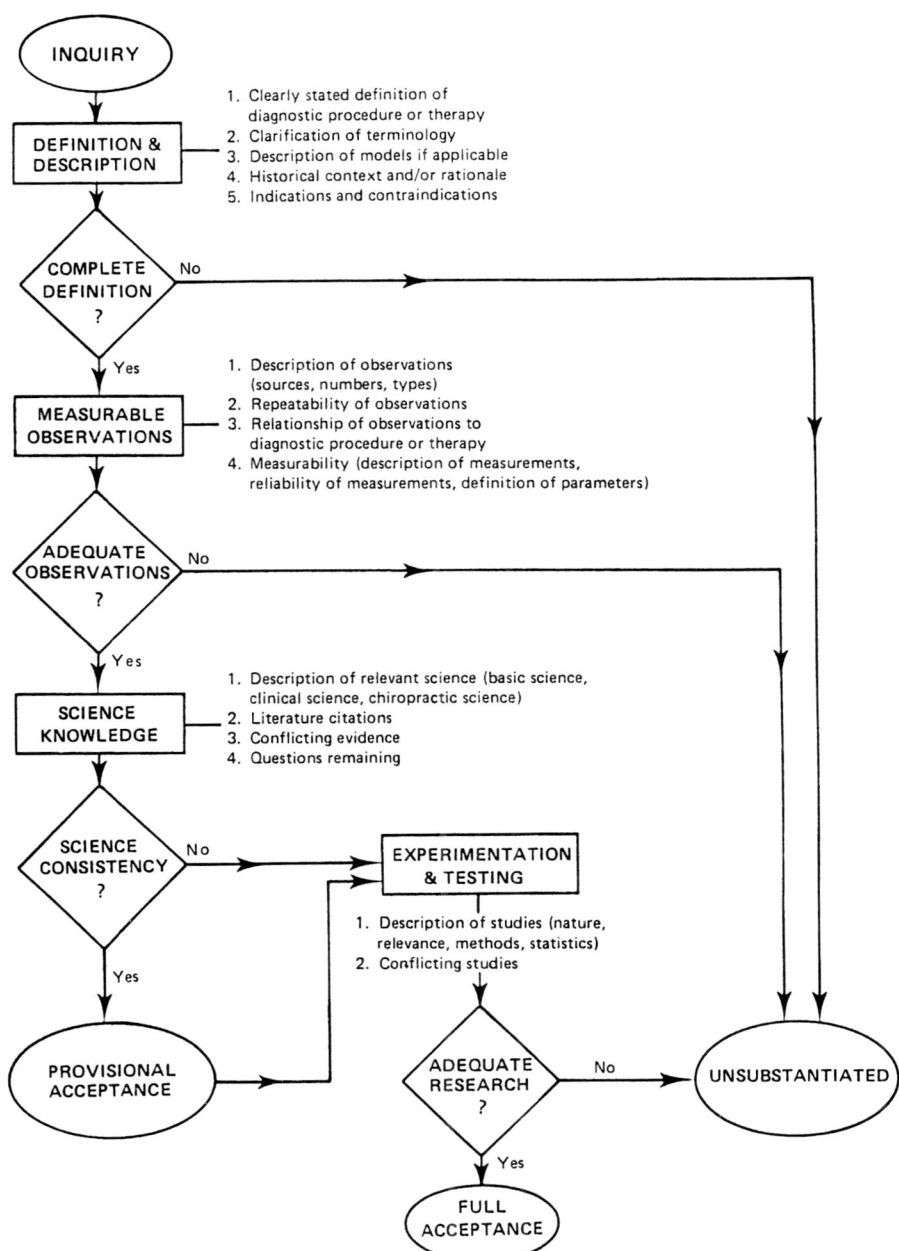

FIGURE 3.
Kaminski's protocol for technique evaluation. (From Kaminski M: *Chiropractic Technique* 2:3, 1990. Used by permission.)

Of course, it is not always easy to interpret surveys such as these. When a doctor purports, for example, to use the "Activator Technique," it is not clear whether the doctor uses the Activator Methods system of analysis or simply uses the percussive device associated with it, perhaps only occasionally. Likewise, the statement that the average doctor practices 5.7 techniques may be interpreted in a number of ways: (1) the av-

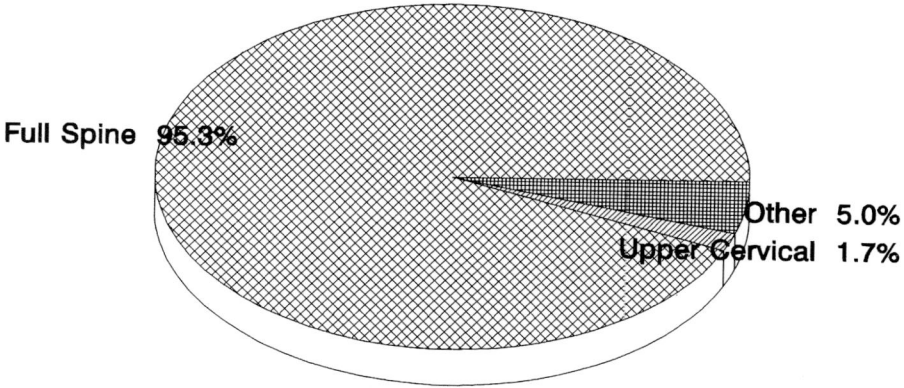

FIGURE 4.
Common chiropractic technique. (Adapted from Christensen MG: *Job Analysis of Chiropractic*. Greeley, Colo, National Board of Chiropractic Examiners, 1993, p 78.)

erage patient is diagnosed or treated during a given office visit with procedures borrowed from 5.7 techniques; (2) individual cases are managed such that one technique is used uniquely, any one of 5.7; or (3) during each office visit, the patient is treated with one specific technique, but which particular technique it is may vary from visit to visit.

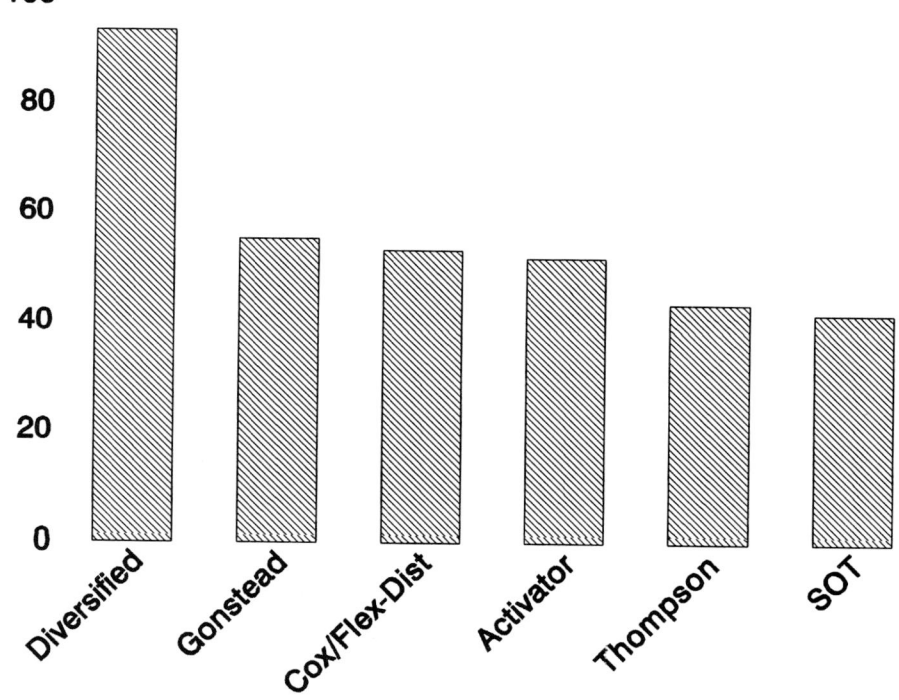

FIGURE 5.
Primary technique approaches. (Adapted from Christensen MG: *Job Analysis of Chiropractic*. Greeley, Colo, National Board of Chiropractic Examiners, 1993, p 150.)

THE CONSENSUS PROCESS

The entire August 1990 issue of *Chiropractic Technique* is devoted to the proceedings of the Consensus Conference of Validation of Chiropractic Methods, held March 2 and 3, 1990, in Seattle. Subsequent annual meetings of the Committee on Research and Education (CORE) of the California Chiropractic Association and its published proceedings have continued the consensus process initiated in Seattle. The Mercy Guidelines document also owes its origin to this same process in that it applies a modified form of the Kaminski protocol to the technique evaluation process and also employs Bartol's classification scheme.[63]

It is hard to overestimate the significance of what happened in Seattle. It marks the moment when the proprietary technique founders and leaders, although they did not exactly cede power to the more college-based and scientifically trained advocates of generic technique, at least agreed to play by the rules of normal science. There was widespread support for the Kaminski protocol, even though no contemporary technique procedure or therapy is particularly close to being validated by its standards. *Chiropractic Technique* editor Bergmann,[64] in his opening remarks, stated: "My expectation for this conference is to see a logical and rational beginning to the validation of chiropractic methods." The point cannot be better stated.

PRACTICE GUIDELINES AND STANDARDS OF CARE

The last few years have witnessed the emergence of practice guidelines and standards of care in chiropractic under the perceived pressure for the profession to come up with standards of care before such standards are quite simply imposed from without, whether by the various governments or the insurance industry.[65] This movement has created a window of opportunity for standardizing the terminology and practice characteristics across the proprietary techniques but has simultaneously provoked a fierce intraprofessional struggle. The frustration and resentment bred in some individuals by the guideline process, aggravating historically entrenched intraprofessional distrust and rivalry, has led to the emergence of not one but several "standards" of care.

As the battle lines keep shifting and organizations scramble to line up support for their positions, the named technique organizations have enjoyed a certain increase in their clout. A recent proposal (from the Congress of Chiropractic State Associations) that there be separate standards of care for each of the technique systems, were it to be taken seriously, would amount to a serious setback for the movement toward more generic and standardized technique. Indeed, relative to the burgeoning movement to rationalize chiropractic technique, it would amount to snatching defeat from the jaws of victory.

MANAGED HEALTH CARE: THE "BLACK BOX" OF TREATMENT

Although it now appears unlikely that the Clinton administration will be able to effect major change in the system of health care at the federal level, the rise of managed care within the existing system and the growing dominance of gatekeepers at all levels foreshadow a whole new method of evaluating chiropractic technique.

From the case manager's point of view (whether on behalf of the federal government, the insurer, a regional buying alliance, the workers compensation system, etc.) it should make little difference what goes on during a chiropractic office visit. There would be several treatment rooms, each designed for a different kind of care: chiropractic, medical, physical therapy, and acupuncture. Patients enter a room, something happens to them in there, and then they leave. The results are quantified with a variety of outcome measures: how patients feel, how they rate their overall treatment, how much it costs, when they are able to return to work.

The treatment rooms themselves, from the case manager's point of view, would be black boxes: patients enter, patients leave, but what goes on inside them is unknown and, what's more, is unimportant. If there is any arena in which chiropractic technique truly merits validation, it is in the high stakes game of managed care, where the winning hand should amount to nothing more than the best clinical results. Ironically, although the profession appears increasingly dissatisfied with worn out phrases such as "Chiropractic works,"[66] such platitudes appear to be the highest truths of the managed care environment.

Unfortunately, there is no guarantee that the chiropractic profession, all the clinical and cost-effectivity studies notwithstanding, will know how to play its cards effectively. In fact, society is not even sure that chiropractic deserves a seat at the gaming table. As long as chiropractors continue to exhibit overwhelming differences in their practice methods and belief structures, as long as chiropractic technique clings to its martial arts character, they risk noninclusion in the process of health care reform. There is one thing for sure: no matter how rapidly the landscape seems to shift, chiropractic will not be allowed to hold onto its idiosyncracies and simultaneously take part in the emerging managed care environment. The price for technique purity and continued indulgence in technique wars will be increased ostracism.

CONCLUSION

Dr. Albert Abrams,[67] considered a quack in his own time by his fellow medical doctors for emphasizing the role of the spine in human health, used these words to warn his colleagues 85 years ago against underestimating chiropractic:

> Others, less scientific but more astute, have determined empirically that manipulation of the spine does sometimes cure conditions which have failed of cure in the hands of experienced physicians. . . . Neither the fury of tongue nor the truculence of pen can gainsay the confidence that these systems of practice have inspired in the community.

Apart from a certain degree of public acceptance, the practice of chiropractic has many things going for it at this time: the Mercy guidelines, the Kaminski protocol, some high-quality journals, annual scientific symposia, growing intraprofessional insistence on scientific rigor, more money available for research, a bent toward generic technique in the colleges, increasing participation of proprietary techniques in consensus conferences and trade journals, a proliferation of comprehensive textbooks, and ongoing participation in interdisciplinary organizations such as the American Back Society. The only way chiropractic could falter in the near future would be by shooting itself in the foot. This could happen. All it would take would be an organized retreat back to technique spectacle, as chiropractors cast a furtive look at the brave new world of managed care—*and blink.*

REFERENCES

1. Palmer DD: *The Chiropractor's Adjuster, the Science, Art and Philosophy of Chiropractic.* Portland, Ore, Portland Printing House, 1910.
2. Stephenson RW: *Chiropractic Textbook.* Davenport, Iowa, Palmer School of Chiropractic, 1927.
3. Manga P: *The Effectiveness and Cost-Effectiveness of Chiropractic Management of Low-Back Pain.* Richmond Hill, Ontario, Canada, Kenilworth Publishing, 1993, p 104.
4. Cherkin D, MacCornack F: Patient evaluations of low back pain care from family physicians and chiropractors. *West J Med* 150:351, 1989.
5. Anderson R, Meeker W, Wirick B, et al: Meta-analysis of randomized clinical trials on manipulation for low back pain. *J Manipulative Physiol Ther* 15:181, 1992.
6. Shekelle P, Adams A, Chassin M, et al: *The Appropriateness of Spinal Manipulation for Low Back Pain: Project Overview and Literature Review.* Santa Monica, Calif, Rand, 1991.
7. Meade TW, Dyer S, Browne W, et al: Low back pain of mechanical origin: Randomized comparison of chiropractic and hospital outpatient treatment. *Br Med J (Clin Res)* 300:1431, 1990.
8. Jansen RD: A survey of American chiropractors' attitudes toward practice standards and the organizations developing them. *Palmer Coll Chiropractic West* 53, 1991.
9. Schumpeter JA: *History of Economic Analysis.* New York, Oxford University Press, 1954, p 1260.
10. Gatterman MI: *Chiropractic Management of Spine-Related Disorders.* Baltimore Md, Williams & Wilkins, 1990.
11. Nelson CF: The cognitive roots of chiropractic theories and techniques. *J Chiropractic Humanities* p 42, 1993.
12. Diggett DM: Commentary: The chiropractic wars. *J Manipulative Physiol Ther* 10:71, 1987.
13. Homola S: *Bonesetting, Chiropractic, and Cultism.* Panama City, Fla, Critique Books, 1963, p 281.
14. Nimmo RL: *The Receptor-Tonus Method.* Granbury, Tex, self-published, 1963.
15. Christensen MG: *Job Analysis of Chiropractic.* Greeley, Colo, National Board of Chiropractic Examiners, 1993, p 150.
16. Bergmann TF: Various forms of chiropractic technique. *Chiropractic Technique* 5:53, 1993.
17. Bartol KM: Algorithm for the categorization of chiropractic technique procedures. *Chiropractic Technique* 4:8, 1992.
18. Montgomery PD, Nelson MJ: Evolution of chiropractic theories of practice and spinal adjustment, 1900–1950. *Chiropract History* 5:71, 1985.

19. Chassen MR: Standards of care in medicine. *Inquiry* 25(winter):437, 1988.
20. Frymoyer JW, Pope MH: Epidemiologic studies of low back pain. *Spine* 5:419, 1980.
21. Liebenson CS: Pathogenesis of chronic back pain. *J Manipulative Physiol Ther* 15:299, 1992.
22. Eisenberg DM, Kessler RC, Foster C, et al: "Unconventional" medicine in the United States. *N Engl J Med* 328:246, 1983.
23. Eaton CB, Eaton DF: *Microeconomics*. New York, WH Freeman, 1988, p 471.
24. Hotelling H: Stability in competition. *Econ J* 39:41, 1929.
25. Boulding K: *Economic Analysis*. New York, Harper & Row, 1966.
26. Gibbons RW: Medical and social protest as part of hidden American history, in Haldeman S (ed): *Principles and Practice of Chiropractic*, ed 2. East Norwalk, Conn, Appleton & Lange, 1992, p 15.
27. Keating JC: Philosophical barriers to technique research in chiropractic. *Chiropractic Technique* 1:23, 1989.
28. Keating JC: Traditional barriers to standards of knowledge production in chiropractic. *Chiropractic Technique* 2:78, 1990.
29. Stonebrink RD: *Evaluation and Manipulative Management of Common Musculoskeletal Disorders*. Portland, Ore, Western States Chiropractic College, 1990.
30. Cooperstein R: Brand name techniques and the confidence gap. *J Chiropractic Educ* 4:89, 1990.
31. Quine WVO: Two dogmas of empiricism, ed 2. Cambridge, Mass, Harvard University Press, 1964.
32. Lawrence DJ: The challenges of teaching technique. *Chiropractic Technique* 1:6, 1989.
33. Kfoury PW, ed: *Catalog of Chiropractic Techniques*. Logan College of Chiropractic, 1977, p 119.
34. Keating JC: The first 85 years: An overview of scientific developments in chiropractic through 1980, in Sweerer J (ed): *Chiropractic Family Practice: A Clinical Manual*. Gaithersburg, Md, Aspen Publishers, 1992, p 1000.
35. Nelson CF: Chiropractic scope of practice. *J Manipulative Physiol Ther* 16:488, 1993.
36. Homola S: Seeking a common denominator in the use of spinal manipulation. *Chiropractic Technique* 4:61, 1992.
37. Herbst A: *Gonstead Chiropractic Science and Art: The Chiropractic Methodology of Clarence S. Gonstead*. Mount Horeb, Wis, Schichi Publications, 1980, p 280.
38. Plaugher G (ed): *Textbook of Clinical Chiropractic: A Specific Biomechanical Approach*. Baltimore, Md, Williams & Wilkins, 1993, p 525.
39. Gitelman R, Fligg B: Diversified technique, in Haldeman S (ed): *Principles and Practice of Chiropractic*, ed 2. New York, Appleton-Century-Crofts, 1992, p 483.
40. States AZ: *Spinal and Pelvic Techniques*. Lombard, Ill, National College of Chiropractic, 1967.
41. Harrison DD: *Chiropractic: The Physics of Spinal Correction. CBP Technique*, Rev. 1994.
42. Pettibon B: *Introduction to Spinal Bio-mechanics*. Tacoma, Wash, Pettibon Spinal Biomechanics Institute, 1989.
43. Logan HB: *Textbook of Logan Basic Methods*. St Louis, Publisher unknown, 1950, p 257.
44. Gillet H, Liekens M: The different types of fixation, in *The Belgian Chiropractic Research Notes*. Huntingon Beach, Calif, Motion Palpation Institute, 1981, p 13.

45. Schafer RC, Faye LJ: *Motion Palpation and Chiropractic Technique.* Huntington Beach, Calif, Motion Palpation Institute, 1989.
46. Leach RA: *The Chiropractic Theories,* ed 2. Baltimore, Md, Williams & Wilkins, 1986, p 234.
47. Triano JJ: The subluxation complex: Outcome measure of chiropractic diagnosis and treatment. *Chiropractic Techique* 2:114, 1990.
48. Giles LGF: *Anatomical Basis of Low Back Pain.* Baltimore Md, Williams & Wilkins, 1990.
49. Deyo R: Epidemiology of low back pain. *Spine* 12:264, 1987.
50. Phillips RB, Schultz GD, Howard B, et al: Posterior osteophytes and low back pain. *Chiropractic Technique* 5:32, 1993.
51. Phillips RB, Howe JW, Bustin G, et al: Stress x-rays and the low back pain patient. *J Manipulative Physiol Ther* 15:127, 1990.
52. De Jarnette MB: *Sacro Occipital Technic.* Nebraska City, Neb, self-published, 1983, p 287.
53. Walther DS: *Applied Kinesiology.* Pueblo, Colo, Systems DC, 1981, vol 1, p 474.
54. VanRumpt R: Directional non-force technique notes. Beverly Hills, Calif, Directional Non-Force Technique, 1987.
55. Schneider MJ: Soft tissue effects of sacroiliac lumbosacral joint manipulation. *Chiropractic Technique* 4:136, 1992.
56. Bennett TJ: *A New Clinical Basis for the Correction of Abnormal Physiology.* Burlingame, Calif, self-published, 1960.
57. Chaitow L: *Soft-Tissue Manipulation.* Rochester, Vt, Healing Arts Press, 1988, p 270.
58. Osterbauer PJ, Fuhr AW: The current status of activator methods chiropractic technique, theory, and training. *Chiropractic Technique* 2:168, 1990.
59. Bartol KM: A model for the categorization of chiropractic treatment procedures. *Chiropractic Technique* 3:78, 1991.
60. Good CJ: An analysis of diversified (lege artis) type adjustments based upon the assisted-resisted model of intervertebral motion unit prestress. *Chiropractic Technique* 4:117, 1992.
61. Kaminski M, Boal R, Gillette RG, et al: A model for the evaluation of chiropractic methods. *J Manipulative Physiol Ther* 10:61, 1987.
62. Kaminski M: Evaluation of chiropractic methods. *Chiropractic Technique* 2:3, 1990.
63. Haldeman S, Chapman-Smith D, Petersen DM (eds): *Guidelines for Chiropractic Quality Assurance and Practice Parameters.* Gaithersburg, Md: Aspen Publishers, 1993, p 222.
64. Bergmann TF: Introduction and opening statement. *Chiropractic Technique* 2:71, 1990.
65. Adams AH, Coulter ID: Consensus methods, clinical guidelines, and the RAND study of chiropractic. *ACA J Chiropractic* 29:50, 1992.
66. Keating JC, Bergmann TF: It works, it works, it works! *Chiropractic Technique* 4:73, 1992.
67. Abrams A: Spondylotherapy: *Physiotherapy of the Spine Based on a Study of Clinical Physiology,* ed 3. San Francisco, Philopolis Press, 1912, p 673.

Advances in Subluxation Terminology and Usage

Meridel I. Gatterman, M.A., D.C.
Research Department, New York Chiropractic College, Seneca Falls, New York

In the past decade we have heard pleas to abandon anachronistic terminology,[1] to seek a common language,[2] and to develop chiropractic nomenclature through consensus.[3] The seriousness of the lack of agreement on terms commonly used by chiropractors has been noted by a number of chiropractic authors. Lawrence[2] states that semantic difficulties have hampered the overall development of chiropractic. He emphasizes that one of the greatest challenges facing the chiropractic profession today is simply to learn how to communicate with one another. Sandoz[4] notes that semantic confusion has caused interdisciplinary misunderstanding, as well as fostered long-standing differences within the chiropractic profession.

At the center of the controversy over terms commonly used by chiropractors is the word subluxation. Not limited exclusively to the chiropractic profession, the term "subluxation" is also used by other disciplines. Within medicine, orthopedic surgeons and radiologists also use the term subluxation.[5] Some of these insist on radiographical evidence of subluxation, whereas others imply that subluxation is a nonmanipulable lesion with obvious misalignment, often requiring surgical repair. Some have argued that chiropractic should abandon the term subluxation because of this ambiguity[6] even though there are those in medicine in addition to other disciplines who use the term to describe the articular lesion that responds to manipulation.[7–10]

In response to the controversy the term subluxation has been included in the consensus process designed to develop nomenclature for the chiropractic profession.[3] An algorithm model (Fig 1) was developed to provide a step-by-step model with expanding representation to include broad geographical areas and philosophical views in the consensus process. A three-member working group reviewed the literature, providing seed definitions and terms for a nine-member nominal consensus panel. Criteria used to evaluate terms and definitions included the uniqueness, occurrence, and origin of the term (Fig 1, box 4). Assessment included origin of the term (appearance of the term in the literature), retrospective variability (uses of the term in the literature), and appropriateness of the continuing usage (the usefulness of the term to the profession) (Fig 1, box 7). Final consensus for the term subluxation at the 84% level was achieved by a 60-member Delphi panel (see Fig 1, diamond 11).

Advances in Chiropractic®, vol. 2
© 1995, Mosby–Year Book, Inc.

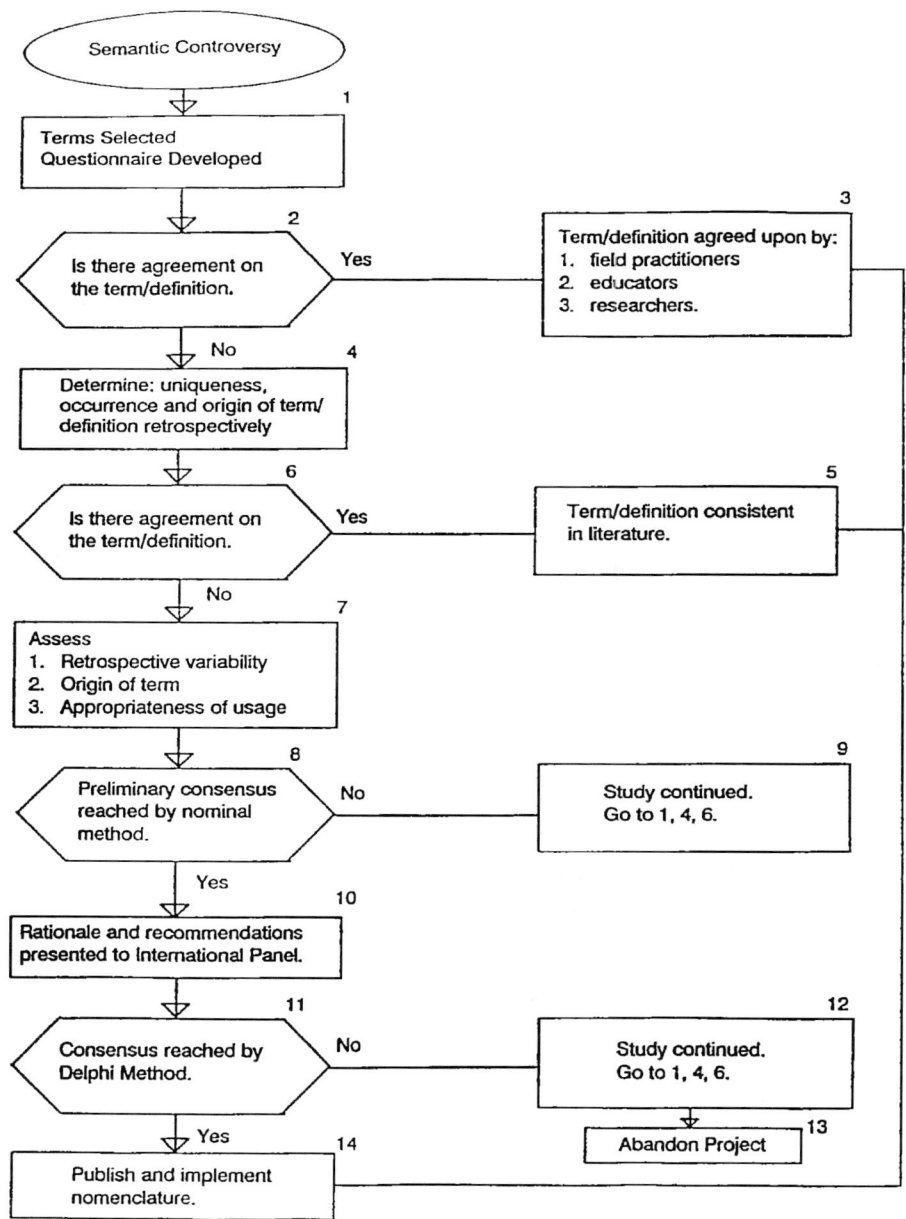

FIGURE 1.
Terminology assessment model. (From Gatterman M, Hansen D: *J Manipulative Physiol Ther* 1994; 17:304. Used by permission.)

SUBLUXATION FIELD OF TERMS

Evaluation of any term includes examining the field with which it is associated. Six terms emerged in the field associated with the term subluxation. Included in the definition of subluxation is the concept of the functional unit of the spine. This three-joint complex, made up of two adjacent vertebrae and their surrounding soft tissues, forms the functional unit of spinal motion. The concept originated with Junghanns, who referred to it as the "bewegunssegment."[11] Mistranslation of bewegungssegment to motor segment[12] by Besemann in 1971 was further confused when the term was modified to "motor unit."[13] Motor unit was then popularized through the National Institute of Neurological and Communicative Disorders and Stroke conference and the subsequent monograph on the Research Status of Spinal Manipulative Therapy published in 1975. The prior use of the term motor unit by physiologists to refer to a single motor neuron and the group of muscle fibers that it innervates has caused confusion when motor unit is used to describe the functional unit of the spine. To clarify the term, chiropractors agreed to return to the literal translation of bewegungssegment (motion segment). Two terms from this conceptual model emerged from the consensus process, one describing the functional unit of the spine and the other applied to movement of other articulations. These were defined as:

- Spinal motion segment—two adjacent vertebrae and the connecting tissues binding them to each other.
- Motion segment—a functional unit made up of the two articulating surfaces and the connecting tissues binding them to each other.

Subluxation as the lesion treated by chiropractors was defined as a motion segment in which alignment, movement integrity, and physiological function are altered even though contact between joint surfaces remains intact. This definition is not unlike the early use of subluxation in the medical literature.

HISTORICAL PERSPECTIVE

Historically the term subluxation appears in the English medical literature in 1746. Terrett[14] notes that this early definition, put forth by Joannes Henricus Hieronymi, is more in keeping with current understanding of the subluxation than early chiropractic definitions. This definition considers decrease in both mobility and pain, as well as malposition: "Subluxation of joints is recognized by lessened motion of joints, by slight change in the position of the articulating bones and pain."[15]

The earliest chiropractic text by Smith et al.[16] describes a subluxated vertebra as differing from a normal vertebra in its field of motion, with its various positions of rest differently located than when it was a normal vertebra and with its field of motion sometimes too great in some directions and too small in others. This emphasis on motion was in contrast to D.D. Palmer's notion that a subluxation is an intervertebral disrelationship amounting to less than a dislocation.[17] Misalignment remained the focus of the chiropractic use of subluxation, culminating in the politically driven radiographic classification of subluxation concocted as the criteria for treatment of patients under Medicare and Medicaid in the United States. Orthopedic surgeons and radiologists reserve the term subluxation for a partial or incomplete articular dislocation secondary to capsular laxity, associated with degenerative joint instability that is demonstrable on radiographs. This, coupled with the questionable reliability of radiographic detection of manipulable subluxations,[18, 19] has led some within the chiropractic profession to suggest that the term subluxation as used for the manipulable lesion be abandoned.[20]

Out of this controversy came the need to differentiate between subluxation amenable to manipulation and subluxations for which manipulation is contraindicated. The definition of subluxation agreed on is broad enough to include the medical concept of subluxation that is severe enough to be visible on x-ray films, as well as the more subtle manipulable subluxation detected by palpation. Manipulable subluxation was further qualified and defined as a subluxation in which altered alignment, movement, and function can be improved by manual thrust procedures. This distinction has been further clarified by Peterson[21] in her discussion of the nonmanipulable subluxation. This review emphasizes the need to differentiate subluxations where manipulation is clearly contraindicated, such as those with evidence of instability, from those in which manipulation is a relative contraindication indicating a different therapeutic approach. A subluxation exhibiting instability may be characterized by severe neurological damage to the spinal cord or nerve roots, incapacitating deformities and pain.[22] Clearly a forceful thrust procedure is contraindicated in the treatment of this type of subluxation. A subluxation in which the mobility of the motion segment is excessive but not so extreme as to be life threatening or require surgery has been referred to as exhibiting hypermobility.[23] Sandoz[24] has noted episodic fixations in motion segments with signs of hypermobility, indicating a subluxation for which manipulation may be appropriate. Although subluxations exhibiting hypermobility must be carefully evaluated, when accompanied by restricted motion in one or another plane, manipulation may be the treatment of choice.

SUBLUXATION-RELATED DYSFUNCTION

The criterion of neurological involvement has been central to the traditional chiropractic concept of subluxation from the beginning of chiropractic. Lantz[25] states that the neurological component of subluxation is for many the cornerstone of chiropractic theory. He has elaborated on this through the model of the vertebral subluxation complex. The vertebral subluxation complex originated as a paradigm shift in the mid-1970s, proposed by Faye to move the emphasis from the misalignment component of subluxation to a more dynamic construct.[26] The vertebral subluxation complex is a heuristic construct that relates current knowledge and experience to a common central conceptual model of dysfunction related to the articular lesion known as subluxation. This construct provides a theoretical model of dysfunction related to the subluxation that is useful in the discussion of the principles of chiropractic and has been defined as a theoretical model of motion segment dysfunction (subluxation) that incorporates the complex interaction of pathological changes in nerve, muscle, ligamentous, vascular, and connective tissue.

The usefulness of a paradigm, in the true scientific sense according to Kuhn,[27] is that it prepares students for membership in the scientific community with which they will later practice. By joining a group who learned the basis of their field from the same concrete models, subsequent practice seldom evokes overt disagreement over fundamentals. Those whose research is based on shared paradigms are committed to the same rules and standards for scientific practice. The subluxation complex provides such a model or paradigm for chiropractic educators and researchers.

CLINICAL MANIFESTATIONS OF SUBLUXATION

The clinical manifestations of the subluxation (articular lesion) are acknowledged in the term "subluxation syndrome," the most common of which is referred pain. Subluxation syndrome is defined as an aggregate of signs and symptoms that relate to pathophysiology or dysfunction of spinal and pelvic motion segments or to peripheral joints.

Although some conditions related to a subluxation etiology have been widely recognized, including sacroiliac (subluxation) syndrome, posterior joint (facet subluxation syndrome), and vertebrogenic headache (upper cervical subluxation syndrome), others such as costovertebral syndrome (rib subluxation) and cervicogenic dorsalgia (cervical subluxation with referred pain into the thoracic region) have not. The aggregate of signs and symptoms related to subluxation of spinal joints varies from region to region in the vertebral column.[28]

The term subluxation syndrome allows for discussion and description of the clinical manifestations of a subluxation, including the signs and symptoms characteristic of subluxation specific to the various joints of the spine and extremities.

METAPHORICAL USE OF SUBLUXATION

Keating[29] regards the continued metaphoric use of subluxation to be harmful to the chiropractic profession and notes that a terminological masquerade may account for some of the continuing interdisciplinary conflict. He states

> A reconsideration of the role of this chiropractic root metaphor is in order. Subluxation has become so overburdened with clinical, political and philosophical meaning and significance for chiropractors that the concept, which once helped to hold a young, besieged profession together, now threatens to strangle the discipline.[29]

Keating[30] calls for consensus on an operational definition of subluxation from which subluxation theories can be tested. Although the subluxation as a metaphor became a rallying point that permitted effective action in the courtroom and the legislatures, he argues that the current emphasis on health care outcomes necessitates an emphasis on rigorous testing to develop standards for detecting subluxation.

OPERATIONALLY DEFINING SUBLUXATION

An operational definition moves beyond the theoretical construct of a term to clearly define a testable component of the theoretical definition.

For example, the component of the consensus definition that states that movement integrity is altered may be operationally defined as "hard end-feel." This may be described as a characteristic of the subluxated motion segment that is detectable through motion palpation. The reliability of this method of detecting altered movement integrity can then be measured. In this manner an operational definition allows for the measurement of the level of agreement between palpators and for determining their ability to detect the variable hard end-feel that is a component of the theoretical definition of subluxation: altered movement integrity. Operational definitions of the identified components of a subluxation must be developed and subjected to rigorous testing if we are to continue using the term subluxation in a meaningful manner.

TERMINOLOGY RELATED TO THE TREATMENT OF SUBLUXATION

Chiropractic treatment has traditionally been directed at restoring the alignment, movement integrity, and physiological function in the subluxated motion segment. The primary chiropractic technique has traditionally used manual procedures to treat the body. As with the term subluxation, much confusion and controversy has surrounded the use of terms and definitions used to describe chiropractic treatment methods. The terms "manual therapy," "manipulation," "mobilization," and "adjustment" were included in the consensus process to differentiate these procedures.

The term manual therapy generated little controversy, but because it was used synonymously with manipulation and spinal manipulative therapy by some to include the broad category of all procedures done by hand, it was included. Manual therapy is defined as procedures by which the hands directly contact the body to treat the articulations and soft tissues.

Of greater importance was the need to differentiate between manipulation and mobilization.[31] Early studies of manipulation did not make the distinction between thrust procedures and those using stretching without thrust to restore joint function. The lack of this distinction produced equivocal data regarding the effectiveness of manual thrust procedures. Later studies where manipulation was defined as a thrust procedure demonstrated the greater effectiveness of this method, for example, in the treatment of mechanical low back pain, making the distinction important.

Based on the 1991 Rand study[32] of spinal manipulation that defined manipulation as a thrust procedure, the following definition was agreed on: a manual procedure that involves a directed thrust to move a joint past the physiological range of motion without exceeding the anatomical limit.

The nonthrust stretching procedure was then designated as mobilization and defined as movement applied singularly or repetitively within or at the physiological range of joint motion, without imparting a thrust or impulse, with the goal of restoring joint mobility.

Next to the word subluxation the term "adjustment" has sparked the most heated debate. It was agreed that chiropractors applying the adjustment intend to influence more than joint mechanics and related pain. Neurophysiological function was therefore included in the definition of adjustment. Adjustment was broadly defined so as not to exclude those procedures routinely used by chiropractors that fall outside the thrust technique category. Although some believed that the definition of adjustment should be restricted to specific short-lever, high-velocity, low-amplitude, thrust techniques it was agreed to define the term to include reflex and thrust procedures, that is any chiropractic therapeutic procedure that uses controlled force, leverage, direction, amplitude, and velocity directed at specific joints or anatomical regions. Chiropractors commonly use such procedures to influence joint and neurophysiological function. (This definition is not meant to imply that neurophysiological effects do not occur with manipulation).

TABLE 1.
Percent Agreement

Field 1: Articular functional units
   88%—Motion segment: A functional unit made up of the two adjacent articulating surfaces and the connecting tissues binding them to each other.
   83%—Spinal motion segment: Two adjacent vertebrae and the connecting tissues binding them to each other.
Field 2: The lesion treated by chiropractors
   84%—Subluxation: A motion segment in which alignment, movement integrity, and physiological function are altered even though contact between joint surfaces remains intact.
   81%—Manipulable subluxation: A subluxation in which altered alignment, movement, and function can be improved by manual thrust procedures.
   82%—Subluxation complex: A theoretical model of motion segment dysfunction (subluxation) that incorporates the complex interaction of pathological changes in nerve, muscle, ligamentous, vascular, and connective tissues.
   83%—Subluxation syndrome: An aggregate of signs and symptoms that relate to pathophysiology or dysfunction of spinal and pelvic motion segments or to peripheral joints.
Field 3: Treatment procedures used by chiropractors
   91%—Manual therapy: Procedures by which the hands directly contact the body to treat the articulations and soft tissues.
   91%—Manipulation: A manual procedure that involves a directed thrust to move a joint past the physiological range of motion without exceeding the anatomical limit.
   88%—Mobilization: Movement applied singularly or repetitively within or at the physiological range of joint motion without imparting a thrust or impulse, with the goal of restoring joint mobility.
   87%—Adjustment: Any chiropractic therapeutic procedure that uses controlled force, leverage, direction, amplitude, and velocity directed at specific joints or anatomical regions. Chiropractors commonly use such procedures to influence joint and neurophysiological function.

CONCLUSION

If we are to achieve a true nomenclature by which to continue discourse about the primary lesion treated by chiropractors, we must go beyond the simplistic definition of subluxation as "a partial or incomplete dislocation," as put forth by D.D. Palmer, and consider the complexities that surround this concept. Although consensus has been reached on 10 terms central to the concept of subluxation (Table 1), adoption of the terms to form a nomenclature that serves as a true vehicle for greater understanding is contingent on compliance in the use of agreed-on terms. Holding to sectarian terms fosters dogma, whether chiropractic or medical, and will not help to provide better care for our patients. True advances in subluxation terminology and usage are contingent on cooperation and integration of the terms agreed on through the consensus process. As further knowledge is gained through scientific evidence, terms will evolve and change. It is time to speak the same language and adopt a consensus-based nomenclature.

REFERENCES

1. Bryner P: Isn't it time to abandon anachronistic terminology? *J Aust Chiropr Assoc* 17:53–58, 1987.
2. Lawrence D: Toward a common language [editorial]. *J Manipulative Physiol Ther* 11:1–2, 1988.
3. Gatterman M, Hansen D: Development of chiropractic nomenclature through consensus. *J Manipulative Physiol Ther* 17:302–309, 1994.
4. Sandoz R: The natural history of spinal degenerative lesion. *Ann Swiss Chiropr Assoc* 9:149–192, 1989.
5. Watkins RJ: Subluxation terminology since 1746. *Can Chiropr Assoc* 4:20–23, 1968.
6. Brantingham JW: A critical look at the subluxation hypothesis. *J Manipulative Physiol Ther* 11:130–132, 1988.
7. Turek SL: *Orthopedics Principles and Their Application*, ed 3. Philadelphia, JB Lippincott, 1977, p 1469.
8. Basmajian JV: *Manipulation, Traction and Massage*, ed 3. Baltimore, Williams & Wilkins, 1988, p 142.
9. Keim HA, Kirkaldy-Willis WH: Low back pain. *Clin Symp* 39:1–32, 1987.
10. Daly JM, Frame PS, Rapoza PA: Sacroiliac subluxation: A common treatable cause of low back pain in pregnancy. *Fam Pract Res J* 11:149–159, 1991.
11. Schmorl G, Junghanns H: *The Human Spine in Health and Disease*, ed 2. New York. Grune & Stratton, 1971, pp 37–39.
12. Gatterman MI: Lost in translation. *J Can Chiropr Assoc* 22–31, 1978.
13. Drum DC: The vertebral motor unit and intervertebral foramen. *J Can Chiropr Assoc* 22–30, 1975.
14. Terrett A: The search for the subluxation: An investigation of medical literature to 1985. *Chiropr Hist* 729–733, 1987.
15. Hieronymi JH: De Luxations et Subluxationibus [thesis]. Jenae, British Museum Catalogue, vol 103, p 666, no 7306.i12 (18) and 7306.i10(9).
16. Smith OG, Langworthy SM, Paxson MC: *Modernized Chiropractic*. Cedar Rapids, Iowa, Lawrence Press, 1906, vol 1, p 26.
17. Palmer DD: *The Chiropractor's Adjustor*, Portland, 1910.
18. Phillips RB: Plain film radiography in chiropractic. *J Manipulative Physiol Ther* 15:47–50, 1992.

19. Taylor JAM: Full spine radiography: A review. *J Manipulative Physiol Ther* 3:87–92, 1993.
20. Hubka MJ: Another critical look at the subluxation hypothesis. *Chiropr Technique* 2:27–29, 1990.
21. Peterson C: The non-manipulable subluxation. In Gatterman MI (ed). *Foundations of Chiropractic: Subluxation*, St Louis, Mosby, 1994.
22. White AA, Panjabi MM: *Clinical Biomechanics of the Spine*. Philadelphia, JB Lippincott, 1978 p 192.
23. McGregor M, Mior SA: Anatomical and functional perspectives of the cervical spine: II. The "hypermobile" cervical. *J Can Chiropr Assoc* 33:177–183, 1989.
24. Sandoz R: The natural history of a spinal degenerative lesion. *Ann Swiss Chiropr Assoc* 9:149–192, 1989.
25. Lantz C: The vertebral subluxation complex: 2. The neuropathological and myopathological components. *Chiropr Res J* 1:19–37, 1990.
26. Gatterman MI: *Chiropractic Management of Spine Related Disorders*. Baltimore, Williams & Wilkins, 1990, p 40.
27. Kuhn TS: *The Structure of Scientific Revolutions*, ed 2. Chicago, Illinois University Press, 1970.
28. Gatterman MI: *Foundations of Chiropractic: Subluxation*. St Louis, Mosby, 1994, Part 3.
29. Keating JC: Science and politics and the subluxation. *Am J Chiropr Med* 1:107–110, 1988.
30. Keating JC: *Toward a Philosophy of the Science of Chiropractic*. Stockton, Calif, Stockton Foundation for Chiropractic Research, pp 113–121.
31. Mierau D, Cassidy JD, Bowes V, et al: Manipulation and mobilization of the third metacarpophalangeal joint. *Manual Med* 3:135–140, 1988.
32. Shekelle PG, Adams AH, Chassin MR, et al: *The Appropriateness of Spinal Manipulation for Low Back Pain and Project Overview and Literature*. Santa Monica, Calif, Kevier, Rand Monograph no R-4025/1 CCR-FCER.

Description and Analysis of Activator Methods Chiropractic Technique

Paul J. Osterbauer, D.C., M.P.H.
Director of Research Activator Methods, Inc., Phoenix, Arizona

Arlan W. Fuhr, D.C.
President, Activator Methods, Inc., Phoenix, Arizona

Tony S. Keller, Ph.D.
Assistant Professor of Mechanical Engineering, University of Vermont, Burlington, Vermont

Perhaps no other technique has been the focus of as much overwhelming scrutiny and controversy as Activator Methods Chiropractic Technique (AMCT). Until recently, the main question of whether a specific treatment is effective for a particular patient with a given condition has been neglected.[1,2] However, developments in health care reform have put the process of technology assessment and dissemination on the fast track. This chapter serves as a follow-up to an appraisal published in 1990.[3,4] It reviews recent research efforts of Activator Methods, Inc. (AMI) and speculates about the future of what has become known as mechanical force manually assisted (MFMA) chiropractic adjusting procedures.

HISTORY

The Activator Method (AM) of chiropractic analysis and low-force spinal adjusting technique originated in Redwood Falls, Minnesota in 1965 through the collaborative efforts of Warren C. Lee, D.C. (graduate of Northwestern College of Chiropractic, 1941) and Arlan W. Fuhr, D.C. (graduate of Logan Basic College of Chiropractic, 1961). Since then, the procedure has become a major chiropractic clinical method and is now used to some extent by approximately 28,000 doctors of chiropractic throughout the world. Recent surveys by the National Board of Chiropractic Examiners show that the AM is one of the four most frequently used procedures in the United States and Canada (Fig 1).[5,6] In Europe, it is estimated that the technique is used in 14% of cases.[7]

The evolution of AMCT has involved a gradual integration of the theories and methods of chiropractic pioneers such as Logan, Derefield, and Van Rumpt. Both Drs. Lee and Fuhr were grounded in the concepts of the Logan Basic Technique. Lee had furthered his chiropractic education by

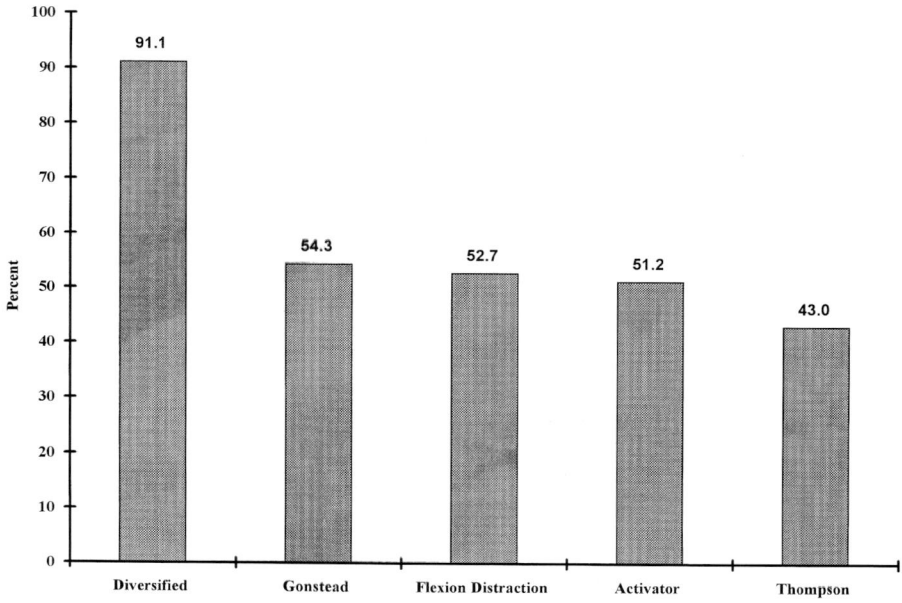

FIGURE 1.
Five of the most commonly used techniques among U.S. chiropractors.

completing a 1-year residency at the Logan College of Chiropractic, where he developed interests in the structural unity of the skeletal system and the effects of gravity on the spinal column. To these seminal ideas were added the leg-length (LL) measurement methods of subluxation-detection by the Derefields and the light toggle-recoil thumb thrusts of the Directional Nonforce Technique developed by Richard Van Rumpt, D.C.

The AM instrument originated from a combination of earlier adjusting devices and a dental impacter used to split wisdom teeth. The Activator instrument was developed to increase control of the speed, force, and direction of adjustive thrusts and to reduce physical stress on clinicians. The modern Activator adjusting instrument (AAI) is the product of many modifications over the years and makes use of a hammer-anvil effect to produce a safe, reliable, and controlled force to osseous spinal structures. The instrument is listed with the U.S. Food and Drug Administration pursuant to the Medical Practices Devices Act.

The first AM field seminar was conducted in Minnesota in 1967. From this modest beginning, a worldwide postgraduate educational program has evolved. Seminars and instructional workshops in AMCT have been conducted throughout the United States and in Canada, Australia, and Europe. AMCT procedures are taught at most U.S. chiropractic colleges, which are approved by the Council on Chiropractic Education (Table 1); participation in these seminars typically qualifies the doctor for license-renewal credits.

After many years of teaching the Activator concepts of subluxation detection, and instrument adjusting (Table 2), a new phase of development was initiated in 1985 when AMI was awarded a grant from the Small Business Innovative Research Grants program of the National Institutes of Health. The award was made to study the safety and effectiveness of

TABLE 1.
Accredited Colleges and Type of Instructional Offerings in AMCT*

Cleveland Chiropractic College, Kansas City: Elective course
Life Chiropractic College: Elective and postgraduate courses
Life Chiropractic College–West: Elective and postgraduate courses
Logan College of Chiropractic: Elective course
New York Chiropractic College: Elective course
Palmer College of Chiropractic: Elective and postgraduate courses
Palmer College of Chiropractic–West: Elective course
Parker College of Chiropractic: Elective course
*From Osterbauer PJ, Fuhr AW: *Chiropr Technique* 1990; 24:173. Used by permission.

the mechanical adjusting instrument on osseous tissues, resulting in two scientific papers published in the *Journal of Manipulative and Physiological Therapeutics*.[8,9]

This increasing interest in scientific activities led to the appointment in 1987 of Paul J. Osterbauer, D.C., M.P.H., a 1986 graduate of the Northwestern College of Chiropractic, to serve as Director of Research of AMI. In this role, Dr. Osterbauer initiated a program of clinical investigations concerning the reliability of leg-length methods of subluxation detection, including the isolation tests developed by Lee and Fuhr.[10–12]

TABLE 2.
Definition of Unique Terms

Activator adjusting instrument (AAI): A mechanical force manually assisted chiropractic adjusting instrument capable of providing a dynamic thrust. It also provides a controlled force of adjustment with a precise contact with a specific line of drive.
Pelvic deficiency (PD): Leg length deficiency (LLD) originally thought to be caused by a posterior inferior rotation and torque of the ilium on the same side, observed when a patient is in a prone, non-weight-bearing position. Current opinion implicates uneven muscle tone about the spine and pelvis via complex tonic postural reflex mechanisms. This is not to be confused with anisomelia.
Functional short leg: See pelvic deficiency.
Isolation test: A specific active movement by the patient to assist in locating and evaluating the subluxated joints of the spine or extremities by eliciting changes in leg alignment reactivity (LAR).
Line of drive (LOD): The angle at which the AAI contacts the articulations to be adjusted.
Reactive leg: See pelvic deficiency.
Pressure test: Light pressure applied to the articulation thought to cause LAR.
Subluxation: Clinical signs and symptoms thought to relate to pathophysiology or dysfunction of spinal motion segments or to peripheral joints that may be amenable to adjustive procedures.

Osterbauer has also guided the organization toward more active involvement in the chiropractic profession's expanding research community. Since 1987, AMI has participated in the research meetings of the California Chiropractic Foundation (Conference on Research and Education), the Consortium for Chiropractic Research, the Foundation for Chiropractic Education and Research (International Conference on Spinal Manipulation), and the several Consensus Conferences on Chiropractic Methods sponsored by the ACA Council on Technic. Concurrently, AMI has conducted a variety of clinical investigations. These studies have yielded numerous papers in the referred scientific literature and conference presentations and have inspired others to study the value of AMCT.[13] Interest in studying AMCT has resulted in interdisciplinary collaboration with the Departments of Bio-Engineering and Exercise Science and Sport of Arizona State University, the Harrington Arthritis Research Center, and the Department of Mechanical Engineering at the University of Vermont and the Vermont Space Grant Consortium in conjunction with the National Aeronautics and Space Administration.

One of the visions of AMCT has been standardization of analysis and treatment of patients with similar conditions. This concept has taken on new meaning in view of managed care. Patients have come to expect higher standardization of care, which has been difficult in the chiropractic profession, because most doctors are in solo practice and come from various schools of thought.

The profession has not been required to undergo the credentialing process until recently by preferred provider organizations (PPOs). To meet this need, AMI began familiarizing seminar attendees with the process of credentialing. Those who attend two or more seminars are eligible to take an examination to become "proficiency rated." Doctors who attend and pass the basic test can qualify to take the Advanced Proficiency Test. The names and addresses of proficiency- and advanced proficiency–rated doctors are maintained in a data base, allowing rapid referrals to qualified practitioners for patients who desire AMCT. In 1994, an estimated 15,000 patient referrals were made to doctors of chiropractic in North America, Europe, and Australia.

Like many health care treatment forms, despite research and standardization efforts, AM practice is largely empirically based. To ensure the most current and widely tested procedures, doctors are encouraged to submit technique observations and adjusting procedures that they have found useful in practice. The tests are sent to a review committee of Activator instructors for testing in their offices. Testing procedures that receive favorable reviews are incorporated into the course work in the following year.

Since the paper on the current status of AMCT was published in 1990, the AMCT seminar program has been divided into three sections, or tracks. Table 3 and Figure 2 provide an overview of the course content for the 12-hour weekend seminar

Today, AMCT is one of the most extensively studied low-force procedures in the profession, yielding a "promising to established" rating at the 1992 Mercy Center Consensus Conference.[14] A similar rating was agreed on by a consensus panel commissioned by the Canadian Chiropractic Association.[15] However, AMCT procedures of subluxation detec-

TABLE 3.
AMCT Course Content

Section	Content
Track 1	Basics of leg prone check
	Isolation tests (pelvis to occiput)
	Manipulation/adjusting procedures (pelvis to occiput)
Track 2	Review of prone leg check
	Isolation tests and adjusting procedures (continued)
Track 3	Isolation tests and manipulation/adjusting procedure (continued)
	Case management treatment algorithms (see Fig 2)
	Outcome assessments
	Credentialing for managed care requirements

tion and chiropractic adjusting have not been scientifically validated,[3] a characteristic these procedures share with many clinical methods across health care disciplines.

Although AMCT health assessment and intervention are among the most widely studied chiropractic procedures in the scientific literature, no estimate for overall efficacy and effectiveness of these procedures are available at this time. Some of the questions concerning AMCT remaining to be tested appear in Table 4. Since 1980, AMI has been committed to continued investigation of the methods of chiropractic practice generally and to the study of AMCT chiropractic procedures in particular. We hope that these early efforts will inspire other doctors of chiropractic to persevere in the scientific investigation of the chiropractic art for the betterment of our patients and profession.

DIAGNOSTIC PROCEDURES

BACKGROUND OF THE CHIROPRACTIC SUBLUXATION

Functional Short Leg

Altered neuromuscular function has been identified as one of the characteristics of the chiropractic subluxation or functional spinal lesion (see Table 2).[16] Others include:

1. Pain
2. Static malposition
3. Altered flexibility
4. Altered physical performance
5. Systemic symptoms

A common method of identifying possible spinal or pelvic dysfunction used by chiropractors[17-19] and others[20] involves observing changes in LL alignment or LL reactivity.[21] It has been hypothesized that subluxated synovial joints (usually of the spine) are characterized by heightened motor thresholds,[22,23] hyperactive tonic neck reflexes* (postural reflexes),[24]

---

*Modification of muscle tone in both right and left halves of the body (trunk and extremities) on movement of the head and neck.

or both. The altered neuromuscular function is thought to result in unilateral paraspinal muscular contraction, which creates a physiological shortening of the leg. The putative lesion may have its origin in the spine or pelvis due to macrotrauma, microtrauma, or excessive foot pronation or may be the result of a true anatomically short leg (anisomelia).[25-28]

Recently the concept of pelvic torsion as a source of LL discrepancy (LLD) has been challenged by Cooperstein.[29] He observed that analytically the amount of pelvic torsion required to cause a 0.6-cm LLD would be associated with a 1.3-cm luxation of the pubic symphysis. With the

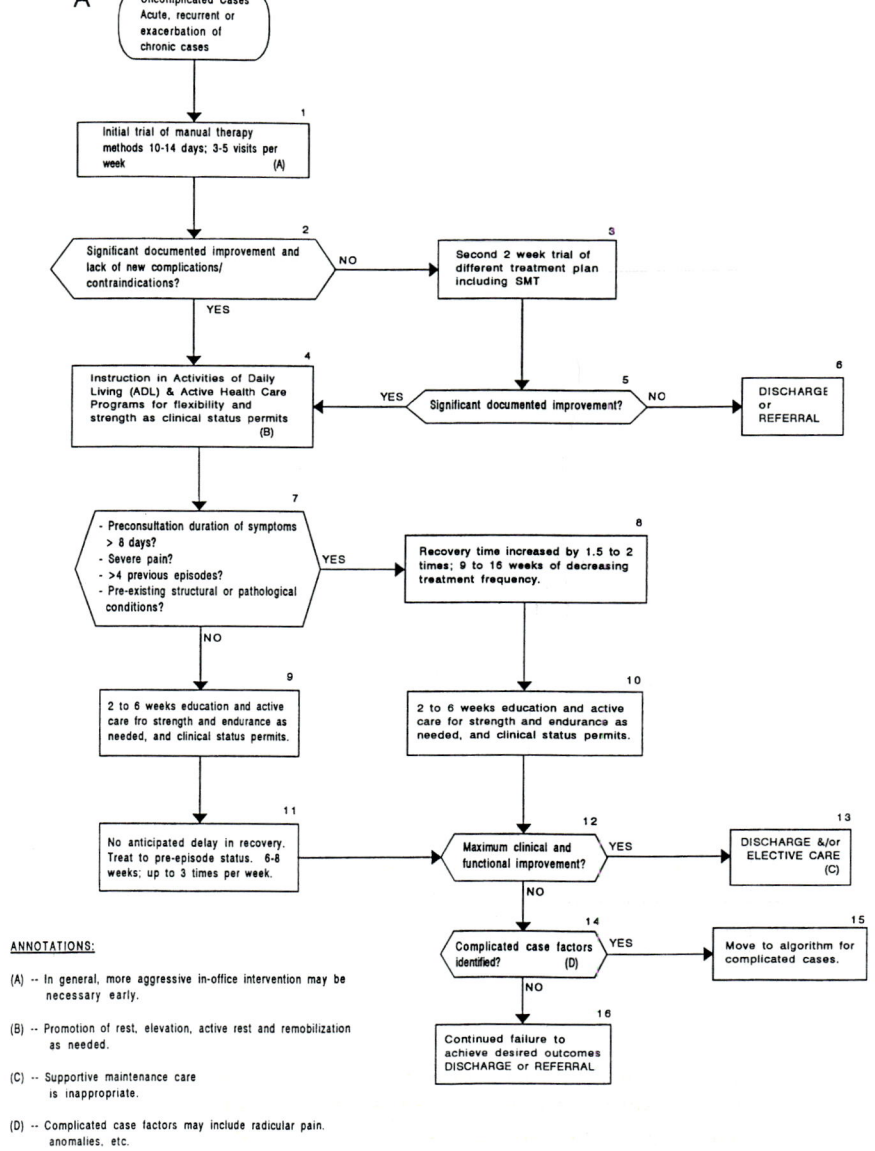

FIGURE 2.
A, acute treatment algorithm.

B

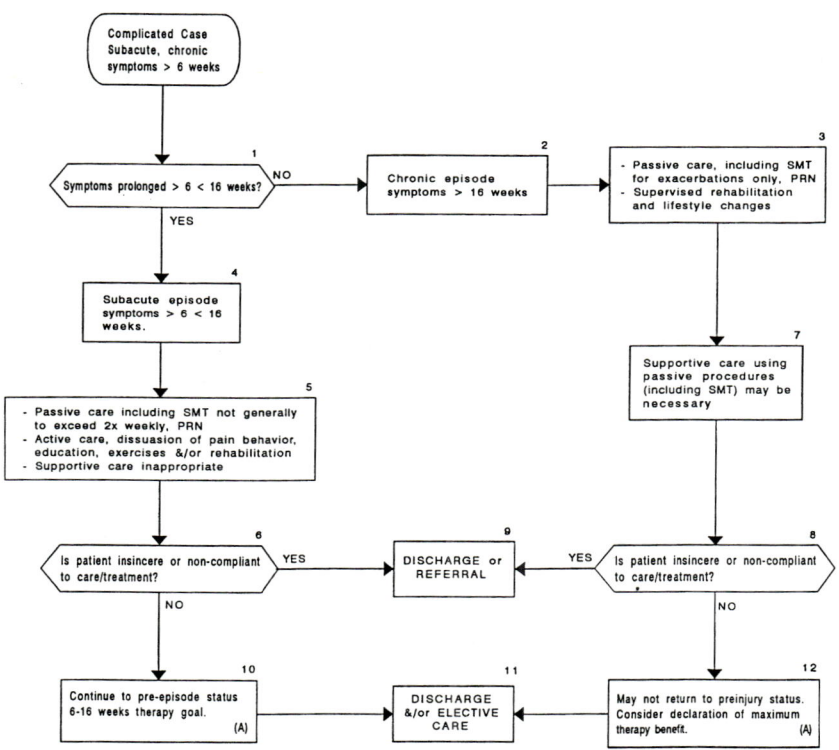

FIGURE 2 (cont.).
B, chronic treatment algorithm. (Courtesy of Activator Methods, Inc., Phoenix.)

advent of biomechanical research, the true cause of these observations may be uncovered.

Significance of Anisomelia as a Contributor to LL Reactivity

Many reviews of the clinical importance of anisomelia appear in the literature.[30-34] However, the importance of the effects of anisomelia with regard to low back pain (LBP) remain controversial (Fig 3).[34-36] Biomechanical evidence exists that anisomelia leads to measurable alterations in posture (static spinal alignment) (Fig 4). Heel and ischial lifts were used to treat a group of patients with chronic LBP who failed to respond to other types of conservative care using electromyography (EMG) to monitor the effectiveness of placement. The results indicated that lift placement via EMG was more accurate than radiographical methods of assess-

TABLE 4.
Testable Questions Concerning AMCT*

Reliability	How reproducible are the variety of AMCT analytic procedures across time and among well-trained (and novice) practitioners?
Concurrent validity	How well or poorly do AMCT isolation tests for subluxation detection co-vary with other spinal assessment/lesion detection strategies (e.g., is LL inequality related to palpable joint fixations or to joint pain)?
Social validity	Are changes in isolation test results correlated with changes in patients' (and significant others') perceptions of the severity of their conditions?
Trial validity	Do relative LL evaluations and isolation test findings reliably change as a function of remediation methods (e.g., AAI and/or manual adjustments, physiotherapy modalities, and exercise regimens)?
Clinical utility	Does spinal manipulation with the AAI produce significant changes in patients' health status? How well does AMCT manipulation compare with other forms of spinal manipulation and with other types of health care intervention? Is AMCT cost effective?

*From Osterbauer PJ, Fuhr AW: *Chiropr Technique* 1990; 2:168–175. Used by permission.

ing pelvic tilt/sacral unleveling.[37] In a later study, Vink and Kamphaisen[38] demonstrated a strong, positive, linear relationship between the angle of pelvic tilt measured by an external girdle and potentiometers and an artificially induced LLD using a board of known thickness in asymptomatic subjects (Fig 5, A). However, the relationship between LLD and paraspinal muscle activity (evaluated by rectified/averaged EMG) was only slightly positive until the LLD reached 34.4 mm (Fig 5, B). At this point, muscle activity increased sharply, indicating that the force required to maintain posture may be partially compensated mechanically (via anteroposterior and lateral curves) for small LLDs not requiring muscular stress exertion to counter the movement caused by LLD.

This evidence suggests that relatively large LLDs are required to elicit a neuromuscular response. If such a response was prolonged or was accompanied by performing stressful tasks, it could lead to symptoms. A recent epidemiological study supports this notion. Soukka et al.[36] sampled 594 people employed as truck drivers, office workers, and clerks. These individuals were asked whether they had ever suffered from LBP, whether they had experienced pain in the last year, and whether their LBP was disabling. Then they were examined for LLD. The authors concluded that there was no increased risk of LBP for a LLD of 10 to 20 mm and that this association appears weak or questionable. An important feature of this study is that it controlled for factors such as height, weight, sex, occupation, and age. Table 5 summarizes the characteristics of the previous studies. The incidence of true anatomical LLD of greater than 1

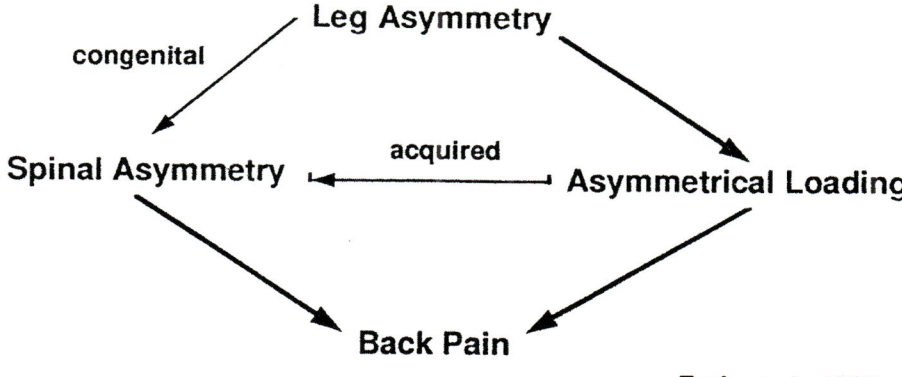

FIGURE 3.
Hypothetical relationship between LLD, lumbar facet orientation, and LBP. (From Froh R, Yong-Hing K, Cassidy JD, et al: *Spine* 1988; 13:325–327. Used by permission.)

cm has been estimated to occur in as much as 15% to 30% of the population.[32, 34, 38]

In the experience of AMCT practitioners, the mere presence of a true LLD does not seem to be related to symptoms. Patients with anisomelia often exhibit leg alignment reactivity that responds to manipulation/ad-

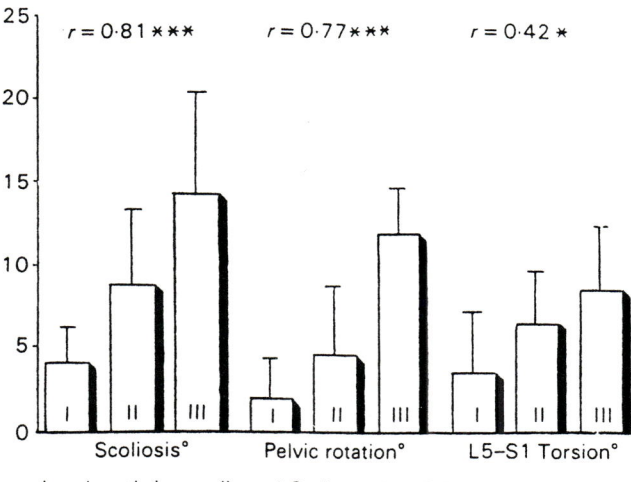

FIGURE 4.
Lumbar pelvic tilt scoliosis, pelvic rotation, and trigonometrically calculated torsion of the L-5 to S-1 segment (means) in groups with different degrees of LL discrepancy in 288 patients with chronic LBP symptoms. (From Friberg O: *Clin Biomechanics* 2:211–219, 1987. Used by permission.)

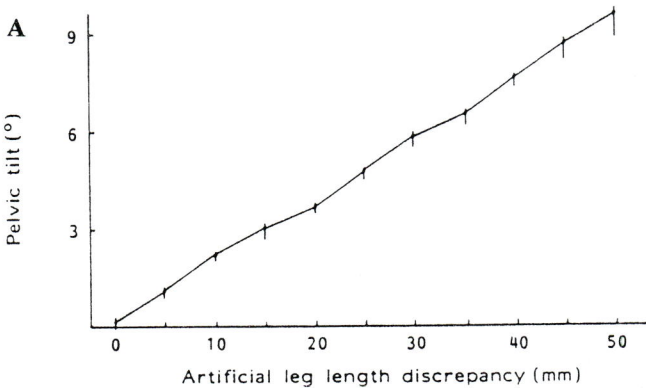

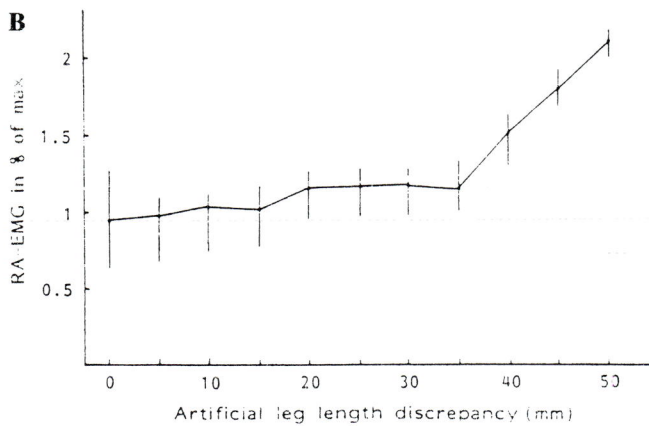

FIGURE 5.
A, increase in pelvic tilt in degrees for different artificial LLDs. The vertical line around each point is the standard deviaion. B, the increase in rectified/averaged EMG for different artificial LLDs for an electrode located 30 mm right from the spinous process of L-3 averaged more than 10 subjects. The rectified/averaged EMG is presented as a percentage of the rectified/averaged EMG during a maximal extension against resistance. The vertical line around each point is the standard deviation. (From Vink P, Kamphaisen HAC: *Clin Biomech* 1989; 4:115–117. Used by permission.)

justment. In the process, the patient's symptoms may abate. Heel lifts should be considered in the management of chronic, unresponsive cases, especially if LLD is excessive (e.g., >20 mm) or where patients perform (biomechanically) stressful tasks.

Eliciting LL Reactivity via Isolation and Pressure Testing
Procedures for eliciting leg alignment reactivity (or possible subluxations) have been termed "isolation" and "pressure" tests (see Table 2) and involve stimulation (via manual pressure or movements of the patient) of the joints of the spine, pelvis, and extremities (Table 6). Relative equalization of leg length following manipulation/adjustment is interpreted as a successful intervention and a sign that heightened reflexes are normalized.

If it is suspected that a component of the patient's condition involves a subluxation complex, the patient is screened for subluxations, observing for prone leg alignment reactivity after isolation testing procedures (Table 7). The first step is observing for discrepancy at the malleoli or heels. Next, the process of isolation testing is initiated, beginning at the knees, followed systematically by the pelvic motion segments, and proceeding caudally to the lumbar, thoracic, and cervical regions (see Table 6). After each stress test or isolation maneuver, the resulting LLs are compared. If one of the legs appears to shorten, a subluxation is believed to exist for the motion segment tested. To determine which side of the patient to adjust, flex the legs to 90 degrees and reobserve. If the initial short leg lengthens while being flexed to a 90-degree position the motion segment may be adjusted via pisiform or AAI in the plane of the joint on the same side as the initially observed short leg. If the leg shortens while being flexed to a 90-degree position, the motion segment is adjusted on the side opposite of the initial short leg. This protocol is intended to provide the clinician with a plan and a starting point that can be modified as necessary.

Validity and Reliability of LLD Evaluation

The theory of functional LLD and reactivity, like many others in chiropractic, is based on clinical observations. The connection between symptoms, testing procedures, and disease processes remains to be explored. One of the main reasons for this lack of understanding is that the measurement of LLD, as it is used in the field, is only moderately reliable under the best of circumstances[10, 11, 40] and poor in others,[21] with a range of $0.05 < K < 0.55$. By conservative estimates, a K value of 0 to 0.4 is considered marginal reproducibility, 0.4 to 0.75 is considered good reproducibility, and greater than 0.76 is considered excellent.[40] The differences in study outcomes may be explained by at least three factors: in Haas's case,[21, 42] a very low prevalence of positive test results might be anticipated because his sample contained relatively healthy subjects and they might not be expected to be reactive; accommodation of the response to multiple (12) pressure-testing stimuli; and potential examiner bias in the case of Youngquist et al.[10, 43]

DeWitt et al.[12] have attempted study of LLD validity using sensitive kinematic measurements. Preliminary study has shown that heel position movement during pressure and isolation tests is highly individualistic between patients and controls. (See Table 6 for a summary of study design features.) Reactivity has been recorded during pressure tests, sham tests, and adjustments in a person known to exhibit a great deal of reactivity. In this case, changes of as much as 0.75 cm were noted. LL reactivity may be a normal physiological phenomenon or may take on importance in some patients with various conditions (pathophysiological). Future studies are planned to determine the clinical utility of LLD reactivity.[44] Based on the findings and limitations of the previous studies, the clinical usefulness of the prone leg check and isolation/pressure tests used by themselves as indicators of subluxation require further investigation.[31, 45]

With regard to the clinical entity known as subluxation, the reliability of most procedures used to detect them is, at best, about 50% beyond

TABLE 5.
Citations: LLD Assessment

	Haas et al.[21]	Haas et al.[42]	Youngquist et al.[10]	Dewitt et al.[12]	Vink and Kamphaisen[38]	Friberg[33]	Froh et al.[35]	Soukka et al.[36]
Gold standard/ comparison	None, redundant measures (3)	None	None	Optoelectric motion analysis system	Electrogoniometer, heel lifts of known height	X-ray assessment of LLD was used and is considered a gold standard	X-ray assessment of LLD was used and is considered a gold standard	X-ray assessment with standardized procedure
Blinding procedure	Double blind	Double blind	Single blind	None, observational pilot study	Not mentioned, descriptive pilot study	Unstated	Unstated	Unstated
Sample/ spectrum of patients	42 asymptomatic and mildly symptomatic students	42 asymptomatic and mildly symptomatic students	72 patients with a history of C-1 subluxation	5 controls, 5 patients	10 asymptomatic males	359 young Finnish military conscripts, male controls, and 798 with symptoms such as LBP, hip pain, or sciatica	Patients (N = 40, 29 men, 11 women, mean age, 43.8 yr); may be inadequate to detect a significant difference	594 surveyed of 35 to 54-yr-old truck drivers (men), clerks, office cleaners (women) from Helsinki.

| Analysis | Kappa concordance statistic, odds ratio to determine the likelihood of identifying an association between the pressure-testing stimulus and LL reactivity | Kappa concordance statistic, odds ratio (relative risk) to determine the likelihood of identifying an association between the pressure-testing/adjustive stimuli and LL reactivity. | Kappa concordance statistic | Descriptive analysis and analysis of variance (ANOVA) | Descriptive analysis | Factors related to LBP in addition to LLD and were not controlled for (e.g., obesity, degree of exposure to high risk activities, height, weight) | Correlation coefficients were used to determine the strength of association between LLD and facet orientation; significant, may have required ANOVA vs. a t test | Logistic regression model tested the association between the LLD and LBP |

TABLE 6.
Selected Isolation and Pressure Test Procedures

Motion Segment	Procedure	Observations
Knees	Stroke the lateral and medial aspect of the knee joints	Equalization of LL
Pelvis		
Posterior/inferior posterior superior iliac spine (PSIS)	Push the PSIS anterior and superior on the short leg side	Equalization of LL
Anterior/superior PSIS	Pull the anterior superior iliac spine (ASIS) posterior and inferior	Equalization of LL
Superior/inferior pubic articulations	Instruct patient to squeeze knees together	Initial "short leg" appears to shorten
Lumbar		
L-5	Instruct patient to place arm of "short leg" across low back	Initial "short leg" appears to shorten
L-2	Instruct patient to place both arms across low back	Initial "short leg" appears to shorten
Thoracic		
T-12	Instruct patient to place arm of "short leg" over head	Initial "short leg" appears to shorten
T-8	Instruct patient to place both arms over head	Initial "short leg" appears to shorten
T-6	Instruct patient to turn head toward the initial "short leg" side	Initial "short leg" retracts
Cervical		
C-7	Patient returns head to neutral position	Initial "short leg" retracts
C-5	Patient looks up	Initial "short leg" appears to shorten
C-1	Patient tucks chin	Initial "short leg" appears to shorten

chance agreement. Pain over bony prominences and soft tissue appears to be the most reproducible finding; for these, K values are between 0.55 and 0.90 and 0.40 and 0.78, respectively. Reliability coefficients for various methods of detecting segmental abnormalities are summarized in Table 8.[10, 42, 46–48] In the face of uncertainty, clinicians have the responsibility to best serve their patients' needs based on their collective private experiences and the information available.

TREATMENT PROCEDURES

Innovation, with or without appropriate scientific testing of the hypotheses, is often met with resistance. This resistance is augmented by lack

TABLE 7.
Performance of the Prone Leg Check

Straight leg alignment analysis
  To perform this procedure:
  1. Position patient prone, arms to the side and palms facing the ceiling.
  2. Determine if a difference is present in leg alignment before touching patient.
  3. Place the palms of your hands over the patient's lateral malleoli and bring the patient's legs together until the heels touch to form a horizontal plane. Then release the heels before proceeding.
  4. Remove supination by placing your thumbs under the heel of each shoe, with your index finger posterior to the lateral malleoli and middle finger anterior to the lateral malleoli.
  5. Remove plantarflexion by applying steady, headward pressure to the soles of the patient's shoes.
  6. Note the side that shortens or feels spongy on the first evaluation. The leg that retracts or appears shorter is used as a reference for further tests.
Flexed leg alignment analysis
  To perform this procedure:
  1. Gently raise both legs to a 90-degree angle using your middle finger as a fulcrum along the edge of the sole to stabilize the feet, then level out the soles.
  2. At 90 degrees, place your thumbs on the soles of the shoes and index fingers along the edge of the soles to stabilize the feet, and then level out the soles (see Table 4).

of controlled studies or, sometimes, in spite of them. Although some believe that MFMA procedures should not be considered appropriate,[49] other authors[50, 51] have suggested their use in cases where forceful adjusting may be contraindicated, as in patients at risk for vertebral artery syndrome and for patients with bone-weakening diseases (metastatic carcinoma to the bone). For additional information see Appendix 1.

TABLE 8.
Summary of Reliability for Selected Chiropractic Assessment Procedures

Method	Reliability	Rating
Osseous pain	0.55–0.90	Fair to excellent
Soft tissue pain	0.40–0.78	Fair to good
Prone leg check	0.28–0.55	Poor to moderate
Thermal devices	0–0.50	Poor to moderate
Active motion palpation	0–0.47	Poor to moderate
Misalignment palpation	0–0.28	Poor

Some believe the main disadvantages of standard spinal manipulation/adjustment are that the line of drive and amount of force are difficult to control. However, recent work by Triano et al.[16] suggest that skills at delivering spinal manipulative therapy (SMT) are attainable and that reproducible maneuvers are possible in skilled hands. The AAI provides a high-speed thrust that is easier to control in terms of force and direction. Three variables are controlled at the discretion of the clinician using the AAI. First, the amount of instrument preload over the patients' skin must be made with care. Ideally it is about the same pressure that one could tolerate over the eye. The gripping action of the rubber tip of the instrument against the patient is also an additional source of uncontrolled shearing loads. The extent of these loads compared with the uniaxial impulse set up by the spring action of the instrument are unknown at this time. Second, the line of drive is intended to correspond with the average plane of the joints in a motion segment. Experience suggests that when the instrument is aligned with the average plane of the joints, the impulse has the greatest potential to induce movement in the motion segments. Third, the excursion of the stylus is controlled by an adjustable collar. The excursion ranges from 0 to just more than 5.5 mm. Lower settings are used on infants, patients with osteoporosis or very tender areas.

An adjustment is delivered by holding the AAI in the palm of the hand with the index and third fingers around the lower handle and placing the butt end (opposite the stylus) against the hypothenar eminence. Next, the lower handle is slowly squeezed against the piece braced against the thumb until it releases with an impulse. Only one impulse is recommended per motion segment.

CLINICAL STUDIES OF MFMA PROCEDURES

The clinical effects of MFMA procedures have been the subject of study and have included two randomized controlled clinical trials (RCTs), five descriptive outcome studies, and a number of case reports. Conditions for which the effects have been studied range from chronic sciatica, mechanical LBP, acute neck injuries, extremity injuries, and elevated blood pressure. Tables 9 and 10 summarize these studies based on four qualities of evidence: outcome measures, patient characteristics, blinding, and methods of analysis.

Randomized Controlled Trials

In one of the first pilot studies comparing two forms of manipulation, Gemmell[52] randomly allocated 30 patients with acute LBP to Meric (n = 16) and Activator (n = 14) treatment groups. Posterior to anterior adjustments were delivered to patients as they lay prone; contacts were made on the mammillary processes of segments exhibiting palpable tenderness and a loss of end-feel. Based on the primary outcome measure of pain reduction, the investigator was unable to distinguish between the different kinds of treatment ($p = 0.415$). Unfortunately, several possible explanations exist that might explain these results: (1) neither treatment was effective (the reduction in pain resulted from regression to the mean or patient-doctor interaction, (2) both treatments were equally effective in reducing the level of pain in the short term, and (3) the sample size was not adequate to detect a statistically significant difference between groups. Also, because the person recording the data was also the treating doctor, the two groups may have been subconsciously treated differently by the doctor. A secondary outcome measure included the patient's level of comfort during the adjustment.[53] Anecdotally, a greater level of comfort was reported with the Activator-adjusted group. The added level of comfort reported may be the result of (1) the rapid delivery of the Activator thrust (<20 msec vs. 100 msec for the Meric procedure), (2) differences in intended preload, or (3) the lower amplitude of thrust force produced by the AAI.

Yates et al.[13] reported a pilot study using randomization of patients with mildly elevated blood pressure (>130/90 mm Hg) and anxiety states. These patients were monitored in three groups using the State-Trait Anxiety Inventory. The first group received Activator adjustments from T-1 to T-5. The second group received sham adjustments with the instrument set in a position to deliver the minimal amount of force, with no excursion of the stylus. The third group received no treatment. Short-term reductions ($p < 0.05$) in systolic and diastolic pressures were noted on the adjusted but not the sham-adjusted and no treatment groups. Although alternative explanations for the results are possible, the authors concluded that this study lent support to the hypothesis that manipulation of the thoracic spine with the AAI significantly reduces diastolic and systolic blood pressures when compared with the placebo and control groups. The long-lasting effects of chiropractic treatment on elevated blood pressure remain to be investigated, and these short-term effects have yet to be replicated.

CASE SERIES

Mechanical LBP

Richards et al.[54] cited the treatment of two patients with sciatic neuropathy and lumbar disk herniation. Clinically significant reductions in pain and restoration of function were noted within 2 weeks of treatment onset, with a treatment protocol consisting of combined MFMA adjusting, pelvic blocking, high-volt galvanic current, and exercise. Comparable effects were noted in a similar case using MFMA and a video-assisted stretching program[55] and other studies using flexion-distraction technique[56] and diversified rotary manipulation.[57] Although firm conclusions cannot be made regarding the efficacy of any one procedure, the similarities in patient responsiveness across treatments warrants further study. Until then, these treatment history results can serve as an estimate of the type of response to expect in similar patients.

Findings similar to those just cited were noted in the treatment of two geriatric patients with chronic mechanical LBP, both of whom were treated with MFMA.[58] The patients' LBP decreased 50% to 75% within the first 2 weeks of care when compared with a 3-week baseline (no treatment). An increase in the patients' functioning (via the Oswestry LBP disability questionnaire) and a reduction in the number and severity of positive provocation test results were also noted (Fig 6).

SIJS

Ten patients with chronic SIJS were treated solely with MFMA procedures over the course of 6 weeks.[59] Significant differences were noted in

TABLE 9.
Citations: RCTs and Sciatica*

	RCTs		Sciatia			
	Yates et al.[13]	Gemmell[53]	Richards et al.[54]	Osterbauer and Fuhr[55]	Cox and Shreiner[56]	Quon et al.[57]
Outcome measures	BP (e.g., sphygmomanometer); variability in the BP of this sample across several visits is unknown	VAS	SOAP notes; this study was conducted before the advent of outcome measures	VAS, Oswestry low BP disability questionnaire	VAS, examination findings, survey	Narrative format; this study was conducted before the advent of outcome measures
Blinding procedure	Single blind	Single blind	None, because this was a retrospective case study	None, case report	Unstated	None reported
Sample spectrum of patients	Patients from a chiropractic practice with a history of low BP on a previous visit	30 patients seen in a private chiropractic practice in Oklahoma with acute low BP	Two cases were chosen from a private practice in suburban Ohio	One case was chosen from a private practice in suburban Phoenix	576 patients with low BP and sciatica at 30 private chiropractic offices	One case was chosen from a private practice in tertiary care, orthopedic setting, Saskatchewan, Canada; susceptible to selection bias

| Analysis | ANOVA with posthoc comparisons to determine differences between groups | Yes, paired t test | Descriptive analysis was performed; multiple interventions make it impossible to ascribe the patients' response to any one treatment; however, the treatments are commonly used in combination, and the results reflect what probably occurs "in the field" | Descriptive analysis | Descriptive analysis was performed; multiple interventions make it impossible to ascribe the patients' response to any one treatment; however, the treatments are commonly used in combination, and the results reflect what probably occurs "in the field" | Descriptive case report |

*BP = blood pressure; VAS = Visual Analogue Scale; SOAP = subjective, objective, assessment, and plan.

TABLE 10.
Citations: Mechanical Low BP and SIJS*

	Mechanical Low BP (Osterbauer et al.[58])	Osterbauer et al.[59]	Herzog et al.[60]	SIJS Herzog et al.[61]	Cassidy et al.[63]	Greenman[64]	Neck; Low Back, and SIJ Problems (Osterbauer et al.[65])
Outcome measures	VAS, and Oswestry low BP disability questionnaire	VAS, ROM, orthopedic tests	VAS, Oswestry, gait analysis, motion palpation	VAS, Oswestry, gait analysis, motion palpation	SOAP notes this study was conducted before the advent of outcome measures	SOAP notes this study was conducted before the advent of outcome measures.	ROM, finite helical axis (kinematic function of the head and neck) VAS
Blinding procedure	No, quasiexperimental approach, case series	None, observational pilot study	Unstated, single case pilot study	Unstated, single case pilot study	Unstated	Unstated	None
Sample/spectrum of patients	Two geriatric patients seen in chiropractic practices in Massachusetts and Missouri	10 consecutive patients with SIJS seeking care from a DC	One case was chosen from a private practice in Calgary, AB, Canada; susceptible to selection bias	11 adults (5 women, 6 men) with a history of chronic low BP from a local chiropractic practice	69 cases of SIJS were chosen from a private practice in a tertiary care, orthopedic setting, Saskatchewan, Canada	Case report from a private osteopathic practice	10 consecutive whiplash patients reporting to chiropractic practices in suburban Phoenix

| Analysis | Time series analysis, baseline and treatment phase, symptoms vs. time | t tests were performed; ANOVA was performed to determine prebaseline/posttreatment significance | Descriptive analysis | Descriptive analysis, time series | Chi-square analysis was used | Descriptive | t test, possibility of finding statistically significant before and after differences by pure chance; multiple interventions make it impossible to ascribe the patients' response to any one treatment; however, the treatments are commonly used in combination, and the results reflect what probably occurs "in the field" |

*SIJS = sacroiliac joint syndrome: ROM = range of motion.

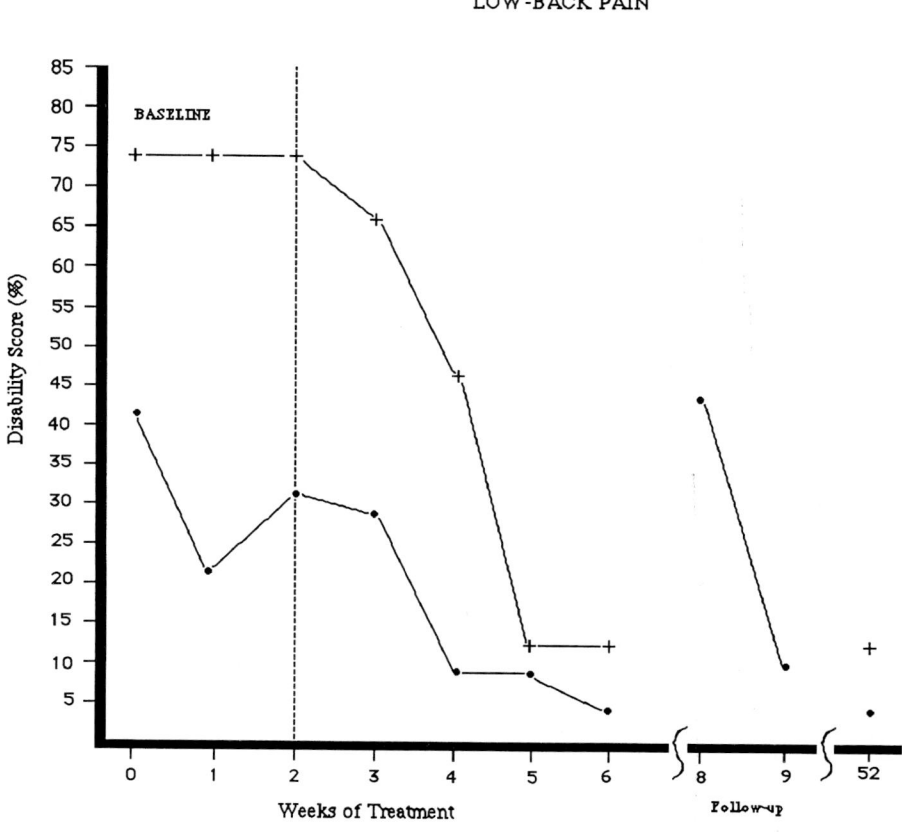

FIGURE 6.
Modified Oswestry disability index scores vs. time in two geriatric patients with chronic mechanical LBP. The baseline includes three data points during which the patients were not receiving treatment.

the Visual Analogue Scale (VAS)-reported average level of pain ($t = 2.3$; $p < 0.05$), Oswestry scores ($t = 2.3$, $p < 0.05$)* and the number of positive orthopedic test results (Fischer's exact probability test, $p = 0.025$–0.045). Control comparisons were not collected, and measures of gait, postural sway, and joint stiffness demonstrated no changes. These results differ from the conclusions of Herzog et al.[60, 61] Some possible explanations for this are found in Table 11, as outlined by Herzog and Conway.[62] However, the clinical results are similar to several studies using long lever rotary manipulation[60, 63] and muscle energy techniques.[64] For a comparison of study methodologies, see Table 10.

Whiplash Syndrome

Osterbauer et al.[65] studied 10 whiplash patients treated for 6 weeks using an ensemble of MFMA, interferential current, medications (analgesics and muscle relaxants), or combination thereof. Significant reductions

---

*Although these values may be thought to reflect α-inflation, they were confirmed at another time using ANOVA and are available from the author on request.

TABLE 11.
Summary of Gait Analysis Studies

Methods	Herzog et al.[60-62]	Osterbauer et al.[59]
Control of walking speed patients with sacroiliac syndrome	Yes	No, self-selected pace (to typify problems).
Number of observations	30–40	10
Force plate hidden	Yes	No
Time frame of test	Before and after gait analysis, 6 weeks of treatment immediately after treatment	Gait analysis before and after
Intervention	Long-lever, side posture rotary manipulation	MFMA procedures
Ground reaction force symmetry index	Yes	Yes

were noted in the average level of neck pain (VAS) ($t = 3.15$; $p < 0.05$), and increases in global range of motion ($t = 5.68$; $p < 0.0001$) were observed. In addition, finite helical axis parameters were monitored and found to return to a more normal level over the course of treatment.[66]

CASE REPORTS

Several case reports have appeared detailing successful treatment of patients with the AAI for a tear of the medial meniscus confirmed on magnetic resonance imaging,[67] frozen shoulder,[51,68] plantar fasciitis,[69] chronic sciatica,[55] otitis media,[70] and Bell's palsy.[71] Although positive, the results of these case reports and observational case series should be interpreted with caution, because the effects of the patient-doctor encounter are powerful regardless of the treatment.[72] The reports, however, supply supportive data necessary for designing more rigorous studies and documenting the kinds of complaints and outcomes encountered in field doctors' offices.

ROLE OF KINEMATICS IN CHIROPRACTIC MANIPULATION/ADJUSTMENT

Knowledge of spine segment motion patterns (kinematics) and associated forces and moments (kinetics) is of fundamental interest to understanding (1) creep and vibration response of the spine, (2) the role of spinal implants in mechanical load sharing, and (3) the response of the spine to externally applied forces such as (chiropractic) manipulation/adjustment. (For a brief review of biomechanics of the normal and pathological spine, see Appendix 2.)

Although chiropractic treatments are generally considered to be therapeutic, very little is understood about the source of the positive treatment effects associated with manipulation, mobilization therapy, or adjustive therapy. Possible therapeutic mechanisms include realignment of vertebral bodies, mobilization of spinal joints, relaxation of back musculature through reflex pathways, production of a respiratory burst, cavitation (causing a temporary increase in joint space and omnidirectional ROM), release of inflammatory agents within the body, and coactivation of mechanically sensitive somatic afferents.[4, 73–77] To understand the biomechanical consequences of spinal manipulation more fully, researchers are currently focusing on quantifying the applied forces associated with spinal manipulation and response of the spine to these forces.

The central objective of AMCT is toward a comprehensive approach to diagnosis and treatment. The current impetus is to better characterize popular subjective assessments such as motion palpation and the prone leg check to improve their reliability and ultimately determine their clinical utility.

VERTEBRAL FORCES AND MOVEMENTS DURING SPINAL MANIPULATION AND MOBILIZATION

Two primary categories of manual therapy are used to treat patients with back problems: manipulation/adjustment and mobilization. In addition to manual manipulation/adjustment, clinicians are also currently using mechanical devices such as table drop pieces and moving stylus instruments to mechanically assist and control the application of force. Manipulation/adjustment involves the application of a thrusting force to a specific part of a spine in a well-defined direction. In contrast, mobilization generally involves slower nonspecific oscillatory movements directed toward multiple segments of the spine.

In commonly used chiropractic procedures such as posteroanterior mobilization, spinal stiffness or the load/displacement response is often of interest. Although neither the relationship between pain and posteroanterior stiffness nor the effect of treatment on spinal stiffness has been objectively demonstrated, a common recommendation is that the therapist take note of the stiffness felt during mobilization.[48, 76–79]

In principle, an unstable segment should exhibit increased displacement or decreased stiffness, whereas a stiffened segment should exhibit decreased displacement compared with adjacent segments.[80] The displacement of a vertebra and the resistance to the displacement during mobilization, therefore, are potentially very useful in spinal diagnosis and to establish effective treatment protocols. During manipulation and mobilization procedures, posteroanterior forces can range from 50 to 800 N, depending on the procedure used.[9, 73, 76, 77, 81–91] In general, the higher peak forces (550–800 N) have been reported for SMT of sacroiliac joint and thoracic fixations, respectively. Peak forces as high as 200 to 300 N have also been reported during cervical adjustments (Table 12).[91] Preload forces during these procedures can be as low as 20 N or as high as 200 N. In vivo stiffness (load/deformation) characteristics of the spine are less well understood primarily because of the difficulties associated with obtaining precise measurement of the displacements of the spinal segments.

Efforts to estimate the in vivo displacement behavior of spinal segments during manipulation and low-frequency mobilization using surface

TABLE 12.
Reported Manipulation Loads†

	Forces				Moments			
	AP	Ax	Tr	Mag	AP	Ax	Tr	Mag
	lb				ft-lb			
Cervical	18	29	27	43.5	125	52	202	244
Thoracic	120	10	10	120.8	—‡	—	—	—
Lumbopelvic	60	—	—	—	—	—	—	—

*From Triano JJ: *J Manipulative Physiol Ther* 1992; 15:71–75. Used by permission.
†AP = anteroposterior; Ax = longitudinal spinal axis; Tr = transverse; Mag = load magnitude.
‡Not measured/reported.

displacement transducers* or mathematical models[87] indicate that the normal spine may exhibit a posteroanterior displacement of about 2 to 10 mm per 100 N of applied load, corresponding to a stiffness of about 10 to 50 kN/m, presuming no deformation of the laminae, which remains to be determined. Using an intervertebral motion device (IMD) attached to pins inserted into the L3 to L4 spinous processes of a young, male subject, Nathan and Keller[90] reported that posteroanterior impulses (72 N) applied to the spinous process of adjacent vertebrae (L-2 to T-11) produced axial displacements, posteroanterior shear displacements, and flexion/extension rotations of 1.6 mm, 0.5 mm, and 0.9 degrees, respectively. These authors also noted that IMD-based motion patterns differed when similar measurements were performed on two patients diagnosed with L-4 to L-5 degenerative disk disease and L-5 retrospondylolisthesis. Subsequent Fourier spectrum analysis* of the mechanical impedance (force/velocity) response at the impulse sites indicated that the stiffness of the human spine was frequency dependent, exhibiting a maximum posteroanterior stiffness of 62 kN/m (T-11) to 124 kN/m (L-2) at a frequency of about 100 Hz. Lee and Svensson[88] also observed that the posteroanterior stiffness of the lumbosacral spine was greater for dynamic mobilization at 0.5 to 1.0 Hz compared with mobilization at quasistatic loading rates (0.05 Hz). Thus, the dynamic stiffness of the lumbar spine appears to be much greater than that realized using slow cyclic or quasistatic loading rates.

NEW METHODS OF CHARACTERIZATION OF THE DYNAMIC MECHANICAL PROPERTIES OF THE SPINE

Recent studies performed at the University of Vermont have focused on the dynamic characterization of human thoracolumbar spinal motion and stiffness characteristics using a low-force, moving stylus–type mechani-

---

*References 76, 77, 81, 85, 87, 88.
*Time-domain signals can be converted to the frequency-domain signals using a Fast Fourier Transform (FFT).

cal instrument, the AAI. The basic premise underlying this work is the notion that the intrinsic mechanical behavior of the human spine can be determined by quantifying the motion response of various portions of the spine to a known force input. The AAI used in these studies was modified to include a load cell and accelerometer (impedance head), which was used to measure the input force and acceleration response characteristics of the spine (acceleration) (Fig 7, A). The AAI delivers a short-duration (<20-msec) impulse to the spine and is characterized by two primary force peaks (Fig 7, B). Depending on the force setting, the first peak is about twofold to fourfold greater in amplitude but is always shorter in duration than the second peak (Fig 7, C).

The AAI device was recently used to deliver posteroanterior thrusts to the spinous processes (T-7, T-9, T-11 to S-2) of 11 subjects: 5 men (26.8 years, SD 7.8) and 6 women (24.5 years, SD 3.7) with no previous history of LBP or spine-related surgery.[90] Five repeated impulses were delivered at 10 spinal levels at the end of the expiration of breath, and force (F) and acceleration (a) signals were sampled at 50 kHz using a 12-bit alternating/direct (A/D) converter for 160 msec. The effects of any direct current (DC) offset in the F and a signals were removed by applying the FFT to each signal, setting the DC term to 0 and applying the inverse FFT. The acceleration-time signal was integrated using Simpson's rule to derive the impulse velocity. A force window (50 msec, 2,500 samples wide) was applied to the zeroed force-time signal. Posteroanterior impedance was calculated at each discrete frequency, as the ratio of FFT(force)/FFT(velocity), along with the phase difference between the force and velocity. This analytical procedure is summarized in Figure 8.

For each spinal level, ensemble-averaged impedance and phase plots were derived from the five trials. Three impedance and stiffness parameters were identified for each impedance curve: first peak (peak1), (2) first minimum (min1 or max mobility), and (3) second peak (peak2); together with the frequency (f) at which each occurred (Fig 9). These frequency peaks/valley were readily identified and were always associated with a rapid change in phase angle (±45 degrees), which is the amount the response (velocity) lags behind the input (force). At resonance (min1) the spine is −45 degrees out of phase. The posteroanterior dynamic stiffness was calculated as the product of impedance and circular frequency ($2\pi f$).

Figure 10 graphically illustrates the variation in the maximum (peak2) impedance (mean + SD) obtained for five of the female subjects (one woman not shown) and five male subjects. The maximum posteroanterior impedance of the thoracolumbar spine ranged from 200 to 800 N/m for levels T-7 to S-2 and occurred between 70 and 100 Hz. Most subjects (both men and women) exhibited a bimodal impedance distribution: higher posteroanterior impedance at spinal levels T-11 to T-12 and L-3 to L-4 when compared with other levels. For the five repeated impulses, variances (100 * SD/mean) in the impedance data tended to be about 25% to 50%.

In both the thoracic and the lumbar regions the male subjects tend to be stiffer (higher impedance) than the female subjects at the first, lowest frequency (peak1 = 20–30 Hz), but were less stiff at higher frequencies (Fig 11). Statistically significant differences ($p < 0.05$ indicated by * in

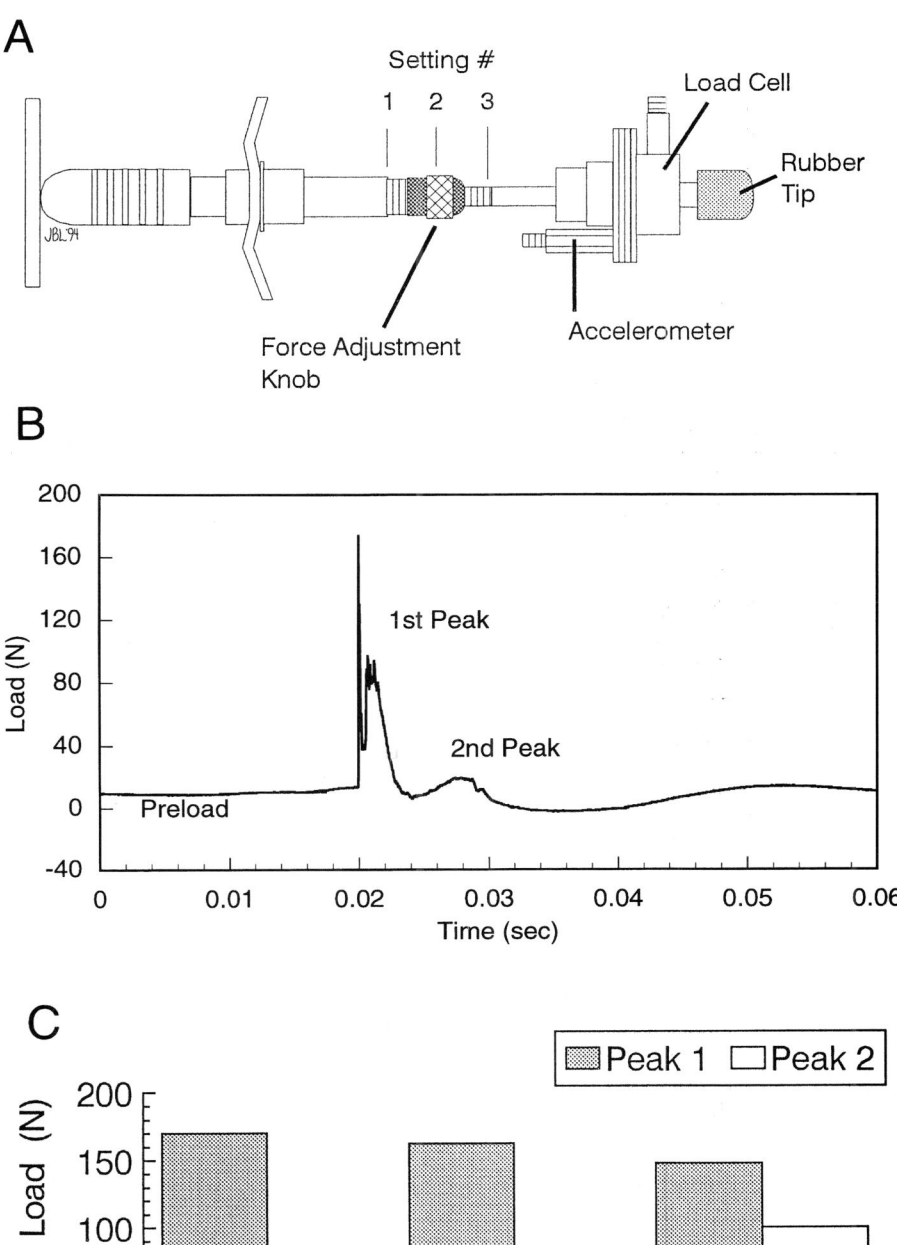

FIGURE 7.
A, AAI device and impedance head − load cell + accelerometer. **B,** typical posteroanterior impulse load-time history obtained from the AAI device for the lumbar spine of a young, male subject. The impulse singal is characterized by two primary peaks, which rapidly damp out within about 5 msec of the first peak. **C,** variation in first impulse peak and second impulse peak load magnitudes obtained for each of the three force adjustment positions illustrated in **A.**

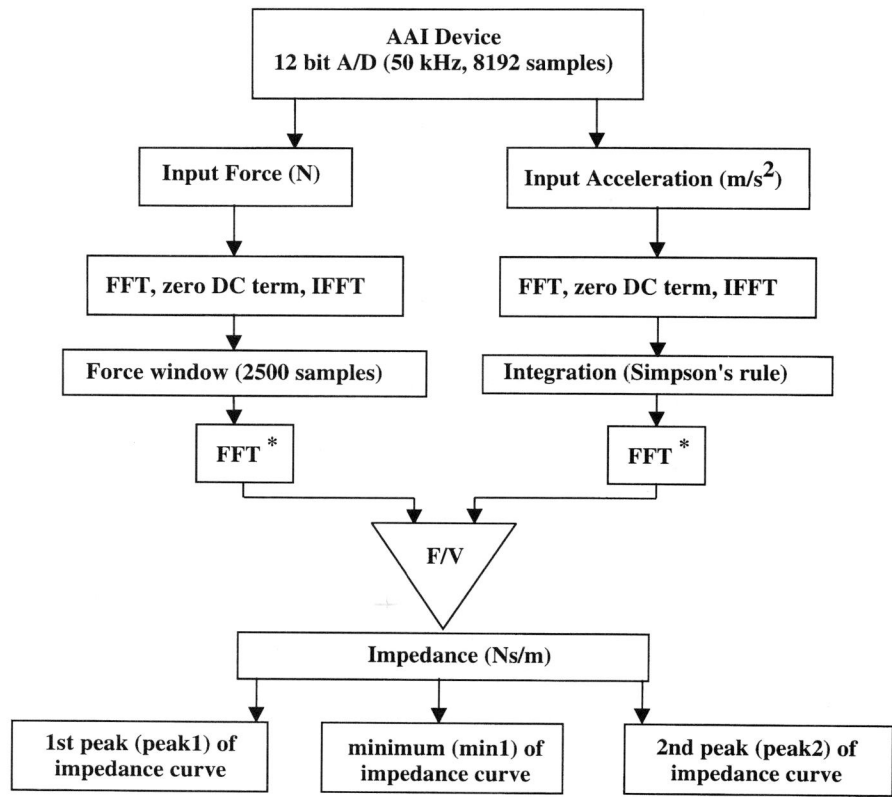

FIGURE 8.
Summary of the driving point impedance data acquisition and analysis procedure.

Fig 11) in mobility between men and women were noted, particularly for frequencies corresponding to the maximum mobility (*min1* = 40–50 Hz) and minimum mobility (*peak2* = 70–80 Hz).

Women exhibited greater *min1* stiffness (21–42 kN/m) and consequently had lower mobility at all levels tested compared with the male subjects (16–23 kN/m). An analysis of variance indicated that there were statistically significant *min1* impedance and stiffness differences between the males and females. For most subjects (both men and women) the lumbar region exhibited a higher *min1* impedance and stiffness when compared with the thoracic region.

MECHANICAL IMPULSE FOR SPINAL DIAGNOSIS AND THERAPY

An increasing body of evidence suggests that the musculoskeletal system may respond most efficiently to specific frequency components of mechanical signals,[92,93] suggesting that dynamic mechanical stimuli may be more effective than static stimuli. This is consistent with the notion that

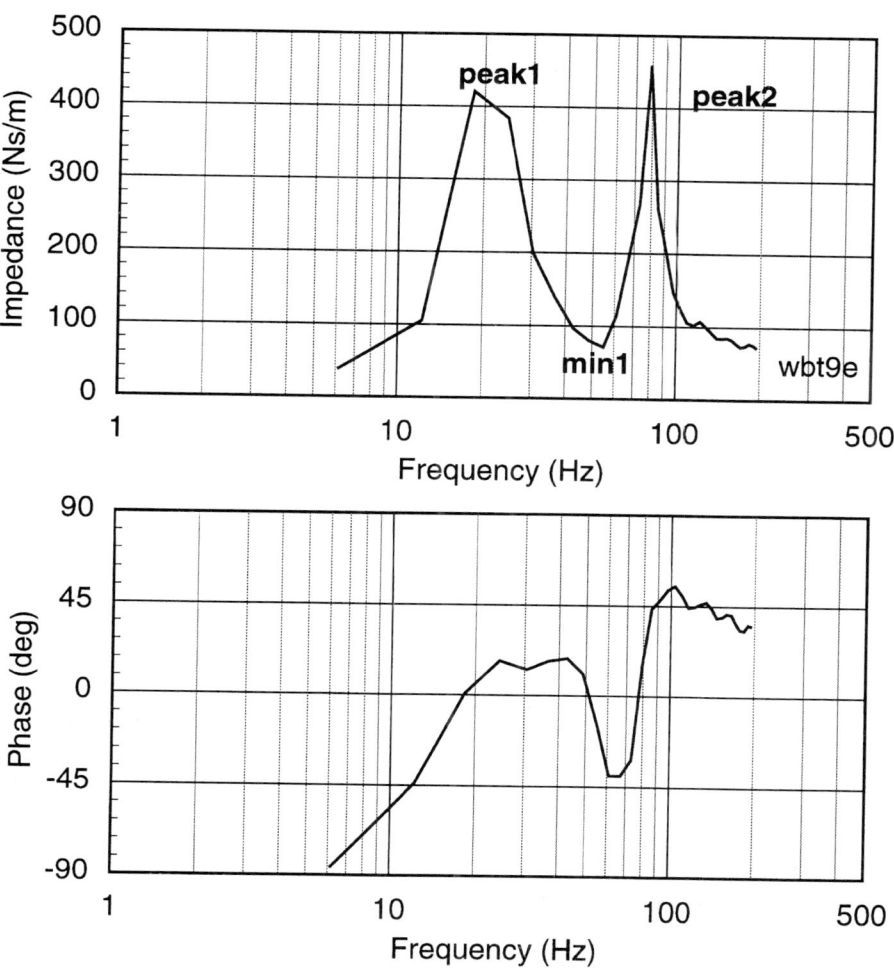

FIGURE 9.
Driving point impedance (top) and phase (bottom) profiles are shown for a typical subject. Three parameters were identified for each impedance curve: (1) first peak (peak1), (2) first minimum (min1, or max mobility), and (3) second peak (peak2, or max impedance); together with the frequency (f) at which each occurred.

chiropractic manipulation/adjustment has therapeutic effects on the musculoskeletal system. As discussed earlier, the effects of chiropractic manipulations/adjustment have generally been hypothesized to result from biomechanical mechanisms or mechanical coactivation of paraspinal tissues; see the reviews by Gillette[74] and Zusman[75] and studies on mechanical impedance, which indicate that the thoracolumbar spine exhibits a maximum mobility of 40 to 50 Hz and is least mobile for frequencies centered around 70 to 90 Hz. An interesting hypothesis, therefore, is the notion that both magnitude and frequency content of manual and mechanical thrusting manipulations are critical elements in determining therapeutic effects of these procedures.

Information concerning the biomechanical response of the spine to

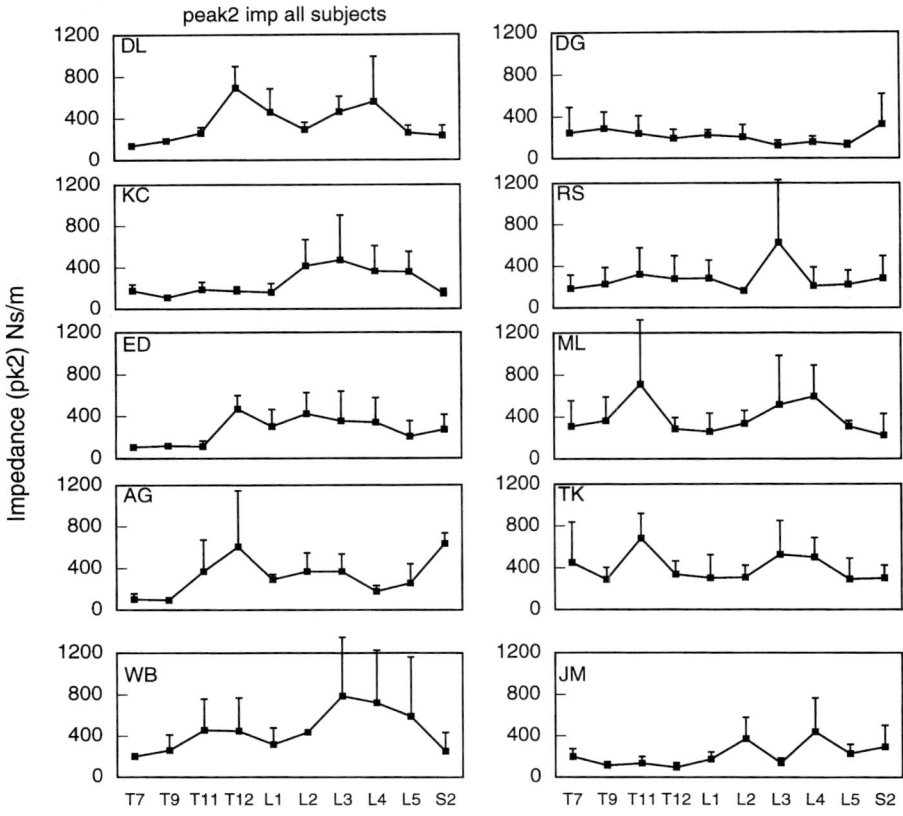

FIGURE 10.
Variation (mean, SD) in the maximum impedance (*peak2* in Fig 4) obtained for five of the female subjects (one woman not shown) and the five male subjects. See Figure 11 for definition of *peak2*.

short-duration posteroanterior impulsive or harmonic oscillations is generally lacking in the literature. However, such information is very important, because these types of motion occur during chiropractic manipulations, as well as daily activities such as walking and lifting tasks. Consequently, additional analyses of the dynamic mechanical response of the spine are needed and may provide important new information concerning the acute viscoelastic behavior of the spinal column. Driving point impedance measurements appear promising as a noninvasive analytical technique for identifying the mechanical behavior of the human spine.

FUTURE PERSPECTIVE: COMPUTER-ASSISTED MANIPULATION

Computers are now commonplace in health care, particularly in critical care areas in both large and small hospitals where the computer can speed up communications, laboratory analysis, and diagnoses and in many cases help to reduce the length of stay of a patient. They are used for a

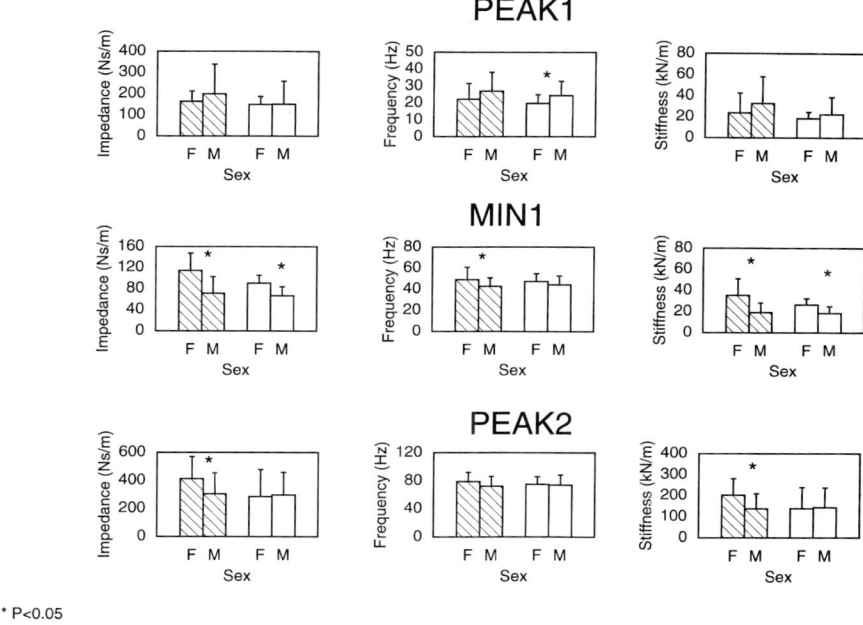

FIGURE 11.
These graphs illustrate the differences in spinal impedance *(left)*, frequency *(middle)*, and stiffness *(right)* for the combined thoracic levels and combined lumbar levels of the male and female subjects corresponding to peak1 *(top)*, min1 *(middle)* and peak2 *(bottom)* regions of the impedance curves. (See Fig 11 for peak1, min1, and peak2 definitions.)

wide range of applications, including the microprocessor that controls bedside equipment and miniframe or mainframe computers, which are an integral part of dedicated critical care systems. The notion of computer-assisted manipulation therefore is timely.

For successful and routine clinical use of spine biomechanical analyses, a given method should be noninvasive, reproducible, inexpensive, simple to operate, and painless in application. The impedance measurement and analysis procedure described here appear to satisfy these requirements. With the use of mechanical devices such as the AAI, impedance measurements may be used to evaluate the dynamic stiffness characteristics of the spine while prescribing treatment. Such procedures, therefore, may be potentially useful to evaluate the biomechanical effectiveness of various manipulative/adjustment, surgical, and rehabilitative procedures.

CONCLUSION

AMCT has been taught and presented as a system of chiropractic analysis and treatment for a variety of neuromusculoskeletal conditions for the past 30 years. During this time, investigation has been initiated on both the analysis and treatment procedures. This participation in the scientific process has changed the way AMCT is presented to the field. The emphasis has shifted from making unsubstantiated claims to a realistic assessment of the strengths and limitations of the evidence. The result has been the elimination of unjustified claims, which have been common in chiropractic for the past 100 years. Although the process of critical assessment is often difficult to balance with the practical demands of patient care, an effort is made to help field practitioners meet the needs of their patients.

Work concerning the reliability and validity of the prone leg check and MFMA adjusting procedure is still in its early stages. The results of interexaminer reliability studies of the prone leg check, like many other methods of chiropractic analysis, exhibit only "fair" to "moderate" reliability. New motion analysis technology is allowing the precise measurement of the reactive leg phenomenon and will hopefully lead to a better understanding of the physiological process behind the clinical observations and ultimately clinical utility.

Advancing technology is also enabling quantification of the mechanical properties of the manipulation/adjustment, as well as characterizing the spine's biomechanical response impulsive loads. Not only is this useful in defending malpractice cases, but this type of analysis may lead to the development of new diagnostic tools to supplement traditional methods of analysis. Although clinical studies of AMCT include two RCTs, numerous case series, and reports suggesting at least parity with the effectiveness of other treatment methods, much more work is needed to replicate the findings and determine the effectiveness of MFMA adjusting procedures in specific cases.

REFERENCES

1. Nelson CF: Five steps to your own technique: The Nelson method. *J Manipulative Physiol Ther* 16:115–117, 1993.
2. Bergmann TF: Various forms of chiropractic technique. *Chiropr Technique* 5:53–55, 1993.
3. Osterbauer PJ, Fuhr AW: The current status of Activator Methods Chiropractic Technique, theory, and training. *Chiropr Technique* 2:168–175, 1990.
4. Osterbauer PJ, Fuhr AW, Hildebrandt RW: Mechanical force manually adjusted short lever chiropractic adjustment. *J Manipulative Physiol Ther* 15:309–317, 1992.
5. Christensen MG, Delle Morgan DR: Job analysis of chiropractic: A project report, survey analysis and summary of the practice of chiropractic within the United States. Greeley, Colo, National Board of Chiropractic Examiners, 1993, pp 78–79.
6. Christensen MG, Delle Morgan DR: Job analysis of chiropractic: A project report, survey analysis and summary of the practice of chiropractic within Canada. Greeley, Colo, National Board of Chiropractic Examiners, 1993, p 108.
7. Pedersen P: A survey of chiropractic practice in Europe. *Eur J Chiropr* 42:3–28, 1994.
8. Fuhr AW, Smith DB: Accuracy of piezoelectric accelerometers measuring displacement of a spinal adjusting instrument. *J Manipulative Physiol Ther* 9:15–21, 1986.

9. Smith DB, Fuhr AW, Davis BP: Skin accelerometer displacement and relative bone movement of adjacent vertebrae in response to chiropractic percussion thrusts. *J Manipulative Physiol Ther* 12:26–37, 1989.
10. Youngquist MW, Fuhr AW, Osterbauer PJ: Interexaminer reliability of an upper cervical isolation test. *J Manipulative Physiol Ther* 12:93–97, 1989.
11. Fuhr AW, Osterbauer PJ: Interexaminer reliability of relative leg length evaluations in the prone extended position. *Chiropr Technique* 1:13–18, 1989.
12. Dewitt JK, Osterbauer PJ, Stelmach GE, et al: Optoelectric measurement of changes in leg length inequality resulting from isolation tests. *J Manipulative Physiol Ther* 17:530–538, 1994.
13. Yates RG, Lamping DL, Abram NL, et al: Effects of chiropractic treatment on blood pressure and anxiety: A randomized controlled trial. *J Manipulative Physiol Ther* 11:484–488, 1988.
14. Haldeman S, Chapman-Smith D, Petersen DM Jr (eds): *Guidelines for chiropractic quality assurance and practice parameters: Proceedings of the Mercy Center Consensus Conference.* Gaithersburg, Md, Aspen, 1993, pp 108–109.
15. Henderson D, Chapman-Smith D, Mior S, et al: Clinical guidelines for chiropractic practice in Canada. *J Can Chiropr Assoc* 38(suppl):110, 1994.
16. Triano JJ: The biomechanics of the chiropractic adjustment. *J Manipulative Physiol Ther* 15:71–75, 1992.
17. Keck WF: A method of chiropractic analysis. *Natl Chiropr Assoc J* pp 1–6, 1958.
18. Van Rumpt R: Directional non-force technique notes. In *Directional Non-Force Technique.* Beverly Hills, Calif, 1987.
19. Thompson C: *Technique Reference Manual.* Thompson Educational Workshops. Ill, SM & Williams Manufacturing, 1987.
20. Heyman WC: Considerations of a diagnostic test for sacroiliac (innominate lesions). *J Am Osteopath Assoc* 67:1013–1017, 1968.
21. Haas M, Peterson D, Panzer D, et al: Reactivity of leg alignment to articular pressure testing: Evaluation for a diagnostic test using a randomized crossover clinical trial approach. *J Manipulative Physiol Ther* 16:220–227, 1993.
22. Sandoz RW: Some reflex phenomena associated with spinal derangements and adjustments. *Ann Swiss Chiropr Assoc* 7:45–65, 1981.
23. Slosberg M: Activator Methods isolation tests. *Today's Chiropr* 16:41–43, 1987.
24. Nansel DD, Waldorf T, Cooperstein R: Effect of cervical spinal adjustments on lumbar paraspinal muscle tone: Evidence for facilitation of intersegmental tonic neck reflexes. *J Manipulative Physiol Ther* 16:91–95, 1993.
25. Carver W: *Chiropractic Analysis.* Self-published, 1923.
26. Filson RM, Johnson G: Logan system of body mechanics assessment. *Chiropr Technique* 6:98–103, 1994.
27. Sandoz R: Principles underlying the prescription of shoe lifts. *Ann Swiss Chiropr Assoc* 9:50–89, 1989.
28. Denslow JS, Chace JA, Gardener DL, et al: Mechanical stresses in the human lumbar spine and pelvis. *J Am Osteopath Assoc* 61:705–712, 1962.
29. Cooperstein R: Functional leg length inequality: Geometric analysis and an alternative muscular model. The Proceedings of the 8th Annual CORE, Monterey, Calif, June 18–20, 1993, pp 202–203.
30. Triano JJ: Interaction of spinal biomechanics and physiology. In Haldeman Scott (ed): *Principle and Practice of Chiropractic,* ed 2. Norwalk, Conn, Appleton & Lange, 1992, pp 225–255.
31. Manello DM: Leg length inequality. *J Manipulative Physiol Ther* 15:576–590, 1992.

32. Lawrence DJ: Chiropractic concepts of the short leg: A critical review. *J Manipulative Physiol Ther* 8:157–161, 1985.
33. Friberg O: Clinical symptoms and biomechanics of lumbar spine and hip joint in leg length inequality. *Spine* 8:643–651, 1983.
34. Giles LGF, Taylor JR: Lumbar spine structural changes associated with leg length inequality. *Spine* 7:159–162, 1983.
35. Froh R, Yong-Hing K, Cassidy JD, et al: The relationship between leg length discrepancy and lumbar facet orientation. *Spine* 13:325–327, 1988.
36. Soukka A, Alaranta H, Tallroth KAJ, et al: Leg-length inequality in people of working age. *Spine* 16:429–431, 1991.
37. Triano JJ: Objective electromyographic evidence for use and effects of lift therapy. *J Manipulative Physiol Ther* 6:13–16, 1983.
38. Vink P, Kamphaisen HAC: Leg length inequality, pelvic tilt and lumbar back muscle activity during standing. *Clin Biomech* 4:115–117, 1989.
39. Specht DL, De Boer KF: Anatomical leg length inequality, scoliosis and lordotic curve in unselected clinic patients. *J Manipulative Physiol Ther* 14:368–375, 1991.
40. DeBoer KF, Harmon FA, Savoic S, et al: Inter and intraexaminer reliability of leg length differential measurements: A preliminary study. *J Manipulative Physiol Ther* 6:61–66, 1983.
41. Rosner B: *Fundamentals of Biostatistics*, ed 2. Boston, PWS, 1986.
42. Haas M, Peterson D, Rothman EH, et al: Responsiveness of leg alignment changes associated with articular pressure testing to spinal manipulation: The use of a randomized clinical trial design to evaluate a diagnostic test with a dichotomous outcome. *J Manipulative Physiol Ther* 16:306–311, 1993.
43. Haas M: The reliability of reliability. *J Manipulative Physiol Ther* 14:199–208, 1991.
44. DeWitt JK: Heel position changes demonstrated by a highly reactive patient associated with isolation tests and adjustments: A technical report. Tempe, Ariz, Arizona State University, July 1994.
45. Mootz RD, Hansen DT, Adams AH: The value of leg length inequality and specific contact short level adjusting in chiropractic practice: Results of a consensus process by chiropractic expert panels. *Chiropr Technique* 16:220–227, 1993.
46. Keating JC, Bergmann TF, Jacobs GE, et al: Interexaminer reliability of eight evaluative dimensions of lumbar segmental abnormality. *J Manipulative Physiol Ther* 13:463–470, 1990.
47. Boline PD, Haas M, Meyer JJ, et al: Interexaminer reliability of eight evaluative dimensions of lumbar segmental abnormality: II. *J Manipulative Physiol Ther* 16:363–374, 1993.
48. Panzer DM: The reliability of motion palpation. *J Manipulative Physiol Ther* 15:518–524, 1992.
49. Nykoliation J: Letter to the editor. *J Manipulative Physiol Ther* 15:211–221, 1992.
50. Byfield D: Cervical spine: Manipulative skill and performance considerations. *Eur J Chiropr* 39:45–52, 1991.
51. Polkinghorn BS: Chiropractic treatment of frozen shoulder associated with mixed metastatic carcinoma. *Chiropr Technique*, in press.
52. Gemmell H: The immediate effort of Activator versus meric adjustment on acute LBP: A random controlled trial. *J Manipulative Physiol Ther*, in press.
53. Gemmell H: Personal communication, 1995.
54. Richards GL, Thompson JS, Osterbauer PJ, et al: Low force chiropractic care of two patients with sciatic neuropathy and lumbar disc herniation. *Am J Chiropr Med* 3:25–32, 1990.

55. Osterbauer PJ, Fuhr AW: Treatment of chronic sciatica by mechanical force manually assisted, short-level adjusting and a video assisted stretching program: A quantitative case report. *Proceedings of the California Chiropractic Foundation's Seventh Annual Conference on Research and Education*, Palm Springs, Calif, June 19–21, 1992, pp 293–295.
56. Cox J, Schreiner S: Chiropractic manipulation in low back and sciatica: Statistical data on the diagnosis, treatment and response of 576 consecutive cases. *J Manipulative Physiol Ther* 7:1–11, 1984.
57. Quon JA, Cassidy JD, O'Connor SM: Lumbar intervertebral disc herniation: Treatment by rotational manipulation. *J Manipulative Physiol Ther* 12:220–227, 1989.
58. Osterbauer PJ, DeVita T, Ward LE, et al: Chiropractic treatment of chronic mechanical low back pain in a geriatric population: a practitioner-scientist protocol. Proceedings of the FCER's Third Annual International Conference on Spinal Manipulation. Washington, DC, April 12–13, 1991, pp 230–231.
59. Osterbauer PJ, DeBoer KF, Widmaier RS, et al: Treatment and biomechanical assessment of patients with chronic sacroiliac joint syndrome. *J Manipulative Physiol Ther* 16:82–90, 1993.
60. Herzog W, Nigg BM, Robinson RO, et al: Quantifying the effects of spinal manipulating on gait, using patients with low back pain: A pilot study. *J Manipulative Physiol Ther* 10:295–299, 1987.
61. Herzog W, Nigg BM, Read LJ: Quantifying the effects of spinal manipulations on gait using patients with low back pain. *J Manipulative Physiol Ther* 11:151–157, 1988.
62. Herzog W, Conway PJ: Gait analysis of sacroiliac patients. *J Manipulative Physiol Ther* 17:124–127, 1994.
63. Cassidy JD, Kirkaldy-Willis WH, McGregor M: Spinal manipulation for the treatment of chronic low back and leg pain: An observational study. In Buerger AA, Greenman PE (eds): *Empirical Approaches to the Validation of Spinal Manipulative Therapy*. Springfield, Ill, Charles Thomas, 1985, pp 119–148.
64. Greenman PE: Innominate shear in the sacroiliac syndrome. *Manual Med* 2:114–121, 1986.
65. Osterbauer PJ, Derickson KL, Peles JD, et al: Three-dimensional head kinematics and clinical outcome of patients with neck injury treated with spinal manipulative therapy: A pilot study. *J Manipulative Physiol Ther* 15:501–511, 1992.
66. Woltring HJ, Derickson KL, Osterbauer PJ, et al: Instantaneous helical axis estimation from 3-D video data in neck kinematics for whiplash diagnostics. *J Biomech* 27:1415–1432, 1994.
67. Polkinghorn BS: Conservative treatment of torn medial meniscus via mechanical force, manually assisted chiropractic adjusting procedures. Proceedings of the Consortium for Chiropractic Research's Eighth Annual Conference on Research and Education, Monterey, Calif, June 18–20, 1993, p 166.
68. Polkinghorn BS: Chiropractic treatment of frozen shoulder syndrome (adhesive capsulitis) utilizing mechanical force manually assisted short lever adjusting procedures. *Chiropr Technique*, in press.
69. Polkinghorn BS: Posterior calcaneal subluxation: An important consideration in chiropractic treatment of plantar fasciitis. *Chiropr Sports Med*, in press.
70. Phillips NJ: Vertebral subluxation and otitis media: A case study. *Chiropractic* 8:38–39, 1992.
71. Frach JP, Osterbauer PJ: Chiropractic treatment of Bell's palsy by mechani-

cal force, manually assisted chiropractic adjusting and high-voltage electrotherapy: A report of two cases. *J Manipulative Physiol Ther* 15:596–598, 1992.
72. Triano JJ, McGregor M, et al: Manipulative therapy vs. education programs in chronic low back pain. Proceedings of the 1994 International Society for the Study of the L-Spine, Seattle, June 21–25, 1994, p 36.
73. Brennan PC, Triano JJ, McGregor M, et al: Enhanced neutrophil respiratory burst as a biological marker for manipulation forces: Duration of the effect and association with substance P and tumor necrosis factor. *J Manipulative Physiol Ther* 15:83–89, 1992.
74. Gillette RG: Potential antinociceptive effects of high-level somatic stimulation—chiropractic manipulation therapy may coactivate both tonic and phasic analgesic systems. Some recent neurophysiological evidence. *Trans Pacific Consort Chiropr Res* 1986; 1(A4):1–9.
75. Zusman M: Spinal manipulative therapy: Review of some proposed mechanisms and a new hypothesis. *Aus J Physiotherapy* 32:89–99, 1986.
76. Lee M, Svensson NL: Measurement of stiffness during simulated spinal physiotherapy. *Clin Phys Physiol Meas* 11:201–207, 1990.
77. Herzog W, Conway PJ, Kawchuk GN, et al: Forces exerted during spinal manipulative therapy. *Spine* 18:1206–1212, 1993.
78. Magerey ME: Selection of passive treatment techniques. Proceedings of the Fourth Biennial Conference of the Manipulative Therapists Association of Australia, 1985, pp 298–320.
79. Maitland GD: *Vertebral Manipulation*, ed 5. New York, Butterworths, 1986.
80. Pipher WL: Clinical instability of the lumbar spine. *J Manipulative Physiol Ther* 13:482–485, 1990.
81. Thompson R: Measurements of relative intervertebral displacements in the lumbar spine during application of a PAIVM. Postgraduate dissertation, Melbourne, Lincoln Institute of Health Science, 1983.
82. Hessel BW, Herzog W, Conway PIW, et al: Experimental measurement of the force exerted during spinal manipulation using the Thompson technique. *J Manipulative Physiol Ther* 13:448–453, 1990.
83. Herzog W: Biomechanical studies of spinal manipulative therapy. *J Can Chiropr Assoc* 35:156–164, 1991.
84. Kawchuk GN, Herzog W, Hasler EM: Forces generated during spinal manipulative therapy of the cervical spine. *J Manipulative Physiol Ther* 15:275–278, 1992.
85. Lee RYW, Evans JH: Load-displacement-time characteristics of the spine under posteroanterior mobilization. *Aust J Physiother* 38:115–123, 1992.
86. Gal JM, Herzog W, Kawchuk G, et al: Movements of vertebrae during PA adjustment to unembalmed cadavers. Proceedings of the 1993 International Conference on Spinal Manipulation, Montreal, Foundation of Chiropractic Education and Research, 1993, p 15.
87. Herzog W, Gal J, Conway P, et al: Vertebral movement during spinal manipulative therapy. Proceedings of the 1993 International Conference on Spinal Manipulation, Montreal, Foundation of Chiropractic Education and Research, 1993, p 14.
88. Lee M, Svensson NL: Effect of loading frequency response of the spine to lumbar posteroanterior forces. *J Manipulative Physiol Ther* 16:439–446, 1993.
89. Lee M, Lau H, Lau T: Sagittal plane rotation of the pelvis during lumbar posteroanterior loading. *J Manipulative Physiol Ther* 17:149–155, 1994.
90. Nathan M, Keller TS: Measurement and analysis of the *in vivo* posteroante-

rior impulse response of the human thoraco-lumbar spine. A feasibility study. *J Manipulative Physiol Ther* 17:431–441, 1994.
91. Wood J, Adams AA, Hansmeier D: Force and time characteristics of Pierce technique cervical adjustments. *J Chiropr Res Clin Invest* 9:39–44, 1994.
92. Rubin CT, Lanyon LE: Osteoregulatory nature of mechanical stimuli: Function as a determinant for adaptive remodeling in bone. *J Orthop Res* 5:300–310, 1987.
93. Hansson TH, Keller TS: Osteoporosis of the spine. In Wiesel S, Weinstein J, Herkowitz H, et al (eds): *The Lumbar Spine*, ed 2. Philadelphia, WB Saunders, (in press).
94. Nachemson A: Lumbar spine instability: A critical update and symposium summary. *Spine* 10:290–291, 1985.
95. Kazarian LE: Dynamic response characteristics of the human vertebral column. *Acta Orthop Scand* 146(suppl):1–186, 1972.
96. Keller TS, Holm SH, Hansson TH, et al: The dependence of intervertebral disc mechanical properties on physiologic conditions. *Spine* 15:751–761, 1990.
97. Volkmann R: Scoliosis. In *Handbuch der allgemeinen und speciellen Chirurgie*. Stuttgart, Verlag von Ferdinand Enke, 1882.
98. Krag MH, Cohen MC, Haugh LD, et al: Body height change during upright and recumbent posture. *Spine* 15:202–207, 1990.
99. Adams MA, Dolan P, Hutton WC: Diurnal variations in stresses on the lumbar spine. *Spine* 12:130–137, 1987.
100. Wing P, Tsang I, Gagnon F, et al: Diurnal changes in profile shape and range of motion of the back. *Spine* 17:761–766, 1992.
101. Tyrell AR, Reilley T, Troup JDG: Circadian variation in stature and the effects of spinal loading. *Spine* 10:161–164, 1985.
102. Eklund JAE, Corlett EN: Shrinkage as a measure of the effect of load on the spine. *Spine* 9:189–194, 1984.
103. Eklund JA: Industrial seating and spinal loading. Ph.D. Diss. Nottingham, UK, University of Nottingham, 1986.
104. Kazarian LE: Creep characteristics of the human spinal column. *Acta Orthop Scand* 6:3–18, 1975.
105. Burns ML, Kaleps I, Kazarian LE: Analysis of compressive creep behaviour of the vertebral unit subjected to a uniform axial loading using exact parametric solution equations of Kelvin-solid models: I. Human intervertebral joints. *J Biomech* 17:113–130, 1984.
106. Keller TS, Spengler DM, Hansson TH: Mechanical behavior of the human lumbar spine: I. Creep analysis during static compressive loading. *J Orthop Res* 5:467–478, 1987.
107. Keller TS, Hansson TH, Holm SH, et al: In vivo creep behavior of the normal and degenerated porcine intervertebral disk: A preliminary report. *J Spinal Disorders* 4:267–278, 1989.
108. Keller TS, Hansson TH, Abram AC, et al: Regional variations in the compressive properties of lumbar vertebral trabeculae: Effects of disc degeneration. *Spine* 14:1012–1019, 1989.
109. Keller TS, Ziv I, Moeljanto E, et al: Interdependence of lumbar disc and subdiscal bone properties: A report of the normal and degenerated spine. *J Spinal Disorders* 6:106–113, 1993.
110. Sandover J: Dynamic loading as a possible source of low-back disorders. *Spine* 8:652–658, 1983.
111. Quandieu P, Pellieux L: Study in situ et in vivo of the acceleration of lumbar vertebrae of a primate exposed to vibration in the z-axis. *J Biomech* 15:985–1006, 1982.

112. Hagena FW, Wirth CJ, Piehler J, et al: In vivo experiments on the response of the human spine to sinusoidal Gz vibration. AGARD Conference on Backache and Back Discomfort, 1985, AGARD-CP-378.
113. Panjabi MM, Andersson GB, Jorneus L, et al: In vivo measurements of spinal column vibrations. *J Bone Joint Surg (Am)* 68A:695–702, 1986.
114. Pope MH, Wilder DG, Jorneus L, et al: The response of the seated human to sinusoidal vibration and impact. *J Biomech Eng* 109:279–284, 1987.
115. Ray J, Keller T, Magnusson M, et al: In vivo measurements of lumbar spine transmissibility in the upright human subject. *Trans Int Soc Lumbar Spine* p 4, 1991.

SUGGESTED READINGS

Activator Methods approved for federal grant. *J Chiropr* 22(8):21, 1985.
Bonci AS, Fuhr AW, Smith DB: Accuracy of piezoelectric accelerometers measuring displacement of a spinal adjusting instrument [letter]. *J Manipulative Physiol Ther* 10:133–135, 1987.
Byfield D: Cervical spine: Manipulative skill and performance considerations. *Eur J Chiropr* 39:45–52, 1991.
Christensen MG, Delle Morgan DR: Job analysis of chiropractic: A project report, survey analysis and summary of the practice of chiropractic within the United States. Greeley, Colo, National Board of Chiropractic Examiners, 1993, pp 78–79.
Cleveland CS: A clarification of the use of the "Activator technique" in chiropractic research [letter]. *Am Chiropr* July–August 1983; 24–25.
Danelius B, DeBoer KF: Inter & interexaminer reliability of leg length differential measurements: A preliminary study [letter]. *J Manipulative Physiol Ther* 10:132–133, 1987.
Dewitt J, Osterbauer P, Stelmach G, et al: Optoelectric measurement of leg length changes during isolation tests. Proceedings of the Consortium for Chiropractic Research's Eighth Annual Conference on Research and Education, Monterey, Calif, June 18–20, 1993, pp 156–157.
Dewitt JK, Osterbauer PJ, Stelmach GE, et al: Optoelectric measurement of leg length inequalities before, during, and after isolation tests. Proceedings of the 1994 International Conference on Spinal Manipulation, Palm Springs, Calif, June 10–11, 1994, pp 24–25.
Dewitt JK, Osterbauer PJ, Stelmach GE, et al: Optoelectric measurement of changes in leg length inequality resulting from isolation tests. *J Manipulative Physiol Ther* 17:530–538, 1994.
Duell ML: The force of the activator adjusting instrument. *Digest Chiropr Econ* 27(3):54–59, 1984.
Frach JP, Osterbauer PJ, Fuhr AW: Treatment of Bell's palsy by mechanical force, manually assisted chiropractic adjusting and high-voltage electrotherapy. *J Manipulative Physiol Ther* 15:596–598, 1992.
Fuhr AW: Activator Methods. *Today's Chiropr* 12:16–19, 1983.
Fuhr AW: Activator Methods technique. *Today's Chiropr* 15:77–78, 1986.
Fuhr AW: *Activator Methods Chiropractic Technique Seminar Work Book*, 1987, Activator Methods, Phoenix.
Fuhr AW: *Seminar Workbook, College Edition*. Phoenix, Activator Methods, 1989.
Fuhr AW: Presentation to the Panel on Short and Long Lever, Non-Specified Contact Chiropractic Adjusting. Proceedings of the California Chiropractic Foundation's Seventh Annual Conference on Research and Education, Palm Springs, Calif, June 19–21, 1992, pp 256–257.
Fuhr AW: Biomechanical studies of spinal manipulative therapy: quantifying the

movements of vertebral bodies during SMT [letter]. *J Can Chiropr Assoc* 38:166–167, 1994.

Fuhr AW, Osterbauer PJ: Interexaminer reliability of relative leg length evaluations in the prone extended position. *Chiropr Technique* 1:13–18, 1989.

Fuhr AW, Osterbauer PJ: A clinical approach to the validation of Activator Methods Chiropractic Technique. Proceedings of the FCER's Third Annual International Conference on Spinal Manipulation, Washington, DC, April 12–13, 1991, p 349.

Fuhr AW, Osterbauer PJ: Short lever mechanical force, manually-assisted adjusting: The Activator instrument. Proceedings of the Consortium for Chiropractic Research's Sixth Annual Conference on Research and Education, Monterey, Calif, June 21–23, 1991, p 352.

Fuhr AW, Osterbauer PJ: Strategies for the detection of neuro-mechanical dysfunction: Acitvator Methods' isolation procedures prone leg check. Proceedings of the Consortium for Chiropractic Research's Sixth Annual Conference on Research and Education, Monterey, Calif, June 21–23, 1991, pp 59–60.

Fuhr AW, Smith DB: Accuracy of piezoelectric accelerometers measuring displacement of a spinal adjusting instrument. *J Manipulative Physiol Ther* 9:15–21, 1986.

Haas M, Peterson D, Jaggar DH, et al: Interexaminer reliability of relative leg-length evaluations in the prone, extended position [letter]. *Chiropr Technique* 1:150–153, 1989.

Haas M, Peterson D, Panzer D, et al: Reactivity of leg alignment to articular pressure testing: evaluation of a diagnostic test using a randomized crossover clinical trial approach. *J Manipulative Physiol Ther* 16:220–227, 1993.

Haas M, Peterson D, Rothman EH, et al: Responsiveness of leg alignment changes associated with articular pressure testing to spinal manipulation: the use of a randomized clinical trial design to evaluate a diagnostic test with a dichotomous outcome. *J Manipulative Physiol Ther* 16:306–311, 1993.

Haldeman S, Chapman-Smith D, Petersen DM Jr (eds): *Guidelines for Chiropractic Quality Assurance and Practice Parameters: Proceedings of the Mercy Center Consensus Conference.* Gaithersburg, Md, Aspen, 1993, pp 108–109.

Henderson D, Chapman-Smith D, Mior S, Vernon H: Clinical guidelines for chiropractic practice in Canada. *J Can Chiropr Assoc* 38(suppl):110, 1994.

Henningham M: Activator adjusting for acute torticollis. *Chiropr J Aust* 2:13–14, 1982.

Herzog W, Conway PJ: Gait analysis of sacroiliac patients [comment]. *J Manipulative Physiol Ther* 17:124–127, 1994.

Herzog W, Kawchuk GN, Conway PJ: Relationship between preload and peak forces during spinal manipulative treatments. *J Neuromusculoskeletal System* 1:52–58, 1993.

Kawchuk GN, Herzog W: Biomechanical characterization (fingerprinting) of five novel methods of cervical spine manipulation. *J Manipulative Physiol Ther* 16:573–577, 1993.

Keller T, Nathan M, Kaigle A: Measurement and analysis of interspinous kinematics. Proceedings of the 1993 International Conference on Spinal Manipulation, Foundation for Chiropractic Education and Research of Arlington, Va, Montreal, April 30–May 1, 1993, pp 51–55.

Keller TS, Lehneman JB: *Dependence of the Delivered Force on the Force Setting on the Activator Adjusting Instrument. Technical Report.* Activator Methods, Phoenix, 1994.

Lee WC, Fuhr AW: Non-force technique in lumbosacral syndrome. *J Clin Chiropr* 1:4–12, 1976.

Lee WC, Fuhr AW: Activator methods. In Kfoury PW (ed): *Catalog of Chiroprac-*

tic Techniques: An Overview of Current Chiropractic Methods. Chesterfield, Mo, Logan College of Chiropractic, 1977, pp 21–22.

Nathan M, Keller TS: Measurement and analysis of the in vivo posteroanterior impulse response of the human thoraco-lumbar spine. A feasibility study. *J Manipulative Physiol Ther* 17:431–444, 1994.

Nathan M, Lehneman JB, Keller TS: The dynamic response of the human spine to low amplitude high velocity posteroanterior thrusts. The Proceedings of the 1994 International Conference on Spinal Manipulation, Palm Spring, Calif, June 10–11, 1994, p 87.

Nykoliation J: Effects of chiropractic treatment on blood pressure and anxiety: A randomized and controlled trial [letter; comment]. *J Manipulative Physiol Ther* 13:113, 1990.

Osterbauer PJ: Interexaminer reliability of relative leg-length evaluations in the prone, extended position [letter]. *Chiropr Technique* 1:150–153, 1989.

Osterbauer PJ, DeBoer KF, Widmaier RS, et al: Treatment and biomechanical assessment of patients with chronic sacroiliac joint syndrome. *J Manipulative Physiol Ther* 1993; 16:82–90.

Osterbauer PJ, Derickson KL, Peles JD, et al: Three-dimensional head kinematics and clinical outcome of patients with neck injury treated with spinal manipulative therapy: A pilot study. *J Manipulative Physiol Ther* 15:501–511, 1992. (Published erratum appears in *J Manipulative Physiol Ther* 15(9).)

Osterbauer PJ, DeVita T, Fuhr AW: Chiropractic treatment of chronic mechanical low back pain in a geriatric population: a practitioner-scientist protocol. Proceedings of the FCER's Third Annual International Conference on Spinal Manipulation, Washington, DC, April 12–13, 1991, pp 230–231.

Osterbauer PJ, Fuhr AW: The current status of Activator Methods Chiropractic Technique, theory, and training. *Chiropr Techique* 2:168–175, 1990.

Osterbauer PJ, Fuhr AW: Treatment of chronic sciatica by mechanical force manually aasisted, short level adjusting and a video assisted stretching program: A quantitative case report. Proceedings of the California Chiropractic Foundation's Seventh Annual Conference on Research and Education, Palm Springs, Calif, June 19–21, 1992, pp 293–295.

Osterbauer PJ, Fuhr AW: Motion analysis as a means to objectify changes in apparent (prone) leg length inequality. Proceedings of the California Chiropractic Foundation's Seventh Annual Conference on Research and Education, Palm Springs, Calif, June 19–21, 1992, pp 291–292.

Osterbauer PJ, Fuhr AW, Hildebrandt RW: Mechanical force, manually assisted, short lever chiropractic adjustment. *J Manipulative Physiol Ther* 15:309–317, 1992.

Osterbauer PJ, Fuhr AW, Nykoliation J: Effects of chiropractic treatment on blood pressure and anxiety: A randomized and controlled trial [letter; comment]. *J Manipulative Physiol Ther* 14:74–75, 1991.

Peters RE: Facet syndrome. *Eur J Chiropr* 32:85–102, 1984.

Phillips NJ: Vertebral subluxation and otitis media: A case study. *Chiropractic* 8:38–39, 1992.

Polkinghorn BS: Conservative treatment of torn medial meniscus via mechanical force, manually assisted chiropractic adjusting procedures. Proceedings of the Consortium for Chiropractic Research's Eighth Annual Conference on Research and Education, Monterey, Calif, June 18–20, 1993, p 166.

Polinghorn BS: Conservative treatment of torn medial meniscus via mechanical force, manually assisted short lever chiropractic adjusting procedures. *J Manipulative Physiol Ther* 17:474–484, 1994.

Polkinghorn BS: Chiropractic treatment of frozen shoulder associated with mixed metastalic carcinoma. *Chiropr Technique*, in press.

Polkinghorn BS: Posterior calcaneal subluxation: An important consideration in chiro treatment of plantar fasciitis. *Chiropr Sports Med*, in press.

Polkinghorn BS: Chiropractic treatment of frozen shoulder syndrome (adhesive capsulitis) utilizing mechanical force manually assisted short lever adjusting procedures. *Chiropr Technique*, in press.

Richards D, Nykoliation J: Effects of chiropractic treatment on blood pressure and anxiety: A randomized and controlled trial [letter; comment]. *J Manipulative Physiol Ther* 14:74–77, 1991.

Richards D: Effects of chiropractic treatment on blood pressure and anxiety: A randomized and controlled trial [letter; comment]. *J Manipulative Physiol Ther* 15:210–212, 1992.

Richards GL, Thompson JS, Osterbauer PJ, et al: Low force chiropractic care of two patients with sciatic neuropathy and lumbar disc herniation. *Am J Chiropr Med* 3:25–32, 1990.

Slosberg M: Activator Methods: Isolation tests. *Today's Chiropr* 16:41–43, 1987.

Slosberg M: Activator Methods: An update and review. *Today's Chiropr* 17:17–19, 1988.

Slosberg M: Activator methods: An update and review: II. *Today's Chiropr* 17:83, 1988.

Slosberg M, Haas M: Reactivity of leg alignment to articular pressure testing: evaluation of a diagnostic test using a randomized crossover clinical trial approach [letter]. *J Manipulative Physiol Ther* 17:497–498, 1994.

Smith DB, Fuhr AW, Davis BP: Skin accelerometer displacement and relative bone movement of adjacent vertebrae in response to chiropractic percussion thrusts. *J Manipulative Physiol Ther* 12:26–37, 1989.

Thomas RJ, Salem T, Nance J, et al: Ligamentous changes in the rat spine following repeated adjustments: A pilot study. Proceedings of the FCER's Second Annual International Conference on Spinal Manipulation, Washington, DC, May 12, 1990, pp 122–123.

Triano JJ: Accuracy of piezoelectric accelerometers measuring displacement of a spinal adjusting instrument [letter]. *J Manipulative Physiol Ther* 9:286–288, 1986.

Triano JJ: Skin accelerometer displacement and relative bone movement of adjacent vertebrae in response to chiropractic percussion thrusts [letter]. *J Manipulative Physiol Ther* 12:406–411, 1989.

Venkataraman S, Yamaguchi GT, Osterbauer PJ, et al: Evaluating mechanical force manually assisted short lever adjusting using an anthropomorphic model. Proceedings of the Fourth International Conference on Spinal Manipulation, Chicago, May 15–17, 1992, p 136.

Venkataraman S, Yamaguchi G, Osterbauer PJ, et al: Evaluating mechanical force manually assisted short lever adjusting using an anthropomorphic model. Proceedings of the Foundation for Chiropractic Research's 1993 International Conference on Spinal Manipulation, Montreal, April 30–May 1, p 13.

Yates RG, Lamping DL, Abram NL, et al: Effects of chiropractic treatment on blood pressure and anxiety: a randomized controlled trial. *J Manipulative Physiol Ther* 11:484–488, 1988.

Youngquist MW, Fuhr AW, Osterbauer PJ: Interexaminer reliability of an upper cervical isolation test. *J Manipulative Physiol Ther* 12:93–97, 1989.

Appendix 1

ACTIVATOR METHODS CHIROPRACTIC TECHNIQUE SUMMARY

The rationale for these adjustments is based on Logan's theory of pelvic torsion and static misalignments resulting from a short leg. Originally the contact points and lines of drive were intended to "realign" the joint in question (e.g., if a segment is inferior, the line of drive is the opposite). In reality the misalignment may or may not actually be present. What occurs in the process of the adjustment is that the joint is perturbed, which is propagated in the kinematic chain. In the following outline, the contact points and lines of drive have been preserved, because the experience of people familiar with the technique suggests that the correct line of drive seems to improve results. These await further research to determine if an optimal line drive exists.

It is recommended that the Activator adjusting instrument (AAI) be used in adjusting procedures only after receiving proper instruction from a chiropractic college that teaches Activator Methods Chiropratic Techniques (AMCT) or after attending an AMCT seminar. With regard to contraindications to care, please see the Mercy Conference Guidelines in Haldeman et al.[14]

1. *Name of procedure:* Pelvic pattern and pubic bone adjustment.
2. *Areas affected may include:* sacrum, sacroiliac joint, pelvic deficiency/functional short leg, sacroiliac syndrome/involvement, low back pain, neck pain, inguinal pain, bilaterally depending on the results of pressure testing.
3. *Listings:* Palmer: anterior superior ilium, posterior inferior ilium, inferior-superior pubic bone.
4. *Contraindications:* Bruises over contact points, fractures, serious trauma, and capillary fragility.
5. *Patient's position:* Prone.
6. *Special equipment:* AAI, adjusting table with face slot.
7. *Doctor's position:* Next to patient facing cephalad
8. *Contact and indifferent hands:* The primary hand holds the AAI; the secondary hand is used to locate the contact point.
9. *Setup:* Place the tip of the AAI on the contact point with very light force (<0.5 kg).

10. *Contacts:*
    For an anterior-superior ilium:
    a. Contact the posterior base of the sacrum; the line of drive (LOD) is anterior to inferior (in the plane of the sacroiliac joint).
    b. Contact the crest of the ilium; the line of drive is inferior and medial.
    c. Contact the inferior portion of the ischial tuberosity; the LOD is anterior to inferior.
    For a posterior-inferior ilium:
    a. Contact the spine of the ischium; the LOD is posterior, superior, and lateral.
    b. Contact under the sacrotuberous ligament; the LOD is posterior, superior, and lateral (toward the sacroiliac joint).
    c. Contact the right portion of the iliac fossa for the gluteus medius, LOD is anterior to superior.
    For a superior pubic bone:
    Contact the superior portion of the involved pubis; the line of drive is straight inferior.
    For an inferior pubic bone:
    Contact the inferior portion of the involved pubis; the line of drive is straight superior.

LUMBAR SPINE

1. *Name of procedure:* Lumbar rotational adjustment
2. *Areas affected can include:* Lumbar spine and musculature sacroiliac joint, leg pain/sciatica.
3. *Listing (Houston, rotation of vertebral body):* Right or left rotated (RR, LR) vertebra.
4. *Contraindications:* Bruises over contact points, fractures, serious trauma, and capillary fragility.
5. *Patient position:* Prone.
6. *Special equipment:* AAI, adjusting table with face slot.
7. *Doctor's position:* Next to patient facing cephalad.
8. *Contact and indifferent hands:* The primary hand holds the activator, the secondary hand is used to palpate the contact point.
9. *Setup:* Place the tip of the AAI on the contact point with very light force (<0.5 kg).
10. *Contacts:* Mamillary process of the affected joint; LOD is anterior-superior in the plane of the facets.

THORACIC SPINE AND RIBS

1. *Name of procedure:* Thoracic/rib rotatory adjustment.
2. *Areas affected can include:* Middorsal, intrascapular pain, T-12 pain, low back pain (LBP) and sacroiliac referred pain, and rib pain.
3. *Listings (Houston, rotation of vertebral body):* RR/LR thoracic vertebra.
4. *Contraindications:* Bruises over contact points, fractures, serious trauma, and capillary fragility.

5. *Patient position:* Prone.
6. *Special equipment:* AAI, adjusting table with face slot.
7. *Doctor's position:* Next to patient facing cephalad.
8. *Contact and indifferent hands:* The primary hand holds the AAI; the secondary hand is used to palpate the contact point.
9. *Setup:* Place the tip of the AAI on the contact point with very light force (<0.5 kg).
10. *Contacts:* Transverse process of the affected side, rib on the opposite side; LOD is anterior-superior for the TP and anterior-inferior for the rib head on the opposite side.

CERVICAL SPINE

1. *Name of procedure:* Cervical rotation adjustment.
2. *Areas affected can include:* Neck pain, headaches, shoulder pain, and midback pain.
3. *Listings (Houston, rotation of vertebral body):* RR/LR cervical vertebrae, lateral C-1.
4. *Contraindications:* Bruises over contact points, fractures, serious trauma, and capillary fragility.
5. *Patient position:* Prone.
6. *Special equipment:* AAI, adjusting table with face slot.
7. *Doctor's position:* Next to patient facing cephalad.
8. *Contact and indifferent hands:* The primary hand holds the AAI, the secondary hand is used to palpate and locate the contact point and the LOD is the articular pillar or lateral mass of the joint in question.
9. *Setup:* Place the tip of the AAI on the contact point with very light force (less than one pound).
10. *Contacts:* For C-7 to C-2:

    Pedicle lamina junction articular pillars of the affected side; LOD is anterior-superior.

    For C-1: Contact the lateral aspect of C-1; LOD is lateral to medial.

    For occiput: Contact the inferior nuchal line of the occiput; LOD is anterior.

Appendix 2

KINEMATIC AND BIOMECHANICAL BEHAVIOR OF THE NORMAL AND PATHOLOGICAL SPINE

The systematic study of the mechanics of manipulation/adjustment is in its early stages. Lines of investigation using the Activator Methods, Inc. (AMI) approach begun by Smith and Fuhr[8, 9] in the middle to late 1980s have continued at the University of Vermont and the University of Calgary.[83, 90] The following section begins by reviewing the kinematic and biomechanical properties of the healthy and pathological spine. This describes a new method of characterizing mechanical properties of the spine derived from various manipulation/adjustment procedures and speculates about how this new knowledge may lead to innovations in diagnosis and treament of spinal disorders.

The spinal column combines an intricate architectural arrangement of bone, muscle, and soft tissue components to form a structure of mechanical, as well as physiological, significance. Not only does the spinal column serve to protect the spinal cord, but it also transmits, attenuates, and distributes the static (time-in varying) and dynamic (time varying) forces associated with daily activities. Although the spinal column provides the structures for load transmission and attenuation, the pathways for load transmission and attenuation may be greatly altered during voluntary (postural changes) and involuntary (fatigue) activities, producing unstable and pathological changes to the kinematic behavior of the spinal column. Segmental instability and pathological conditions of the spine are believed to produce abnormal patterns of motion and forces, which may also play a significant role in the cause of low back pain (LBP).[93] The ability to quantify in vivo spine segment motion, or *kinematics*, is therefore of clinical significance in terms of both diagnosis and treatment of spinal disorders and LBP.

The S-shaped spine can be considered as a column of relatively rigid vertebrae punctuated by intervertebral disks that are very flexible. The 24 articulating vertebrae are divided into 7 cervical, 12 thoracic, and 5 lumbar regions. The intervening 23 intervertebral disks account for 20%

to 30% of spinal length and are responsible for the majority of spinal motion. Fluid flows in or out of the disks, causing an alteration in the height, shape, and stiffness of the disks. The mechanical response of the disks (and to a lesser extent the vertebrae) are dependent on the rate, duration, and mode of loading. Such behavior indicates that the spine is *viscoelastic*. Experimentally, the viscoelastic mechanical behavior of the spine can be evaluated using both static and dynamic tests. An example of the static mechanical testing of the spine is *creep*, whereas dynamic mechanical tests include *oscillation* and *impact*.

CREEP

Experimental investigations have shown that over short periods, the disks are partially elastic, that is, they deform when a load is applied and return to their original height when the load is removed.[95] Over long periods, however, the disks are viscous and exhibit a slow and progressive deformation described as creep.[96] Physiological compressive forces, due to weight bearing and muscular contraction, create an imbalance in the equilibrium water content and stresses within the disk such that the rate of height change decreases over time until a new steady-state equilibrium is reached. A change in psoture from recumbent to upright, therefore, produces a decrease in body height. Such changes have been noted as early as 1882,[97] and over the years, experimental studies measuring body height changes during the day have made it an established fact.[98] Changes in height have been referred to as diurnal change,[99,100] circadian variation,[101] or spinal shrinkage[102] and are approximately 16 to 20 mm (1% of stature) in young adults. Approximately equal decreases in body height occur during both standing and sitting postures, indicating that the majority of this body height loss originates in the intervertebral disks.[103]

The static viscoelastic properties of the intervertebral disks have been extensively studied and modeled.[96,104–107] The principal mechanical parameters calculated during static tests are the creep compliance ($1/E$) and viscosity coefficient (η), which can be obtained by mathematically modeling the spine as a simple three-parameter, linear solid composed of spring (elastic) elements and dashpot (viscous) elements. The equations of motion associated with the serial and parallel arrangements of these viscous and elastic (viscoelastic) elements may also be used in conjunction with experimental data to compute the creep compliance and viscosity coefficients associated with the static mechanical behavior of a particular spinal column (Fig 12).

Creep characteristics of the spine are closely dependent on the load magnitude, as well as aging and degeneration processes.[96,106,107] A link between degenerative changes in the intervertebral disks and the mechanical behavior of the underlying vertebral bone has also been observed.[108] This has been hypothesized to reflect the fact that the properties of ligaments, disks, and bone in the spine are interrelated and stems from biomechanical considerations of load sharing by these structures.[109] The notion that disks, ligaments, and vertebral bone properties are interdependent has important implications for the etiologies of degenerative processes in the spine.

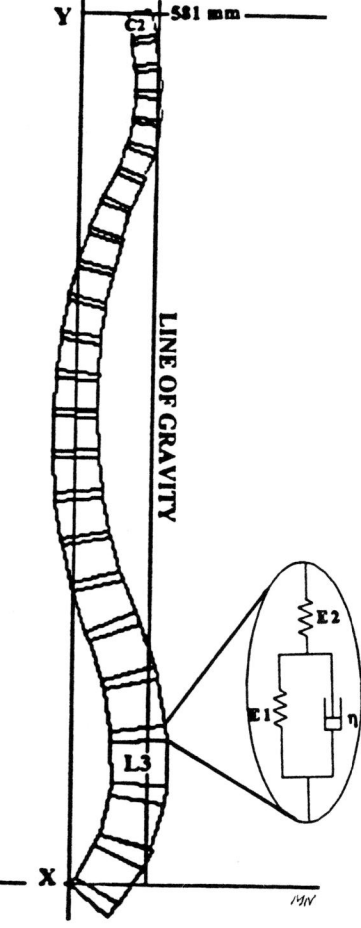

FIGURE 12.
Schematic diagram of the spine illustrating the three parameter solid model of the intervertebral disk. In the model (inset) E1, E2, and η correspond to the viscous modules, elastic modules, and viscosity coefficient, respectively, of the intervertebral disk. These parameters can be used to characterize viscoelastic behavior of the spine.

OSCILLATION

Perhaps less well studied is the dynamic viscoelastic response of the spine, which is associated with activities that impose oscillatory accelerations, velocities, forces, and displacements on the spine. Chronic exposure to mechanical oscillations, or *vibrations*, is hypothesized to produce pathological changes to the spine and may be linked to LBP.[110] As a result, numerous in vivo acceleration, displacement, and force measurements in the human and animal spine have been performed using both noninvasive and invasive measurement techniques.[111–115] Most of these studies have focused on harmonic (e.g., sinusoidal) oscillations of a given frequency. The principal mechanical parameters calculated in such tests generally include *transmissibility* and *mechanical impedance*. Transmissibility is the ratio of the output signal (displacement, force, and acceleration), whereas the mechanical impedance is the ratio of the transmitted force and the velocity. If the velocity is measured at the point of force application, the ratio is called the driving-point impedance. A lower impedance value implies that the intervertebral joints are easier to excite and capable of larger motions and storage of larger amounts of energy, whereas the opposite holds for transmissibility.[104] Identification of the frequency of maximum mobility (natural frequency) of the thoracolumbar spine is important, therefore, because lower forces can be used to excite a mechanical structure when applied at its natural frequency. Analogous to the creep compliance, equations that describe the vibratory response of linear mechanical systems can be derived and used with experimentally determined velocity and force data to compute stiffness (complex modules) and damping coefficients.

Principles of Quality Management in Chiropractic Practice

Grant C. Iannelli, B.S., D.C., D.A.A.P.M., C.P.H.Q.
Associate Professor of Clinics, Quality Assurance Coordinator, National College of Chiropractic, Lombard, Illinois

HISTORY OF QUALITY MANAGEMENT IN HEALTH CARE

Chiropractic has begun the process of documenting quality care. As a less visible ambulatory health care provider, chiropractic was previously not a participant in the early attempts to document quality of care. Others in the ambulatory arena have been much more productive and have begun to reap the benefits of having quality programs. The importance can be seen in three areas: economically, as the percentage of the health care dollar paying for ambulatory services has increased each year[1]; politically, as the federal government becomes more involved in determining health care policy; and ethically, with the consumer becoming more educated about what quality health care is, practitioners are obligated to provide care at that level, or consumers will go elsewhere.

In recent years, increased societal concern over the spiraling cost of medical care has resulted in the shift of many treatments from inpatient to the ambulatory setting, often with no established program to assess the quality of care delivered. R. Heather Palmer, a noted specialist in ambulatory health care quality, challenged ambulatory health care providers in 1988 to develop uniform quality requirements that would satisfy all external reviewers. She saw quality in the ambulatory arena as being difficult to assess, having a nonexistent data base, and having no standards or criteria.[2] At that time, she was absolutely correct. Without a data base or standards, reviewers have no reference for guidance.

DEFINITIONS

Before we embark on a discussion of quality management in chiropractic practice, several terms must first be defined. Quality assurance (QA) is defined as an ongoing program designed to objectively and systematically monitor and evaluate the quality and appropriateness of patient care, pursue opportunities to improve care, and resolve identified problems.[3] Quality management (QM) is the totality of ways in which quality can be achieved and includes three processes: quality planning, quality control, and quality improvement. QM as used in this chapter is synonymous with

Advances in Chiropractic®, vol. 2
© 1995, Mosby–Year Book, Inc.

terms such as continuous quality improvement (CQI), total quality management (TQM), and total quality (TQ).

The term "quality" is not as easily defined. Previously the health care literature has provided no consistent definition. Community Health Network, Inc., managed contractually by Methodist Hospital of Indiana, Inc., adapted and adopted a 1974 Institute of Medicine policy statement in which the primary goal of a QA system was proposed to be "health care that effectively betters the health status and satisfaction of the population, within the resources that society and individuals have chosen to spend for that care."[1,4] A survey of 282 health care professionals on the topic of a quality ambulatory health care program yielded 98 different responses! A composite definition representing the combined judgment of nearly 80% of the 281 respondents was:

Quality ambulatory health care—

- meets the expectations of (pleases) the patients,
- is enhanced and demonstrated by an effective quality assurance program,
- is dependent upon the excellence of the provider staff, and
- is enabled by an accurate, timely, and complete medical record system.[5]

Another discussion of quality focused on five major components that are common to most definitions[6]:

- Effectiveness
- Acceptability to patient
- Accessibility/availability
- Efficiency/appropriateness
- Continuity of care

Avedis Donabedian, to some the "father of modern QA," assessed quality on the basis of structure, process, and outcomes of care. Structure describes the resources used for health care. It includes such things as facilities, equipment, staffing, finances, and organizational arrangements. Process involves what is done for or to the patient, including how the physician uses resources and knowledge for patient care. Outcome is simply, "Is the problem for which the patient sought care reduced or eliminated?"[7,8]

According to Miller,[1] "Both the development of the ambulatory care program and the evaluation [quality assurance] of that program can be based on the dimensions of quality included in the definition." This is why it is important for each facility or institution to define "quality" according to such characteristics. For the purposes of this text, quality will be defined as *meeting or exceeding customer expectations, needs, preferences, and values.* Once "quality" has been defined, assessing and documenting its presence or absence, and then striving to improve it is the mandate of the QM program.

QUALITY IN HEALTH CARE: 1860s–1990s

To discuss the development of quality in the health care environment, we should first explore its roots. QA had its origins with Florence Nightingale in the early 1860s when she called for a uniform format for collecting and evaluating hospital mortality statistics. In this century, QA came to the forefront when the Joint Commission on Accreditation of Hospitals (JCAH) was formed in 1951. The JCAH mandated that hospitals have an active QA program to become accredited. Then in the 1960s, the federal government required that any hospital receiving federal monies must be accredited. This explains how QA became an operating department in all hospitals. Still, before the boom in ambulatory services in the 1980s, QA was not a part of ambulatory care.

In 1976, the Joint Commission expanded their horizons and included accreditation of ambulatory facilities in their scope. Subsequently, accreditation was also offered by the Accreditation Association for Ambulatory Health Care (AAAHC). In 1987, the Joint Commission outlined the use of the monitoring and evaluation process (a QA tool) in an ambulatory setting.[9] In 1988, the JCAH updated the language in the *Ambulatory Health Care Standards Manual,* becoming more specific and requiring the use of a 10-step monitoring and evaluation process.[10] Recently the Joint Commission mandated the evaluation of clinical performance outcomes as part of the ambulatory accreditation process, shifting the emphasis to the *continuous assessment and improvement of quality.*[11, 12]

Currently the Joint Commission accredits more than 5,300 hospitals, as well as about 300 free-standing ambulatory facilities,[13] and is seen as a major force in the movement toward health care quality. With an increasing number of managed care providers requiring facilities to be accredited, the Joint Commission's latest requirement has forced many ambulatory providers to implement complete QA programs to renew accreditation or become accredited and thus maintain provider status with managed care networks. It can be seen how, once again, accrediting agencies have stimulated the development of QA programs, this time in the ambulatory setting.

Since the 1970s, QA has drawn increasing attention to the issue of quality in health care. Even with this emphasis, many refused to jump on the QA bandwagon. QA was often compartmentalized, ineffective, or punitive in its corrective actions and was weakly supported by management. This "failure" of QA led many to explore the area of QM.

QM had its beginnings in industry in the 1950s when Joseph M. Juran and W. Edwards Deming brought their QM concepts to Japan after World War II in an attempt to improve the quality of Japan's industrial output. Deming's use of statistical controls for quality, as well as his *Fourteen Points of Management Obligations,*[14] brought about changes to management practices in Japan that then spread worldwide. Juran[15] broadened the focus of QM beyond production to include management functions, which he termed the *Juran trilogy:* quality planning, quality control, and quality improvement. Quality planning is an organization's process of identifying its customers and their needs and developing products or services to meet those needs. Quality control is the management process that evaluates actual performance against expected performance and takes action on the difference. Quality improvement is a process in which an organization selectively identifies and implements change to improve a product or service. Quality improvement usually includes the following activities[16]:

- Project nomination
- Project selection
- Project team development
- Diagnostic and remedial team activities

Table 1 lists the basic characteristics that differentiate QA from QM.
Although still in its infancy, QM in health care has had limited acceptance. This raises the fundamental question, "Why do we need QM?" To establish the need for QM, we will review a number of reasons for its incorporation, as well as obstacles that must be overcome if QM is to flourish.

TABLE 1.
Distinctions Between QA and QM*

Quality Assurance	Quality Management
Organized according to organizational structure	Organized according to patient care processes
Leadership rarely comes from the top management and is usually delegated to a few	Leadership from the top is essential and responsibility for quality is delegated to all
Conflicts over the definition of quality	Quality equals customer satisfaction
Little guidance, and consequently little similarity, in quantitative methods or reporting	Quantitative methods and reporting based on accepted statistical principles
Detection orientation	Prevention orientation
Thresholds for evaluation (data points)	Control limits (data ranges)
Adversarial: Indicators that met thresholds for evaluation too easily led to questions such as, Who is responsible and what should be done to them?	Collegial: Variation causes the questions: Why did it happen (chance vs special cause), and how can we work together to improve it?
Focused primarily on problem resolution	Focused primarily on continuous improvement
Rarely integrated determination of quality with efficiency (cost)	Quality cost measurement an integral part of evaluating processes

*From Bliersbach CM: *The NAHQ Guide to Quality Management*, ed 3. Skokie, Ill, National Association for Healthcare Quality, 1993, p 23. Used by permission.

The primary goal of QM in health care is the continuous improvement of patient care. From an ethical viewpoint, there can be no argument of the need for QM. After all, if QM is practiced in the manufacturing of some of the most mundane products, why would we not want to practice it when dealing with the care of human beings?

Financial concerns also dictate the necessity for QM. There is little dispute that the United States has a health care cost crisis, driven by overutilization, waste, fraud, and abuse. As efforts to contain health care costs increase, the need for effective measurement of quality will also increase.

Both corporate and case law uphold the fact that the governing board is ultimately responsible for the quality of care offered in a health care organization. From a legal perspective, therefore, the need for effective QM and its link to risk management are of the utmost importance.

At the organizational level, implementing QM will meet with some resistance, because it is natural to resist change. In general, change is frightening and raises anxiety about one's job security. Management from the top down must exhibit total commitment to QM to overcome this fear.

Finally, regulatory considerations make a strong case for QM. Virtually all regulatory and voluntary accrediting agencies require quality assessment in some form.

Although there are obstacles to assessing and improving quality, there are ethical, financial, legal, organizational, and regulatory considerations for continuing to develop more sophisticated means for assessing and improving quality. The following discussion of QM activities in chiropractic and other ambulatory professions culminates in methods of incorporating QM into everyday practice.

QUALITY MANAGEMENT IN AMBULATORY HEALTH CARE

CHIROPRACTIC ATTEMPTS

With the release of the proceedings of the Mercy Center Consensus Conference entitled *Guidelines for Chiropractic Quality Assurance and Practice Parameters*,[17] the chiropractic profession has taken an enormous step toward facilitating quality care by the practitioner. This document lists 307 individual recommendations (guidelines) agreed on by the consensus of the 35 Commission members (all chiropractors from various fields of expertise) present at the conference. Although the guidelines form a starting point in the development of standards of care, they do not address the documentation of quality assurance in the profession. The profession must now add this element to its list of priorities.

Chiropractic's efforts before now have been negligible. Before my previous publication on this topic in 1993,[18] the one published study on QA in a chiropractic setting was by Josef Bohm in 1991. He[19] is to be commended for his attempt to document the quality of care rendered by interns for four conditions, two musculoskeletal and two organic, at two teaching clinics. Using the "tracer method,"[20] Bohm compared interns' performance against arbitrary protocols for the conditions of cervical syndrome, repetitive motion, elevated blood pressure, and diabetes mellitus. His conclusion appears eminently sensible, noting that interns perform best when rendering care for spinal conditions. Unfortunately, as a result of sampling via randomly choosing only the first file, then sequentially reviewing files until reaching his sample size of 50, there is the possibility that the unspecified block of time during the collection period may represent an aberration in quality of care. In addition, the use of tracers for analyzing quality of care has fallen out of favor because it depends on only a few illnesses to detect poor quality of care in an institution. If an institution performs well in these areas but poorly in others, the tracer method would not detect the poor quality of care. This is especially important because studies have shown that good performance in one area of care does not predict good performance in another.[21]

OTHER AMBULATORY QUALITY MANAGEMENT ATTEMPTS

Other ambulatory health care professions have been more productive than the chiropractic profession.[1, 22-31] However, we are not alone in our previously minimal attempts. In the Veterans Administration medical centers (which provide primarily inpatient care affiliated with academic institutions), the concept of QA in the ambulatory setting was unaddressed as recently as 1989. In addition, no educational program to teach QA to the students, interns, or residents was available.[32]

Conversely, much has been written in the area of ambulatory nursing. Developments included standards for well children receiving health services in public health clinics in Ohio; several unit-based QA programs to evaluate the nursing component of ambulatory care, some including goals, development of the evaluation model, evaluation methods, audit worksheets and reports, feedback mechanisms, committee organizations, identification of standards, outcome indicators, monitoring tools and problem identification sheets; as well as a specific approach to conducting QA activities (AmbuQual), which is discussed in detail later.[1, 17, 18, 21, 26] Although these citations may serve a nursing unit well in establishing a QA program, with the exception of Miller's AmbuQual system, they are not specific enough or broad enough for use in a multidisciplinary primary care facility.

Other departmental QA programs have included an infection control QA monitoring program used in the 143 outpatient clinics of the University of California–Davis Medical Center, measurement of patient satisfaction with outpatient rehabilitation services, tracking and solution of a specific problem in a dialysis unit, patient education on drug use in an ambulatory pharmacy department, an evaluative framework for assessing Medical Care Classification Systems (coding systems for tracking ambulatory care), and an ambulatory drug utilization review system and experiences in monitoring patients taking theophylline.[19, 20, 22-25] Another project involved a two-tiered system for ambulatory chart review that was used by three Minnesota HMOs. Although the sampling process used was appropriate, the conclusion that the review system was "unusually efficient" must be questioned, because the physician reviewers rejected three possible "care problems" identified by initial screening for every "problem" they reviewed.[33] Again, although these articles identify practical ideas that can be implemented in specific settings, none describe a generic system that can be used in a multidisciplinary setting.

AMBUQUAL QUALITY MANAGEMENT SYSTEM

In a series of papers and texts dating from 1987 through 1993, Dale Benson, Jane Miller, and others documented the structured approach to QM in the ambulatory setting known as AmbuQual. AmbuQual is a computer-supported ambulatory QM system developed at Methodist Hospital of Indiana, Inc. in Indianapolis and its three associated community health centers (Community Health Network). It uses as its framework 10 critical components, or *ambulatory care parameters,* that reflect quality care. The parameters are generalizable—applicable to a wide variety of ambulatory settings, yet functional; each is a behaviorally based measure of the quality of care that has a direct effect on a patient's health. The 10 parameters have been weighted to identify their impact on the patient's health. Table 2 lists the parameters and their weights.

Each parameter is divided into four functional subdivisions, which are then evaluated by scoring several indicators. Each indicator receives a numerical score based on review of its related data source or sources. The scores are compared with predetermined thresholds to determine whether a deficiency exists and corrective action is required. The indicator scores and their associated subdivisions are weighted in a manner similar to the parameter weights. The computer program applies the appropriate weighting to the indicator scores, then generates numerical scores for each parameter. Finally, a composite program quality score, the *program quality index* (PQI), is generated based on the parameters' scores times their weights.[34–39]

The AmbuQual approach has not gone unnoticed. Not only was it documented in use in homeless health care at the People's Health Center in Indianapolis,[40] but it was also used by the University Physicians, Inc.

TABLE 2.
AmbuQual Ambulatory Care Parameters*

Parameter Name	Weight
Provider staff performance	1.90
Support staff performance	1.10
Continuity of care	0.90
Medical record system	0.70
Patient risk minimization	0.70
Patient satisfaction	0.60
Patient compliance	1.30
Access to care	0.90
Appropriateness of service	1.40
Organizational performance	0.50

*From Benson DS, Miller JA: *AmbuQual® II: An Ambulatory Quality Assurance and Quality Management System.* Indianapolis, Methodist Hospital of Indiana, 1993. Used by permission.

at the University of Arizona College of Medicine.[41] In addition, a study at the Community Health Network centers and the University of Colorado Health Sciences Center conducted before and after the introduction of AmbuQual at each site revealed statistically significant increases in providers' awareness of QA activity and attitudes about QA processes and their effectiveness.[42]

Although QA and QM have been in the forefront of the medical ambulatory arena, in chiropractic, prior to 1988, there was no organized program in place in any of the chiropractic educational institutions or in any documented in the private sector. At that time the administration of The National College of Chiropractic recognized the need for a program to document and improve the quality of care rendered to patients, satisfy outside review organizations, and begin the process of establishing standards of care. For these reasons, in 1989 the administration chose to implement a quality assurance program to encompass the entire clinics domain. After available programs and systems were reviewed, the AmbuQual system was chosen for implementation. What follows is the method of implementation of the program at The National College Chiropractic Clinics and recommendations for how the system can be utilized in other settings.

QUALITY MANAGEMENT ACTIVITIES

AMBUQUAL IMPLEMENTATION

One of the attractive features of AmbuQual is its step-by-step documentation. By following the steps listed in the manual (Table 3), implementation of the AmbuQual system was perceived to be straightforward and uncomplicated.[31] These steps have been slightly modified to reflect the lines of authority present in my institution.

Initially a written quality assurance plan was drafted and approved (Appendix 1) The plan listed the objectives, organization, and scope of the QA program. The plan and organizational structure were patterned after the AmbuQual documentation. After approving the plan, the president appointed a QA coordinator and formed two committees within the QA program: the Quality Management Group (QMG) (Table 4), and the Quality Assurance Committee (QAC) (Table 5).

The QMG reviews 1 of the 10 *ambulatory care parameters* and its related *indicators* each month. Table 6 identifies all of the indicators that make up the four aspects of one of the parameters, provider staff performance. It identifies into which of the three levels of implementation (basic, intermediate, or advanced) each indicator is assigned. It also lists each indicator's relative weight. Table 7 is a printout of 3 of the 13 basic level indicators. As a part of the monthly parameter review process, the QMG approves the *standards* for each indicator, adapting them to our setting; sets *QIP (quality improvement plan) levels* for each indicator (thresholds defined as being deficient that require taking corrective action); plans data sources for quantifying the indicators; and identifies a manager responsible for each indicator. The QMG keeps 1 month ahead of the QAC's review schedule. In the course of 1 year, all 10 parameters are reviewed and approved by the QMG.

TABLE 3.
AmbuQual Implementation Steps*

I. The governing body (president)
   A. Receives orientation to AmbuQual
   B. Commissions the use of the AmbuQual program
   C. Appoints coordinator, quality management group and quality assurance committee
II. The coordinator
   A. Chooses the level of implementation
   B. Identifies the quality assurance secretary
   C. Arranges for AmbuQual orientation for quality management group and quality assurance committee
   D. Facilitates acceptance of AmbuQual
   E. Reviews minutes of meetings and enters scores into computer
III. The quality management group
   A. Receives orientation to AmbuQual
   B. Selects order for parameter review
   C. Reviews and adapts generic indicators chart for first parameter
   D. Continues to review and adapt one parameter per month
IV. The quality assurance committee
   A. Receives orientation to AmbuQual
   B. Follows agenda prepared and distributed by the chair (coordinator) for first parameter review
   C. Begins monthly parameter review

*From Benson DS, Miller JA: AmbuQual® II: An Ambulatory Quality Assurance and Quality Management System. Indianapolis, Methodist Hospital of Indiana, 1993, p 78. Used by permission.

The QAC also meets monthly to score the parameter and indicators that the QMG had previously reviewed. Before the meeting, each indicator is assigned to a QAC member, who is responsible for data collection and reporting to the Committee as a whole. If the indicator's data source is quantitative, the score is entered directly into the computer system.

TABLE 4.
Quality Management Group (QMG) Membership*

Chief of clinics staff (chairperson)
QA program coordinator
Clinics business administrator
Director—National College Chiropractic Center
Director—National College Chiropractic Clinic, Chicago
Director—National College Chiropractic Clinic, Aurora, Ill
Supervisor—Salvation Army Clinics
Faculty/specialty practice representative

*From The National College Chiropractic Clinics, Lombard, Ill, 1994, unpublished data.

TABLE 5.
Quality Assurance Committee (QAC) Membership*

QA program coordinator (chairperson)
Clinician representative
Allied health representative (e.g. physical therapist, nutritionist, radiologist, laboratory director)
Technical support staff representative (e.g., research or clinical laboratory staff, radiology staff)
Clerical support staff representative (e.g., cashier, receptionist, medical records clerk, billing clerk)
Administrative staff representative

*From The National College Chiropractic Clinics, Lombard, Ill, 1994, unpublished data.

TABLE 6.
AmbuQual Indicator Implementation Chart*

	Implementation Level		
	Basic	Intermediate	Advanced
Parameter No. 1: Provider staff performance			
Aspect A: Credentials and provider staff systems			
1.30 Indicator 1: Credentials—education, training, and professional experience		X	X
1.30 Indicator 2: Credentials—current certification and licensure (rev 2/94)	X	X	X
0.80 Indicator 3: Job descriptions (rev 2/94)	X	X	X
0.80 Indicator 4: Personnel performance evaluation system (rev 2/94)	X	X	X
0.80 Indicator 5: Continuing education—policy			X
1.00 Indicator 6: Peer review audit system (rev 2/94)	X	X	X
1.00 Indicator 7: Provider staff protocols			X
1.00 Indicator 8: Provider policies and procedures		X	X
Aspect B: Current competence			
0.50 Indicator 1: Health status			X
1.50 Indicator 2: Review of privileges			X
1.00 Indicator 3: Continuing education—units earned			X
1.00 Indicator 4: Personnel performance evaluation system—results		X	X
Aspect C: Clinical performance			
1.40 Indicator 1: Accurate clinical diagnosis (rev 2/94)	X	X	X

1.40 Indicator 2: Correct clinical treatment (rev 2/94)	X	X	X
1.10 Indicator 3: General clinical performance (rev 2/94)	X	X	X
0.70 Indicator 4: Internal referral performance (rev 2/94)	X	X	X
0.40 Indicator 5: Health maintenance performance		X	X
1.00 Indicator 6: Treatment goals, follow-up (rev 2/94)	X	X	X
1.00 Indicator 7: Elective care utilization (rev 2/94)	X	X	X
1.00 Indicator 8: Policies and procedures utilized		X	X
Aspect D: Clinical effectiveness			
1.00 Indicator 1: Mechanical low back pain (rev 2/94)	X	X	X
1.00 Indicator 2: Mechanical neck pain (rev 2/94)	X	X	X
1.00 Indicator 3: Shoulder impingement (rev 2/94)	X	X	X
1.00 Indicator 4: Condition no. 4		X	X
1.00 Indicator 5: Condition no. 5		X	X
1.00 Indicator 6: Condition no. 6		X	X
1.00 Indicator 7: Condition no. 7			X
1.00 Indicator 8: Condition no. 8			X

*From The National College Chiropractic Clinics, Lombard, Ill, 1994.

For qualitative indicators, the Committee votes on how well the standard is fulfilled and how any deficiencies would impact on the health of patients. By using the qualitative voting forms provided by AmbuQual (Fig 1), the qualitative vote is converted into a numerical score according to the following process:

Based on an indicator's data presented at the QAC meeting, members decide how much the standard (goal) is fulfilled (left column) and what impact any deficiency would have on the health of patients (right column). Those decisions are then converted by the QA secretary into a numerical score using the scoring guidelines at the bottom. It should be noted that the score for "complete fulfillment" would be doubled, to equal 100. Otherwise, the fulfillment scores are added to the impact scores for each member, then divided by the number of votes to yield the average score, which is then entered into the AmbuQual system.

Anytime an indicator scores below the approved QIP level, a memorandum known as a QIP (Fig 2) is sent to the appropriate manager, notifying them of the deficiency and suggesting corrective actions necessary. The QIPs are tracked by the computer system, allowing for systematic follow-up of deficiencies.

The duties of the QA coordinator include creating the meeting agendas of both committees, serving as a member of the QMG, and chairing the QAC. In addition, the coordinator is responsible for maintaining the computerized AmbuQual tracking system.

TABLE 7.
Parameter 1 Indicator Chart*

Parameter 1:	**Provider staff performance**
Aspect A:	**Credentials and provider staff systems**
Indicator 6:	**Peer review audit system (rev 2/94)**
Standard:	There is a current, functional, accurate, and complete procedure describing how each provider staff group performs the peer audit. The procedure includes a mechanism for review and feedback of audit results. Audits are carried out as planned.
QIP level:	85
Data source:	Provider performance audit policy/procedure
Weight:	1.00
Scoring:	Qualitative; consider procedure and utilization; QA Committee votes.
Responsibility:	Dr. Iannelli
Aspect C:	**Clinical performance**
Indicator 1:	Accurate clinical diagnosis (rev 2/94)
Standard:	The subjective and objective data in the current medical records adequately substantiate the clinical diagnoses made by the provider staff.
QIP Level:	80
Data Source:	Performance audit
Weight:	1.40
Scoring:	Quantitative (computer).
Responsibility:	Dr. Kuehner
Indicator 2:	**Correct clinical treatment (rev 2/94)**
Standard:	The diagnostic and therapeutic treatment plans are consistent with the diagnoses and current medical knowledge and practice patterns.
QIP Level:	90
Data source:	Performance audit
Weight:	1.40
Scoring:	Quantitative (computer).
Responsibility:	Dr. Iannelli

*From The National College Chiropractic Clinics, Lombard, Ill, 1994.

As parameters were approved, data sources had to be created. This required implementation of physician performance (peer review) audits of the medical records and patient satisfaction audits. Although not provided in the AmbuQual documentation, additional resources were available from Methodist Hospital of Indiana, Inc., which simplified the implementation of these audits.[43,44]

PHYSICIAN PERFORMANCE AUDIT

The physician performance audit that was developed at The National College Chiropractic Clinics was patterned after the process in place at the

Goal Fulfillment	Probable Impact of Deficiencies on Patient Care
AmbuQual® Qualitative Scoring Indicator#_____ Initials:_____	
☐ ☐ Completely fulfilled, no deficiencies	
☐ ☐ Nearly fulfilled	☐ ☐ Minimal impact: "Paper or technical requirement."
☐ ☐ More than half fulfilled	☐ ☐ Moderate impact: "Should be improved."
☐ ☐ Half fulfilled	
☐ ☐ Less than half fulfilled	☐ ☐ Significant impact: Worrisome; Important omissions."
☐ ☐ Barely fulfilled	☐ ☐ Critical impact: "Urgent; Must be promptly corrected; Severe compromise."
☐ ☐ Not fulfilled at all 11/92	

Impacts (right column on form) are defined as follows:

Minimal: thinking that deficiency relates to a paper or technical requirement; is of relatively little significance.

Moderate: thinking that situation should be improved to promote optimal patient care or center efficiency.

Significant: thinking that situation is worrisome. There are important omissions occurring in patient care or center operations.

Critical: thinking that situation is urgent and must be promptly corrected.

Goal Fulfillment	Probable Impact of Deficiencies on Patient Care
50 Completely fulfilled, no deficiencies	
45 Nearly fulfilled	45 Minimal impact: paper or technical requirement
35 More than half fulfilled	30 Moderate impact: should be improved
25 Half fulfilled	15 Significant impact; worrisome; important omissions
15 Less than half fulfilled	0 Critical impact; urgent, must be promptly corrected; severe compromise
5 Barely fulfilled	
0 Not fulfilled at all 11/92	

FIGURE 1.
AmbuQual qualitative scoring form. This form is used by members of the Quality Assurance Committee to score indicators whose data source is not quantitative. (From Benson DS, Miller JA: *AmbuQual® II: An Ambulatory Quality Assurance and Quality Management System*. Indianapolis, Methodist Hospital of Indiana, 1993, pp 98, 116. Used by permission.)

Community Health Network Centers in Indianapolis.[45] It is an ongoing audit of the overall performance of the practitioner staff and provides up to 25% of the data required for the AmbuQual system.[34] The audit is peer review, in which each practitioner is responsible for auditing another practitioner's performance. Although the audit looks mainly at the "pro-

AMBUQUAL
Quality Improvement Plan

1. _____ Date ___/___/___ QIP# _____
   Name of Organization / Dept / Division   Assigned   (optional)

2. _____ _____
   Manager Responsible for QIP   Job Title

3. QIP Description for Computerized Log:

   |_|_|_|_|_|_|_|_|_|_|_|_|_|_|_|_|_|_|_|_|_|_|_|_|_|_|_|_|_|_|_|_|_|_|_|_|_|_|_|_|
   (Description can be no longer than 40 characters long)

4. Related AMBUQUAL Indicator # _____ Performance or Effectiveness Goal _____
   _____
   _____

5. Indicator Score _____ Related QIP Level (threshold) _____

6. QIP Narrative Description (reason for QIP)
   _____
   _____

7. QA Committee's Recommendations for QIP Resolution (optional) _____
   _____

8. Target Date for Resolution ___/___/___ X_____
                                            (QA Committee Chair's Signature)

   ┌──┐
   │ 9. RESOLUTION   │
   │   Review Date ___/___/___ Indicator Score____ At/Above QIP Level = Resolved ____ │
   │   Below QIP Level = Director's QIP ____ │
   │   Review Date ___/___/___ Indicator Score____ At/Above QIP Level = Resolved ____ │
   │   Below QIP Level = Governing Body's QIP ____ │
   │   Governing Body QIP Decision _____ │
   │   Review Date ___/___/___   │
   │   X_____   │
   │   (QA Committee Chair's Signature)   │
   └──┘

10. Distribution:
    1) Copy to Manager Responsible
    2) Copy to Head of Initiating Organization / Dept or Division
    3) Original and Copy of all updates to QA Document File

   This Document is for PEER REVIEW purposes and is priviledged under:
                      - Indiana Code 34-4-12.
              _____
              (other applicable State Confidential Priviledged Information Act)

FIGURE 2.
AmbuQual quality improvement plan (QIP). This memorandum is completed and sent to the responsible manager whenever an indicator's score falls below the QIP level (described in text). (From Benson DS, Miller JA: *AmbuQual® II: An Ambulatory Quality Assurance and Quality Management System.* Indianapolis, Methodist Hospital of Indiana, 1993, 163. Used by permission.)

cess" of care—whether or not the practitioner followed the correct steps in providing care—it can also track outcomes if the appropriate questions are utilized.

The medical record is used as the data source for the performance audit. Because the auditor is not in the room during the patient encounter, the visit must be evaluated by reviewing the information contained within the medical record. If a visit is well documented, there is usually no problem in establishing quality care. However, an incomplete medical record gives insufficient data to determine quality and may infer that incomplete (poor quality) care was rendered. The medical record must be able to provide accurate, complete, and timely information at the time a medical judgment is made, which makes medical record documentation a critical issue. Thus, it is appropriate to rely on the medical record for a peer review performance audit.

Van Osdol[45] compiled a list of audit principles that he found to be important and helpful:

1. *Use explicit criteria as much as possible.* Using predetermined, defined criteria makes the audit more reliable and objective than using implicit criteria.
2. *Clinical protocols are an effective framework for explicit criteria.* Protocols are written standards for common problems that guide practitioners through appropriate data base collection, patient treatment, and patient education.
3. *Identify "critical elements" as audit criteria in the clinical protocol.* Critical protocol elements are those elements that, if they are not in compliance, clearly indicate suboptimal care. These elements are necessary to confirm the diagnosis, establish the prognosis, rule out other significant problems, or influence treatment.
4. *The audit should be timely.* Practitioner performance is more likely to be influenced if the audit feedback is as concurrent as possible. For this reason, the emphasis of the audit should be on the most recent visit, although a general chart review may be conducted as well. The charts selected for review should be for patients most recently seen, which allows feedback to come in time to correct deficiencies that can benefit specific patients.
5. *The audit should be random.* Charts should be selected randomly by date and time, not by specific diagnosis. A totally random chart selection system will enable the auditor to review charts of patients not only on whom diagnoses have been made but also on whom diagnoses should have been made.
6. *The audit should not be time consuming or expensive.* Audit only enough charts to get a sufficient sample from each practitioner. A 1% sample (1 out of every 100 visits) appears to be sufficient. It should usually take 10 minutes or less to review a chart. The major expense in the audit is the time of the practitioners involved in doing the audit. Therefore, it is important to minimize their time spent. This can be facilitated by having well-trained clerical support.
7. *All practitioners should participate in the audits and in the development of audit standards.* By involving the practitioners in the development of the standards (criteria) by which they will ultimately be audited, the paranoia can be taken out of the audit process. Practitioners are more likely to comply with standards they have helped to write.

8. *Feedback from the audit should lead to correction of deficiencies by changing the behavior of the practitioner.* Providers should review and discuss their own audit results. An awareness of one's performance compared with the performance of one's peers is often all that is needed to improve patient care behavior. Providers should also be able to contest the audit results, because these disagreements can lead to better understanding of the standards or changes in the standards.

The National College Chiropractic Clinics Physician Performance Audit was implemented in 1990 and revised in 1991 to its current version (Appendix 2). It is a continuous process, with each physician auditing another physician for 2 months at a time on a rotating schedule. Refer to the procedure for details on its implementation.

The questions on the performance audit have been developed over the past 4 years and may change as the emphasis or needs of the organization change. Questions are developed through the AmbuQual QM process; as an indicator is added to the AmbuQual system that uses the chart review as its data source, a question must be developed and added to the audit form. Although it may be preferable to print audit forms in large quantities, printing too many at a time may prevent the timely modification of the questions. For this reason, we try to print no more than a 6-month supply of audit forms at a time. The audit currently contains 29 questions and requires 5 to 10 minutes to complete but could easily be expanded to 40 to 50 questions if needed and still be completed in a timely manner. Figure 3 is the most recent audit form. Figure 4 is the form that provides practitioners the ability to offer feedback on audit results. Table 8 is a partial printout of the audit results after entry into the AmbuQual system. This printout tabulates the audit results for eight of the current questions in use. The AmbuQual software generates this site- and date-specific report, then compiles the scores to generate the system score. Although it took approximately 2 years to fully implement this performance audit, the results have provided considerable feedback to practitioners, who have then made significant behavioral changes.

PATIENT SATISFACTION AUDIT

Instruments to measure customer (patient) satisfaction have existed for years, even in the field of ambulatory health care. Many formats exist, including mail questionnaires; telephone, exit, and home interviews; and focus groups. Each method has its own advantages and disadvantages.

The patient satisfaction audit system described here is taken from the Community Health Network centers in Indianapolis[46] and is unique in that patients respond to questions according to the school system grading matrix (A, B, C, D, and F). Hence, it is called the *Give Us A Grade Program.*

Because patient satisfaction is an important component to quality care (AmbuQual assigns it to its own parameter), assessing satisfaction is an important activity. In addition, a functional plan to follow up on dissatisfied patients is needed to ensure continuing improvement in the level of quality in the program. Other issues that relate to quality care, such as accessibility and compliance, can also be evaluated by means of a patient

NATIONAL COLLEGE CHIROPRACTIC CLINICS
PRACTITIONER PERFORMANCE AUDIT

Center_____ Chart #_____ Date of Visit_____ Practitioner_____

ACUTE/CHRONIC PROBLEM CARE   Yes   No   NA   Comments
Problem/#Title_____
1. Was the subjective data adequate?   ____   ____ ____ _____
2. Was the objective data adequate?   ____   ____ ____ _____
3. Was the assessment adequate?   ____   ____ ____ _____
4. Were the diagnostic procedures adequate?   ____   ____ ____ _____
5. Was recommended therapy indicated and appropriate
    for the stated condition?   ____   ____ ____ _____
6. Does the plan contain appropriate initial short and
    long term goals?   ____   ____ ____ _____
7. Are treatment goals reviewed/revised according
    to their expiration dates?   ____   ____ ____ _____
8. Was a consultation requested if indicated?   ____   ____ ____ _____
9. Was the patient referred to the nutritionist if
    indicated?   ____   ____ ____ _____
10. Was the patient referred to rehabilitation if
    indicated?   ____   ____ ____ _____
11. Was the patient referred to electrodiagnosis if
    indicated?   ____   ____ ____ _____
12. Was the patient referred to ergonomics if indicated?   ____   ____ ____ _____
13. Was the patient referred to orthopedics if indicated?   ____   ____ ____ _____
14. Was the patient referred to family practice if
    indicated?   ____   ____ ____ _____
15. If appropriate, was the patient placed on elective
    care?   ____   ____ ____ _____
16. Does a progress note indicate the patient received
    patient education, including explanation of diagnosis?   ____   ____ ____ _____
17. If the patient received a new therapy, does SOAP note
    indicate specific pt. ed. was given about therapy?   ____   ____ ____ _____
18. MECHANICAL LOW BACK PAIN: Has the initial treatment
    goal been achieved within 3 weeks?   ____   ____ ____ _____
19. MECHANICAL NECK PAIN: Has the initial treatment goal
    been achieved within 3 weeks?   ____   ____ ____ _____
20. SHOULDER IMPINGEMENT: Has the initial treatment goal
    been achieved within 6 weeks?   ____   ____ ____ _____

MEDICAL RECORDS
21. Does the Problem List contain all significant clinical
    impressions?   ____   ____ ____ _____
22. Does the Problem List accurately indicate if problems
    are active or resolved?   ____   ____ ____ _____
23. Were all entires in the record legible?   ____   ____ ____ _____
24. Does the progress note follow SOAP format?   ____   ____ ____ _____
25. Do all therapy/plan orders bear the clinician's
    signature and date?   ____   ____ ____ _____

CONTINUITY OF CARE
26. If ordered, was consultation/referral carried out?   ____   ____ ____ _____
27. Are all abnormal laboratory, imaging and specialty
    procedure results adequately followed up?   ____   ____ ____ _____
28. Are test results available for tests ordered on
    previous visit? (NA if 1 wk since last visit)   ____   ____ ____ _____
29. Was the patient seen by the same provider/group on 8
    out of the 10 most recent visits (within 6 months)?   ____   ____ ____ _____

4/10/92

FIGURE 3.

Physician performance audit form. This questionnaire is completed by the auditing practitioner by reviewing the chart specified by the medical records staff. (From The National College Chiropractic Clinics, Lombard, Ill, 1994, unpublished data.)

NATIONAL COLLEGE CHIROPRACTIC CLINICS
PRACTITIONER PERFORMANCE AUDIT FEEDBACK

Center______ Chart#______ Date of Visit______ Practitioner______

AUDIT RESULTS

____ No questions about care/documentation

____ Questions about care/documentation #______

PRACTITIONER REVIEW # Reason

____ Agree should improve care/documentation

____ Disagree should improve care/documentation

Practitioner Date

CLINIC DIRECTOR'S REVIEW # Reason

____ No questions about care/documentation

____ Questions about care/documentation

Clinic Director Date

CLINICAL STAFF REVIEW # Reason

____ Agree should improve care/documentation

____ No questions about care/documentation

Clinic Director Date

FIGURE 4.
Physician performance audit feedback form. This form accompanies the audit form, and provides the audited practitioner with a mechanism for disagreeing with the audit results. (From The National College Chiropractic Clinics, Lombard, Ill, 1994.)

audit system. The patient becomes the data source for questions such as waiting times, patient education, and compliance to home instructions.

The "Give Us A Grade" program is a form of exit interview. As the cashier computes the final charges, the patient is asked to complete a grade card. (Virtually all persons have an understanding of the public school grading system.) The cards are 5 by 7 in., with a picture of a school-marm and one of 28 question sets on the front and a comment/name space

TABLE 8.
Physician Performance Audit Results: National College Chiropractic Clinics: Total Site Report April 1–June 30, 1994*

Parameter/ Indicator	Performance Audit Question	Yes	No	Score (%)
1.C.1	1. Were the subjective data adequate?	52	12	81%
1.C.1	2. Were the objective data adequate?	55	9	86%
1.C.1	3. Was the assessment adequate?	47	13	78%
1.C.2	4. Were the diagnostic procedures adequate?	32	4	89%
1.C.2	5. Was recommended therapy indicated and appropriate for the stated condition?	48	15	76%
4.C.7	6. Does the plan contain appropriate short- and long-term goals?	28	32	47%
4.C.8	7. Are treatment goals reviewed/revised according to their expiration dates?	39	21	65%
9.D.1	8. Was a consultation requested if indicated?	5	0	100%

*From The National College Chiropractic Clinics, Lombard, Ill, 1994, unpublished data.

on the back (Fig 5). New patients are given two cards: a "new patient card" and a random card from the general system. Each card asks for grades for one area relating to patient satisfaction. Although the card asks only one set of questions for each patient encounter, the overall system will interview about a 100% sample of the current patient population. Each of the 28 question sets will be answered many times. This system also ensures that all patients will have an opportunity to respond at some point.

One modification our organization has made to the program is to have the cashier hand each person a set of five cards (unless the patient has already completed two sets of five cards during that survey period) instead of only one card per visit. This change was implemented after patients became hesitant to complete a single card on more than three or four visits during the month. This way, all patients respond to a maximum of 10 questions during two visits and then are not asked to complete any additional questionnaires during that month. Once patients have completed their responses, they place the completed cards in the collection box next to the cashier window. At the end of the day, the cards are reviewed by either the office manager or clinic director for comments and problems that require immediate attention. Any action taken as a result of a complaint or comment is noted on the survey form. The cards are then sent to the QA coordinator for processing.

At the end of the survey period, results are computed and tabulated for entry into the AmbuQual system. Survey results include tabulations and transcribed comments, complaints, and resulting action and are reported to the QMG, QA committee, and clinical staff.

Surveys are conducted at each clinic at least twice annually. Survey

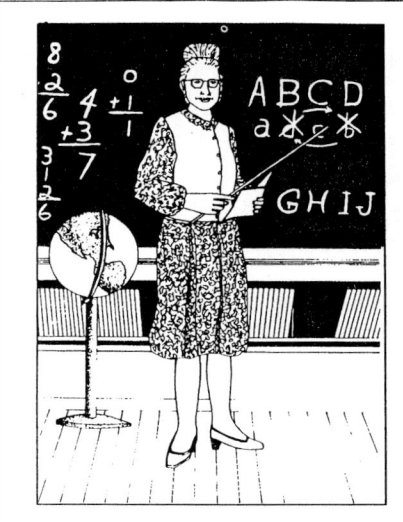

FIGURE 5.
Patient satisfaction audit ("Give Us A Grade") card. This card, 1 out of 28, asks the patient to "give a grade" on their satisfaction with their doctor. The cards are printed on the front *(top)* with the questions chosen for the patient satisfaction audit and on the back *(bottom)* with a space for other comments, and name, address, and telephone information. (From Benson DS, Van Osdol WR: *Quality Audit Systems.* Indianapolis, Methodist Hospital of Indiana, 1987, pp 46–51. Used by permission.)

periods are 1 month. The survey schedule is set by the QA coordinator. Question content is determined by the chief of clinics staff or the QMG and is based on the data needs of the AmbuQual system. The questions relate primarily to the parameters of patient satisfaction, patient compliance, and access to care. Appendix 3 lists the questions currently in use in the "Give Us A Grade Program" at The National College Chiropractic Clinics.

With this system, it is possible to obtain data from more patients than with other satisfaction instruments. It is relatively quick, adding little time to a patient's visit. Patients are not requested to take anything home to be mailed back (or forgotten). It reinforces to the patients that their opinions count and that should they have a problem, there is a way to let the organization know about it. During the 4 years that we have performed the audits, we consistently find patients who use the comment section on the back of the cards, making both positive and negative remarks. Patients also express gratitude that they are even being asked their opinion. The "Give Us A Grade Program" has proved to be an effective tool to mea-

TABLE 9.
Parameter 1 Score Report*

	Last Update	Score	Weight	Description
1.A.2	03/10/94	100	1.30	Credentials—current certification and licensure (rev 2/94)
1.A.3	03/10/94	90	0.80	Job descriptions (rev 2/94)
1.A.4	03/10/94	39	0.80	Personnel performance evaluation system (rev 2/94)
1.A.6	03/10/94	79	1.00	Peer review audit system (rev 2/94)
Aspect A		**80**	**0.50**	**Credentials and provider staff systems**
1.C.1	06/30/94	85	1.40	Accurate clinical diagnosis (rev 2/94)
1.C.2	06/30/94	83	1.40	Correct clinical treatment (rev 2/94)
1.C.3	06/30/94	65	1.10	General clinical performance (rev 2/94)
1.C.4	06/30/94	63	0.70	Internal referral performance (rev 2/94)
1.C.6	06/30/94	62	1.00	Treatment goals, follow-up (rev 2/94)
1.C.7	06/30/94	87	1.00	Elective care utilization (rev 2/94)
Aspect C		**76**	**1.25**	**Clinical performance**
1.D.1	06/30/94	68	1.00	Mechanical low back pain (rev 2/94)
1.D.2	06/30/94	51	1.00	Mechanical neck pain (rev 2/94)
1.D.3	06/30/94	75	1.00	Shoulder impingement (rev 2/94)
Aspect D		**65**	**1.75**	**Clinical effectiveness**
Parameter 1		71	1.90	Provider staff performance

*From The National College Chiropractic Clinics, Lombard, Ill, 1994.

sure patient satisfaction and has allowed us to identify not only problem areas within our organization that are in need of intervention but also shining stars (personnel/departments) that deserve commendation.

AMBUQUAL SYSTEM SCORING

As each parameter is scored and new data sources quantified, the computer system rescores the entire program, applying the appropriate weighting to the scores (Table 9), generating a revised PQI, a quantitative summation of the quality of the program (Table 10). It is derived from the average score of the 10 ambulatory care parameters times their weights and is a number from 0 to 100. Although Benson and Miller admit the scores are only a rough approximation of an organization's actual performance and they stress repeatedly to "not take the scores too seriously," the scores are useful in monitoring trends. Scores going down indicate deficiencies that management must deal with. Scores that remain level may be improved by management emphasizing performances in those areas. A score trending upward is responding to an increased level of quality, resulting in the potential to improve patients' health.[34] An example of how a quality issue can affect the PQI follows:

Assume a newly hired practitioner does not document adequate histories and physical examinations. A chart audit determines that the number of files with accurate history, physical examination, and diagnosis is 20% less than the previous audit. The indicator score for "accurate diagnosis" decreases by 20 points. Because of the indicator's weighting (1.40) and because there are four other indicators for that aspect, the clinical performance aspect score drops 3 points. Because the clinical performance aspect is weighted 1.25, the provider staff performance parameter score decreases by 4 points. Because of the parameter's weight (1.90), the net effect on the PQI is a 1-point drop.

TABLE 10.
Program Quality Index (PQI) Report*

Parameter	Score	Weight	Description
1	71	1.90	Provider staff performance
2	92	1.10	Support staff performance
3	72	0.90	Continuity of care
4	52	0.70	Medical record system
5	33	0.70	Patient risk minimization
6	90	0.60	Patient satisfaction
7	83	1.30	Patient compliance
8	68	0.90	Accessibility
9	52	1.40	Appropriateness of service
10	49	0.50	Organizational performance

PQI 68

*From The National College Chiropractic Clinics, Lombard, Ill, 1994.

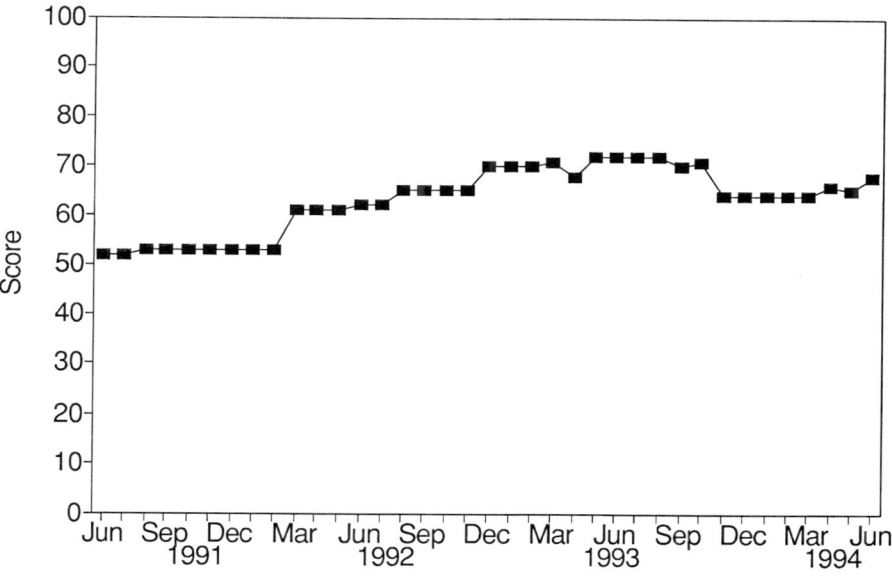

FIGURE 6.
The National College Chiropractic Clinics Performance Quality Index (PQI) graph. Monthly PQI scores obtained from the computerized AmbuQual system are charted for the 3-year period 1991 to 1994. The PQI changes each time indicator scores change. On a monthly basis, the indicators for a given parameter are scored, as well as any deficient indicators that have been recalled for review by the system. (From The National College Chiropractic Clinics, Lombard, Ill, 1994, unpublished data.)

IMPLEMENTATION ISSUES

Initially several indicators were modified to conform to a chiropractic setting. Drug-related indicators were deleted. Strict medical records indicators related to the problem list and progress notes were created. The initial "committee" style performance audit process outlined in Van Osdol's text had to be converted to the continuous version previously described.

Implementation of the program identified several deficiencies in our clinics. Examples of deficiencies in "systems" would include the lack of written procedures, job descriptions, and safety inspections. Examples of deficiencies in "processes" would include poor provider documentation of patient education and treatment goals and poor continuity of provider care. Through corrective actions (writing the missing procedures, retraining clinicians in documentation protocols, etc.) these deficiencies were resolved, ultimately improving the PQI. Monthly PQI scores for the past 3 years are graphically represented on Figure 6.

CONCLUSION

Using a standardized system designed for the medical ambulatory health care arena in a chiropractic setting has not been a difficult task. Given the fact that only 7 indicators out of 80 currently in use required significant revision, deletion, or creation, AmbuQual proved itself to be highly adaptable. Even though there are different professions involved in ambulatory health care, through AmbuQual it can be seen that chiropractic shares many problems with our counterparts. In addition, our experiences in implementing AmbuQual appear to mirror those documented in other professions.[47-52]

Other chiropractic organizations have become involved in the AmbuQual movement. I have provided information about this program to numerous practitioners across the country. Currently there are at least two other chiropractic colleges, one chiropractic PPO, and one private practitioner operating four clinics who are using AmbuQual. It is important to note that its flexibility is what makes AmbuQual well suited for use in our profession. It is not necessary to operate AmbuQual with multiple committees, employees, and levels of bureaucracy unless they are already present! What follows is a scenario for implementing AmbuQual in a private practice setting.

The QA plan can be pared down dramatically. The components that must remain are the identification of the responsible authority (this could be the solo practitioner), the scope of services (what is done for/to patients in the practice), and the organizational structure. It is not necessary to have any committees unless there are personnel to assign as members. One alternative is to have a single blended committee made up of managers and staff. This single committee can serve both functions: standard review and development and data collection. In an even smaller setting, a solo practitioner with an employee could manage the process.

The one activity that requires cooperation between practitioners is the performance audit. For a solo practitioner to implement the audit, it is necessary to team up with other practitioners (at least two). The practitioners can trade off and audit each other's charts on a rotating schedule. There are already chiropractors who have formed these "peer review groups" to obtain privileges with managed care networks. The evidence is in: QM works!

This is just the beginning for quality management in chiropractic. Although we have identified and filled a need for documenting quality by implementing a standardized system, more must be done. Specific changes in indicator scores as a result of changing clinical behaviors must be documented. As we speak, the technology of quality management continues to move forward. Now is the time for others in chiropractic to begin endeavors in managing quality. It is altruistically valuable for all ambulatory health care professions to make strides in this area before outsiders require it of us.

REFERENCES

1. Miller JA: Monitoring practice: An ambulatory care example, in Schroeder P (ed): *The Encyclopedia of Nursing Care Quality*. Rockville, Md, Aspen Publishers, 1991, vol III, pp 127–147.
2. Palmer RH: The challenges and prospects for quality assessment and assurance in ambulatory care. *Inquiry* 25:119–131, 1988.
3. Joint Commission on Accreditation of Healthcare Organizations: *Joint Com-*

mission Accreditation Manual for Hospitals, 1990. Chicago, Joint Commission, 1989, p 211.
4. Institute of Medicine: Advancing the Quality of Health Care: Key Issues and Fundamental Principles. Washington DC, National Academy of Sciences, 1974, pp 1–2.
5. Benson DS: Quality in ambulatory care: The two minute demonstration. J Qual Assur 13(3):8–12, 1991.
6. Benson DS, Flanagan E, Hill KL, et al: Quality Assurance in Ambulatory Care. Chicago, Joint Commission on Accreditation of Hospitals, 1987, p 3.
7. Batalden PB, O'Connor JP: Quality Assurance in Ambulatory Care. Rockville, Md, Aspen Publishers, 1980, p 3.
8. Donabedian A: Evaluating the quality of medical care. Milbank Memorial Fund Q 44:166–206, 1966.
9. Joint Commission Staff: Monitoring and evaluation of the quality and appropriateness of care: An ambulatory health care example. QRB 13:26–30, 1987.
10. Koska MT: Push is on for ambulatory quality assurance. Hospitals 62:66, 1988.
11. Joint Commission Staff: Accreditation Manual for Ambulatory Health Care. Chicago, Joint Commission on Accreditation of Healthcare Organizations, 1992, p 1.
12. Miller JA: Personal communication, 1993.
13. Joint Commission Staff: Personal communication, 1994.
14. Deming WE: Out of the Crisis. Cambridge, Mass, MIT Press, 1982.
15. Juran JM: Juran on Leadership for Quality: An Executive Handbook. New York, Free Press, 1989.
16. Bliersbach, CM: The NAHQ Guide to Quality Management, ed 3. Skokie, Ill, National Association for Healthcare Quality, 1993, p 32.
17. Haldeman S, Chapman-Smith D, Petersen DM: Guidelines for Chiropractic Quality Assurance and Practice Parameters. Gaithersburg, Md, Aspen Publishers, 1993.
18. Iannelli GC: Application of a standardized quality assurance program (AmbuQual) in a multi-doctor chiropractic clinic system. J Neuromusculoskeletal System 1:1–9, 1993.
19. Bohm J: Health care quality assurance: Tracer analysis in quality assessment of ambulatory care provided by two out patient teaching clinics. J Manipulative Physiol Ther 14:249–254, 1991.
20. Kessner DM, Kalk CE, Singer J: Assessing health quality—the case for tracers. N Engl J Med 288:189–193, 1973.
21. Saywell RM, Bean JA, Redman RW, et al: Examination of physician team performance in six processes of care. QRB 10:385–392, 1984.
22. Hastings CE: Measuring quality in ambulatory care nursing. J Nurs Adm 17(4):12–20, 1987.
23. Lane K, Peppe KK: Editor's choice. Where are the standards? J Pediatr Nurs 2:291–294, 1987.
24. Bradford M, Flynn NM: Ambulatory care infection control quality assurance monitoring. Am J Infect Control 16:21A–28A, 1988.
25. Davis D, Hobbs G: Measuring outpatient satisfaction with rehabilitation services. QRB 15:192–197, 1989.
26. Gates RA, Przykucki JM: Improving practice in ambulatory care: Development of an ambulatory nursing QA program. J Nurs Qual Assur 3:36–48, 1989.
27. Caro DH: Medical care classification systems in the ambulatory care environment: An evaluative framework. J Med Syst 14:283–296, 1990.
28. Koecheler JA, Sfeir TL, Wilson B: Outcome-focused counseling program for

quality assurance in ambulatory care. *Am J Hosp Pharm* 47:2020–2022, 1990.
29. Sims TW: Nephrology nursing consult: Case study. Quality assurance works. *ANNA J* 17:258, 1990.
30. DeNeef P, Ellsworth A, Schneeweiss R: A system for drug utilization review in ambulatory care. *J Fam Pract* 32:607–612, 1991.
31. Betta PA: Developing a successful ambulatory QA program. *Nurs Manage* 23(4):31–33, 1992.
32. Bennett WG, Delafield JP, Mishra SK, et al: Quality assurance in ambulatory care. *Acad Med* 64(10 suppl):S22–S27, 1989.
33. Solberg LI, Peterson KE, Ellis RW, et al: The Minnesota Project: A focused approach to ambulatory quality assessment. *Inquiry* 27:359–367, 1990.
34. Benson DS, Gartner C, Anderson JG, et al: The ambulatory care parameter: A structured approach to quality assurance in the ambulatory care setting. *QRB* 13:51–55, 1987.
35. Benson DS, Miller JA: *Quality Assurance for Primary Care Centers*. Indianapolis, Methodist Hospital of Indiana, 1988.
36. Benson DS, Miller JA: *AmbuQual® II: An Ambulatory Quality Assurance and Quality Management System*. Indianapolis, Methodist Hospital of Indiana, 1993.
37. Miller JA: Evaluating structure, process and outcome indicators in ambulatory care: The AmbuQual approach. *J Nurs Qual Assur* 4:40–47, 1989.
38. Anderson JG, Benson DS, Schweer HM, et al: AmbuQual: A computer-supported system for the measurement and evaluation of quality in ambulatory care settings. *J Ambulatory Care Manage* 12:27–33, 1989.
39. Benson DS: System measures ambulatory care quality. *Physician Exec* pp 15–20, March–April 1990.
40. Watt J, Miller JA: Quality assurance in homeless health care. *Streetreach* pp 4–5, spring–summer 1990.
41. Warren BH: Ambulatory quality assurance in the academic medical center. *Group Pract J* pp 54–60, July–August 1990.
42. Main DS, Fried RA, Benson DS, et al: Changes in knowledge and attitudes following implementation of a structured ambulatory quality assurance system. *J Ambulatory Care Manage* 15:71–76, 1992.
43. Benson DS, Van Osdol WR: *Quality audit systems for primary care centers*. Indianapolis, Methodist Hospital of Indiana, 1987.
44. Van Osdol WR, Johnston PE: *Quality Medical Records for Primary Care Centers*. Indianapolis, Methodist Hospital of Indiana, 1989.
45. Van Osdol WR: The performance audit, in Benson DS, Van Osdol WR: *Quality Audit Systems for Primary Care Centers*. Indianapolis, Methodist Hospital of Indiana, 1987, pp 53–77.
46. Timm VL: The patient satisfaction audit, in Benson DS, Van Osdol WR: *Quality Audit Systems for Primary Care Centers*. Indianapolis, Methodist Hospital of Indiana, 1987, pp 43–51.
47. Fried RA: Experiences with AmbuQual-User. Paper presented at Methodist Hospital of Indiana AmbuQual Users' Conference, Indianapolis, October 1990.
48. Pickering P: The AmbuQual QA meeting. Paper presented at Methodist Hospital of Indiana, AmbuQual Users' Conference, Indanapolis, October 1990.
49. LoPresti J: Implementation and innovation—user presentation. Paper presented at Methodist Hospital of Indiana, AmbuQual Users' Conference, Indianapolis, October 1991.
50. Gottlieb A: Common problems and solutions—user presentation. Paper presented at Methodist Hospital of Indiana, AmbuQual Users' Conference, Indianapolis, October 1992.

51. Bushman D: Implementation and innovation—user presentation. Paper presented at Methodist Hospital of Indiana, AmbuQual Users' Conference, Indianapolis, October 1992.
52. Gray-Jones T: Data collection techniques—user presentation. Paper presented at Methodist Hospital of Indiana, AmbuQual Users' Conference, Indianapolis, October 1992.

Appendix 1*

National College Chiropractic Clinics Quality Assurance Plan*

I. Objectives
   A. Purpose of the quality assurance (QA) program
   B. Objectives of the QA program
II. Organization
   A. QA program coordinator
   B. Quality management group (QMG)
   C. QA committee
III. Scope (parameters)
IV. Mechanisms for overseeing program effectiveness
   A. Computer tracking and referral to higher authority
   B. Report to the College administration
   C. Annual program review
V. Confidentiality
   A. Activity reporting
   B. Access to QA data
   C. Information requests
   D. Subpoena exemption
VI. Retention of records
   A. Minutes of meetings
   B. Departmental activity reports
   C. Monthly QA reports
   D. Practice profiles

I. OBJECTIVES
   A. Purpose
      The National College Chiropractic Clinics purpose is to perform appropriate health care delivery that, within available resources, is optimal and consistent with achievable therapeutic goals. For services not supplied by the clinics, appropriate brokering of health care through allied professionals will be carried out. The QA program developed by the College is designed to enhance the care provided to patients through a system of ongoing monitoring

---

*Adapted from The National College Chiropractic Clinics, Lombard, Ill.

and evaluation of important aspects of patient care. Opportunities to improve the quality of patient care and clinical performance will be pursued and problems that are identified will be resolved.

B. Objectives
The objectives of the National College Chiropractic Clinics Quality Assurance Program are as follows:
1. To conduct monitoring and evaluation activities of health care delivery on a planned, systematic and ongoing basis.
2. To carry out a comprehensive program that incorporates consideration of the important aspects of patient care provided by all clinic departments.
3. To use indicators and thresholds for evaluation that are based on current clinical standards of care, are agreed on by clinical staff and are acceptable to the College.
4. To review indicators, thresholds and standards annually.
5. To take appropriate actions to resolve identified problems.
6. To ensure through continuous monitoring that improvements in care and performance are sustained.
7. To share the information, strengths, and weaknesses derived from monitoring and evaluation activities with all clinical departments and services and with the College administration.
8. To document and report quality assurance activities to staff and administration in a manner that substantiates the effectiveness of the program.
9. To comply with the quality assurance standards set by those bodies responsible for ascertaining the existence of an ongoing and effective quality assurance program.
10. To provide staff education about quality assurance activities on a regular, periodic basis.

II. ORGANIZATION
A. QA program Coordinator
The QA program coordinator is recommended by the chief of clinics staff, appointed by the president (or his or her designee) and has the following primary responsibilities:
1. To provide assistance to and monitor the performance of all personnel designated to be involved in quality assurance activities.
2. To provide training for clinical and support personnel in the areas of quality assurance procedures, including indicator development, data retrieval and analysis, preparation of reports and confidentiality.
3. As directed by the QA committee, to assist heads of departments and clinic directors in the investigation of problems and incidents, and in determining actions for remediation when appropriate, and in the preparation of quality improvement plans (QIPs).
4. To request any employee or professional member of the clinics' staff to complete and file incident reports with the QA committee, including copies to the chief of clinics staff and the appropriate clinic director.

5. To implement the AmbuQual (or other selected system) quality assurance system of ongoing monitoring and evaluation.
6. To conduct meetings of the QA committee as provided for in II.C.3.
7. To assist the chief of clinics staff in preparing a quality assurance budget to be included as part of the clinics' administrative services budget.
8. To take necessary steps to assure the confidentiality of all quality assurance data and reports.
9. To work in a collegial and cooperative manner with all faculty and support staff for the most effective and efficient attainment of the College's mission.

B. QM Group
   1. Membership
      The QMG is composed of the following persons:
      a. Chief of clinics staff (Chairperson)
      b. QA program coordinator
      c. Clinics business administrator
      d. Director–Lombard Chiropractic Clinic NCCC
      e. Director–Chicago General Health Service NCCC—C
      f. Director–Aurora Chiropractic Clinic NCCC—A
      g. Supervisor–Salvation Army Clinics
      h. One representative of the specialty practice/academic faculty

      The QMG shall have a recording secretary (not a member).
   2. Responsibilities of QMG
      The QMG is responsible for the following:
      a. Development of *indicators* to be monitored
         An indicator is what is monitored to determine how well an organization is doing on an aspect of care. Each level of AmbuQual (for example) suggests various indicators which could be monitored for each parameter. Each indicator has been determined to be important to monitor as a part of the quality assurance program, has its own clinically valid standard and has the potential to impact the health of the patient. The QMG should affirm that these indicators are appropriate for the program. The QMG is also encouraged to develop new site-specific indicators that reflect the unique characteristics of the program.
      b. Affirmation or revision of *standards* on an annual basis
         A standard is the performance expectation defined for a particular indicator. AmbuQual standards are proposed for each of the indicators. Standard affirmation or revision is a critical activity in the start-up of AmbuQual. Standards for each indicator in each parameter must be modified or affirmed by the QMG before the Quality Assurance Committee can review the clinics' performance in relation to them.
      c. Affirmation or revision of QIP levels
         In AmbuQual, a threshold is called the QIP Level. The

threshold for evaluation (QIP level) states, in advance, the acceptable margin of error in meeting a particular standard. Performance below the QIP (threshold) level is defined as unacceptable performance and requires problem solving activity. Performance at or above the QIP level is understood to be acceptable at that particular point in time. No problem evaluation or solving activity is required, whereas performance below it mandates intervention. AmbuQual suggests initial QIP levels. These QIP levels must be affirmed or revised by the QMG. As the level of quality, as monitored by specific indicators, rises, the QMG can adjust the QIP level upward to increase performance expectations.

d. Development of data sources necessary for AmbuQual
 The data sources required by AmbuQual include, but are not limited to, audit systems such as provider performance audits and patient satisfaction surveys. Data source development is a major responsibility of the QMG during the implementation of AmbuQual.

e. Assignment of indicator responsibility
 For each indicator a specific person in management (clinical staff or administrative staff) is assigned responsibility for the standard associated with the indicator. That person is ultimately responsible for the performance on that standard. One of the duties of the QMG in AmbuQual is to determine the management responsibility for each indicator and standard. Data collection rests with the members of the Quality Assurance Committee.

f. Resolution of problems identified by the Quality Assurance Committee
 QIPs are generated by the Quality Assurance Committee if the actual performance doesn't meet the QIP level. The QIP is forwarded to the manager previously assigned the responsibility for that particular indicator and standard. It is the responsibility of the member of management receiving the QIP to see that the problem identified is resolved.

C. QA committee
  1. Committee membership
  The membership of the QA committee is recommended by the chief of clinics staff and appointed by the president (or his or her designee). Members of the committee are as follows:
  a. QA coordinator (chairperson)
  b. One clinician
  c. One "allied health" representative (e.g., physical therapist, nutritionist, radiologist, laboratory director)
  d. Two "support staff" members:
   i. one technical (e.g., research or clinical laboratory staff, radiology staff)
   ii. one clerical (e.g., cashier, receptionist, medical records clerk)

e. One administrative staff member
   The QA committee shall have a recording secretary (not a member) unless also appointed as a member under C.1.
2. Term of office
   The term of committee membership is 1 year. Members may serve consecutive terms at the discretion of the president.
3. Meetings and agenda
   The committee meets once monthly. Extra meetings may be called by the chairperson. The agenda for each meeting is developed by the chairperson using the predetermined AmbuQual format. The agenda is circulated to committee members in advance of the meeting. On the agenda, members are assigned items to review before the meeting. At the meeting, members are asked to report on their agenda items and help identify any related patient care problems.
4. Systematic program review
   Using the AmbuQual system the committee reviews, on a cyclical basis, the entire clinical care program of the National College Clinics.
5. Authority
   The committee has the authority to:
   a. Score qualitative indicators.
   b. Identify problems and assign responsibility and priority for resolving these problems by issuing QIPs.
   c. Determine whether problems documented on QIP's have been adequately resolved.
6. QIP
   The AmbuQual QIP is used to document all significant patient care problems. The QA committee chairperson initiates the QIP. QIPs may be generated automatically if the indicator is below the predetermined QIP level.
7. Minutes
   A secretary records minutes and circulates these to the QA committee, the QMG, and the president of the College (or his or her designee).

I. SCOPE
During an AmbuQual cycle, which is expected to take 12 months to complete, the entire clinical care program (including all 10 ambulatory care parameters and their related aspects of care) is reviewed.

II. MECHANISM FOR OVERSEEING QA PROGRAM EFFECTIVENESS
   A. Computer Tracking and Referral to Higher Authority
      1. The QIP system
         All new QIPs are entered into the computer for tracking. On a monthly basis the Quality Assurance Program Committee secretary generates a computerized list of QIPs and their status—complete, incomplete, director's QIP, and governing body QIP. This list is distributed to the quality assurance program coordinator, the chief of clinics staff, and the president of the College (or his or her designee).

A QIP that has not been resolved 3 months past its target date automatically becomes a director's QIP. The chief of clinics staff is given 1 year to resolve the QIP.

A QIP that is not solved at the director's QIP level in 1 year automatically becomes a governing body QIP. The president (or his or her designee) then makes the ultimate decision regarding what will be done in relationship to that particular QIP.

2. QIP resolution

Only the QA committee is authorized to declare that a QIP has been resolved. This is done by collecting data subsequent to the changes implemented as a result of the QIP and rescoring the indicator related to the QIP.

3. QIP cancellation

Only the president (or his or her designee) has the authority to determine that a QIP will not be resolved. The president (or his or her designee) may rely on the recommendation from the QMG and may choose to leave the QIP unresolved, change the QIP level, change the standard for that particular indicator, or delete the indicator from the AmbuQual Quality Assurance Program.

B. Report to the College administration

On a quarterly basis, the chief of clinics staff reports to the president (or his or her designee) regarding the level of quality in the National College Chiropractic Clinics. The report includes current scores for the performance quality index (PQI) and the 10 parameters, as well as the current status of all outstanding QIPs.

C. Annual Program Review

Annually, a review of the effectiveness of The National College Chiropractic Clinics QA program will be accomplished. The chief of clinics staff will ensure that the review is accomplished. The review will be done by seeking input from QA committee members, the QMG, other staff members, and the College administration.

The results of the annual quality assurance program review will be submitted to the president (or his or her designee).

III. CONFIDENTIALITY

A. Activity Reporting

All departmental quality assurance activities will be reported to the QA committee. The minutes of the QA committee meetings will reflect such reports. Departmental reports will be secured in each department with a copy in the Quality Assurance Program coordinator's office.

B. Access to QA Data

QA data and reports will be accessible only to those participating in the QA program and those bodies responsible for ascertaining the existence of an ongoing and effective QA program. Individual elements related to resolving an identified problem may be disclosed to individuals who need to know to resolve it. Those individuals are bound by the appropriate requirements of confidentiality.

C. Information Requests
All quality assurance information is exempt from public access. Any requests for quality assurance information from attorneys, health insurance companies, patients or their families, or consumer groups must be submitted in writing to the chief of clinics staff, who will then issue an appropriate denial.

D. Subpoena Exemption
In general, quality assurance records are exempt from subpoena, are never released outside the authorized channels of the clinics, and are not included in any way in the patients' medical records.

IV. RETENTION OF RECORDS

A. Minutes of Meetings
All transcribed minutes of meetings will be kept permanently either in their original form or on microfilm.

B. Departmental Activity Reports
Quality assurance activity reports, as submitted to the QA committee, will be kept for 3 years from the date of the annual report they are incorporated into, either in their original form or on microfilm.

C. Monthly QA Reports
Monthly reports from the QA committee, as well as completed worksheets, will be retained for 3 years from the date of the annual report they are incorporated into, either in their original form or on microfilm.

D. Practice Profiles
Profiles of practice generated from quality assurance activities will be kept permanently, either in their original form or on microfilm.

Appendix 2*

Procedure: Physician Performance Audit

PURPOSE

The purpose of the physician performance audit is to evaluate and monitor the clinical performance of the practitioners.

DESCRIPTION

I. Chart selection
   A. The medical records department shall select every 100th consecutive chart for each practitioner to be audited.
   B. Charts should be selected for audit as they are returned to the department after the patient's visit. The quality assurance (QA) coordinator may specify certain charts that are to be included in the audit.
   C. Each practitioner will be assigned to audit one other practitioner for 2-month periods.
   D. The QA coordinator will be responsible for generating a rotation schedule for the auditors.
   E. The medical records department will complete the top sections of the audit form and feedback form, indicating the clinic, chart number, date of visit, and practitioner.
   F. The audit forms will be forwarded in an interoffice mailing envelope to the person currently auditing that practitioner.

II. Chart audit procedure
   A. It is the responsibility of the auditor to complete the chart audit within 5 working days after receiving the audit forms. Auditors who must travel to another site may choose to perform all audits for a 1-month period at one time but no later than 5 days after the month has expired.
   B. The auditor will request the medical records department to pull the charts for audit. If more than five charts are to be audited at one time, the records department should be given 24 hours advance notice.
   C. The chart should be audited for both the index visit and a general review for the past 12 months using the performance audit criteria.

---

*Adapted from The National College Chiropractic Clinics, Lombard, Ill.

D. Each question on the audit form should be answered as follows:
   1. If a deficiency/question of care is found, the auditor should check "NO." A brief explanation should be listed in the "comments" area.
   2. If the chart is in compliance, the "yes" should be checked.
   3. If the question is not applicable to the visit or general review, "NA" should be checked.

III. Audit feedback
   A. After completion of the audit form, the auditor will complete the first section of the practitioner performance audit feedback form.
      1. If there are no deficiencies/questions about care, check the appropriate line.
      2. If there are deficiencies/questions about care, check the appropriate line and enter the numbers of the questions involved.
      3. The auditor will return the chart and audit forms to medical records.
      4. Medical records will forward the top copy of the audit form to the QA coordinator. The other copies of the audit form and the feedback form are to be forwarded to the practitioner who was audited using an interoffice mailing envelope.
   B. The practitioner who was audited will review the audit results within 2 working days.
      1. If the practitioner agrees with the deficiency/question about care, he or she should check the line for "agree should improve."
      2. If the practitioner disagrees with the auditor, he or she should check "disagree" and enter the appropriate numbers and the reason for disagreement.
      3. The practitioner should then sign on the appropriate line and enter the date.
      4. The audit form and the feedback form should be placed back in the interoffice mail envelope and sent to the QA coordinator.
   C. The QA coordinator will review the results of the audit.
      1. If there are no disagreements about the audit, the results are recorded. One copy of the audit form should be returned to the practitioner who was audited.
      2. If there has been a disagreement, the results in question are not recorded. The audit forms will be forwarded to the practitioner's clinic director for review.
   D. The clinic director will review any disagreements.
      1. If the clinic director finds no deficiencies/questions about care, he or she should check the appropriate line on the feedback form. The forms are then returned to the QA coordinator, who will record the results.
      2. If the clinic director also has questions about care, the appropriate line should be checked, and the chart should be taken to the clinical staff.
   E. Questions about care by both the auditor and the clinic director

should be reviewed by the clinical provider staff at monthly meetings.
1. The practitioner who has been audited should be kept anonymous, if possible.
2. The questions about care and reasons for disagreement should be presented to the staff by the clinic director.
3. At the end of the discussion, the clinic director should ask for a vote by the practitioners on each disputed question to determine either "agree should improve" or "no questions about care."
4. The clinic director should then sign on the appropriate line on the feedback form and enter the date.
5. The audit forms should then be returned to the QA coordinator and the chart returned to medical records.
F. The QA coordinator will review the action taken by the clinical provider staff.
1. The results from the audit will be recorded.
2. One copy of the completed audit form will be returned to the practitioner who was audited.
IV. Audit statistics
A. The QA coordinator will keep statistics on the audit as follows:
1. Number "yes," "no," and "NA," and percent of compliance for each audit question. (# yes / (# yes + # no)) × 100% = percent compliance
a. Total for all clinics
b. Individual claims
c. Each physician
2. Statistics are to be compiled quarterly for each location.
3. Statistics are to include year-to-date (last 12 months) and most recent quarter.
B. The statistical summary will be sent to each provider quarterly and will be reviewed at a physician staff meeting each quarter.

Appendix 3*

"Give Us A Grade" Patient Satisfaction Audit Questions*

The facility
   Card 1. Give us a grade for
        Clean building
        Easy to find where to go
        Rooms neat, picked up
        Comfort while here

The appointment process
   Card 2. Give us a grade for
        Getting an appointment to see the doctor
        How nice the appointment people were

Waiting time
   Card 3. Give us a grade on your wait after you got here
        In the waiting room
        In the examination/treatment room

The fiscal process
   Card 4. Give us a grade on
        What you pay to see the doctor
        How clear the bill is
        The way we collect money

Satisfaction with staff
   Card 5. Give the *doctor* in charge of your care a grade on
        Understanding what you said
        Taking enough time with you
        Telling you what you needed to know
        Being careful and helpful
   Card 6. Give the *intern* assisting with your care a grade on
        Understanding what you said
        Taking enough time with you
        Telling you what you needed to know
        Being careful and helpful

---

*From The National College Chiropractic Clinics, Lombard, Ill. Used by permission.

Card 7. Give our *receptionist* a grade on
  Understanding what you said
  Taking enough time with you
  Telling you what you needed to know
  Being careful and helpful
Card 8. Give our *cashier* a grade on
  Understanding what you said
  Taking enough time with you
  Telling you what you needed to know
  Being careful and helpful
Card 9. Give us a grade on how well your privacy was respected

Satisfaction with health outcome
Card 10. Give us a grade on how much better your health is after you come to the Health Center

Participation in development of health care plan
Card 11. Give our doctor and staff grades for
  Listening to you
  Using your ideas
  Taking your way of living into plans for your health

Patient education activity
Card 12. Give us a grade for teaching you about your treatment
  Why it is necessary
  What to expect from it
  Give us a grade for teaching you about new things to do at home to help your health (things like using ice, exercise and special diets)
Card 13. Give us a grade for
  Teaching you about how to take care of your health
  How helpful the handouts are in understanding your health condition
Card 14. Give us a grade for how well our doctor or intern taught you
  About your condition
  What to do for better health

Patient concerns understood by physician
Card 15. Give us a grade on how well the doctor understood you

Patient compliance
Card 16. Give *yourself* a grade for
  Doing what the doctor and intern told you to do the last time you were here
  Coming back when the doctor told you
Card 17. Has the doctor told you to change any of your health habits (like smoking, drinking, exercise, diet, cancer check, safety or other)?
  If yes, give yourself a grade for how well you are doing.

Trust in health care staff
Card 18. Give us a grade for how easy it is to tell the doctor things that are hard to talk about.
Card 19. Give us a grade to show how much you feel the staff cares about you and your health.

Grade 20. Give us a grade to show how much you feel you can trust the staff (not counting the doctor).

Card 21. Give us a grade on how much you feel you can trust your doctor.

New patients

Card 22. Were you given a new patient brochure today?

If you were very sick or in much pain when you called to make an appointment, were you offered an appointment within 24 hours?

If you needed an appointment for regular health care, were you offered an appointment within 7 days?

Access to care

Card 23. Answer one of the following questions:

If you were very sick or in much pain when you called to make an appointment, were you offered an appointment within 24 hours?

If you came in for regular health care, were you offered an appointment within 3 days?

Card 24. Give us a grade for

When you need to reach the doctor, how easy is it for you to talk with him or her on the day you call?

Card 25. Give us a grade for

How easy is it to reach a staff doctor any time of the day or night when someone is sick or hurt?

Or check one

____never tried ____did not know I could

Card 26. How did you get to the health center? (circle one)

Bus
Walk
Your car
Friend's car
Cab
Other

Give us a grade for how easy it is for you to get to the health center

Card 27. How did you first hear about the health center? (circle one)

Family   Television
Friend   Yellow pages
Newspaper   Outreach
Poster   Radio
Other_____

Availability

Card 28. Give us a grade on how well you like the clinic hours

Assessing Clinical Research Material: The Clinician's Role and Responsibility

Marion McGregor, B.Sc., D.C., F.C.C.S.(C), M.Sc.
Research Consultant, Private Practice, Richardson, Texas

THE CASE

Mrs. B.T. is a 42-year-old laborer who hurt her back while lifting her 18-kg daughter 6 months ago. She has not returned to work since her injury. She has come to you complaining of a dull ache in her low back. On examination you find tenderness to palpation in the left paraspinal region between L-1 and L-4. You treat Mrs. B.T. three times per week for 2 weeks using spinal manipulation/adjustments to the areas of concern and apply ultrasound and low-volt stimulation as needed. She reports that at the end of 2 weeks she feels temporarily better after each treatment but is in her usual pain state by the next day. On the basis of the relief she has received to date, you continue your treatment for another 10 weeks. At that time an independent medical examination (IME) is requested by her insurance company. The independent examiner denies benefits for the past 6 weeks of treatment, and the insurance company requires Mrs. B.T. to seek care at a rehabilitation center. Mrs. B.T. acknowledges that her relief through your treatment was only temporary and follows the insurance company's directions. She refuses to pay her bill to you, stating that she was only doing as she was told in the belief that her insurance company agreed with your treatment plan. You have lost the patient and potentially the monies owed from the last 18 office visits.

The patient is described by the independent examiner as chronic. She acknowledges that the patient had never had chiropractic care and allows the initial 2 weeks of this alternative passive care. Noting some temporary improvement, she also allows for the second 2 weeks as a trial for continued improvement. She states, however, that at that time you should have realized that the patient's temporary relief from chiropractic manipulations/adjustments was unchanged and that the patient had reached maximum therapeutic benefit. The change then, should have been made from passive to active care. You strongly disagree with the examiner, having had patients like Mrs. B.T. who have been successfully cared for by your procedures before. You want to know the basis of the IME report.

On inquiring, you are informed that the IME physician based her report on the scientific clinical literature in the area, as well as clinical judgment. You ask to see the scientific literature[1,2] that formed the basis of the IME physician's judgment.

You are familiar with the first reference,[1] and recall that it stated that in chronic low back cases, more than 70% were helped by manipulation. You are unfamiliar with the second[2] but have a hard time understanding how these two papers could be used to formulate the decision that has been made.

In the indemnity, casualty, and preventive care market of the past, this would have been an unusual circumstance for the clinician. Questions regarding physician care of patients were rarer. Independently practicing doctors in all health care disciplines were considered the single best authorities on their own patients. The changes in health care policy within even the last 10 years have been significant and confusing to many providers. To some, it appears that the shift has moved from the physician as the authority to the insurer as the authority.

The changes have come about for two reasons. The first is the great concern today regarding cost-effective health care.[3,4] The second is the advancement and popularity of clinical research methods as tools for understanding "appropriate" and "useful" health care.[5-7] Politicians and policy makers have been drawn to the scientific literature to find an approach that may be ethically pleasing in providing cost-effective, high-quality patient care.

This overall shift in the health care paradigm has been referred to as "evidence-based medicine."[6] Although the term "medicine" is used, it nonetheless impacts all of health care delivery. The term for the clinician essentially means using the available clinical science literature to update decision making for alternatives in patient care. It is no longer reasonable to rely on what was taught or observed during chiropractic college training. How then, will you as a chiropractor be able to work effectively within the newly emerging evidence-based health care paradigm? Suddenly important is the acquisition of a skill never required before: appraising the value of clinical literature.

Not long ago, a colleague[8] conducted an informal survey to determine how six of his chiropractic peers might react to being asked to assess a piece of clinical chiropractic literature. The following quote from one of those polled seems to speak for many field doctors:

> In all honesty, as much as I might want to use the tables to correlate the reading material, they are not "user friendly" and I do not have the time to go back and forth in order to validate the article. . . . I would rather have the article explained and critiqued for me.

THE PAST

In the past, clinicians of all kinds have relied on others to tell them what the scientific literature says. As noted in the previous quote, the reasons have included lack of time for sorting out the details of a given study, a concern for his or her ability to appropriately assess research, and feeling overwhelmed by the tremendous amounts of information that come from the journals each month.

Lack of time is a common and reasonable concern for busy practitioners who would rather leave their reading to someone else. That "someone else" has generally been entrusted with providing the short version of lengthy and complex original research reports. Often that someone else is one of three common sources in private practice: colleagues, product information (sales representatives and mail), and textbooks.

COLLEAGUES

Informal collegial contact is an important source of information used by everyone. A colleague may provide news regarding meetings he or she has attended or provide additional information about a difficult patient case. Various professional peers will have read research information and may be excited to share what they have read. If that information is to be useful, the reliability of the source must be known.

In the same study undertaken to determine the response of a sample of field practitioners to appraising literature, the six practitioners were asked to read an article dealing with sudden infant death syndrome (SIDS)[9] and write down their impressions. Three of their responses are provided:

> 1. At that rate, the atlas inversion and proving of such a theory certainly solidifies, and could be a major contributing factor in acceptance of examining infants shortly after birth for the vertebral subluxation complex.
> 2. The concept of atlas inversion frightened me as a practicing manipulator from a malpractice standpoint, since I do not know many fellow chiropractors, myself included, who routinely x-ray for "atlas inversion." How many SIDS deaths might be caused by inappropriate upper cervical manipulations to correct the so-called "birth canal trauma subluxation"?
> 3. The conclusion it draws [that SIDS may be due to a misalignment of the atlas], I'm sure would get any chiropractor excited. But we must realize that this study also says that SIDS is associated with *hypermobility* which is *not* a chiropractically treatable condition, and in fact could indicate that chiropractic would be contraindicated here.

The interpretations depicted here are so diverse that a clinician would receive an extremely different perspective of this paper dependent on who of his or her colleagues actually read it. Further, all three of the quotes assumed that the results of this study could reflect on experience in his or her own practice situations. It may be pertinent at this time, however, to mention that this was a cadaver study, fraught with all of the expected difficulties in trying to conclude anything about real life clinical practice.

A list of the comments provided by four of the six practitioners when asked about the sample size in the study they read follows*:

1. "Views were performed on *74 infants* following death, 50 of which met the criteria."

---

*Note: Emphasis has been added.

2. "You can't just have 58 *patients* in a study."
3. "Small *(n = 46)* subject number tends to weaken the significance."
4. "*Seventeen patients* is not enough for objective research."

The process of allowing colleagues to do your reading for you is obviously problematic. The conclusions drawn may be inappropriate and lead to change in practice behavior, where the information does not substantiate it. As in the case just discussed, even the "facts" of a research article may be misread. It behooves the practitioner to formulate his or her own judgment when provided with scientific clinical evidence or risk-making decisions based, in part, on hearsay.

PRODUCT INFORMATION

Almost every practitioner can relate to the amount of unsolicited product-related information that comes into the office each week. Sometimes the information comes in the mail, and sometimes the "detail" sales representatives come to the office to discuss their products. Claims such as "scientifically based" or "research shows" are important statements used to assure the clinician that the product they are being asked to buy and sometimes sell to their patients are valuable and do what is claimed. How reliable is this information? As with any industry, the reliability of the statements made can be extremely variable.

Take, for example, a piece of promotional material that came to my office a few years ago. The ad discussed garlic supplementation. The manufacturer, among other claims, stated that garlic was related to "reduction of total serum lipids and specific in LDL [low density lipoprotein] VLDL's [very low density lipoprotein's] while increasing the beneficial HDL's" [high-density lipoprotein's] and recommended a dosage of "1–3 tablets with meals" with a tablet strength of "400 mg raw garlic concentrate." Intrigued by the possibility and having heard favorable things about garlic before, I considered the claim.

Anticipating a purchase, most manufacturers are more than willing to provide you with the clinical scientific references that are used for their advertisements. If they are not willing or able to supply these, the busy clinician should be wary of further consideration of the claims being made. In the previous case, happily, there was already a reference number beside the statement. Although the actual reference had not been supplied, a call to the manufacturer yielded the source.

The reference related to an article in the journal *Atherosclerosis* from 1981 entitled "The Effect of Fried Versus Raw Garlic on Fibrinolytic Activity in Man." Although I was surprised that the title did not relate directly to HDL, LDL, and VLDL, another part of the ad did state "increases fibrinolytic activity," so I decided to read the article. Several things of interest were quickly apparent.

First, the journal had listed this article as a "preliminary note," indicating that the research was in its infancy. Although potentially valuable to a researcher, it was perhaps not valuable to the clinician. In fact, in the two experiments listed, the sample size was quite small, with 10 subjects in each receiving raw garlic. Next, it was found that the article was written by members of a medical college in India. Although the article did not specify, it can be assumed that the patients used in the study were also from India. There was no discussion regarding the potential similarity between the dietary habits of the patients used in this study compared with those in North America and what impact the interaction between current diet and the additional administration of garlic might have. Finally, in the methods section, the authors stated that the garlic was provided at doses of 0.5 g/kg of body weight. For a 74.91-kg man, that would mean that 74.91 kg × 500 mg/kg = 37,455 mg of garlic were provided at least daily to each subject during the study period! (The article states that patients were given the garlic "during meals" for the second experiment but does not specify how many meals.) Relating that back to the original ad, that would mean that clinic patients would have to take 37,455 mg/ 400 mg = 93.64, or about 94 of the manufacturer's tablets per day to mimic the minimum experimental dose!

When making a decision that may affect your practice overhead (e.g., buying new equipment or maintaining inventory) or your therapeutic recommendations to patients, the source of claims such as "scientifically proven" supporting anything you are seriously considering should not be left for others to assess.

TEXTBOOKS

Having spoken to professionals in past years about where they primarily retrieve information they find useful, another common response is the textbook. However, compiling literature for textbooks can be a complicated business, and errors, even by those with the best of intentions, occur regardless. An example of such an error, for which an erratum has since been requested, occurred a few years ago. A line in a chapter of a textbook[11] read as follows:

> Dabert, Freeman, and Weis commented that the incidence of hemmorhage complications of spinal adjustments on patients receiving anticoagulation therapy varies from 3.5% to 48%.[20]

In this case, careful reading would have helped the judicious reader determine that a misprint may have occurred. The range of values "3.5% to 48%" implies more than one study having been conducted for the relationship between spinal adjustments and anticoagulation therapy. Given a widespread concern for rare but important complications to manipulation, it would be surprising if a body of studies implying this particular problem were not more substantially well known. Reference 20 in the text turned out to be a case report contained in a letter to the editor.[12] In the comment section, the actual statement relating to the textbook quote read, "The incidence of hemorrhagic complications from anticoagulation therapy varies from 3.5% to 48%."

Although the sensible practitioner will always use the facts in the case history to define careful and safe treatment, it is clear that the error, relating manipulation/adjustment to all complications from anticoagulation therapy, overstates the problem. The difference is even more compelling when considered as evidence, for example, in a malpractice case. The practitioner who understands and uses original source literature correctly is in a much better position to make clear and appropriate decisions for his or her patient than the one who relies on second-hand information.

Feeling "overwhelmed," however, is common, especially in light of the prospect of having to find and read all original research material published monthly in one's field of interest. It is a dilemma shared by every health discipline and deservedly so. In a study conducted in 1989, a chiropractic college library was checked for the amount of reading material that would have to be consumed for a practitioner to keep up with all of the information available to him or her each month that was considered pertinent to chiropractic. A random sample of 10 out of 400 journals contained in the library was searched for the number of editorials, reports, papers, letters, and chapters. On average, there were 14.4 pieces of literature to be consumed per journal. If we extrapolate from this, if a clinician were actually trying to keep up with all of the journal literature considered important by a chiropractic college library (remembering that this is limited by topic matter) and that clinician were completely caught up at the current time, and he or she read one article per day for one year, the same clinician would be almost 1 century behind in his or her reading at the end of that year.[13]

The information pool has not gotten smaller. If anything, it has increased. Articles pertinent to chiropractic are found in a huge variety of clinical journals, both within and outside of the profession.

Further, a tremendous number of chiropractic professionals feel uneducated in the skills required to efficiently and effectively read research to find what is useful and be able to discard the rest. Students, anxious to become clinicians, have considered courses in research subordinate to their goals for practice. Now, as evidence-based care begins to affect individual practices, research is no longer one more technical hurdle to jump. Rather, it is a component of the busy clinician's daily life. Clinical science articles are used to make decisions for the appropriateness of care, if not by the practitioner, then by outside agencies that have the ability to impact the physician's practice.

THE PRESENT

To become efficient at reading clinical scientific literature without becoming overwhelmed, one must collect and process certain key pieces of information. Although relatively basic, they are nonetheless vital to triage what should be read from what can be read. In the triage process the following steps are taken:

1. Defining the reading purpose and finding the source most likely to satisfy the purpose
2. Separating fact from opinion
3. Appraising the applicability of information from the facts

DEFINING THE READING PURPOSE AND FINDING A SOURCE

Because it is virtually impossible to keep up with all of the clinical literature available, it is important that the practitioner have a clear understanding of his or her purpose in reading. There are essentially two major objectives to resourcing information.

The first objective is to search out news, such as practice opportunities; conference and seminar topics, times, and locations; ideas and thoughts on practice management type of procedures; and information regarding the activities of various members of the profession. Although some of these data may be found in clinical science journals, for the most part, trade magazines and newspapers fulfill this role.

The second objective is to search for information on patient care. This may relate to a potential change in treatment that either the clinician or an outside agency is considering, the value of a diagnostic test, or an expectation of patient outcome. Such information is found in peer-reviewed clinical scientific journals. These journals have an editorial board whose members' names and sometimes credentials are published. It is to a subset of the editorial board that every original research article is submitted for peer review. Also published in peer-reviewed journals is a set of instructions to authors. Authors are usually requested to send a number of copies of their work in a particular and structured format to the chief editor. The number of copies required is usually related to the number of members of the peer review team that can be expected to read the submitted manuscript.

The peer review process, although admittedly imperfect,[14-16] is currently the best vehicle available to assure some baseline clinical-scientific standard that can be expected from what is read. The notion is based on the assumption that a consensus of peers, knowledgeable in the clinical discipline and its scientific foundations, judging the clarity and viability of the work done, will minimize the reporting of spurious or frivolous opinion. This is dependent, of course, on the standards of the journal and the quality of the editorial board itself. A quick look at the members of the board and a survey of a few articles that survived their review usually suffice in providing material from which an appropriate judgment of the journal can be made.

In addition to peer review, a journal may be indexed. The indexing of a journal is extremely important, because it means that the title, author or authors, journal volume, date, and pages of each article it contains will be listed so that a reader can find a publication without having to go through journal after journal in search of his or her areas of interest. Typically articles are indexed by both subject and author. This means, of course, that if the reader is interested only in treatments for "chronic low back pain" as might pertain to Mrs. B.T. or remembers an article of importance but knows only the author, he or she would not have to turn pages aimlessly or go through the year-end indexes of multiple journals that might contain the research of concern. Rather, a search of the index would pick up only those references likely to be wanted, and the reader could go directly to the source. Each indexing system has a set of criteria by which it judges those journals (and sometimes other materials) it is willing to include. One of the most famous indexing systems is *Index Medicus*. It includes a huge array of journals that have met its particular (and stringent) standards. It can be accessed both by hand, in the form of searching its published lists of articles, and by computer, directly and through various services. A local medical science librarian can be very helpful in aiding the practitioner to access the information it contains.

An indexing system currently dedicated to what will be of interest to chiropractic is a system called CHIROLARS. This is a computer-based index that the practitioner can subscribe to, to search topics that are likely to be relevant, in particular, to chiropractic.

It is rare that a clinician will have time to sit down and read any journal from cover to cover. Further, much of what is in a journal for any given month may not be of value for the practitioner or his or her patient. Subscriptions to journals therefore are typically based on a relatively consistent high yield of quality articles of interest per issue. However, even journals that can be expected to consistently yield a good number of articles pertinent to the clinician's needs will also contain publications that are not useful. It is the reader's job to sort out what is useful from what is not. Many journal editors are kind enough to label their contents in such a way as to help the reader decide whether an article is applicable to the reader's current practice situation. Publications listed as "pilot studies" and "preliminary reports," for example, are research papers discussing early work that requires further validation before the practical clinical merit can be determined. The reader, however, is ultimately responsible for judging the practical value of what he or she has read. Happily, there are criteria, which will be discussed later, that help the busy clinician make appropriate use of what is available.

SEPARATING FACT FROM OPINION

The first step in judging the practical value of what might be read is to separate fact from opinion. Because most readers are quite capable of formulating their own opinions, facts should be found and read first. Additional opinions by the author of the article and others may be of interest and provide an alternative perspective, time permitting.

For many busy readers, the abstract of a research article (in some circles this is referred to as the summary) is a great source from which to decide how useful the research will be. With the advent of structured abstracts (where specific information is required under specific headings), the reader's job is made substantially easier. In this case, important facts are easily found and highlighted. Unfortunately, structured abstracts are not always used. Where they are not, the material contained is largely up to the author. A wonderful example of how different perspectives of a single study can be abstracted is provided by the following. All three quotes are from abstracts of the same study, published in different journals:

1. "Manual therapy showed a faster and larger improvement in physical functioning compared to the other three therapies."[17]
2. "Difference in effectiveness between physiotherapy and manual therapy could not be shown. A substantial part of the effect of manual therapy and physiotherapy appeared to be due to nonspecific (placebo) effects."[18]
3. "Improvement in the main complaint was larger with manipulative therapy (4.5) than with physiotherapy (3.8) after 12 months' follow up (difference 0.9; 95% confidence interval 0.1 to 1.7). Manipulative therapy also gave larger improvements in physical functioning (difference 0.6; −0.1 to 1.3)."[19]

Although this information appears discouragingly disparate, none of the versions of text is necessarily inaccurate. The resolution of this dilemma is an understanding of the difference between fact and opinion. The numbers obtained as results can typically be considered facts. The interpretation of their meaning, although usually based on statistical criteria, is generally an expression of an opinion based on the facts.

The abstract provides the reader with what the author believes is pertinent information to the study. It provides an understanding of the purpose of the research and may provide some facts, such as numerical results. If, however, the reader relies only on the abstract for his or her impression of the contents of the article, he or she abdicates his or her opinion in favor of the author's. As noted earlier, even from the same study, authors can view various aspects of their work differently. The reader's impression should, at least initially, be created by the facts alone.

Where then, are the facts? Virtually all research articles are partitioned into sections: the *introduction, methods, results,* and *discussion.* The introduction lays the foundation for the work that has been done, and the discussion is the author's or authors' perspective of the results. The material used to shape both the introduction and the discussion are at the discretion of the author or authors involved. As such, most of the information contained in these sections can be considered opinion. To the extent that they are realistically available, the facts for a given clinical research article are contained in the methods and results sections.

APPRAISING THE APPLICABILITY OF THE INFORMATION FROM THE FACTS

It is the material in the methods and results sections of a publication that must be used to judge value and applicability to practice. It is also this material that a great number of consumers of clinical literature have avoided as being too complicated and too cumbersome. Understanding how to read clinical science literature has become more and more immediately important to practice, with the establishment of practice guidelines and the popularity of IMEs. These previously underread sections in literature have been significantly elevated in value. Thus, the field clinician is now required to understand the skills of assessing them. Happily and contrary to popular belief, these skills are actually based more on common sense than anything else. With a little understanding of the nomenclature and a critical eye, obvious difficulties in research articles become readily apparent.

To begin, the methods and results section of the clinical scientific paper essentially has the following overall structure:

1. Population
2. Sample
3. Initial assessment
4. Time/treatment
5. Final assessment
6. Analysis

Discussion of the relevant things to look for will be limited to articles dealing with the efficacy and effectiveness of treatment. Due to the scope that can effectively be covered in a single chapter, this appraisal procedure is further limited to only features thought to be the most significant of the many issues that could be addressed within the given structure. Although not meant to be exhaustive, it is intended to help the reader to see some of the important elements and potential problems within clinical science articles that he or she might select to read. To obtain more detail regarding this topic and appraise others such as diagnosis and prognosis, the reader can be directed to a host of books, two of which are included in the reference list.[5, 7]

Population
This is the group to whom the study is attempting to generalize. The population may be as broad as "all people on earth" or may be limited to, for example, "all male workers' compensation claimants between the ages of 25 and 45 who have had low back pain of 6 months' to 20 years' duration and also have leg pain but whose leg pain is not neurological in nature." The population is usually not stated. The information about the population is gathered from the available description of the sample.

Sample
The sample is the group of patients (in research they are called "subjects") who are actually in the study. The limitations on who is allowed in the study are referred to as the "inclusion and exclusion criteria." These limitations also define the population to which the study may be generalized. The reading clinician's patient would be considered a potential member of the population. The clinician's task is to assess whether his or her patient's characteristics actually match those of the people used in the study. An example of where the characteristics may differ was discussed earlier with respect to the application of the "garlic" article.[10] In that experiment subjects with dietary habits potentially significantly different from those in North America were given huge quantities of raw and fried garlic, and fibrolytic affects were observed. The applicability of giving garlic tablets to a North American patient without consideration of the dietary differences must be seriously questioned.

Beyond the characteristics of the sample patients, two more things may be worth looking for when one is reading this part of the methods section. The first is how the sample was drawn. This is basically to find out how they collected people to come into the study. Were they all volunteers? Volunteers may be more enthusiastic participants than average patients. The results of a study could end up reflecting the enthusiasm and motivation of the volunteers more than an actual treatment result; in trying to generalize to your patient, the results in your office may not be as good.

The best way to collect people for study is by using a "random draw." Technically this means that every patient in the population from which the sample is taken has a mathematically equal chance of being selected to participate. If the population is "the whole world" or even "all North Americans with chronic LBP of 6 months' duration whose leg pain is not neurological in nature," obtaining a random draw is clearly unfeasible.

As a result, samples are typically drawn in a more haphazard manner from available patients in available study clinics. Again, what is most important is that the members of the sample actually appear to represent the patient you are thinking about applying the information to.

Another key as to whether the sample is fair is an understanding of how many patients who were asked to participate actually agreed to do so. If only 10% asked actually said yes to being part of the sample, that 10% may have unique characteristics that make them different from the typical office patient you see. It is equally helpful to look at the numbers of patients who finished the study. It is typical to hope that 80% of those who started in the sample actually made it all the way to the end of the trial. If a large proportion of subjects left part way through, the study procedures, for example, may have been uncomfortable for them, and your patients may not wish to engage in the therapeutic or diagnostic procedures either. Also, if too many subjects drop out of the study, just as if too few enter, or if they all are volunteers, the sample of patients remaining is less likely to represent the population (or your patient) well. This can occur, for example, when a disorder (e.g., low back pain) is found in a wide range of age groups. If at the completion of the study most of the elderly patients dropped out and only the young remained, the study is unlikely to be applicable to your 75-year-old patient.

Initial Assessment

Every clinical research study, regardless of purpose, does some kind of baseline estimate of both patient characteristics (defining the sample as mentioned earlier), and *outcome measures*. Outcome measures are simply clinical tools used to determine the success or failure of treatment. In an article that discusses a particular therapy, an outcome measure may be something like "perceived pain by the patient." That is, on the initial assessment, before anything is done, the researcher would measure the amount of pain the patient was in. A typical way of doing this is with the visual analogue scale. This is simply a 100-mm line on which the patient marks an X to indicate how much pain he or she is currently in.[20] Clearly if one is trying to determine the therapeutic benefit of treatment, knowing how much pain a patient is in before as opposed to after treatment is important.

One must consider a few things when appraising this part of the methods. The most important is that the outcome measures are valid. Validity simply means that it measures what it actually intends to measure. Although it may be beyond the intent of most readers to search through yet more literature to find out if the outcome measures used in a study are valid, much can be gleened by simply looking at what those measures are. For example, a visual analogue scale may not measure pain itself and would therefore not be considered a valid measure of pain, but it certainly seems to measure *perceived* pain. For perceived pain the visual analogue scale would be considered to have validity.

Another illustration of what might be considered when one is evaluating the validity of the initial assessment is provided by a look at an article published not too long ago dealing with change in lumbar disk herniation fragment size with conservative treatment.[21] One outcome measure was "disk fragment size." For the initial assessment, the researchers chose to use diagnostic computed tomography (CT) scans to get a good view of the disk. Clearly this is reasonable. Unfortunately, the authors did not specify just how the measurements were made. Is this important?

Consider, for a moment, the alternatives. A pencil and ruler could have been used to measure length and width, but disk fragments do not typically occur in well-defined geometrical shapes. Any area measurement would be fraught with problems. One of the best ways to measure this outcome might be volumetric. This requires specific information on the views taken. Because the procedures used were not mentioned in the text, it is difficult for the reader to be assured that the assessment tool was valid.

This example also relates well to the second issue for this portion of the methods section, that is, the reliability of the outcome measurement. Authors of articles should provide the reader with a sense of the qualifications of study personnel involved, as well as the reliability of different qualified personnel in measuring outcomes. Reliability here is simply the assurance that different assessors will find the same result, given the same clinical situation. With respect to the example, neither the study personnel and their qualifications nor any assurance that the measurement of disk fragment size was reliable was provided.

If the initial assessment tools (outcome measures) have not been shown to be reliable and valid, the reader has no basis for believing that a change as a result of therapy really exists. To observe change (the success of treatment), one requires a clear baseline of stable measures that make sense.

Time and Treatment

In technical terms, time and treatment are considered the *intervention*. The means by which the intervention is provided in a study of treatments gives a good indication of the strength of the study design.

The first consideration is the temporal (time) direction of the study. The researcher will be taking either a *prospective* look at a treatment regimen or a *retrospective* look. Retrospective means that the researcher is looking back on his or her cases after already having completed treatment. Contrary to the belief that "hindsight is 20/20," retrospective studies are considered to provide the weakest possible evidence for how valuable a treatment might be. The reason is that when we as clinicians look back on our work with patients, we can rationalize a multitude of reasons for any given outcome. It is easy to build a case for our favorite belief, true or not, given the outcome of the case and a whole case file full of data to select from. Case reports are typically considered retrospective. There is a prospective form of case report, called an "N of 1" study, that is, where a single patient, with a relatively stable condition, who consents to be studied, is alternately provided and withdrawn from treatment, which if well designed, can provide more useful information than the usual case report.[7]

Prospective investigations are considered to yield much better quality evidence. In these, the researcher begins with his or her belief, then tests that belief and watches to see if it is supported by the clinical outcome (instead of, as stated earlier, supporting a belief with material that is already there). In other words, in prospective studies, experimental observation of the patient begins before that patient is given a treatment. The efficient consumer of clinical research publications is prudent to limit serious consideration to only those studies that are prospective in nature.

Having determined whether the clinical investigation was prospective or retrospective and eliminating (for the sake of time and value of information) the retrospective ones, the reader must address another issue: whether in the prospective study the patient chose his or her treatment or the researcher chose the treatment.

When the patient chooses the treatment he or she will undergo and this treatment is compared with either other treatments chosen by other patients or to patients who, in the same circumstances, have chosen no treatment at all, this is called a *cohort study*.[7] The name is less important than what is implied by the design. When a patient self-selects his or her care in a research project, the choice may be based on a factor outside of the researcher's control that may inadvertently bias the results. For example, if a researcher were to compare a well-publicized but expensive new treatment for ulcers with an older, conservative, less expensive standard, it may be that a larger proportion of patients who are economically well off choose the newer treatment. As a result of being more economically well off, those patients' overall health may be better than that of the poorer patients in the less expensive standard. The less expensive standard, then, may provide a less convincing treatment result, not because it is actually less effective but because the patients had more health problems to start with.

It is best, then, if the researcher chooses who goes into which treatment. Because the researcher already has a preconceived notion that he or she is testing, the method by which the choice is made must circumvent this bias. The best way to do this is by what is referred to as *random allocation*. Like random sampling, random allocation means that every patient has a mathematically equal opportunity of being placed in any of the treatment groups. Although it is possible still to accidentally have, as earlier, for example, a higher than expected proportion of well-off patients in one of the treatment groups (this is known technically as *failure of the randomization procedure*), especially if the overall sample size for the study is small, this method provides the greatest assurance that the groups will have roughly equal characteristics. A prospective investigation of treatment effects using random allocation of patients to more than one treatment group is called a *randomized clinical trial* (RCT). This kind of study provides the strongest, least biased, evidence available regarding comparatively how well a treatment might work.

Because randomized clinical trials are clearly the most effective form of clinical research methodology, why doesn't everyone just do those? The answer is threefold: feasibility, funding, and ethics. Any or all of these factors may result in a lesser quality study design being chosen.

Sometimes the degree of suspicion that a new treatment may be effective is simply not high enough to justify support of a large-scale RCT. That is the reason the literature contains pilot studies and preliminary reports. These are the works that researchers build on to support the need for an RCT. Also, RCTs are incredibly time and people intensive. To assure strong and unbiased procedures, a good research team is required to shepherd the project to produce useful results. This requires substantial funding, which is often extremely difficult to obtain. Even a relatively small randomized clinical trial may cost well into the hundreds of thousands of dollars to assure that the appropriate staff and facilities are available when necessary. Finally, there are times when a newer treatment (or the decision to have no treatment) may be suspected of resulting in harm to the patient. It would be unethical for a researcher to randomize patients to a group when harm might occur. Taking these issues into consideration, the reader should look for prospective investigations where the strongest ethical and feasible method of patient allocation has been used to assign patients to treatment groups.

Finally, it is important for the reader to know that clinical studies may address either *efficacy* or *effectiveness* of treatments tested. When a study looks at efficacy, it is looking for results under very controlled experimental conditions that may not apply to practice. There may be a treatment effect, but under the conditions of a regular office setting such as that of the reader's the effect may be much smaller or nonexistent. This is because the rigorous control of the research environment may not be generalizable to the real world, where patients may be uncompliant or have complicating factors that interfere with treatment success. Effectiveness studies, on the other hand, allow more typical practice circumstances to be included in the design. These are studies that will translate more easily to a typical practice environment. The reader, then, should be aware of which kind of study he or she is looking at and whether the same results can reasonably be expected in his or her own practice situation.

Final Assessment

The final assessment should simply be a repeat of the initial assessment, timed after the treatment or intervention has occurred. That is, the same reliable and valid outcome measures used to check the baseline status of the patient should be used again after treatment to see if the measures are now different. Although this seems intuitively obvious, this consistency of measurement does not always occur. An excellent example is the disk fragment size study that was discussed earlier.[21] The initial assessment was completed via CT scan. On follow-up, apparently, magnetic resonance imaging was used. Because no assurance was provided by the authors that the magnification factors and level of cut were actually comparable, the use of a different technology for the post–time measure is of serious concern in interpreting the results.

Analysis

For clinical research articles looking at treatment results, the analysis usually centers on a comparison of the change in patient status between groups. Usually the investigator and the reader are interested in whether treatment A improved patients more and faster than treatment B. A series of statistical tests might be used to assess this. Common tests include the t test (to search for differences between two groups of patients), analysis of variance (ANOVA) (for differences between more than two groups), and chi-square (to look for differences in category of outcome in different groups of patients). Usually the author will report which test was used, a number associated with the outcome of the test, and a *p value*. The p value is used to decide if the results of a study are *statistically significant* (see later discussion). If the p value is less than 0.05, the statistically assessed difference between groups is considered to be real. As more statistical tests are used on the same sample of subjects, the p value should be set at a more rigorous threshold (a smaller value, e.g., 0.01). A more thorough discussion of what to look for to determine if the statistics in a publication are appropriate is beyond the scope of this chapter. A handbook on statistics for the clinician (e.g., *PDQ Statistics*[22]) that explains the purpose of each test without including too cumbersome a look at the mathematics involved is recommended. What the reader can then do is look up the tests used in the research report and simply answer the question: Does this form of analysis make sense given the purpose of the research?

The clinician can also make good use of the descriptive data in the results section. Along with providing the results of statistical tests, most papers present average scores for before and after treatment or the average difference for an outcome measure between the initial and final assessment. The reader can then judge if a *clinically meaningful* change has occurred. For example, let us say that a test of outcome in a particular study is a change in the straight leg raise test. If the average initial score for a group of patients was 35 degrees and on final assessment the average was 38 degrees, most clinicians would probably agree that a clinically meaningful change had not occurred. Given a large number of subjects in the study and a relatively small range of results, a change of this magnitude might be *statistically significant*, but such a change, although perhaps real, is unlikely to matter much to the patient. It is thus clinically irrelevant. If, on the other hand, the initial assessment provided an average of 35 degrees and the final assessment was 50 degrees, a more convincing argument could be made that an important change for the patient had occurred. Unfortunately, a clinically meaningful result will not always translate to a statistically significant result. A large change may be apparent only in the descriptive statistics and not in the statistical tests, if, for example, too small a number of subjects were used in the experiment and sometimes, if the incorrect statistical tests have been used. The descriptive information, then, provides the reader with the information necessary to decide whether, in context of the rest of the analysis and study design, a change has occurred that may be important to practice. If the sample size is adequate, the statistical tests provide a measure of the probability that the clinical difference is real.

IME LITERATURE SUPPORT FOR THE DECISION ON MRS. B.T.

Referring to the original dilemma, let us apply this skeleton set of rules to appraise the two articles used by the IME physician.[1,2]

GENERALIZING FROM THE SAMPLE TO MRS. B.T.

Potter's[1] Article

From the abstract, it is determined that the sample consists of all patients with low back pain seen by this practitioner or author from early 1974 to December 1975, who were referred from a hospital orthopedic clinic, from specialists in private practice, general practitioners, and chiropractors. No proportions are provided as to how many came from where; thus a sense of the severity cannot be judged. One hundred and twenty-five of the 744 patients considered were classified as "chronic low back pain, no leg involvement." This seems closest to Mrs. B.T.'s situation; however, no definition of chronic is provided. This author also does not classify patients according to time away from work. How important is this? The definition of chronic is known to range, for example, from pain of 7 weeks' to 1 year's duration.[2, 23] It is also believed that patients who have chronic low back pain are different from those who have chronic low back pain and are unable to work. Further, it is known that the longer the duration of the problem for those unable to work, the poorer the prognosis for them ever returning to their jobs.[22] Because all of these were referral cases, it is probable that a fairly significant percentage had had low back pain for quite some time, and many may have stopped working. Unfortunately, without an understanding of how many that might be, generalizing to your current practice situation will be quite difficult.

This study simply described the practitioner's clinical results from usual and customary treatment of patients within his setting who were seen with low back pain over the described time. Concern for the percent who agreed to participate therefore is not applicable.

Article by Manniche et al.[2]

In the methods section is a list of the inclusion/exclusion criteria for patients involved in this study. All patients were referred from general practitioners. Unless your practice includes orthopedic and other referrals, such as those described in Potter's[1] study, the general practice patients from this study are more likely to be typical of your own. Included were patients with "chronic low back pain at rest or associated with back strain for at least 1 year; acute low back pain for the third time or more in the past 6 months, with or without sciatica (pain into the lower limbs); age between 20 and 70 years, inclusive; radiological examination of lumbar spine in the past 2 years" who were able to get to the hospital themselves. Patients were excluded if they had hard neurological signs or had pathological conditions (including "mental illness and inability to cooperate") that may have resulted in an inability to tolerate the exercise program. The median duration of low back pain for this entire sample was 15 years, with the 10th and 90th percentiles listed at 5 and 34 years, respectively. Seventy-eight of the 105 patients included in the study were working at least part time.

With this stronger description of the sample profile, it is somewhat easier to get a sense of where Mrs. B.T. might fit. "Chronic pain" is defined as pain of more than 1 year, although the authors did include a type of recurrent pain (three or more episodes within the past 6 months) as part of their pool and did not discuss how many of each type they had.

Their median duration of pain was listed at 15 years. The term *median* refers to the "middle" number of years. That is, if the pain duration of each patient was lined up in order in one long list, the pain duration in the middle of the pool would be considered the median.

The median is one of three possible estimates of the "middle" value of a sample. The other two are the *mean*, which represents the arithmetic average mentioned earlier; and the *mode*, which represents the most frequently occurring value. For reasons beyond the scope of this chapter, the middle may be best represented by any one of these three methods.*   Because 15 years does fall roughly in the middle between the 10th and 90th percentile (5 years and 34 years, respectively), it is likely that the median is a reasonable representation of the middle in this case.

What does all this mean to your situation with Mrs. B.T.? It is pretty clear that most of the patients with chronic low back pain in this study had pain for significantly longer than Mrs. B.T. In terms of getting rid of chronic low back pain, this means that the prognosis was at least as bad for the patients in the study, as for her. Unfortunately, although the authors of this paper were kind enough to tell the reader how many patients were in some way employed, they did not stratify their methods according to employment. What that means is that after identifying patients, they did not put an equal number of employed/not employed patients in each group and then separately analyze the results of those who were employed vs. those who were not. Because the prognosis is believed to be worse for those who have been unemployed for an extended period, and Mrs. B.T. is in this category, we will still have some difficulty generalizing to the current situation. As more details have been provided, however, we do have a clearer understanding of how well Mrs. B.T. fits than we have from the Potter[1] study. Given the severity of symptoms described, Mrs. B.T. might be expected to do at least as well as the patients in this study.

With respect to the number who agreed to participate, the methods section states that "of 140 patients referred, 105 were entered consecutively after interview and examination." Although it is not totally clear, it does appear that 75% of patients asked did agree to participate and met the inclusion/exclusion criteria.

INITIAL ASSESSMENT

Potter's[1] Article

The outcome measure described is a clinical classification of recovered, much improved, slightly improved, no change, and worse. The classifications are subjective except for the return to work or activity issue. "Recovered" was defined as free of symptoms and return to full activity; "much improved" was defined as "not 100% free of symptoms but functioning normally at work and other activity"; "slightly improved" involved restricted activity and either being willing to live with the prob-

---

*For those who are interested, when the data are representative of a true normal distribution, all three are actually represented by the same number. When a true normal distribution is not found in the sample, the author and statistician must get together to decide what the best estimate of the middle actually is.

lem or being a surgical candidate; "no change" was similar to slightly improved "but intervention may be necessary or even urgent"; and "worse" was defined as aggravation of the patient's symptoms due to treatment. The reliability of this classification system is unknown, and it is obvious from the components of classes just listed that there is much room for discussion as to where various patients might fit. There is no indication of who actually classified the patients. Because a single author is involved and it is a single practice, we can presume that the author classified the patients himself. The potential for bias due to both the subjectivity of the rating system and the subjectivity of the rater is obvious.

Beyond the actual classifications used, it should be noted that the system itself is an attempt to describe patient change. In other words, there is no *actual* initial assessment procedure and no follow-up procedure using the same criteria. We therefore have no estimate of where patients actually began before they were determined, for example, to have "recovered."

Article by Manniche et al.[2]
The initial assessment was made using a new instrument devised by the principal author. Included were a series of three, 11-point box scales used to rate pain (similar to the visual analogue discussed earlier but using boxes instead of a single line), a disability questionnaire consisting of 15 questions dealing with everyday activities and a series of physical impairment tests. Although these seem sensible, no evidence is provided that this assessment system was pretested for reliability or that the numerical rating system used for the assessment was either reliable or valid.

All assessments were completed by a single observer who did not know what treatment was given to the patient. In other words, the observer was blind to the interventions involved. This is important because it guarantees that the observer who assessed the patients could not involve his or her subjective beliefs regarding which treatment should be better and thus influence the results. For example, if the observer knew that a patient was in the "intensive back strengthening" group and disagreed with such intensive exercises, he or she might inadvertently be looking for an aggravation of physical impairment and may observe things that he or she did not look for in the other groups.

The fact that all of this was completed by a single observer is both good and bad. A positive reason for using only one person to do the assessments is that usually a single person will develop his or her own criteria, which will more easily remain consistent from assessment to assessment. That is, the single observer is, within himself or herself, usually more reliable than a group of observers who may be basing their observations of the same criteria on different things even if they are unaware of it.

A good example of how this works (not related to the article) is again the evaluation of a straight leg raise test. A single observer may choose to stop the test as soon as the patient feels pain. From patient to patient and within the same patient after a series of treatments, the criteria for reaching the end point of the test will always be the same. If, on the other hand, there are two observers and one chooses to stop as soon as the patient feels pain, whereas the other looks for the end-feel of the joint and moves as far as patient tolerance will allow, the two observers will get different results on the same patient even though each is reliable within himself or herself.

With this illustration, we also have one of the problems of using a single observer. Which form of the test is the valid one: the point of pain or the end point of motion? The chance of a single observer using a test consistently incorrectly may be higher than the team approach, where at least some team members can be expected to have done the test correctly. In the single rater situation, it may be that the results will be biased simply because of the unusual manner in which the observer has completed the tests. This relates directly to trying to translate the results of this article by Manniche et al.[2] to your private practice. There is no guarantee that you would observe the testing procedures in the same way that the observer in the study did. Not enough information is provided. The results, therefore, might not be the same in a given private practice.

Comparing the two articles, however, in the Manniche et al.[2] investigation, an observable initial assessment was made, and the single rater who did complete the preintervention and postintervention tests was blind to what happened to the patient. This provides greater assurance than does the paper by Potter[1] that the results are objective and can be trusted.

TIME AND TREATMENT

Potter's[1] Article

Although the information is not specifically presented, it would appear that this is a retrospective study. It would seem (although a better description of the methods would be necessary to confirm this) that the author looked back into his files between early 1974 and December of 1975 to see how his patients with low back pain fared. From the discussion section (usually this information is found in the methods), we know that the only intervention used was manipulation. In other words, there is no comparison of techniques. Because this is a retrospective study, the mechanism of patient allocation is not applicable.

The time of treatment was not specified at the outset of this experiment but was a matter of observation. The researcher looked at the number of visits required "in obtaining the best result." How "best" was defined and whether the patient's status (in terms of recovery) deteriorated after the "best result" was obtained are unknown.

Although it is clear that this investigation occurred as an observational study of the cases in a single practitioner's office and in this way would be considered an effectiveness study, the author states in the discussion that the purpose was to assess the role manipulation plays in low back pain care. He notes that because these observations have been made, a "team approach" is being used to aid patients in obtaining relief without surgery. In this sense, the original study could be viewed as looking at efficacy of manipulation. Again, the descriptions are too scant of the details to be certain.

Article by Manniche et al.[2]

This was a prospective study, where patients were randomly allocated (drew lots) to one of three treatments/interventions. The interventions consisted of thermotherapy, massage, and mild exercises for 1 month, an intensive back strengthening program over 3 months, and a modified back strengthening program of one fifth the dose for one half the time over a total of 3 months. No indication is provided as to whether any of these could be considered usual and customary, thus, a sense of efficacy vs. effectiveness cannot be determined. It is clear, however, that the study itself had a much stronger design than the study by Potter.[1]

FINAL ASSESSMENT

Potter's[1] Article

As stated earlier, there was no distinct time point where the study ended for any given patient, and the result at that time was monitored. Rather, the researcher sought to find the time of the "best result" and that was described. Also, as discussed earlier, this study did not have an initial and final assessment per se. The author instead described his perspective on how much change had occurred to that point of maximum improvement.

Article by Manniche et al.[2]

Two "final assessments" occurred in this study. One was directly after the study intervention time (at the 3-month mark), and the second was at a follow-up time of 6 months. As stated earlier, the same tests were used by the same observer for all assessments made. The problems already discussed regarding the assessment tool used and the single observer situation apply here.

ANALYSIS

Potter's[1] Article

Results of the classification of patients according to clinical group are presented in terms of percentages. Means (arithmetic averages) are used to describe the typical number of patient visits required to achieve the best outcome and the typical treatment period. There is, however, no sense of the range of patient visits or treatment period. A sense of the range in which these arithmetic averages fall is important in generalizing to Mrs. B.T.'s case, because the average treatment period for the chronic low back pain patients who had no leg involvement was 19.4 days. If the best outcome occurred in a certain subsample of this group (e.g., the more chronically affected who were also unemployed) after a much longer time, this would provide some support at least for Mrs. B.T.'s length of care and your situation. Unfortunately, these results were not published.

Article by Manniche et al.[2]

The medians and 10th and 90th percentiles for pain, disability and physical impairment ratings are provided in table form for the before treatment time period, after treatment period, and final follow-up time in each group. In this way the reader can make some clinical judgments as to which group or groups did better and when. In addition, statistical tests were run to determine both before-after differences in each group and differences between groups. As per the discussion earlier, these tests can be found in a good text looking at the reasons for using the types of statistics mentioned without getting into the mathematics involved. On doing

TABLE 1.
Characteristics Assessed in
Publications Regarding Treatment
of Mrs. B.T.

1. Population/sample
    Generalizability
    Sampling procedure
    Percent Agreeing to participate
    Sample size
2. Initial assessment
    Reliability
    Validity
3. Time/treatment
    Prospective vs. retrospective
    Random allocation
    Efficacy vs. effectiveness
4. Final assessment
    Consistent with initial
        assessment
5. Analysis
    Appropriate for study design

this, we can see that Manniche et al.[2] made a reasonable choice (given their belief that they had nonparametric data) and that the various tests used support statistically what can be seen in the table providing the medians and percentiles for the different groups at different times. It is also clear from the "clinically important" standpoint that the descriptive results strongly support the use of the intensive back strengthening program.

SUMMARY

The characteristics on which the two articles[1,2] were assessed are provided in Table 1. Although both publications are flawed, it should be pointed out that there is no research project that is perfectly designed and conducted. It is simply not possible when live patients with pain are involved. Much of what happens cannot be controlled or predicted. With respect to the two publications briefly assessed, it is clear that the article by Manniche et al.[2] was the better designed of the two and had a stronger likelihood of providing results that could be trusted in a different clinical setting. Questions of applicability to Mrs. B.T.'s situation can still be asked, however. A better way to decide on which mode of care has the higher likelihood of success is to examine the *preponderance of evidence*.

PREPONDERANCE OF EVIDENCE

As a result of reviewing these two works, you remain unsatisfied with the IME verdict. You question the clear applicability and overall value of both articles used and believe that a further search of the literature may provide evidence closer to your clinical situation and perhaps in your favor. As a result, you use your computer and tap into a service that provides Index Medicus listings. Using the terms "chronic," "low back pain," and "treatment," you come up with a list of relevant articles and check to see what they say. In an informal way you are viewing for yourself what is referred to as the preponderance of evidence. You want to know how much of the literature supports each position and the quality of the literature on both sides. Your browse through Index Medicus yields the following.

A total of nine articles that you are able to retrieve from your college library appear to be relevant to your patient.[24–32] That is, by title, they are studies of treatment effects on patients who have what has been in one way or another classified as chronic low back pain. None of these appears to look at chiropractic treatment. In your search of the chiropractic literature, you are unable by title to identify any clinical trials dealing specifically with chronic low back pain and chiropractic treatment protocols. From discussion with your peers and from your own memory, you finally find two publications looking at chiropractic management.[33, 34] Neither contains the word "chronic" in the title, but you know that some of the patients involved had chronic low back pain. Your total informal sample of articles, then, is 11. Only two deal specifically with chiropractic; the rest seem to deal in large measure with rehabilitative procedures. This is an important observation. The majority of the material that is easily available pertains to something other than your therapy of choice. It will now be meaningful to evaluate the quality of the publications you have found.

Table 2 provides the name of the author, year of publication, and title of the references you have found. After scanning the material you received from the computer search, you notice that the paper by Ongley et al.[28] is a comparison study using injections with and without a single manipulation. Because you are concerned about what has been termed "active care" vs. ongoing manipulation, this article does not apply, and you eliminate it from your assessment.

Table 3 provides the completed worksheet of the factors you believe are important to evaluate the remaining 10 articles. You discover in the process that Newman et al.'s[31] 1978 article is a long-term follow-up of a proportion of patients from the study by Seres and Newman[32] in 1976 and that you can look at them side by side. Because these two articles are concerned with different issues on the same theme, you do not discard one in favor of the other.

On reviewing your worksheet, you are struck by several important points. All of the publications appear to contain patients who fit Mrs. B.T.'s characteristics in terms of age and chronicity. The definition of "chronicity" varies tremendously across the group, and specific age by chronicity results are not available in even a single study. Further, although all of the articles contain patients who were unable to work, the time frames vary, and in some articles these results are not easy to separate out. Because you know that the 6-month time frame that Mrs. B.T. has been off of work is important, this is a problem. Although there are questions about the generalizability of these studies to Mrs. B.T.'s case, this is all of the information you have; therefore, you proceed.

TABLE 2.
Results of an Informal Search of Conservative Care Literature for Chronic Low Back Pain

Author	Yr	Title
Computer search		
Mellin et al.[24]	1993	Outcome of a multimodal treatment, including intensive physical training of patients with chronic low back pain
Kohles et al.[25]	1990	Improved physical performance outcomes after functional restoration treatment in patients with chronic low back pain: early vs. recent training results
Hazard et al.[26]	1989	Functional restoration with behavioral support: a 1-yr prospective study of patients with chronic low back pain
Mayer et al.[27]	1987	A prospective 2-yr study of functional restoration in industrial low back injury: an objective assessment procedure
Ongley et al.[28]	1987	A new approach to the treatment of chronic low back pain
Tollinson et al.[29]	1985	Chronic low back pain: results of treatment at the pain therapy center
Lichter et al.[30]	1984	Treatment of chronic low back pain: a community-based comprehensive return to work physical rehabilitation program
Newman et al.[31]	1978	Multidisciplinary treatment of chronic pain: long-term follow-up of low back pain patients.
Seres and Newman[32]	1976	Results of treatment of chronic low back pain at the Portland Pain Center
Additional search looking specifically at chiropractic care		
Cox and Schreiner[33]	1984	Chiropractic manipulation in low back pain and sciatica: statistical data on the diagnosis, treatment, and response of 576 consecutive cases
Cassidy et al.[34]	1985	Spinal manipulation in the treatment of low back pain

You are surprised by the kind of study designs used. Nine of the 10 studies were prospective[24, 26, 27, 29–34]; however, 7 of the 10 publications have no comparison groups.[24, 29–34] This includes the two articles dealing with chiropractic care. These are simply a description of the cases that have been treated within a particular clinic or clinics. Of those studies where there are groups, random allocation was not used. Rather, the patient or the insurance company by default, made the decision as to where they should be. One study created groups based on the insurance company denying treatment and created a comparison group, where there

TABLE 3.
Worksheet for Informal Search of Active vs. Passive Care in Chronic Low Back Pain

	Mellin et al.[24]	Kohles et al.[25]	Hazard et al.[26]	Mayer et al.[27]
I. Population/sample				
A. Generalizability				
1. Definitive chronicity	Unstated	Unstated	≥4 mo>4 mo	
2. Time off work	48% not working time unknown	Avg 10.9 mo, 10.6 mo for approx 90%	≥4 mo	Avg 12–18 mo; s.d. 14–22 mo
3. Age	Avg 42.8 yr; s.d. 7.2 yr	Avg 37.1, 38.2 yrs	Avg 37–40 yr; s.d. 4.3–10.8 yr	Avg 38–44 yr; s.d. 9.1–9.3 yr
B. Sampling procedure volunteers/random	All patients treated between 1988–1989	Consecutive patients	Patients refusing not enrolled	Consecutively referred in
C. Percent agreeing to participate	194/261 enough follow-up data	Not applicable	87/90	127/199
D. Sample size	194	1984: 45; 1987: 57	59 Grads, 5 do†; 17 comparison	116 treated; 72 not; 11 do†

II. Initial assessment				
A. Reliable	Some standard	Unstated, some probably	Unstated, some standard	Some standard
B. Valid; makes sense	Yes	Yes	Yes	Yes
III. Time/treatment	4-wk inpatient; multi/active	3 wk; multi/active	3 wk; multi/active	3 wk; multi/active
A. Prospective/ retrospective	Prospective	Retrospective	Prospective	Prospective
B. Random allocation	No groups	No	No	No
C. Efficacy/ effectiveness	Effectiveness	Effectiveness	Effectiveness	Effectiveness
IV. Final assessment (same as initial)	Yes	Yes	Yes	Follow-up: 1–2 yr by telephone
V. Analysis (Test matches design)	Descriptive information in addition to modeling	Mostly descriptive	Mostly descriptive	Mostly descriptive
VI. Results of interest to Mrs. B.T.	52% Working on admission 56% working at 12 mos follow-up	Both groups: Greater functional capacity ending 3-wk program Early ed: Perhaps benefitted later group	1 yr follow-up 81% return to work: grads 40%; do† 29%: Comparison group	85%–87% return to work in treatment group, and 39% in comparison group Some initial character differences

*WC = Workers' compensation.
†do = dropouts.
‡Max improv = return to prepain state or point where treatment no longer provides relief.
§RTF = return to function.

	Tollinson et al.[29]	Lichter et al.[30]	Newman et al.[31]	Seres and Newman[32]	Cox and Schreiner[33]	Cassidy et al.[34]
	Avg 32 Mos Range 5–96 mo	>3 mo	Avg 6.3 yr Range 2–25 yrs	Avg 5.7 yr Range 1–25 yr	Unclear	>6 mo
	72/100 WC*; avg 22 mo (1–77)	93/120 WC*; time unknown	Unstated	Majority had open claims	Unstated	All unable to go about normal activity
	Avg 42.6 yr; range 19–66 yr	Avg 37 yr; s.d. 7 yr	Avg 44.6 yr; range 17–62 yr	Avg 45 yr	Avg 43.4 yr; range 13–86 yr	Avg 42 yr; range 16–79 yr
	Consecutive patients	Consecutive files	Invited, geographic basis	Consecutively treated	Consecutive patients from 23 DCs	Referred in
	Unstated	120/350 met all analysis criteria	Unstated	Represents 65% of admissions	Unstated	Not applicable
	100	120	36	100	576	285

Col 1	Col 2	Col 3	Col 4	Col 5	Col 6
Unstated, some probably Yes	Unstated, some standard Yes	Unstated, some probably Yes	Unstated, some standard Yes	Unstated, some probably Yes	Unstated Yes
Avg 25 days; multi/active Prospective	4 wk minimum; multi/active Prospective	Avg 3 wk; multi/active Prospective	Avg 3 wk; multi/active Prospective	Avg 42.8 days; max improv‡ Passive/prospective	Avg approx 7 treatments Passive/prospective
No groups Effectiveness At least some	No groups Effectiveness For work status: yes	No groups Effectiveness Yes	No groups Effectiveness Yes	No groups Effectiveness Unstated; dependent-survey questions	No groups Effectiveness Yes
Descriptive	Descriptive	Mostly descriptive	Descriptive	Descriptive	Mostly descriptive
Increase of 66% working or attending school compared with start of study	54/93 return to work within 12 mo and were considered a success	Two thirds remained unemployed. Graphs show unemployed did consistently worse. Gains in physical functioning	3 mo f/u, 80% no longer seek medical care. Recommended claim closure in 75% seen at follow-up	Mean days to maximum improv‡ 42.8 (18.6 treatments)	Approx 75%–90% posterior facet and/or SI syndrome RTF§. Unstable posterior facet: significantly more treatment needed; avg 8.9 and fewer RTF§

appears to be a pretreatment difference with respect to the use of opiates.[27] Usage was found to be 15% for those in the treatment group and 48% for those in the comparison group. The effect that widespread opiate use might have on a return to work outcome is unknown, but this may be a confounder (something unrelated to the treatments tested that may alter the outcome) to the results reported.

Eight of the 10 studies used a multidisciplinary, active treatment approach,[24–27, 29–32] whereas the last 2, of course, used manipulation and an apparently passive approach.[33, 34] Although the reliability of at least some of the outcome measures is unknown, for the most part the assessments make sense. Return to work rates were fairly easy to find in the results sections of most of the studies surveyed. Although there were significant methodological problems with all of the publications, five of the eight studies using a multidisciplinary active treatment approach showed increased numbers of people who returned to work.[26, 27, 29, 30, 32] One study had essentially the same number working on admission to their program as at completion,[24] and two had no separate analysis of the return to work issue.[31, 25] Both studies involving manipulation showed patient improvement, and one indicated that for posterior facet or sacroiliac problems, approximately 75% to 90% of patients improved to the point of returning to work or normal activity.[34] This same publication noted that "unstable" posterior facet joints required significantly more treatments to achieve the final outcome. The amount of time given to treatment in all studies ranged or averaged from 2 to 4 weeks to the point at which the results were available.

What does all of this mean to Mrs. B.T.? Although the evidence is substantially less than optimal, a greater amount of positive information was found looking at the multidisciplinary active approach. Although the two chiropractic articles did indeed suggest benefit, the time frame for this approach was substantially less than the one you used. You are disappointed, but it is clear that your brief and informal look at the literature will not support your position for the IME decision. You therefore decide not to proceed further.

Although the problem with Mrs. B.T. still bothers you, you are now concerned with a new issue. If decisions are to be made in health care, first according to scientific evidence, then the preponderance of evidence, and, finally, by consensus, and your brief look at your own situation is any indication of what the quality of the clinical literature relevant to at least this patient is like, you fear that many decisions are being based on significantly flawed research. You are not alone in this concern. In fact, the authors of a recent publication discussing the results of Agency for Health Care Policy and Research's involvement in PORT (Patient Outcomes Research Teams) projects were surprised to discover that when reviewing the literature "studies often failed even the simplest tests of quality with regard to design."[4] Unlike your informal look at clinical publications from peer-reviewed and indexed literature, PORT projects use a very formal and rigorous approach to try to survey all of the relevant material, distill this down to the usable and useful information, and make graded judgments based on quality. This is, of course, a considerably challenging task.

Although you are comforted that even formal searches have difficulty getting clear answers to clinical situations, you recognize that what is needed is more research with stronger methods. You remember that many publications are to provide documentation that will aid research in progressing but that much of this kind of information cannot yet be used to make changes in clinical practice. With this in mind, as well as your ability to evaluate the facts in clinical research publications, you can cut down the amount of reading necessary to keep up with what is going on in patient care.

This does not mean that you can avoid reading altogether—quite the contrary. With the information boom and electronic availability of resource material, the clinician today is expected to be aware of developments in his or her field. The clinician today is expected to practice, based on a judicious look at what is available and to make wise decisions regarding change in practice as information from clinical studies unfold. It is, as stated earlier, a new and required skill.

REFERENCES

1. Potter GE: A study of 744 cases of neck and back pain treated with spinal manipulation. *J Can Chiropr Assoc* 21:154–156, 1977.
2. Manniche C, Hesselsoe Bentzen L, et al: Clinical trial of intensive muscle training for chronic low back pain. *Lancet* 2:1473–1476, 1988.
3. Lave JR, Pashos CL, Anderson GF, et al: Costing medical care: Using Medicare administrative data. *Med Care* 32:JS77–JS89, 1994.
4. Maklan CW, Greene R, Cummings MA: Methodological challenges and innovations in patient outcomes research. *Med Care* 32:JS13–JS21, 1994.
5. Eddy DM: *A Manual for Assessing Health Practices and Designing Practice Policies: The Explicit Approach.* Pennsylvania, American College of Physicians, 1992.
6. Evidence-Based Medicine Working Group: Evidence-based medicine: A new approach to teaching the practice of medicine. *JAMA* 268:2420–2425, 1992.
7. Sackett DL, Haynes RB, Guyatt GH, et al: *Clinical Epidemiology: A Basic Science for Clinical Medicine,* ed 2. Boston, Little, Brown, 1991.
8. McGregor M, Sportelli L: Statistics for the clinician. Workshop at the 1993 International Conference on Spinal Manipulation, Montreal, Quebec, April 1993.
9. Schneier M, Burns RE. Atlanto-occipital hypermobility in sudden infant death syndrome. *Chiropr J Chiropr Res Clin Invest* 7:33–38, 1991.
10. Chutani SK, Bordia A. Preliminary note: The effect of fried versus raw garlic on fibrolytic activity in man. *Atherosclerosis* 38:417–421, 1981.
11. Gatterman MI: Standards for contraindications to spinal manipulative therapy, in Vear HJ (ed): *Chiropractic Standards of Practice and Quality of Care.* Gaithersburg, Md, Aspen, 1992, pp 221–238.
12. Dabert O, Freeman DG, Weis AJ: Spinal meningeal hematoma, warfarin therapy and chiropractic adjustment. *JAMA* 214:2058, 1970.
13. McGregor M, Mior SA: Critical appraisal of journal literature pertinent to chiropractic. Paper presented at the Fourth Annual Meeting of the International Chiropractic Academy on the Study of Back Pain, St Louis, October 1989.
14. Chalmers TC, Frank CS, Reitman D: Minimizing the three stages of publication bias. *JAMA* 263:1392–1395, 1990.

15. Cullen DJ, MacAulay A: Consistency between peer reviewers for a clinical specialty journal. *Acad Med* 67:856–859, 1992.
16. Strayhorn J Jr, McDermott JF, Tanguay P: An intervention to improve the reliability of manuscript reviews for the *Journal of the American Academy of Child and Adolescent Psychiatry*. *Am J Psychiatry* 150:947–952, 1993.
17. Koes BW, Bouter LM, vanMameren H, et al: A blinded randomized clinical trial of manual therapy and physiotherapy for chronic back and neck complaints: Physical outcome measures. *J Manipulative Physiol Ther* 1:16–23, 1992.
18. Koes BW, Bouter LM, vanMameren H, et al: The effectiveness of manual therapy, physiotherapy, and treatment by the general practitioner for nonspecific back and neck complaints: A randomized clinical trial. *Spine* 17:28–41, 1992.
19. Koes BW, Bouter LM, vanMameren H, et al: Randomised clinical trial of manipulative therapy and physiotherapy for persistent back and neck complaints: Results of a one year follow-up. *BMJ* 304:601–605, 1992.
20. Huskisson EC: Measurement of pain. *Lancet* 2:1127–1131, 1974.
21. Saal JA, Saal JS, Herzog JR: The natural history of lumbar intervertebral disc extrusions treated nonoperatively. *Spine* 15:683–686, 1990.
22. Norman GR, Streiner DL: *PDQ Statistics*. Toronto, BC Decker, 1986.
23. Frymoyer JW, Nachemson A: Natural history of low back disorders, in Frymoyer JW (ed): *The Adult Spine: Principles and Practice*. New York, Raven Press, 1991, pp 1537–1550.
24. Mellin G, Harkapaa K, Vanharanta H, et al: Outcome of a multimodal treatment including intensive physical training of patients with chronic low-back pain. *Spine* 18:825–829, 1993.
25. Kohles S, Barnes D, Gatchel RJ, et al: Improved physical performance outcomes after functional restoration treatment in patients with chronic low-back pain: Early versus recent training results. *Spine* 15:1321–1324, 1990.
26. Hazard RG, Fenwick JW, Kalisch SM, et al: Functional restoration with behavioral support: A one-year prospective study of patients with chronic low-back pain. *Spine* 14:157–161, 1989.
27. Mayer TG, Gatchel RJ, Mayer J, et al: A prospective two-year study of functional restoration in industrial low back injury: An objective assessment procedure. *JAMA* 258:1763–1767, 1987.
28. Ongley MJ, Klein RG, Dorman TA, et al: A new approach to the treatment of chronic low back pain. *Lancet* 2:143–146, 1987.
29. Tollinson CD, Kriegel ML, Downie GR: Chronic low back pain: Results of treatment at the pain therapy center. *South Med J* 78:1291–1295, 1985.
30. Lichter RL, Hewson JK, Radke SJ, et al: Treatment of chronic low-back pain: A community-based comprehensive return-to-work physical rehabilitation program. *Clin Orthop* 190:115–123, 1984.
31. Newman RI, Seres JL, Yospe LP, et al: Multidisciplinary treatment of chronic pain: Long-term follow-up of low-back pain patients. *Pain* 4:283–292, 1978.
32. Seres JL, Newman RI: Results of treatment of chronic low-back pain at the Portland Pain Center. *J Neurosurg* 45:32–36, 1976.
33. Cox JM, Shreiner S: Chiropractic manipulation in low back pain and sciatica: Statistical data on the diagnosis, treatment and response of 576 consecutive cases. *J Manipulative Physiol Ther* 7:1–11, 1984.
34. Cassidy JD, Kirkaldy-Willis WH, McGregor M: Spinal manipulation in the treatment of low-back pain, in Buerger AA, Greenman PE (eds): *Empirical Approaches to the Validation of Spinal Manipulation*. Springfield, Ill, Charles C Thomas, 1985, pp 119–148.

Physician-Patient Interactions

Robert C. Shiel, Ph.D.
Associate Professor, National College of Chiropractic, Lombard, Illinois

Patient compliance with therapeutic regimens is a well-documented health issue and also a prolific area of research. From 1990 to 1994 more than 2,000 articles focusing on the physician-patient interaction appeared in the referenced journals. In some of the articles the focus is on what the physician should do; others examine the role of the ideal patient; others talk of the structure of the relationship between physician and patient. These articles ask the questions: What is the patient's experience? What is the physician's role? What are the structures of the relationship between physician and patient? What is the effect of the social context in which these relationships take place?

Unfortunately, even with the attention that it receives, the research on patient behavior identifies that the percentage of patients that are compliant and do what the physician asks is very low.[1] Virtually nobody does everything the physician asks. On the other side, the percentage of patients that are entirely noncompliant and do nothing that the physician asks appears to be on the rise. Even when health care providers arrive at a correct diagnosis and devise appropriate management plans, they are often frustrated by unsatisfactory outcomes resulting from patient noncompliance. The efficacy of any treatment depends on the appropriateness of the treatment and the extent to which patients adhere to the recommended regimen. The consequences of noncompliance with a prescribed treatment may provoke exacerbation and progression of the disability, development of secondary complications, medical emergencies, or unnecessary prescription. In general, noncompliance often leads to failure of treatment.

Research suggests that noncompliance is an endemic problem. Hulka et al.[2] found that 50% of patients did not follow referral advice, 75% did not keep follow-up appointments, and 50% suffering from chronic illnesses dropped out of treatment within 1 year. Even with simple medical regimens such as taking prescribed medication, approximately one third of patients can be expected to be noncompliant and where regimens are more demanding even lower compliance rates can be expected. Turk and Rudy[3] note that assuming 100% of the patients who enter a treatment program are committed to adopting the program, there is a drop of 40% to 80% in actual maintenance of these compliant behaviors during the first 6 weeks.

Why are compliance levels so low if the treatment regimen is designed for the patient to relieve discomfort and increase functioning? Resolving this noncompliance is an essential issue in successful health care. But what promotes a successful outcome to the physician-patient encounter where the patient follows through with the treatment plan?

Initially noncompliance was conceptualized as a problem residing within the patient, but researchers looking to determine the patient characteristics that predict noncompliance have not been successful. Demographic variables such as age, sex, race, and marital status are not predictive of compliance with health care recommendations. Similarly, socioeconomic status, occupation, and level of income are also not characteristics that predict compliance. Even more dramatically, there is little evidence that the severity of the illness, the duration of the illness, or the degree of the patient's functional impairment influence the amount of compliance achieved.[2] Outcomes reported by Lay and Spelman[4] suggest that patient compliance levels are remarkably similar even where there are large differences in the amount of apprehension and anxiety experienced. With both high or low levels of anxiety, patients' sick role and preventive health behaviors were similar. Under both conditions, patients not only remember fewer of their physician's instructions but also were less likely to follow the instructions they could recall.

If adherence to the treatment protocol was important only because it determined the amount of specific therapy the patient received, that would be important enough, but there is evidence that adherence levels may directly influence outcome.[5] Horowitz and Horowitz[6] found that patients who comply with treatment, even when that treatment is a placebo, have better health outcomes than poorly adherent patients receiving therapeutic interventions. This suggests that the relationship of the patient to the treatment plan has an impact on the clinical outcome. The connection between compliance and outcome may be greatly influenced by the relationship between physician and patient because adherence to the regimen recommended by the physician has been found to be positively associated with certain characteristics of the physician-patient relationship. Where the physician demonstrates the ability to make the patient feel understood, provide support, and provide a healing climate for the patient, compliance is enhanced.[2, 4, 7] When the patient feels connected to the physician, the patient is more likely to be compliant. When the patient feels connected to what is happening to them, they are more likely to be compliant.

Lack of compliance, on the other hand, is often identified as the result of a poor physician-patient relationship, Smith and Thompson[7] argue that a typical effect of a less than optimal physician-patient relationship is noncompliance and then point to these physician-patient problems as the major cause of treatment failure in many cases. The issue becomes more serious when you take an expanded view of health care. In cases where compliance occurs during active treatment, apparently related to a good physician-patient rapport, posttreatment relapses for many conditions exist and may be viewed as a form of noncompliance. Relapse rates for obesity, substance abuse, and smoking cessation treatment programs all have shown high decay of effect curves after completion of treatment. Approximately 50% of those successfully treated for these problems show relapse by 6 months after treatment. These results appear to hold for chronic pain patients as well. Even when the improvements noted at longer-term follow-up remain statistically significant, a trend of regression toward pretreatment baselines remains.[3]

An understanding of what is happening with patients requires an examination of the physician-patient relationship. Compliance is something that happens in the relationship between physician and patient. It is the patient's response to the physician's directive and is intimately tied to the relationship between the two. How this compliance is viewed and promoted by the physician can have a dramatic impact on patient outcome.

The term compliance suggests a passive role with the patient following the advice and direction of the physician. Hence, the term noncompliance includes an evaluation of the patient that presumes the failure to comply is the fault of the patient. In contrast, the terms cooperation and adherence imply an active and voluntary collaboration between the physician and the patient in a mutually defined and acceptable course of behavior toward health. Cooperation conveys the implication of choice and partnership in treatment planning and implementation. Patients who are adherent act on a consensually agreed on plan that they had had a role in designing.[3]

Therefore, a significant difference between compliance and cooperation exists in the relationship between the physician and patient. Compliance exists in a relationship of unequal power with the patient disinvested from his or her own health care. It implies doing what you are told, following through on the prescription of the physician to act in a particular way.

Cooperation may be more important to achieve than mere compliance. Cooperation implies an active participation on the patient's part. In that active participation, the patient complies with what is happening because he or she is invested in the process of health care. Patients who are cooperating may in some sense be compliant. However, compliant patients do not necessarily cooperate. Individuals may be compliant and still be entirely passive in the process of their health care.

It is then important to note the context in which the compliance occurs. Is it happening in a context of coercion or one of cooperation? How do you build cooperation? To do so an understanding of the roles and interactional sequences of the physician and patient is needed.

PATIENT'S CONTEXT

Although physician and patient may appear to have a common goal of treatment, there are often significant differences in the contexts from which they operate. Health care providers by their training and responsibilities take a somatic view of illness and treatment, whereas patients frequently take a more functional view of their problem. Patients understand the treatment regimen in terms of the ways it will affect their lives. The physician, however, is more likely to think of the treatment plan in terms of the way it will correct or improve the patient's health and functioning. Although this structural definition of physical functioning and the therapy recommendations based on it are designed in the patient's interest, it is not identical to the patient's functional measure of health that is based on how his or her symptoms will affect activities of daily living. Consequently, the physician's prescription is not simply accepted and carried out as ordered. Rather, it is received by the patient in the specific psychosocial context of his or her life and evaluated according to a personal and subjective estimate of appropriateness, then implemented in varying levels and degrees within a particular sociocultural setting.[3]

What are the common elements of that context? Neighbour[8] suggests that a regression toward a more dependent and childlike state is a basic human response to illness. Sick and worried people look to find and endow someone with the power to make it better.

Cassel[9] in his landmark article argues the following:

> People are their roles, and each role has rules. Together, the rules that guide the performance of roles make up a complex set of entitlements and limitations of responsibility and privilege. By middle age, the roles may be so firmly set that disease can lead to the virtual destruction of a person by making the performance of his or her roles impossible. Whether the patient is a doctor who cannot doctor or a mother who cannot mother, he or she is diminished by the loss of function.

When patients come in for treatment, it is important to recognize that not only are they experiencing this physical disruption of their health but they are also experiencing a psychological disruption that is suffering. Suffering a loss of function. People, when they come in to a physician, are feeling out of control in some way. Patients come to their physician precisely because they are feeling out of control in terms of their health care needs. This includes worrying about the problem, not understanding the problem, experiencing some threat to their existence as a person, and some loss of control in their life that translates to some loss of self-esteem.

Cassel[9] states the following:

> Suffering occurs when an impending destruction of the person is perceived; it continues until the threat of disintegration has passed or until the integrity of the person can be restored in some other manner. It follows, then, that although suffering often occurs in the presence of acute pain, softness of breath, or other bodily symptoms, suffering extends beyond the physical. Most generally, suffering can be defined as the state of severe distress associated with events that threaten the intactness of the person.

The details of our day-to-day behavior are taken for granted when healthy. People perceive themselves as healthy by whether they are able to carry out their routine behaviors. Patients decide that they are ill because they cannot perform as usual and thereby suffer the loss of their routine.

Cassel[9] points out this psychological factor:

> It is not possible to treat sickness as something that happens solely to the body without thereby risking damage to the person. An anachronistic division of the human condition into what is medical (having to do with the body) and what is nonmedical (the remainder) has given medicine too narrow a notion of its calling. Because of this division, physicians may, in concentrating on the cure of bodily disease, do things that cause the patient as a person to suffer.

These things are not necessarily intended by the physician. The physician acts out the role of expert based on his or her special knowledge, sets a timetable and agenda to maximize efficiency of service bringing the patient into the context of the physician's routine, establishing the physician's authority over the decision-making process. However, these actions tend to marginalize and disinvest the patient in the process of health care. In addition, from patients' perspective, illness causes them to lose control over their own body and, coupled with the loss of voice over their health care, they inevitably experience a threat to their self-reliance and self-esteem.[10]

Consequently, suffering is enhanced in a physician-patient relationship where the patient is placed in a passive, dependent role where compliance with the "physician's orders" is an engramatically programmed response. The physician maintains an autonomy and professional dominance in a role that defines illness, confers the sick status on the patient, establishes priorities of diagnosis and treatment, and in general assumes a position of dominance in all matters relating to the patient's health status.[10]

When patients are suffering, they are suffering the loss of their routine, of how they identify themselves. They struggle to hold onto the routine. They are under stress, and so they become relatively inflexible because they are doing everything that they can in their routine and because they are defensive and hurting. Two common strategies that patients employ in this circumstance are either to give up control to the doctor and be passive or take an aggressive stance toward the physician through either actively aggressive behavior or passive-aggressive behavior.

In giving up control and taking a passive stance, the patient is very often willing to attempt anything that the physician orders. They are willing to take that one-down position for the security of having someone in control. However, because patients have relinquished control over the symptoms and illness to the physician, they often resist taking responsibility for action in the treatment program or find the responsibilities of a treatment program overwhelming. In these circumstances, it is very easy for physicians to fall into this authoritarian model because patients present themselves as falling apart and in need of rescue. So, the physician attempts to save the patient and starts manipulating and treating.

Initially this may work out, but as the patient starts to feel healthier, a conflict arises. The relationship with the physician promotes a healthier physical functioning but at the same time fosters a lower than acceptable level of self-esteem for the patient. As patients feel healthier, their sense of control returns and they begin to act in ways to regain the autonomy given over to the physician. Without the return of this autonomy, the relationship becomes untenable and may be the cause of patients dropping out of treatment before it is finished.

If, in the relationship with the physician, the patient operates out of the position of low self-esteem, the easiest path to an improved sense of self is through noncompliance or termination of care, which does not require a restructuring of the relationship. As the patient gets healthier, it becomes more and more difficult to stay with the physician. The patient continues care until he or she begins to improve. At the point where the patient is feeling better and the physician feels that treatment could be successful, the patient drops out. The physician wonders, "Why is the patient dropping out? The treatment was working." In fact, the patient is dropping out because the treatment was working. It becomes untenable to stay in the relationship established with the physician, caught in a one-down position, in a passive role, when he or she is feeling better. The patient feels psychologically worse to go to the physician because he or she is feeling physically better. This being the case, it does not matter how simple the treatment plan, how little time it takes to implement, or how few therapy sessions are left. Very often patients withdraw from health care and stop being compliant with health care because, in fact, to do so increases their sense of psychological well-being by divesting themselves of the one-down relationship.

The patient's decisions and reactions are based on a complex assessment and experience of both short- and long-term goals. Both the goal of regaining control and the goal of self-esteem are there. In the crisis of not knowing, the patient focuses on the need of someone to take charge. But as that need recedes, the patient's loss of routine function and loss of autonomy come to the foreground. As the need to regain autonomy becomes more pressing, the patient will often not recognize, be able to clearly identify, or act on the long-term goal of health.

Consequently, as the course of treatment progresses, a struggle ensues over the patient's role in medical decision making that is often characterized as a conflict between autonomy and health and between the values of the patient and the values of the physician but that is rooted in the patient's sense of self.[11] This is often played out in the roles of a paternalistic physician and an autonomous patient as a struggle for control in the relationship. However, to say that all patients demand autonomy is to misrepresent what doctors actually experience. If patients react in a manner to regain autonomy through noncompliance, they are not doing so with this as an expressed, overt agenda.

Of course, this disinvestment from treatment is not in the patient's best interest and results in continued loss of function and diminished capabilities. If it is established as a result of the patient's attempts to be saved and the physician's willingness to take control, it may be avoided by avoiding that scenario in the relationship. Specifically it may be avoided by the physician working to alleviate not only the physical distress but also the loss of control and consequent suffering of the patient.

Cassel[9] notes that patient's recovery from suffering often requires help and identifies that one of the functions of physicians is to lend strength to patients who have lost parts of themselves and can be sustained by the personhood of the physician until their own recovers. Without that added dimension in the relationship, health care becomes much more difficult, frustration elevates for both physician and patient, and the effectiveness of treatment diminishes.

The physician's goal, then, is to increase the level of the patient's sense of autonomy while at the same time directing treatment and to promote patient self-esteem and control to enhance compliance and cooperation.

MODELS OF PHYSICIAN BEHAVIOR

"Psychological, relationship-based factors have always been important in medicine; in fact, most of the earliest medical treatments had little or no biologically based therapeutic value. Indeed, psychological factors were the main therapeutic component of most of medicine until about eight decades ago, when modern scientific medicine became more widespread."[7]

Emanuel and Emanuel[11] identify four different models of physician behavior labeled as paternalistic, informative, interpretive, and deliberative. Each of these models defines the physician's behavior in relationship to the patient. The paternalistic model assumes that there are shared objective criteria for determining what is best for the patient. Consequently, the physician can determine what is in the patient's best interest with limited or no patient participation. Because of the physician's status as expert, it is assumed that the patient will be thankful for decisions made by the physician even if the patient does not agree to them at the time. And in the tension between the patient's autonomy and health, the paternalistic physician's main emphasis is toward the latter, with the assumption that ultimately the autonomy and well-being will not be in conflict.

From this authoritarian stance, physicians pontificate and the patients do what they are told. Patients will often adopt this model because it is the least intrusive, requiring the least investment of time and energy. The physician tells them what to do, does not give them any information about their own health and their own health care, and they do not have to be responsible. The physician is in charge. The physician processes all information and makes decisions on it. Although intrusive on the part of the physician, this model can be viewed as providing the most conservative approach from the point of view of the patient, conservative in that little or nothing is required of the patient. Models requiring more patient input and participation are much more intrusive on the patient's lifestyle.

However, to a large extent, the physician focuses on the diagnosis and treatment and views the patient as inanimate or at least as immobilized to the extent that the patient is unable to contribute actively in the treatment. The frame of reference is one in which the physician does something to the patient that is an application of the many advances in modern health care in which the patient is not expected to understand and therefore would not be able to actively participate. Thus, treatment takes place regardless of the patient's real informed consent and is often taken by the physician as an affirmation of his or her belief that the patient cannot intelligently contribute to his or her own treatment.[10]

In the informative model, the physician's objective is to provide the patient with all relevant information, for the patient to select the medical interventions he or she wants, and for the physician to execute the selected interventions. Ideally patients come to know all the medical information relevant to their disease and the available interventions. Patients then select the interventions that best realize their values. The information model assumes a fairly clear distinction between facts and values. It is the physician's obligation to provide all the available facts, and the patient's values then determine what treatments are worthwhile based on those values. The physician is a technical expert providing the patient with the information necessary to make sound choices and exercise control. An emphasis on the informative model is embodied by the recent adoption of business terms in medicine. Physicians are described as health care providers and patients as consumers. It is also found in the language of patients' rights statements and in rules regarding human experimentation. Possibly the most forceful endorsement of the informative model rests in the ideals inherent in informed consent standards and statements.[11]

The aim of the physician in the interpretive model is to elucidate the patient's values and what he or she actually wants and to help the patient select the available medical interventions that realize these values. The physician's role is essentially the same as the informative model but takes on the additional task of helping the patient to give voice to his or her value system.[11]

The deliberative model directs the physician to explain to the patient the clinical situation and then help clarify the types of values embodied in the available clinical options. The physician's responsibilities and objectives include suggesting why certain health-related values are more worthy and should be aspired to. However, the physician discusses only health-related values, that is, values that affect or are affected by the patient's disease and treatments. To go beyond that boundary would be invasive of the patient's life. The physician recognizes and refrains from entering into the many elements of mortality that are unrelated to the patient's disease or treatment and therefore beyond the scope of the professional relationship. Coercion is avoided, and the patient must define his or her life and select the values to be acted on.[11]

If the physician does not actively promote one of these models, it is likely that the physician will either unconsciously adopt a particular model or follow the model espoused and promoted by the patient. When physicians enter practice and are responsible for patients' care, they naturally feel a strong sense of commitment to their patients. It is often precisely because of this sense of responsibility and caring that the physician takes over the total management of patients' illnesses to the point where the patients have to do nothing. All decisions are made for them. Patients are told what is wrong, they are told what to do and given the necessary medications or instructions, and are then left with the expectation of getting better.[12] In this paternalistic scenario, the patients make no decisions and thus can make no mistakes, and if they do not get better, it is the physician's fault. This effectively disempowers the person and puts him or her into the accepted sickness role. The role of the physician becomes one of what McKay et al.[12] call "oppressive caring," which translates into physician statements such as "I don't have any needs; I can cope with anything; I know what is best; I'll take care of everything; I am the expert, trust me; I have all the answers; I am the physician, I am trained to take over." Yet this omnipotent context of oppressive caring cannot be maintained by the physician. It will eventually inevitably fail because in this role, the physician becomes responsible not only for the treatment but also for the patient. The physician's attempts to control the patient will eventually run up against the patient's need for autonomy or the patient's simple failure to follow through on the orders of the physician. As a result, the physician begins to experience burnout, in what McKay et al.[12] defines as oppressed caring. Here the physician begins to feel: "I don't have any time for myself; I feel hopeless; I can't do anything to help; I've tried everything; the patients demand too much; stop depending on me; no one appreciates my caring; don't I get any privacy." The physician then oscillates between these two extremes, holding to the omnipotent oppressive care until it is no longer possible and then shifting to feeling oppressed. Each of these positions overstates the physician's role, one attributing more power and control to the physician than is real, the other abdicating responsibility. In this sense the physician may play out these polarities of existence as defined by gestalt psychology and creates a win-lose scenario in the relationship with the patient where the patient's sense of well-being and the physician's sense of well-being are in apparent competition.

The resolution of McKay et al.[12] to this impasse is for the physician to develop empowered caring, delineated in statements such as: "I have my own needs and you have yours; let's work together to sort out the problems; are there ways to cope with this? When I choose to give my time, I do so willingly; together we will find the solution; you do what you can and I will help you; your needs are important and so are mine." Here the physician and the patient are mutually active, they respect one another's needs, and they work together to achieve a result. The physician advises the patient, who then decides to accept or reject the advice, and the physician acknowledges that decision. A symbiosis of caregiver and patient roles with a mutual regard is promoted.[12]

The empowered caring of McKay et al.[12] and Emanuel's[11] deliberative model of interaction are quite similar. Both frameworks reject an authoritarian model of physician-patient interaction and direct the physician and the patient to acknowledge themselves and each other as people. Both must work together to maximize outcomes. The physician is directed to acknowledge the patient's humanity and recognize and respect the patient's life and values. Practice models that fail in this regard and thereby objectify patients are associated with increases in recidivism, litigation, and the cost of care, as well as decreases in compliance, beneficial behavioral changes, and overall quality of care.[7]

Freedman[13] further delineates the need for the physician to recognize the patient beyond the illness by making a distinction between the ethic of care and the ethic of rights. The ethic of rights focuses on autonomy, informed consent, and the hierarchy of expert physician imparting information to the less knowledgeable patient. The ethic of care focuses on connection and relationship. Together these define the physician's dual roles of autonomous expert and connected and caring human being.

Whichever model the physician promotes, the mere fact of that acceptance does not bring the patient to act appropriately. The physician not only must be consistent in playing out the role but also must be able to influence the patient to play his or her respective part as well.

NARRATION: THE PATIENT IN PERSONAL CONTEXT

Advances in technology have changed the nature of health care. A greater reliance on laboratory results and machines for diagnosis and treatment has changed perceptions of health and illness along with altering perceptions of the relationship between physician and patient.[14] One of the changes that has resulted is the patient coming to the physician rather than the physician going to the patient.

Rees[15] argues that when a physician saw a patient in his or her own environment, an opportunity to comprehend the total background of the patient's life existed and that the phrase "clinical picture" should refer to more than a photograph of a patient sick in bed. "It is an impressionistic painting of the patient surrounded by his home, his work, his relatives, his friends, his joys, sorrows, hopes and fears."[15] Patients, when seen in their own environment, retain a greater sense of self, conversation with the patient is inseparable from diagnosis and treatment, and the patient's role as a narrator of the illness is crucial. Rees[15] argues that this context is one of the most important elements of care.

With trends toward efficiency of time and place and the increasing complexity of diagnosis and treatment modalities, the patient's role as narrator of his or her own illness has been put aside.

Beckman and Frankel[16] found that physician did not allow patients to complete their opening statement of concern in 69% of visits, interrupting patients after a mean time of 18 seconds. Information was sought almost exclusively through the use of closed-ended, physician-centered questions. Once patients were interrupted, fewer than 2% went on to complete their statements. Their conclusion is premature termination of the patient's initial statement had the effect of making early clinical material the primary diagnostic focus. In a similar context Frankel[17] found that 94% of physician interruptions resulted in the physician taking charge of the conversation.

Yet as Smith and Hoppe[18] point out, every patient has a story that demonstrates the interaction among the biological, psychological, and social components of his or her life. The patient's story emerges in a meaningful, integrated, and complete way that identifies the patient's relationship to his or her illness. The physician's task is to elicit and understand this story, because it provides an introduction to the patient and why he or she is seeking treatment.

Smith and Hoppe's[18] conception of an ideal interview integrates the patient-centered and physician-centered approaches, where the patient leads in the areas or his or her life such as symptoms, concerns, preferences, and values, and the physician leads in areas to technical expertise such as the details of diagnosis.

Smith and Hoppe[18] are making a clear distinction between symmetrical and complementary tasks and encouraging the patient to increase involvement in care, leading to an increase in self-sufficiency as a sharing of power occurs and patient autonomy grows. It is through this type of patient-centered interview that a connection between patient and physician is established because the physician can then express such humanistic attributes as respect and empathy.

Shapiro[19] asserts that stories are a primary means of organizing and making sense of our world and are integral in developing solutions to problems and coping with experience and then argues:

> The classic example of narrative in medicine is the patient history, or medical interview. This is the opportunity for patients to present an account of their illness through the prism of personal experience and values. However, the medical interview has become so structured and analyzed that it runs the risk of becoming simply one more mechanistic tool in the armamentarium of the contemporary physician. Nevertheless, it is through the interview (and subsequent follow-up dialogs) that the physician has the best opportunity to access the subjective, idiosyncratic context in which the presenting symptoms occur.

The story reflects not only the patient's relationship to the present but also his or her association to the past. Cassel[9] states:

> The experiences gathered during one's life are a part of today as well as yesterday. Memories exist in the nostrils and the hands, not only in the mind. A fragrance drifts by, and a memory is evoked. My feet have not forgotten how to roller-skate, and my hands remember skills that I was hardly aware I learned. When these past experiences involve sickness and medical care, they can influence present illness and medical care. They stimulate fear, confidence, physical symptoms, and anguish. It damages people to rob them of their past and deny their memories, or to mock their fears and worries. A person without a past is incomplete.

In addition, every patient has a perceived future. There are events that the patient expects to come to pass. The intrusion of illness alters these perceptions, and the patient may suffer a loss of this expected future, leading to a loss of sense-of-self if a substitute, acceptable expectation is not created. Disease can alter the person's relationship with his or her body. It becomes untrustworthy. This is intensified if the illness comes on without warning, and if the illness persists, the person may feel increasingly vulnerable. "Just as many people have an expanded sense of self as a result of changes in their bodies from exercise, the potential exists for a contraction of the sense through injury to the body."[9]

The patient's story, then, is not a literal recreation of experience. Rather, it is an attempt at construction of a coherent account of how the patient's life came to this point and what might be done to ameliorate the problems. In this context the patient's presentation of the story may be evaluated as either pathogenic or therapeutic. Pathogenic stories promote illness, loss of function, diminishment of the person, and alienate both patient and physician, whereas therapeutic stories promote healing, competence, and a relationship between the patient and others. One goal of using storytelling in health care can be the transformation of the patient's narrative into a story of healing. The patient's telling of the story and the physician's reaction to it may have therapeutic value by restoring the patient's disrupted connectedness, reducing anxiety and guilt, and giving coherence to the patient.[19]

It is important to note that the physician also takes the patient's story and transforms it into a medical narrative. Consequently, two distinct narratives are involved: the patient's original motivating account related to the physician and the medical account, a metastory, constructed by the physician from selected parts of the patient's narrative and from the physical findings. These two versions of the same story can hamper mutual understanding and impede communication. This medical narrative must be retranslated to the patient's context before being returned to the patient with respect to diagnosis, prognosis, and recommendations for treatment. Rees[15] argues that much of the tension in health care encounters stems from a poorly defined narration to patients where physicians too often regard the medical version as the reality and neglect the retelling of the story to the patients in a meaningful way.

The patient narrative reveals the patient's understanding of his or her illness, but it also affects the relationship between physician and patient because it involves both the act of telling the story and the act of responding to it. In valuing the narrative, the physician is not simplistically taking a history but including the patient in a collaborative process of transforming the narrative over time, cocreating a positive outcome from a mutually agreeable position. Consequently, the physician has a responsibility to challenge the patient's story, to look for hidden relationships and meanings, to help the patient gain a momentum and depth, and to draw out a story of therapeutic value.

Emanuel and Emanuel state the following:[11]

> The patient's values are not necessarily fixed and known to the patient. They are often inchoate, and the patient may only partially understand them; they may conflict when applied to specific situations. Consequently, the physician working with the patient must elucidate and make coherent these values. To do this the physician works with the patient to reconstruct the patient's goals and aspirations, commitments and character. At the extreme, the physician must conceive the patient's life as a narrative whole, and from this specify the patient's values and their priority.

LaCombe[20] eloquently pleads, "Let us allow ourselves to become a part of the case history—a part of the stories in which we may play many roles—stories about that moment of sharing, when all defenses are down, when nothing else matters, when the lines of priority are drawn. That is where the greatest reward in medicine can be found.

Finally, it is important to understand the patient's story in the therapeutic triangle of relationships among the physician, patient, and family. The patient's story is not complete without the relationship of the patient to the significant other in his or her life. Epstein and Beckman[21] view the concept of the physician and patient as a dyad, or fundamental unit, in medical care as an illusion, noting that the family is involved in most of what takes place between the physician and patient whether present in the office at the time of the visit or not. Inclusion of the family in both the narrative and in action provides an important resource in assessment and treatment planning beginning with obvious information such as previous family history of the patient's illness to important relationship and support issues such as identifying who in the family is concerned about the problem and what others have done about the problem. The effectiveness of a treatment program can quickly become compromised if a family member who has been involved in care becomes marginalized.

PHYSICIAN AND PATIENT IN RELATIONSHIP

Smith and Thompson[7] contribute the following:

> Balint metaphorically described the physician, in addition to his or her biomedical ministrations, as a "drug" to which the patient may robustly respond. Balint's studies with general practitioners showed that the dosage, form and frequency of administration of the "drug" called "doctor" (i.e., length of appointments, interactions during appointments, and intervals between appointments) have major therapeutic implications for many patients.

There is a potent therapeutic value inherent in good physician-patient relationships. This beneficial aspect of the relationship between physician and patient has sometimes been labeled as a *placebo* effect. However, the term placebo inaccurately implies that this effect is passive and harmless. Good physician-patient relationships have an effect that is active, effective in relieving suffering, and not harmless if misused.[7]

This interaction is characterized by the exchange of information between the physician and the patient. Information exchange occurs, according to linguistic theory,[22] on three different levels referred to as syntax, semantics, and pragmatics. Whereas syntax is the basic structure of the language, the words used, and the sentences constructed, semantics has to do with the meaning of those words, the definitions, and also the variety and subtlety of the different uses of words. Words have many different meanings, and at times, the meaning of what people say is not always clear. Finally, there are the pragmatics of communication, that is, the practical effects of the communication, what happens as a result of the communication. It is the pragmatics of the communications that determine the relationship and that affect the rules or patterns of exchange of information that develop. Your patient's behavior affects you as a physician, and your behavior as a physician affects the patient's behavior.

Quite clearly, patients react to the behaviors and context set by the physician and either fit into their assigned roles or promote a different role. This is also true for physicians. The physician will react to the context set by the patient. Difficult relationships are often a consequence of a breakdown in agreed roles and communication between physician and patient. Schwenk and Romano[23] found that physicians find as many as 10% of all patient interactions to be highly frustrating and suggest that the common causes of the difficult physician-patient relationship include physician expectations that are not met by the relationship, norms that are challenged by the patient's behavior, and patient expectations that are not met by the relationship.

There are two hidden assumptions in the role theory models of doctoring that create problems for physicians. The first is the assumption that the role is monolithic, which creates the debate over how far toward autonomy the physician can go without losing the control of the treatment, creating a win-lose scenario in the context of a zero-sum game where every bit of autonomy that the patient gains is a loss of control for the physician. The second assumption is that if the physician plays the desired role that the patient will play the reciprocal role. This defines the entire relationship at least on a metalevel as complementary, holding the assumption that the patient must follow along and invests a metalevel power with the physician that he or she can control the behavior of the patient through the assumption of the role. Such models also imply that the physician can choose to influence or not influence the patient's choices and behavior. The influence is unescapable!

Whenever the physician communicates a message to the patient, that act is a maneuver that works to define the relationship. By what is said and the way it is said an indication of the sort of relationship desired is communicated. The patient is thereby posed the problem of either accepting or rejecting the physician's maneuver and definition of the relationship.[24] Health care providers are typically seen by patients as powerful figures. In communication with patients, physicians are constantly giving verbal and nonverbal suggestions. Kelly[25] notes that all of these suggestions can be thought of as informal hypnotic communication and can work to enhance or hinder therapeutic outcomes, and much of the art of medicine can be thought of in terms of suggestions given to, received by, and acted on by patients. "Many gifted clinicians have intuitively incorporated therapeutic suggestion into their communication with patients without realizing it, or at least without labeling what they do as therapeutic suggestion."[25]

Haley[24] argues that in the interchange between any two people, they must deal not only with what kind of behavior is to take place between them but how that behavior is to be qualified or labeled. Consequently, two issues arise: what kind of behaviors are to take place in this relationship and who is to control what is to take place in the relationship and thereby control the definition of the relationship. It is not possible for the physician to avoid being involved in this struggle over the definition of the relationship with the patient. Both are constantly involved in defining the relationship or countering the other person's definition.

Watzlawick et al.[22] make the same distinction by identifying two parts to any communication: a report and a command. The report aspect of a message conveys information; the content of the message. This content may be about anything that is communicable regardless of truth or validity. The command aspect, on the other hand, defines the meaning of the message and therefore ultimately determines the nature of the relationship.

In the interaction with patients, two things are always occurring: the content of what is being talked about and the relationship being negotiated. Whenever communication takes place, there is not only the communication of content but also the communication of relationship, what is happening at any moment and the relationship being established.

Haley[24] states:

> A basic rule of communications theory demonstrates the point that is impossible for a person to avoid defining, or taking control of the definition of, his relationship with another. According to this rule, all messages are not only reports but they also influence or command. A statement such as "I feel badly today," is not merely a description of the internal state of the speaker. It also expresses something like "Do something about this," or "Think of me as a person who feels badly."

By "control" Haley[24] does not mean that one takes control of the other person's behavior. The emphasis is not on the struggle to control another person but on the struggle to control the definition of a relationship. Two people inevitably work out together what kind of relationship they have by mutually indicating what kind of behavior is to take place between them. By behaving in a certain way, they define the relationship as one where that type of behavior is to take place. Patients may take on a role of helplessness and control whatever behavior is to take place in the relationship, just as the physician may act authoritarian and insist that the patient behave accordingly. The helpless behavior may influence the physician to respond with authoritarian behavior. If the patient acts helpless, she or he may be taken care of by the physician and in a sense be in the control of the physician, but by acting helpless the patient defines the relationship as one where he or she is taken care of.

There is a fundamental connection between the roles that we play and the relationship we have. The roles stem out of the relationships and are altered by the relationship. Coulter[26] points out, "Roles are locked together by a form of social glue—the rights of one, the patient, are the obligation of the other, the doctor . . . . Roles are mostly defined in terms of the counter role and cannot be defined in isolation—you cannot be a teacher without students, a husband without a wife, a doctor without patients, at least not in the long term."

It is important for physicians to become aware that these roles have a dramatic effect on how patients cooperate and comply. The way in which these roles develop between physician and patient has led to a number of problems in the delivery of health care. On the relationship level a struggle develops in the competition for power and control over the patient's life. The physician takes charge for the good of the patient, and the patient either attempts to regain a sense of autonomy by sabotaging the physician's efforts, or assumes a passive role by regarding control of health care as something outside, having no direct relevance. In either case the patient will be noncompliant with the physician's orders.[10]

The negotiations, or maneuvers of physician and patient, to define the relationship are related to each one's interests and goals in the encounter based on each's needs, desires, concerns, and fears. It is these interests that motivate both the physician and patient. Although physician and patient may have a common interest in the health of the patient, the positions that each takes to achieve goals based on that common interest may not be compatible. A focus on the positions taken will likely lead to a failure to develop cooperation. Fisher and Ury[27] encourage that in any such negotiation it is important to identify the compatible interests behind these opposing positions and to not fall victim to the assumption that because the patient's positions are opposed to the physician's that the patient's interests must also be opposed.

In addition, it is important to recognize that both physician and patient have many interests, not just one. These interests include all aspects of physician and patient as individual human beings.

Fisher and Ury[27] state the following:

> In searching for the basic interests behind a declared position, look particularly for those bedrock concerns which motivate all people. If you can take care of such basic needs, you increase the chance both of reaching agreement and, if an agreement is reached, of the other side's keeping to it. Basic human needs include: security, economic well-being, a sense of belonging, recognition, and control over one's life.

This framework is expressed in the description of Epstein et al.[28] of a patient-centered method of patient interviewing. In this method, the physician's responsibility includes understanding the meaning of the illness for the patient, as well as interpreting it in terms of the medical frame of reference. Based on a shared understanding, the physician works to find common ground with the patient about the problem and its management. To accomplish this, Epstein et al.[28] suggest that the interview use techniques of open-ended questioning, an open-to-closed cone of questioning to progressively narrow the focus of the narrative, facilitation (tell me more about that), clarification (tell me what you mean by that), checking (this is what you said?), and surveying for new problems. The development of this rapport not only increases patient satisfaction by humanization of the physician-patient encounter but also increases the efficiency of data gathering, improves physician outcome, and increases physician satisfaction.

This approach requires a shift from the traditional power balance between physician and patient. Patients are granted the opportunity to express themselves and encouraged to take more control over the process. The goal becomes to create understanding on a person-to-person level and is based on the development of trust and commitment. Finally, it is the patient who validates the patient centeredness of the process.

Changes of this sort give new meaning to concepts such as informed consent. With this approach, informed consent can no longer be viewed as a discrete act that takes place at a circumscribed point in time, usually before treatment, where there is an emphasis on the disclosure of information and the patient is invited to decide whether to accept the physician's recommendations. Rather, informed consent is integrated into the physician-patient relationship at all stages of medical decision making, requiring continuous care by the physician and active participation by the patient.[15]

Rees[15] states:

> What passes as disclosure and consent is so often an attempt by physicians to shape the disclosure process so that patients will comply

with their recommendations. In this manner, informed consent represents a legitimization by the patient of the doctor's unilateral professional decision. Dialogue with patients is not always conducted in the spirit of inviting patients to share with their physicians the burden of decision and is viewed only as a necessary formality to avoid a malpractice suit. [This] undermines the role of the form in the shared decision-making process and perpetuates adversity in the physician-patient relationship.

Turk and Rudy[3] review the treatment literature and suggest that an important step in increasing compliance and, consequently, long-term maintenance of treatment efficacy is to involve the patient in the design and mode of implementing the treatment regimen. They conclude the patient should be engaged as a collaborator in customizing a self-care program to facilitate ongoing performance and that collaborative relationship should focus on the development of a mutually acceptable course of behavior. This facilitates the maintenance of therapeutic gains. Turk and Rudy conclude, "Clinicians and clinical investigators need to acknowledge the problem of nonadherence and address it throughout the treatment program. We need to be proactive rather than reactive if we hope to witness the maintenance of therapeutic gains following treatment of . . . patients."

Attempts by the physician to control the behavior of the patient define the relationship as authoritarian and noncollaborative. In addition, these attempts at control of the content of how the patient acts happen at the expense of control in the relationship. As the physician gets caught up in trying to control what the patient is doing, he or she becomes reactive rather than proactive in the relationship. As a result the patient develops more and more influence over the course of the interaction. Both patient and physician can then become frustrated as the relationship develops poorly. It is the physician's responsibility to direct the relationship not to control the behavior of the patient. Ultimately patients must be responsible for their own behavior.

The inescapable conclusion is that the more doctors try to control patients, the less the control they will have over the structure of the relationship. The corollary to this statement, and a basic principle for physicians to follow is—the more physicians focus on the relationship and attempt to control the relationship with patients, the more influence they will have over the patients. However, this influence comes at the expense of giving up attempts at direct control of patients' actions. Control in the relationship has to do with the rules of interaction and not with any one individual's behavior. The relationship that is established has to do not only with the actions of physician and patient but the meaning of those actions or the context in which they occur.

To improve outcomes, physicians must pay attention to the effect they have on patients. It means a shift of focus away from compliance based on the behavior of the patient toward cooperation based on the relationship. It means an increased awareness of the rules being established on a relationship level between the physician and the patient, an awareness that there is a negotiation going on. It is not an overt or obvious negotiation. It is not a negotiation in a sense of bargaining or bartering. It is a negotiation of the rules of interaction.

The physician can try to make rules explicit and sign a contract with the patient. Here are the rules, I am going to do this, and you are going to do that. However, it is actual development of the rules in the relationship that matter, not making the rules explicit or in getting a moment of compliance to a contract.

Yet, the physician is also responsible for establishing diagnosis and developing and directing the treatment plan if not the behavior of the patient. In this respect the physician by necessity is caught up in content and not relationship. The physician, then, is caught in a dual role of responsibility for the development of the relationship and development of the treatment plan. Both are essential elements of health care. As experts physicians must direct the patient on what to do, but they must also resist becoming invested in getting the patient to comply. To understand the difference in these roles it is helpful to differentiate the different types of interactions that occur.

STRUCTURES IN THE RELATIONSHIP BETWEEN PHYSICIAN AND PATIENT

One of the drawbacks to the modeling schemes just discussed is that they may inadvertently promote viewing the physician-patient relationship as monolithic, with physician and patient continually taking the same ideal stance. The relationship between physician and patient is as complex as any other human interaction. In that context it is helpful to understand, evaluate, and label the varied interactional sequences that exist between physician and patient.

People in relationships are caught in a constant web of action and reaction with no real or distinct breaks between one person's communication and the other's. These ongoing exchanges can quickly become quite complex. However, artificial breaks can be inserted to look at the basic dyads of communication between two people arbitrarily starting with one and looking at the other's response. Communication theory identifies that there are three of these basic kinds of interactional sequences that may occur between people: symmetrical, complementary, and paradoxical.[22]

Complementary interactions are defined as a relationship that is based on the difference between people. Parent-child is complementary, as is teacher-student and physician-patient. The roles are defined by the difference in stance between the two people, and power is shared unequally as a result. If two people are engaged in a complementary interaction, although one is assigned more power than the other, that complementary sequence is maintained because both sides promote it. Physicians are encouraged to take on the role of authority because the patients are acting in need. Patients are encouraged to act more helpless because physicians act out the role of expert. Often the person granted the majority of the power based on the complementary roles has the illusion of increased control in the relationship. However, the reality remains that each person is responsible for and in control of his or her own behavior. Attempts to control the behavior of the other person appear to succeed because the person in the one-down role allows for this definition of the relationship and acts as if the other person has that power. This illusion is maintained as long as both individuals maintain their relative positions, with each person playing out a different role in the interaction.

Complementary interactions have an important place in physician-patient relationships precisely because the physician is the expert. The physician has information about health care that the patient does not have. And, if one of the physician's responsibilities is the education of the patient, the physician must play the teacher role while the patient plays the student.

Although complementary interactions are an essential element of physician-patient relationships, they are not the only part of the relationship. One of the problems seen traditionally with physician-patient relationships is the physician continually maintaining a one-up role and the patient settling into a one-down role. The physician becomes an authoritarian figure, and the patient becomes a passive figure. Good health care is compromised when the patient is so passive. However, this scenario does not develop because physicians are power hungry and love to have control over their patients or because patients are helpless. The danger in complementary interactions is that the complementary nature of the relationship generalizes to all aspects of the relationship. It is invasive and promotes a monolithic one-up and one-down definition of roles in what might be called complementary "creep."

Because part of the physician-patient role is that the physician is the health expert and the patient or student has to listen to the physician's expertise, there is an inherent danger that it will immediately generalize and so become the rule governing behavior in all aspects of the interaction. Because the rules of any relationship begin to develop from the first moment of interaction or even from the first moment of surrogate interaction (the structure of the patient making an appointment for the physician's time and expertise) sets this danger in motion. It is something that physicians must guard against just as strongly as the problems of a symmetrical competition. If a physician gets caught up in a complementary interaction that generalizes to all aspects of the relationship, the patient is encouraged to become entirely dependent. Neighbour[8] suggests that a basic human response to illness may be regression toward a more dependent state, endowing physicians with power, but he also notes that physicians can easily become addicted to the role of expert.

Because the patient is coming in on a one-down position and feeling out of control in his or her life and because the physician is taking some responsibility for putting things back on track by being an expert in health care, the patient will immediately begin to start generalizing the relationship into a complimentary relationship over all its aspects. Physicians find the patient encouraging them to take responsibility, not just responsibility for the diagnosis, treatment plan, and education but for things that the physician has no right taking responsibility for— the patient's behavior and life. It is quite a natural tendency. Patients do not mean to do it; physicians do not mean to do it. It is not a deliberate, conscious act but a path of least resistance in the relationship.

As the physician slides into this ever increasing complementary interaction and lives the illusion of being in control of the patient's life, the potential for partnership deteriorates. The patient becomes increasingly passive and helpless, looking for the physician's input in areas beyond his or her expertise. Patients ask questions such as, "What should I tell my spouse about the problems that I'm having? How can I get them to cooperate with the treatment that you tell me to do?" or making statements such as, "That was too difficult for me to do. I forgot. I didn't have time. Life conspired against me to keep me from doing it."

In attempts to exercise control over the patient, it is very easy for physicians to become overwhelmed by that burden. One reason health care practitioners, psychologists, psychiatrists, and many people in the health community end up experiencing burnout is they end up becoming responsible for their patients' lives. Physicians cannot be responsible for how their patients live their lives. They are responsible for the diagnosis, treatment, and education of the patient. Of course, this is not to say that the physician should not care about the patient's behavior. Just as in education where the teacher is responsible for the quality of the teaching but cannot be responsible for the learning of the student, the physician is responsible for creating an atmosphere conducive to treatment that promotes the patient's participation but ultimately cannot be responsible for the patient following a treatment plan. If the complimentary nature of the relationship generalizes beyond appropriate bounds, however, the physician does attempt to be responsible, and the patient will encourage the physician to take this stand and at times even order the physician to be in charge or make the decisions, creating a no-win paradox for the physician. In addition, the physician is setting himself or herself up for unachievable expectations on the part of the patient, leading to patient dissatisfaction. Running the patient's life is beyond what is possible to do even if the attempts to do so are small. The physician cannot run the patient's life. The belief that this is possible stems from the patient's requests for direction or his or her current willingness to acquiesce to the physician's directives. The reality is that the physician never controls the patient's behavior but can only set a context from which to view that patient's behavior.

The second kind of interactional sequence is symmetrical. Symmetrical interactions are based on the concept of equality: people acting in the same way or doing the same thing. If two individuals exchange pleasantries, mutually support one another, argue with one another, defend themselves against the other, or ignore each other, they are acting in a symmetrical way. Each is doing the same thing that the other is doing. Symmetrical interactions are based on this idea of equality and sameness. The people in the interaction are mirroring each other's behavior. Symmetrical interactions are inherently neither negative nor positive. They may express mutual trust or mutual animosity or cooperation or competition.

The Emanuel-Emanuel[11] deliberative model and the empowered caring of McKay et al.[12] both require that the physician and patient act in symmetrical ways, promoting mutual recognition and responsibility. It is the delineation of the need for symmetrical interactions to obtain successful outcomes that differentiates these approaches from the traditional physician-patient models that viewed the interaction as entirely complementary. This symmetrical interaction is necessary for physician and patient to maintain a sense of self-esteem and for each person's needs to be expressed and met. It is through symmetrical interactions that physician and patient acknowledge one another, cooperation is established, and the patient becomes an active participant who makes an investment in his or her own health care.

If the physician is hoping for cooperation, some form of symmetrical interaction on a human level with that patient must be promoted to get that cooperation. Cooperation requires a symmetrical interaction in some ways. Slaves do not cooperate with masters; that is a contradiction in terms. The oppressed do not cooperate with the people who are oppressing them. They may be compliant, and they may have a choice in being compliant or not, but they are not cooperating. It does not make any sense to talk in those terms. Patients cannot be coerced into cooperating.

Whereas the danger in a complementary interaction is its invasion into other areas of the relationship, the danger in a symmetrical system lies in each side becoming competitive. Symmetrical interactions may deteriorate into what is called symmetrical escalation. Each side, in an attempt to become equal with the other and to be symmetrical, to have an equal stance with the other person, begins to compete. Out of fear of losing control or in an attempt to gain an advantage, competition arises. As each side continues to mirror the behavior of the other, these attempts to maintain or assert control are thwarted. A runaway system develops where each side continually expends more and more energy without breaking the equilibrium. Each side feels compelled to continue the escalation for fear of losing. On a geopolitical level, the nuclear arms race was a good example of such a symmetrical escalation. But whether on an international level between countries or in personal encounters between physician and patient, competition can emerge out of uncertainty and defensiveness in a symmetrical interaction.

Symmetrical encounters take place in the physician-patient interaction as both cooperation and competition. Cooperation exists with equal power sharing and a stable, positive symmetrical sequence in the relationship. Symmetrical escalation in negative terms of confrontation and arguing can certainly happen in a physician-patient interaction where the patient strives for control directly. However, patient noncompliance can also be defined as a competition for control in the relationship and be viewed as an attempt by the patient to act symmetrically with the physician. Patient noncompliant behavior operates as a passive-aggressive stance that serves as the patient's mechanism of competition because the patient is less likely to successfully compete for control directly because of their lack of technical expertise in health care.

The physician's acknowledgment of the patient as a human being and the patient's acknowledgment of the physician as a human being is a symmetrical interaction. Symmetry is essential in the relationship for this validation of the patient's and physician's humanity. If the physician does not validate that experience on the patient's part and does not act symmetrically toward him or her in that respect, the physician is damaging the relationship with the patient and limiting the patient opportunity to incorporate the health care regimen.

From the first moment of the relationship, the physician and patient are negotiating when to be symmetrical and when to be complimentary. Definition of those rules starts right from the beginning, and those rules are constantly being defined and redefined, actively supported or rejected. As the rules become quickly established, the danger of the complimentary interactions invading the relationship and the danger that the symmetrical interactions may develop into competition and escalate are real. These difficulties can be defined as the physician and patient falling into inappropriate complementary roles or inappropriate symmetrical roles. Operating out of a complementary stance in the area of the patient's behavior is inappropriate. A patient must remain autonomous and responsible for himself or herself as a person. Operating out of a symmetrical stance where it should be complementary is failing to take responsibility for health care. Responses to patient behavior should be designed to reestablish the correct boundaries of the relationship. For example, if the patient fails to carry through with a treatment regimen, because the patient is not cooperating, that is, acting symmetrically appropriate, the physician should respond and discuss the failure from a symmetrical stance, exploring the patient's experience and values but not attempting to coerce the patient to follow through, thus reinforcing the need for symmetrical behavior.

What are the correct applications of symmetrical and complimentary interactions with the patient? It is a balance. At times, symmetrical is appropriate. At other times, complimentary is required, and some fluidity between the two must exist. When the physician is involved in diagnosis, treatment, or education, a symmetrical interaction should take place. At all other moments, in all other respects, the relationship needs to be symmetrical. It is important to recognize that this balance must be struck from moment to moment in the interaction. Watzlawick[22] points out that symmetrical and complementary relationship patterns can stabilize each other, and changes from the one to the other pattern and back again are important homeostatic mechanisms. This entails a therapeutic implication that the physician can influence the direction of the relationship and the patient's relationship to their illness by the introduction of symmetry into complementarity or vice versa.

The third type of interaction sequence is paradoxical. This occurs as the result of a confusion between symmetrical and complementary. Symmetrical behavior cannot be demanded because the demand, by definition, is complementary behavior. A paradoxical interaction exists, then, where symmetrical behavior is ordered, hence creating confusion by attempting to promote symmetrical behavior and complementary behavior simultaneously. These paradoxical interactions are often referred to as be-spontaneous paradoxes. One person is ordering another to be spontaneous. But a behavior is not spontaneous if it has just been ordered; it is directed behavior. Once an order is given to someone, that order defines a complementary one-up position. Once ordered, symmetrical behavior becomes impossible.

This happens routinely in the physician-patient relationship on a number of occasions. Whenever the patient directs the physician to give care, a paradox is created for the physician. Who is in charge then? Who directs the care? Whenever the physician directs the patient to cooperate, a paradox is created for the patient. How can the patient maintain self-esteem and a sense of control once his or her autonomy is robbed by the order to cooperate? The patient is placed in a no-win one-down position, with loss of self-esteem with either choice.

Some paradoxes are much more subtle than others. The physician may not even be aware of the fact that there is a paradoxical interaction going on. For the most part, patients will not often explicitly play a one-up position with the physician. The kind of paradoxical interactions promoted by patients will not typically come from the patient standing up and demanding symmetrical behavior; however, that does occasionally occur. What is much more likely to happen, and what is much more subtle, is the patient takes a one-down, helpless position and by so doing directs the physician, "Take care of me!"

Another example of this paradox occurs when the patient offers a symmetrical, intimate relationship either by inquiring about the physician's private life or by making romantic advances toward the physician. These symmetrical interactions are inappropriate to the nature of the relationship, which is appropriately defined as complementary. If the physician responds to the request or invitation (positively or negatively), that response validates the symmetrical context offered by the patient. A positive response negates the professional relationship. A negative response does little better because it becomes defined as the physician's considered choice to a viable question. A response of "No!" in a symmetrical context might leave the patient feeling rejected, ashamed, and embarrassed, making it difficult for him or her to return without loss of face. Or, the patient might then simply wait or lobby for the physician to change that decision. The response in these scenarios should be complimentary.

These advances by the patient may be the result of the patient attempting to seize more control in the relationship by defining it in a more symmetrical way. Whether this is a genuine emotional response or not is irrelevant. In either case validation of the context negates the possibility of an effective physician-patient relationship by restructuring the rules of interaction.

On the physician's side, any attempt to promote an intimate, romantic relationship is inappropriate because the patient is forced to respond to this offer out of the complementary context that preceded it. The patient accepts, then, as the result of following the physician's recommendations as with a treatment prescription. The patient is responding to the complementary context by acting symmetrically in romantic terms as suggested by the physician. The requirement of a significant complementary aspect of the relationship negates the possibility of a symmetrical, romantic relationship. To operate out of both simultaneously, or even to move from one to the next in succession, puts the patient in a paradoxical situation. In addition, because of this initial unequal power sharing in the relationship, the patient is vulnerable and has a right to expect to be protected from the physician. Hence, symmetrical encounters of an intimate nature are considered unethical, and professional ethics codes expect a significant time lapse between the professional relationship and any relationship defined as symmetrical.

As with symmetrical and complementary interactions, paradoxical relationships have appropriate and positive application as well. These therapeutic paradoxes provide a no-lose situation, just as negative paradoxes create a no-win scenario. One of the most powerful of these paradoxes can be described as "symptom prescription." Here, the patient's seemingly disruptive behavior is directed by the physician to continue as a positive element in the treatment program. As a result, if the patient gives up the behavior in an attempt to be noncompliant, cooperation is enhanced by the elimination of the disruptive behavior. If the patient continues the behavior, the patient is compliant with the directive of the physician. For example, if the patient is challenging the treatment plan, the physician may instruct the patient to continue these challenges as a method to direct patient education.[29]

In any relationship there is a mix of symmetrical, complimentary and paradoxical. When one is dealing with patients, it is important to be aware of these interactional sequences. Physicians can benefit by awareness of the nature of the interaction, recognizing the negotiation and maneuvering that occur as the rules of the relationship are defined. It is not just a question of how the physician presents but a question of what rules of interaction are established. The relationship is not defined solely by the physician or the patient; it is defined by the relationship they have with each other.

Act complementary in those essential matters of education of the patient, diagnosis, and treatment plan. In all other respects, act symmetrical. If the patient has been given instructions to engage in a therapy and he or she does not, to tell the patient again (assuming that the patient has not forgotten what was said) or to insist that the patient does it changes the nature of the interaction from one of information giving to one of coercion where the physician attempts to control the behavior of the patient. The result is that either the patient will accept the one-down role and a complementary invasion, leading to a passive patient, or the patient will resist the coercion and a symmetrical escalation for control will begin. In either scenario, the physician has defected from the original model of interaction.

MODELING COOPERATIVE INTERACTIONS: PRISONER'S DILEMMA

Game theory is a method often used to evaluate potential outcomes in structured relationships. A game known as the "prisoner's dilemma" has been used repeatedly as a model to understand human as well as biological systems (Fig 1). The game is based on an interaction between two individuals where each has two options of behavior: cooperate or defect. The value or effectiveness of either possible response depends on a simultaneous choice that the other player makes. The only direction to the game is to be as successful as possible in accumulating points. With the game consisting of repetitive interactions of an undisclosed number, the strategies used and how players conceptualize success are instructive.

A competitive strategy of defection works best as long as the other person is willing to be taken advantage of. Mutually competitive behav-

		Doctor's Choices of Behavior	
		Cooperation	Defection
Patient's Choices of Behavior	Cooperation	Mutual Cooperation Patient receives 3 points Doctor receives 3 points	Patient receives 0 points Doctor receives 5 points for successful defection
	Defection	Patient receives 5 points for successful defection Doctor receives 0 points	Mutual defection Patient receives 1 point Doctor receives 1 point

FIGURE 1.
Prisoner's dilemma applied to physician-patient interactions.

iors, however, produce worse results than mutually cooperative behaviors. Yet, acting in a cooperative way makes the player vulnerable to competitive behavior from the other. Some strategies focus on the short-term success, accumulating points as quickly as possible with little thought of the effect or success of that strategy as the game progresses. When the game is perceived to be near the end or a short-term need to get points becomes pressing, these strategies predominate. Other strategies focus on long-term stability in point accumulation even at the expense of possible short-term gains. These are more likely used where the game appears that it will continue for some time.

The prisoner's dilemma game is an excellent, although abstract, description of the dynamics of physician-patient interactions. Physicians and patients both are interested in maximizing the outcome of the relationship. The physician is trying to be as effective as possible, and the patient is trying to get as healthy as possible. Patients want their health, but this health is a complex combination of many needs that includes both physical and psychological well-being. Physicians want to be effective, but effectiveness holds many different dimensions.

These goals of physician and patient are symbiotic, although not identical. If a physician is concerned for the welfare of his or her patient, the physician's self-interest can be thought of as including this concern for the patient. But this does not necessarily eliminate all potential for conflict between them. Concern for others does not ensure that cooperation will take place.[30] With physicians and patients, as in the prisoner's dilemma game, mutual gain is possible but not inevitable. Defensiveness, uncertainty, fear of vulnerability, a desire for quick results, and anticipation that the relationship will end all promote a strategy to defect. Once defection occurs, the discussion of its appropriateness often follows, along with accusations, blame, coercions, and arguments, all with a dramatic effect on the relationship between the players. As in any relationship, the actions taken work to define that relationship.

Cooperation and noncooperation by physician and patient can be understood as prisoner's dilemma strategies:

> The theoretical game model of cooperation has applications in health care as well. It appears to us that both patients and doctors have been competitive with each other, continually defecting. The patient defects by noncompliance with the healing regimen, with the payoff being maintenance of autonomy, while the doctor defects by maintaining control and authority through refusing to attend to the patient's perceived needs. Each of these positions is safe and reasonable when anticipating noncooperation.[10]

Patient noncooperative behavior may be viewed as a lost opportunity for improved health but may also be experienced by the patient as a won opportunity to feel healthier based on a greater sense of autonomy. Particularly where treatment has been ineffective or is nearing completion, autonomy may become the more dominant motivation. Yet defection to achieve autonomy comes only where that autonomy is not better achieved by cooperation. The more the physician attempts to direct the behavior of the patient, the more likely patient autonomy will be associated with defection.

Within the prisoner's dilemma, as with physicians and patients, strategies to control or direct the choice of the other are not effective. No matter what is said or done, each player continues to act out of self-interest. Self-interest and mutual interest are not necessarily at odds because the prisoner's dilemma is not a zero-sum game. One of the significant principles to emerge from game theory is that cooperation can develop out of a pragmatic strategy for individual success. Because mutual cooperation is desirable but not inevitable, what strategy can promote it? A strategy labeled as tit-for-tat has proved to be the most successful. It operates on two simple rules: On round one of the game, choose cooperation, on every successive round, select the other player's choice from the previous round.

Because of the behavior of the person playing this strategy, it is in the other player's best interest to choose to cooperate, because any other choice will, very quickly (in two rounds of the game), yield a lower score. Thus, it is successful because its success promotes mutual success.

The power of this approach is clear: It offers cooperation, is never the first to defect, always responds immediately to defection, but never seeks revenge. It cannot be taken advantage of, nor will it take advantage of others. It will also never score higher than the other player. It does not define success competitively. Tit-for-tat is effective not because it continues with cooperation as long as the other side does but because its immediate response to defection makes defections by the other side unrewarding. It is the dual strategy of offering cooperation with never initiating defection and the immediate action against defection that promotes stable mutual cooperation.

Players facing the prisoner's dilemma strategy quickly realize that they can do no better than to go along with it. The prisoner's dilemma is a robust strategy because it defines the rules of the relationship, regardless of the choices of player facing it. It is a metastrategy because it never attempts to coerce or take advantage of the choice of the other side. It defines the relationship as one where "I will follow the choices you make." By defining the relationship in this way and acting on that definition, the relationship is encouraged to stabilize with mutual cooperation.

How does tit-for-tat translate to physician and patient? The strategy is based on three basic principles: offer cooperation at the start; make immediate responses to competitive behaviors; and direct those responses to promoting a stable relationship, not to altering the behavior of the other player. The first two principles are straightforward; the third requires some explanation. The significant element of the patient's noncooperative behavior is not the action itself but the potential change in the rules in the relationship that develop because of that choice. Therefore, the doctor's response should be directed to stabilize the relationship. The patient's noncooperative behavior offers a competitive context to the relationship. If the physician stabilizes the relationship as cooperative, the patient's action is unsuccessful at defining the relationship as competitive, and the behavior of the patient takes on a new meaning. No behavior has only one meaning. Meaning derives from the context in which a behavior takes place and the context derives from the relationship. Consequently, the meaning of a patient's behavior lies in the effect it has on the relationship. It follows that physicians should focus on the relationship with patients and not on the content of the patient's behavior. Controlling the rules of the relationship appears to be the key to productive physician-patient interactions.

A number of rules define an interaction as a prisoner's dilemma. One important factor is the relative values of the payoffs in the different cells. If the value of mutual cooperation is higher than defection, there is no reason to not cooperate. Only if defection is viewed as potentially better than mutual cooperation and mutual defection better than being taken advantage of does a prisoner's dilemma exist. Where the payoff for defection is low compared with the gains for cooperation, defection is unlikely. Consequently, where the patient is experiencing a significant loss of control and serious illness, a prisoner's dilemma scenario does not exist. At that point, the patient does better by picking cooperation regardless of the actions of the physician. But as the patient improves and the value of cooperation diminishes relative to competition, a prisoner's dilemma does emerge. Noncooperation, then, becomes a real possibility in the relationship when the patient feels sufficiently healthy, either physically or psychologically, to gain from defection. Because this subjective sense of health will not necessarily be correlated with the patient's need for physical treatment, a prisoner's dilemma scenario is always possible.

Another important factor in the success of a tit-for-tat strategy stems from the anticipation of continued interactions. In any relationship where the future is viewed as relatively unimportant, chances for cooperation are diminished. Players tend to value payoffs less as the time of their obtainment recedes into the future and there is the chance that this future may not occur. Treatment plans that do not offer relief in the immediate future are less likely to get patient cooperation. For these reasons the immediate payoff always counts more than future payoffs. The importance of future payoffs relative to the current behavior is labeled by Axelrod[30] as the "discount parameter." It represents the degree to which the payoff of a future move is less influential or discounted relative to the current move. If the discount parameter is sufficiently high, that is, if the needs of the present moment are in the foreground, the chances for mutual cooperation are diminished. During the early stages of patient care, the patient cannot afford detection due to the loss of future potential treatment. When patients enter treatment, as long as the expectation is that the physician can do something to alleviate the patient's illness in the future, the discount parameter is low and the value for compliance is high.

However, both physician and patient prefer to achieve a given benefit today rather than having to wait for the same benefit until some future time. Physicians are encouraged to defect to achieve short-term results, that is, they will become authoritarian to get immediate results. As long as the future treatment is important enough to the patient, he or she will allow this behavior by the physician. But as the treatment continues and the value of future interactions drops in importance, the payoff for cooperation goes down. This loss of importance can derive from either a physician or patient attitude of disease management, where, once the problem is gone, there is no need to continue care with the physician or by an increased urgency of other needs such as the patient desiring to regain a sense of autonomy lost in a too complementary relationship with the physician. Mutual cooperation will be stable only if the future is sufficiently important relative to the present. Hence, primary care, with an ongoing relationship between physician and patient, provides the environment for the highest rate of patient compliance. The more important the future becomes, the greater the chances of cooperation continuing.

Strategies that are unsuccessful within the prisoner's dilemma provide a mechanism for predicting what will be unsuccessful strategies in the physician-patient relationship. Strategies that begin with defections promote mutual distrust and encourage mutual defection. Strategies that do not respond immediately to defection allow that defection to be successful. In addition, when delayed responses to defection do occur, they are likely to be viewed either as revenge or as unrelated to the initial defection.

Many physicians resort to reason and logic as a strategic response to noncooperation. The assumption is made that an explanation of why cooperation is more beneficial than other behaviors will influence the patient. If it can only be explained to the patient, he or she will have to come around and do what is expected. Information may be necessary for a cooperative patient to behave appropriately, but the education itself does not create the cooperation. Education does not create cooperation because education by its nature establishes a complementary interaction. Cooperation is symmetrical.

When the physician's attempts to persuade the patient by reason and logic fail, the physician may escalate to coercion. Yet, cooperation cannot be coerced. A bribe, a threat, a deal, and an order are attempts at coercion. All are attempts to try to control the patient. Reason and logic fail then, because on the relationship level, they belong to a set of actions that attempts to get the patient to behave in a particular way. As a result, they are a form of coercion, albeit benevolent coercion in the patient's best interest.

With patients, once cooperation is established, reason and logic are wonderful things. Once patients are cooperative, they will be able to successfully use information to become even better patients. But the cooperation must precede the information and education. In a cooperative context, then, reason and logic work well. If, however, reason and logic are presented in a noncooperative context, a fight is encouraged. Competition and debate emerge. A alternate outcome may be continued patient passivity, fostered by the complementary interaction. Here the patient will not use or integrate the information provided.

As Axelrod[30] notes, "Promoting good outcomes is not just a matter of lecturing the players about the fact that there is more to be gained from mutual cooperation than mutual defection. It is also a matter of shaping the characteristics of the interaction so that over the long run there can be a stable evolution of cooperation."

When patients come in for treatment, they are already in a one-down position because they are seeking help. Attempts by the physician to achieve short-term gains by taking advantage of this patient vulnerability lead to a destabilization of the relationship. Attempts to direct the behavior of the patient will make the pattern of responses less predictable. This is true regardless of whether the patient has encouraged the physician to act in this way! Even when the patient is compliant, if the physician takes that as a indication that he or she does not need to promote patient autonomy, it is a defection from cooperation by the physician! Doing well with patients who are willing to abdicate responsibility for their lives by allowing the physician to be authoritarian is eventually a self-defeating process. The lesson is that not being cooperative may look promising at first, but in the long run it will destroy the very environment needed for success. And the physician-patient interaction is likely to deteriorate into either rivalry or accusation and threat as the physician's attempts to control the patient begin to fail.

As the patient begins to regain a sense of autonomy, competition often emerges as a struggle for control over the patient's behaviors. Patients are hesitant to relinquish the often tenuous autonomy that they retain. Physicians are just as hesitant to give up control over what is happening in terms of the therapy. Neither physician nor patient may be viewing his or her own behavior as a form of defection. Each side begins to perceive the other side as having defected first. Physicians often perceive that treatment fails because of the failure of the patient to cooperate. The physician thinks, "Why is that patient resisting? He came to me for help. Why doesn't he just go along and let me help him?" Patients begin to view the physician as not helping. Each feels justified in his or her position as the relationship drifts toward mutual defection. Each side begins to mistrust the other and becomes defensive. Each begins to expect the other to allow a relationship where successful defection is possible.

Some patients take the strategy of always competing and never following the treatment plan. It is not that they have no interest in their own health care. They are coming, they have invested in their health care, but they are not willing to take the risk to cooperate. They do not know how to go about taking that risk; they are on the defensive. It is a safe position in the relationship, a way of maintaining control, albeit at the expense of improved physical health.

Even in the event that both sides cooperate from the beginning, the relationship is not necessarily stable. Without a strategy of response to defections, the relationship remains uncertain even in the face of continuing cooperation. Without a defection by either physician or patient, neither side can be sure of the other's response to that defection and instability develops.

Three strategies are essential in establishing and fostering a cooperative relationship with your patient. Offer cooperation. Make it an immediate response to a noncooperative behavior by the patient, and make that response on a relationship level. Attempts to establish a cooperative relationship require a focus on the relationship and rejection of any attempt to control the patient's behavior. Attempts to control the patient are a defection from a cooperative interaction. Often physicians give up the goal of cooperation for the short-term gains, hoping that it will not meet with resistance. The success achieved will be, at best, only temporary and illusory, because the long-term effect to the relationship is deleterious. The relationship becomes destabilized and drifts toward mutual defection.

Any variation from a tit-for-tat strategy reduces the likelihood of mutual cooperation. Cooperation is advanced by a focus on the relationship and establishing appropriate rules in the relationship. This means, in a sense, a kind of dance between the physician and the patient. How the physician responds to the patient and how the patient responds to the physician defines the relationship. It has nothing to do with specifically the content of how the patient acted or what the patient said or the content of how the physician acted or what the physician said. It has to do with the pragmatic effect of each of those actions on the definition of the relationship. As Haley[24] noted, every behavior operates to determine the rules of the relationship. Physicians cannot *not* influence the relationship and consequently are faced with two options: benevolently manipulate the structure of the relationship to promote cooperation or abdicate control of the relationship to the patient by following the patient's definition of the encounter.

How does the physician establish a stable relationship where the needs of both physician and patient are met? Specifically, what physician behaviors work to promote patient cooperation? How is the momentum of a passive-dependent relationship fostered by the complementary nature of the physician and patient roles overcome?

CONCLUSIONS: DIMENSIONS OF CAREGIVING

What then are the essential issues of the physician in the relationship with the patient? Delbanco[31] identifies seven dimensions of care given by the physician: respect for patient's values, communication and education, coordination and integration of care, physical comfort, emotional support and alleviation of fears and anxieties, involvement of family and friends and continuity and transition, and respect for values.

Epstein et al.[28] name three core functions of the interaction between physician and patient: gathering of data to understand the patient; development of rapport and response to the patient's emotions; and patient education and behavioral management. The development of rapport rests on the physician's ability to respond to the patient's emotions with reflection, legitimation, support, partnership, and respect. These characteristics create what Allen[32] describes as a patient-centered interview where the patient leads the conversation and the physician expresses empathy, sensitivity, and respect toward the patient, which leads to open-ended, emotion-oriented responses that allow the patient to act out of a cooperative role.

These dimensions of care stem from a model of physician-patient interaction based on cooperation rather than confrontation where added dimensions of care evolve from the physician's increased responsibility as both a technical expert and a supportive participant in relationship with the patient. Consequently, a cooperative model takes into account not only the application of technical knowledge but also the complexities of communication with the patient. There is no real alternative to this model because physician and patient cannot escape having an impact on each other in the relationship. In physician-dominated relationships with the focus on the illness, the exercise of physician power necessarily distorts the decision-making and treatment process for both physician and patient by creating a polarization between them.

Patient-centered care is a principle to be followed by the physician to promote cooperation, regardless of the expectations of the patient. Physicians should not defect from maintaining these dimensions of care because of a perception that the patient is helpless or even at the request of the patient. The patient's definition of the relationship is not necessarily a therapeutic one. Such requests and perceptions likely stem from a noncooperative relationship.

With a recognition of the necessity to deal with the relationship to provide for successful outcomes, physicians must master a hierarchy of skills, one building on the next to be successful in promoting and maintaining cooperation. This hierarchy proceeds from acknowledgment of the patient to acceptance to understanding to empathy to flexibility. With each skill there are competing, and tempting, noncooperative options that the physician must avoid.

ACKNOWLEDGMENT VS. DISQUALIFICATION

Acknowledgment of the patient occurs when discussion during the medical visit includes psychosocial topics, thus asserting the patient's existence as a person. These acknowledgments include everything from eye contact and using the patient's name to an exploration of the patient's emotions and values. Bertakis et al.[33] found patients were more satisfied with their health care when the physician made these acknowledgments than when the visit is restricted to biomedical exchanges. The more questions asked of patients regarding psychosocial topics and the fewer questions asked in the biomedical realm, the more satisfied patients appeared.

In addition, the more psychosocial talk the patient engaged in and the less biomedical talk, the more satisfied the patient was. It was also found that the more the physician dominated the talk of the visit, either in actual talk or in directing the context, the less satisfied the patient was. In addition, Ben-Sira[34] noted that the patient's evaluation of the physician's ability to discuss psychological issues will affect the patient's evaluation of the physician's biomedical abilities.

Disqualification is a response to a communication that negates the existence of all or part of that communication—failing to recognize some aspect of the patient as a human being. Often this can occur despite the physician's best attempts at acknowledgment because not all of the patient's experience is immediately obvious to the physician. Any disqualification of the patient, intentional or not, sets the stage for a noncooperative interaction. Either the patient will accept the disqualification based on the need to receive health care, and treat herself or himself as less valuable and less able to contribute, promoting a passive response, or the patient will become passive-aggressive and in some way attempt to regain self-esteem and control through a sabotage of the interaction.

Bowman's[35] comment that the lack of sufficient attention to psychosocial issues may be more related to dissatisfaction than the presence of attention is related to satisfaction is well taken. Failure of the physician to acknowledge the patient may likely promote noncompliance but simply giving recognition to the patient's psychosocial concerns falls far short of the basics needed to engender cooperation. Acknowledgment is important but only an initial step toward promoting cooperation in the relationship with patients. And it is not limited to a cursory acknowledgment of at the beginning of the session but is an ongoing attempt to notice the patient as a person throughout the course of treatment. This requires a constant attention to the patient's humanity, giving recognition and voice to the patient's experience as immediately as possible.

ACCEPTANCE VS. APPROVAL OR DISAPPROVAL

Acceptance becomes possible once the physician gives acknowledgment, or recognition, to the patient's experience. Acceptance, however, is not the same as approval. Approval and disapproval of the actions of the patient are, at base, value judgments of the patient and attempts to directly control the behavior of the patient either to ensure continuation of the current behavior or direct a change to something different. Both the approval and disapproval of the behavior of a patient can create problems in cooperation, because in trying to control the patient, control of the relationship is relinquished.

If the physician's disapproval works, that is, shows an immediate positive effect through the patient being more compliant, chances for cooperation have still been diminished. The relationship becomes less stable in the long term, and the goal of the relationship has changed. The original, symmetrical goal of seeking cooperation is replaced by the complementary goal of trying to seek the physician's approval. If the physician disapproves of the behavior and the patient, the physician is encouraging the patient to seek approval. The rule in the relationship then becomes trying to achieve the physician's approval rather than improving health.

Where the patient is compliant and the physician approves of a patient's behavior, the patient is still caught in this goal of trying to maintain the physician's approval. The patient must now worry about the change in the physician that will ensue as the result of failure. If success meets with approval, it is logical to conclude that failure will meet with disapproval. Hence, the patient is encouraged to be less than truthful to avoid possible recriminations. Patients may worry what the physician will think of them in their failure. The patient may begin hedging on the truth to avoid disapproval. Quite easily the game can become making the physician happy through offering those responses that will elicit approval whether or not they are factually true. The goal of seeking approval is promoted at the expense of the goal of health. It is important to recognize the contradictory nature of these different goals. One will take precedence over the other. Every time the patient is given approval or the patient seeks the physician's approval, the goal of physical well-being is undermined.

Whether the physician intends it to happen or not, patients often operate out of this context. They will seek the physician's approval and encourage the physician to give approval. Physicians can easily capitulate, figuring, what is the harm in a little approval? But the dangers are real. To acquiesce to this definition of the relationship promoted by the patient deters good health care.

This is not to say that a patient should not receive some behavioral reinforcement for health-appropriate actions. However, approval and disapproval are not the appropriate reinforcers for at least two other reasons. First, the approval will not likely be frequent enough or important enough to alter behaviors outside of the physician's office. Second, once active treatment stops, the active reinforcement of the behaviors through approval ceases, and the behavior will extinguish. Consequently, approval acts as a very poor reinforcer. What is an effective reinforcer? Behavioral scientists often argue that the best reinforcers are thoughts carried by patients in their heads. The most appropriate reinforcer is the patient's own recognition of feeling better and increased self-esteem. If the patient does something and feels healthier and more complete as a person because of it, that will be a powerful reinforcer. It is through the relationship with the physician that the patient comes to that recognition.

In place of approving and disapproving, to maintain the appropriate context, the physician must accept whatever behavior the patient presents. In giving acceptance, the physician takes the behavior as a significant description of the patient's experience that must be incorporated into the treatment process. The single exception to this standard is a direct physical threat to the physician by the patient. Such actions render the real possibility of cooperation, based on repeated interactions, untenable, and the physician's best strategy is to immediately disengage from the interaction.

In a cooperative context the patient will be more likely to volunteer a failure of compliance because it does not threaten self-esteem to do so. With acceptance of the patient's experience, the patient's interests hidden behind the positions and actions taken begin to emerge.

UNDERSTANDING VS. PROBING

In the acceptance of the patient's experience, an understanding emerges from the exploration of the full narrative of the patient's illness. With the attempt to discover and listen to the patient narrative, the physician searches for windows of opportunity to ask open-ended questions to elicit patient emotions and promote a patient-centered interview.[36] The physician strives to understand the relationship of the patient to their illness.

When the physician loses sight of the patient narrative, and consequently, the value of the patient's relationship to their illness, the focus of inquiry becomes isolated on the facts. The physician needs to be careful that this pattern does not get established, especially during history collection. Here, the physician, out of necessity, asks many closed-end, factual questions to which the patient dutifully reports. Very easily an expectation may develop that this is how things are done. With this restriction of history collection, the patient in disenfranchised from the information collected. The physician is then engaged in technical procedure of probing for information. As time efficient as it may appear to limit the focus of questioning in this way, because of the patient's reduced investment, responses tend to be more limited with less independent evaluation. Hence, when open-ended questions appear, the patient has little or nothing to say. It is quite easy for physicians to get caught up in probing in a noncooperative relationship. With the patient's reduced involvement and subsequent lack of initiative, this information gathering is experienced as something done to them, not as an opportunity to tell his or her story. The physician experiences the information collection as difficult and the patient as withholding. The physician becomes the only one taking initiative, when, in fact, it is appropriate for the patient to be taking the initiative as well. Very easily, the patient gets caught up in responses of "Yes, doctor" and "No, doctor." Remember, the rules of the relationship are always being negotiated from the outset. How the history is collected has a tremendous effect on what the rules of the relationship are and how the patient will behave thereafter.

The patient needs to be continually offered opportunities to take the initiative and express a narrative. This comes from the physician asking open-ended questions, where the patient is encouraged to volunteer information and ideas. Another way to promote the patient to take initiative that is often overlooked is for the physician to take a moment to simply be quiet, to offer silence. Physicians can get caught up in a pressure to perform that is fostered and intensified by the complementary interactions in the relationship. The physician feels the pressure of having to make something happen and be productive. Under that pressure, the physician will be less aware of the need for the patient to become actively involved. A physician can put in a fine performance and still not have come to an understanding of the patient's narrative or have promoted a cooperative relationship. Ultimately it is not enough to promote that the patient volunteer fact. The physician must promote an investigation of the patient's relationship to the illness and a discovery of the patient's interests in relation to the illness.

EMPATHY VS. REASSURING

Once understanding has taken place, empathy becomes possible. Zinn[37] describes empathy as "a process for understanding an individual's subjective experiences by vicariously sharing that experience while maintaining an observant stance. It is a useful tool in the medical encounter as it provides the physician with a fuller, more personalized view of the patient and it provides the patient with a sense of connectedness to the physician that may allow him/her to more freely express his/her emotional distress."

Bellet and Maloney[38] argue that the accuracy of the physician's empathic response rests in the response of the patient. If the physician's response stimulates and deepens the patient's narrative, the physician's understanding of the patient was correct. They concluded that an important factor in achieving compliance is the perception of the physician's empathy for the patient in his or her illness.

In place of empathy, however, physicians often offer reassurances such as "Don't worry." Although patients work to elicit these reassurances from the physician, they just as often reject them once presented. If the patient is worried, it is unlikely that the physician's directive to do otherwise will succeed. In fact, it is more likely that the patient will experience the reassurance as a directive to change emotions, to stop worrying. Because patients will not likely succeed at this attempt, they may continue to worry despite the physician's directive to stop. Consequently, reassuring does not work; it only makes the patient more nervous or more worried.

Beyond that, reassurance serves as an attempt to control the patient, directing him or her to behave differently. A dependent patient may crave the physician's authoritarian stance, but this will not promote cooperation. Reassuring sets up a rule that the physician makes it better for the patient. The physician is then taking a complimentary stance in a place that should be symmetrical. The physician cannot possibly control the patient's worry. To reassure the patient and say, "Don't worry," is tantamount to saying, "This is the way you are and it's wrong. You should change. You're worried and you shouldn't be. Stop doing it!" The attempt to control the patient's behavior will lead to loss of control over the relationship and reduced effectiveness.

It is true that the physician would like the patient to feel reassured. The patient should not be kept in suspense of the treatment plan or predictable outcomes. Certainly the physician wants the patient to come to a sense that it will be all right and that progress is being made. Rather than trying to reassure the patient and eliminate his or her worry, physicians do much better by being empathetic and understanding the patient experience of worry. Let the patient know that it is okay to be worried. If the patient is worried about what is going to happen, the physician can say, "It's all right to be worried about what's going to happen. That's natural and that's understandable." Patients need to be able to discover and experience reassurance on their own, not as something told to them by the physician. The patient may be told, "It might not be until you start noticing the effects of treatment and when you are feeling better that your worry will entirely go away." If the patient can see the course of treatment and see what is going to happen and the physician can describe the course of treatment to the patient, the patient may become reassured. By being empathic and understanding of their worry and seeing it as reasonable, the physician can reassure patients in the process. It is by accepting patients and empathizing with their experience that allows them to be reassured.

RESPECT VS. ADVICE

Coercion may be defined as any attempt to control the behavior of the patient. There are many different types of coercion such as threats, bribes, and even reason. Approval and disapproval are varieties of coercion; advice is another.

Patients ask for advice all the time. If the physician gives advice, an interesting cycle is likely to develop called the "Why-don't-you? Yes-but" game.[29] When patients ask for and receive advice, very often they dispute that the advice will be successful. They then proceed to ask for another piece of advice. The physician's advice is continually discounted, the physician's effectiveness is diminished, and the physician is flunked out. Giving advice assumes that patients have been unable to explore the different options available in their own lives, that they have failed to carry through due to lack of knowledge about living. The physician acts as guru, imparting wisdom. What is more likely, however, is that the patient has rejected all reasonable options because he or she finds difficulty or fault with each. The physician's response to the patient's request, then, is walking into a setup.

Physicians do have a responsibility to give prescriptions to patients. Whether that prescription is an exercise regimen, a diet, a medication, or a vitamin supplement, it lies within the narrow definition of the physician's expertise. Advice goes beyond prescription and tells patients how they should behave, think, or feel. It is an attempt to direct the patient's life. Advice is at best misdirected and at worst arrogant on the part of the physician. What kind of relationship is established as a result? It is not a cooperative or therapeutic relationship. When the physician gives the patient advice, he or she is overstepping the bounds of the cooperative relationship. Complementary behavior is invading what should be a symmetrical interaction. There is a tremendous momentum to take that complimentary interaction past where it belongs in terms of giving prescription and move it and generalize it into giving advice. That is the danger of any kind of complimentary interaction; it generalizes. The more the physician attempts to control or direct the patient's behavior, the more control over the relationship is lost and the more control the patient gains over the definition of the relationship.

Out of respect for the patient as a person, the physician should stick to prescription and avoid advice. Where advice is requested, refrain from offering it. If the patients asks, "How am I going to explain this to my spouse?" any direct answer is likely to promote trouble. A better response is, "I wish I could tell you how to relate to your spouse but you know the relationship you have much better than I do. What have you thought about saying? What do you think are likely responses? What do you think will work?" The physician can collect patients' feedback and encourage them to answer the question for themselves. It is easy to give advice but much more difficult to help patients express their own thoughts and feelings.

The physician must respect patients' ability to come to terms with their illness. The physician cannot save them from that. Coercions are at best successful for a brief period. After that, the coercion must be escalated to maintain the effect. Repeated escalations of coercion eventually bring the relationship to a dead end. The physician can no longer reasonably escalate, and the patient is no longer affected. Alternatively, the physician must respect that patients are ultimately responsible to run their own life. The physician can set the necessary preconditions for change, but the patient has to do the change. The patient needs to take the initiative. The physician can only set a context for change through an appropriate definition of the relationship. The patient needs to take an active role in making that change occur.

FLEXIBILITY VS. DEFENSIVENESS

The physician must seek to understand the patient's interests and how he or she relates to care. Patient noncompliance can be seen as an expression of the patient's hidden interests that need to be incorporated into care. Failure to identify these interests lead to defensiveness by both the physician and patient where each side often views the other's defense as an attack. To take a defensive stance is, in fact, to invite attack because it defines the relationship in terms of attack and defense. To do nothing is to allow the maneuver to define the relationship as attack and defense. Consequently, defense, or inaction in the face of defense, always leads to noncooperation.

In response to a defensive stance by the patient, the physician should make an immediate response to redefine the patient's behavior within the context of cooperation. No behavior has only one meaning. The meaning is established by the context out of which the behavior is viewed. Patients are often ambivalent about the meaning of their reactions to the physician, particularly when the relationship is still in the process of forming. The physician may select any context to view the patient's behavior that fits. It is the physician's response that ultimately assigns meaning to the patient's action. The physician makes an immediate response to stabilize the relationship by reestablishing cooperation.

Watzlawick et al.[29] state, "To reframe, then, means to change the conceptual and/or emotional setting or viewpoint in relation to which a situation is experienced and to place it in another frame which fits the 'facts' of the same concrete situation equally well or even better, and thereby changes its entire meaning."

Although not all patient attitudes and interests are acceptable, particularly when they are presented in a competitive framework, the physician can refrain from competing with the patient and establish a common ground by mirroring that part of the patient's attitude that is acceptable. It becomes the physician's responsibility to transform, as much as possible, the attitudes of the patient into the therapeutic process, both affirming them and putting them in a cooperative framework.

REFERENCES

1. Sbarbaro JA: The patient-physician relationship: Compliance revisited. *Ann Allergy* 64:325–331, 1990.
2. Hulka BS, Cassel JC, Kupper LL, et al: Communication, compliance and concordance between physicians and patients with prescribed medications. *Am J Public Health* 66:847–853, 1976.
3. Turk D, Rudy T: Neglected topics in the treatment of chronic pain patients—relapse, noncompliance, and adherence enhancement. *Pain* 44:5–28, 1991.
4. Lay P, Spelman MS: Communication in an outpatient setting. *Br J Soc Clin Psychol* 4:115–120, 1965.
5. Epstein LH, Cluss PA: A behavioral medicine perspective on adherence to long-term medical regimens. *J Consult Clin Psychol* 50:950–971, 1982.
6. Horowitz R, Horowitz M: Adherence to treatment and health outcomes. *Arch Intern Med* 153:1863–1868, 1993.
7. Smith TC, Thompson TL: The inherent, powerful therapeutic value of a good physician-patient relationship. *Psychosomatics* 34:166–170, 1993.
8. Neighbour R: Paternalism or autonomy. *Practitioner* 236:860–864, 1992.
9. Cassel EJ: The nature of suffering and the goals of medicine. *N Engl J Med* 306:639–645, 1982.
10. Shiel RC, Baker JA: Resolving noncompliance in patient care. *J Manipulative Physiol Ther* 6:37–40, 1983.
11. Emanuel EJ, Emanuel LL: Four models of the physician-patient relationship. *JAMA* 267:2221–2226, 1992.
12. McKay B, Forbes JA, Bourner K: Empowerment in general practice: The trilogies of caring. *Aust Fam Physician* 19:513, 516–520, 1990.
13. Freedman A: The physician-patient relationship and the ethic of care. *Can Med Assoc J* 148:1037–1043, 1993.
14. Metzger NJ: Improving communication in health care: The uses of literature. *Second Opinion* 17:55–77, 1992.
15. Rees AM: Communication in the physician-patient relationship. *Bull Med Library Assoc* 81(1):1–10, 1993.
16. Beckman HB, Frankel RM: The effect of physician behavior on the collection of data. *Ann Intern Med* 101:692–696, 1984.
17. Frankel RM: From sentence to sentence: Understanding the medical encounter through microinteractional analysis. *Discourse Process* 7:135–170, 1984.
18. Smith RC, Hoppe RB: The patient's story: Integrating the patient- and physician-centered approaches to interviewing. *Ann Intern Med* 115:470–477, 1991.
19. Shapiro J: The use of narrative in the doctor-patient encounter. *Fam Systems Med* 11:47–53, 1993.
20. LaCombe MA: Living the patient's story. *Ann Intern Med* 113:890–891, 1991.
21. Epstein RM, Beckman HB: Health care reform and patient-physician communication. *Am Fam Physician* 49:1718–1720, 1994.
22. Watzlawick P, Beavin JH, Jackson DD: *Pragmatics of Human Communication.* New York, WW Norton, 1981.
23. Schwenk TL, Romano SE: Managing the difficult physician-patient relationship. *Am Fam Physician* 46:1503–1509, 1992.
24. Haley J: *Strategies of Psychotherapy.* New York, Grune & Stratton, 1963.
25. Kelly RB: Art of therapeutic communication. *J Fam Pract* 32:13, 1991.

26. Coulter ID: The physician, the patient, and the person: The humanistic challenge. *J Chiropr Humanities* 1:9–20, 1993.
27. Fisher R, Ury W: *Getting to Yes.* Boston, Houghton Mifflin, 1981.
28. Epstein RM, Campbell TL, Cohen-Cole SA, et al: Perspectives of patient-doctor communication. *J Fam Pract* 37:377–388, 1993.
29. Watzlawick P, Weakland J, Fisch R: *Change: Principles of problem formation and problem resolution.* New York, WW Norton, 1974.
30. Axelrod R: *The Evolution of Cooperation.* Basic Books, 1984.
31. Delbanco TL: Enriching the doctor-patient relationship by inviting the patient's perspective. *Ann Intern Med* 116:414–418, 1992.
32. Allen TW: Patient involvement key to enhancing doctor-patient relationship. *J Am Osteopath Assoc* 92:690, 695, 1992.
33. Bertakis KD, Roter D, Putman SM: The relationship of physician medical interview style to patient satisfaction. *J Fam Pract* 32:175–181, 1991.
34. Ben-Sira Z: Stress potential and esotericity of health problems: The significance of the physician's affective behavior. *Med Care* 29:414–424, 1982.
35. Bowman MA: Good physician-patient relationship—improved patient outcome? *J Fam Pract* 32:135–136, 1991.
36. Branch WT, Malik TK: Using windows of opportunities in brief interviews to understand patients' concerns. *JAMA* 269:1667–1668, 1993.
37. Zinn W: The empathic physician. *Arch Intern Med* 153:306–312, 1993.
38. Bellet PS, Maloney MJ: The importance of empathy as an interviewing skill in medicine. *JAMA* 266:1831–1832, 1991.

Applications of Quality Assurance in Chiropractic Practice

Daniel T. Hansen, D.C.
Private practice, Olympia, Washington; Medical Director, Chiropractic Network Services, Lynnwood, Washington

John J. Triano, D.C., M.A.
Private Practice, Texas Back Institute, Plano, Texas; Board of Advisors, Institute of Spine and Biomedical Research, Plano, Texas

---

> Quality . . . Every man is tasked to make his life, even in its details, worthy of the contemplation of his most elevated and critical hour.
> Henry David Thoreau (1854)

Health care delivery and its costs are a topic in every corporate board room across North America. Their objective is to seek accountability and value in the health-related products they purchase. In Miami, a large trucking firm sends questionnaires to local physicians asking for detailed information about their training, fees, and malpractice history. In Philadelphia, a large teaching hospital distributes a special report each month detailing the cost to the hospital for every patient case by diagnosis-related group (DRG) for individual physicians. In Rochester, provider profiles of patient satisfaction are used to select those with the best performance for awarding future contracts.[1] Health maintenance organizations (HMOs) and independent practice associations routinely perform audits of outpatient facility patient charts and conduct patient satisfaction surveys assessing reported and perceived quality of the medical intervention.[2, 3] These are not draconian scenarios drawn from some future dominated by a national health insurance plan. Rather, they are actual programs functioning as a part of our current multifaceted and pluralistic delivery system. Are they new to the 1990s? No, some of them have been around for more than 10 years.

Health reform's initial steps have used costs as the catalyst to initiate changes with only minimal interest on the effect on quality of service. That emphasis is now changing. Relman[4] states that this is "a new era of assessment and accountability . . . [that] is the third and latest—but probably not the last—phase of our efforts to achieve an equitable health care system, of satisfactory quality, at a price we can afford." How quality is assessed and how information on the quality of care delivered is to be used form the current social and political challenges.[5]

The market, not just the academics, is changing. The shift is fueled by competition, transfer of financial risk from the payer to provider and potentially to the patient. Employer demands for cost containment and regulatory initiatives now serve as the implements of change.[6] Effects of the new standards are being felt by an increasing proportion of practitioners and likely will affect better than 50% of the patient care administered by the year 2000.[7] Berwick and Knapp[5] suggest that with the modern changes, important questions emerge. Physicians and patients wonder about the sanctity of the doctor-patient relationship; patient advocates fear that needed care may be sacrificed at the altar of dollars saved; patients ask if the lowest cost care is really the best; and purchasers of care for groups agonize over which choice offers the best service for their clients. Answering these concerns requires a means to evaluate the relative quality of services.

Quality management (QM) programs, to be successful, must involve all parties and cause them to interact in the development and implementation of programs that make sense socially and individually. "Society is searching for better answers to complex questions that relate to resource allocation, medical decision making and the role of the patient. [Society is] asking the [health] professions to meet this challenge."[8] This chapter will take the reader through quality assessment and quality assurance (QA) applications and implementation strategies. The purpose is to define some of the quality attributes that may be directed at the chiropractic discipline and how quality may be assured in both the reimbursement and delivery arenas. The assessment of quality will be examined from the perspective of its potential impact within social policy and on the doctor-patient relationship.

QM is a fledgling aspect for our discipline. The chapter includes some QA checklists and worksheets as guides for use in chiropractice practices. The need for QA specialists in the chiropractic profession and for the emergence of college-based QA training programs is also discussed.

HISTORICAL AND SOCIAL PERSPECTIVES

To many, the apparent speed with which reform has been implemented and the accompanying political turmoil suggest a weak foundation. Despite false starts and rapidly changing objectives in the political arena, the fundamental steps for public policy decisions and implementation in health care have been tested over the course of the past 40 years. In fact, many of the concepts from demonstration projects on managed care principles are being applied now with impetus from business, industry, and local governments, including the notions of high quality of care and lower cost. Instrumental to these ideals have been the techniques of provider credentialing of closed panels, precertification, concurrent and retrospective review of services, guidelines of care, and critical pathways.[3]

Yesterday's practice was guided and protected by the guild mentality.[9] The professional associations (e.g., American Chiropractic Association [ACA], International Chiropractic Association [ICA], American Medical Association [AMA]) were expected to provide paternal recommendations on usual and customary practice. The characteristics of health care practice under that era are (1) patient choice of provider, (2) solo/small group practices, (3) fee for services, and (4) insurance competition for subscribers. Competition for subscribers offered an environment that promoted development of different policy benefits as a means of attracting premium generated revenues. In a domino effect, the result was a blending of competition and regulation that fostered cost-inflating incentives for use of services that were insensitive to real demand or need, forming a positive feedback. The current evidence of a system of health care out of control has been the spiraling increase in practice variations across the country without commensurate differences in clinical outcomes.

The response has been a sequence of efforts on the part of government and payers to restrict access to providers and services while ensuring a minimum level of quality. Experimentation with credentialing of limited or closed panels of providers appeared as early as 1929 with the Ross Loos project in Los Angeles. Other successful efforts include the Group Health Association in Washington, D.C. (1935), Kaiser Permanente of the 1930s, and the Group Health Cooperative of Puget Sound (1945). Even the possibility of single-payer options on a large scale has been demonstrated through the Federal Employees Health Benefits Program, which began in 1960.[10]

Evaluation of health care services for therapeutic necessity is perhaps the first formal step toward the guidelines and treatment protocols of today. In 1962, the establishment of the Medicare law through the Health Care Financing Administration (HCFA) gave statutory authorization for utilization review. Health insurance plan managers gradually adopted and further developed utilization review methods and applications to ultimately include precertification, concurrent procedures, and retrospective procedures.[9] A further reinforcement for review of provider services was added to the statutes in 1987 when mechanisms to financially penalize providers who administer services not found to be therapeutically necessary were sanctioned. The next major step required criteria for the circumstances under which review of services is to occur. Drawing on advisory publications ranging back into the 1970s, the Americans with Disabilities Act of 1990[11, 12] set limitations on the purview of medical procedures. Although specific procedures and technologies are not addressed by the statute, the criteria for clinical decisions makes it clear that the issues of validity, reliability, and relevance to critical job tasks are relevant concerns.

Quality in health care through the 1960s and 1970s was ordained by physicians and hospitals. These central figures in health care closed ranks as a guild and applied, controlled, and evaluated their own performance. Careers in health care became popularized as much for their economic potential and self-interest as their altruistic position and noble commitments.[20] The decisions of need for diagnostic tests, therapeutic measures, hospitalization, or surgery were relegated to physician discretion with little likelihood of review. Management trends often were learned through peer interaction, from pharmaceutical and surgical hardware detailers, and from the published literature.[21] Peer oversight was loosely structured through specialty rounds and consultation with recognized community experts. QA was a buzz term limited to radiography, clinical laboratory, and pharmacology, with no insight to applications involving direct doctor-patient interaction.

Public entitlements (e.g., Medicare and Medicaid) and the advent of government and consumer watchdogs precipitated social pressures in the late 1970s and through the 1980s for stronger emphasis on QA. In the delivery of medical care, this took shape in the form of peer review organizations (PROs), a precursor to the much more sophisticated quality management firms of the 1990s. Health care practitioners found their clinical judgments being reviewed and sometimes reversed for issues of cost and quality by those outside the sanctity of their guild. The peer review organizations, insurance company medical directors, and claims reviewers would examine recorded details of a medical case to implicitly determine issues of appropriateness. Early review activity was nothing more than contrasting practice activities against a colleague's clinical hunches.

In the 1980s, irreconcilable evidence of unexplained practice variations was identified showing wasteful practices and procedures that failed to enhance patient benefit.[22] Finding their way into the public domain, these reports have forced the issue for provider accountability and the quality of care. The full scope of impact from these social pressures have taken longer to influence policy changes for the chiropractic profession. The early changes from the federal entitlements had less effect because of the preexisting constraints imposed by the Medicare definitions of 1974. The HCFA already had targeted chiropractic services for review based on x-ray criteria and frequency of services.

The use of second opinions on chiropractic claims have emerged, particularly in the domains of indemnity, casualty, and workers' compensation insurance to adjudicate chiropractic claims where there was question of necessity of care. File reviewers included nurse practitioners, medical physicians, and chiropractors. Second opinion examiners, which became known as independent medical examiners (IMEs) or independent chiropractic examiners (ICEs) were typically chiropractors who made themselves available for such activity. This kind of review quickly became controversial and caused significant action in the courts of law and state legislatures.

In contrast, this same period saw the emergence of an industry that developed technologies to prove chiropractic necessity and to be more convincing before a judge or jury. Technologies such as Moire's photography, plethysmography, videofluoroscopy, thermography, surface electrode electromyography, muscle strength analysis, spatial analysis, computerized x-ray analysis, and other high technology–high cost procedures were developed. Founded on the notion that documentation of a symptom or physiological/pathological change equated to necessity to treat, they were marketed often before there was much testing for reliability or validity.[23] This notion and the technologies it fostered are now beginning to clash with the health care industry's movement into technology assessments, outcome assessments, and the purchasing public's measure of accountability.

The concept of peer review in the chiropractic profession was foisted on the system as a defensive strategy primarily through the dominant national and state chiropractic associations. The controversy over the control of the review process and what constitutes a peer has had beneficial effect. Ultimately manuals and training exercises were created, driving toward cohesive peer review functions that mimicked those arising out of the peer review organizations (PROs) movement for the HCFA Medicare payment system. Through this process, individual claims of doctors would be evaluated according to norms or values either established by the PRO, implicitly by their reviewers, or, where possible, from application of flexible but evidence-based criteria. The review groups would pass their recommendations to the payer for action. During this pre-1990s era, there was no attention given to cause corrective action or physician improvement. Typically the action was to pay the claim, adjust the fee, or refuse the claim.

During the decades of the 1970s and 1980s, a parallel recognition of quality as a means to savings and increased market share was occurring in manufacturing industries based on input and influence of the customers. The health care industry has been the latest to grasp customer-driven concepts of QM. Early professional arrogance resounded across the entire health care community: "I'm the doctor, I know what is best for my patients!" A chiropractic version has been, "My technique requires special training; don't pass judgment on my patient care without my specialized and unique training!" The public is growing more intolerant of such practices and attitudes when they are unaccompanied by evidence of effectiveness.

The banner of quality of health care has now been formally adopted by academics and professionals in epidemiology and public health,[13] clinical disciplines,[14,15] and public agencies.[16] Each group is attempting to supply a defensible and credible basis for governing routine health practices. While health professionals are struggling under the imposition of restrictions, managed care organizations (MCOs) and third-party payers are quickly incorporating these guidelines. Through the National Commission on Quality Assurance (NCQA),[17] Joint Commission on Accreditation of Healthcare Organizations (JCAHO)[18] and the Health Plan Employer Data and Information Set version 2.0 (HEDIS-2),[19] policies have been implemented to govern and certify organizations that sponsor health care delivery on a managed and discounted basis. Major insurers or independent HMOs are accredited following these guidelines. NCQA and HEDIS-2 are the benchmarks by which these organizations are graded and permitted to expand their business. In turn, they pass performance expectations on to their panel providers.

QA requirements have achieved substantial penetration into the mechanisms of health care reform. It behooves each practicing doctor of chiropractic to become aware of the QA process, its benefits, and its liabilities as they select their future practice styles: (1) independence, (2) group, (3) network/panel participation, or (4) integrated practice settings.

The 1990s may come to be known as the dawning of the "era of accountability." The "watchdog" function has expanded to include government, employers, insurance, and managed care companies (even those that are physician run) due mostly to upward spiraling health costs while the general health of the American public remains static. One strategy of

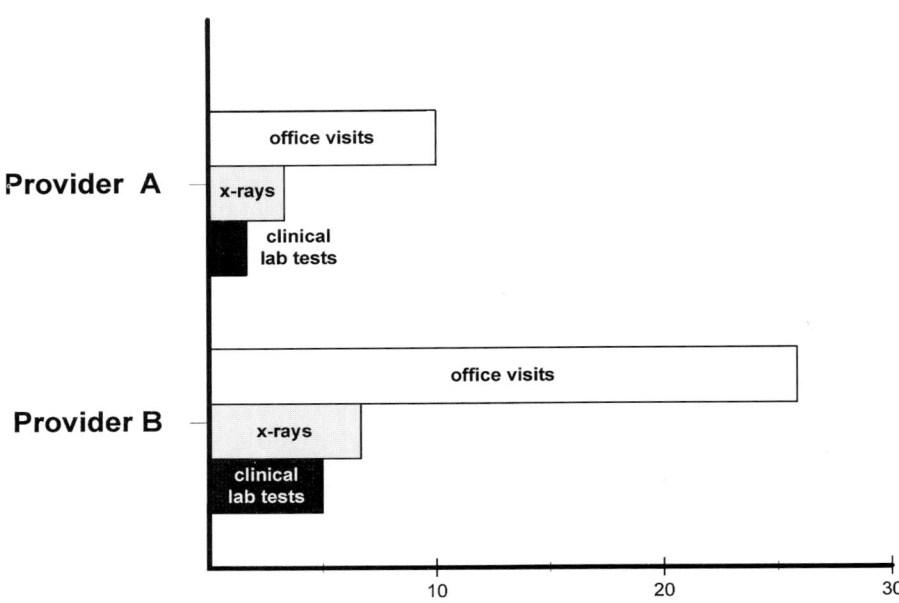

FIGURE 1.
Provider profile: services per patient per year.

health care reform is simply to make public a grading system of provider performance. Categories include physician (i.e., M.D. or D.C.) selection, adequacy of facilities, availability of medical staff, patient waiting time, and warmth of clinic staff. Provider profiles (Fig 1) allow anyone to essentially "shop" for a quality doctor or hospital. Such data are espoused by managed care organizations in "credentialing" physicians, hospitals, durable medical goods, and ancillary services.[24]

The prospect of provider profiling and limited panel enrollment of providers has caused significant anxiety within the chiropractic profession. Neither of the principal national organizations for the profession have established a position or plan of action in response to the social emphasis on quality of care. Neither have the associations become a clearinghouse for quality of care issues or to serve as a platform for affecting health policy and advancing chiropractic leadership on socially responsible issues.[25]

In contrast, since the early to mid-1980s, medical and specialty organizations have energetically engaged this issue, and their momentum has not wavered.[26] The American medical guilds have set out to prepare physicians and clinics for impending changes that emphasize cost controls and improved quality. They have published physician guidebooks to deal with QA and improvement issues and to prepare them for coping with the diverse elements of managed care.[27, 28]

DEFINING QUALITY

Traditionally physicians have been reluctant to define quality. In part, the physician-patient relationship was unequal; the physician held sway by nature of his or her technical knowledge and skill. Each physician exercised flexible definitions of quality for each patient without consideration of whether the cumulative results of health care delivery was more or less effective than that of other care givers. Researchers, practitioners, and trade organizations have been struggling with their definitions of quality, searching for a common basis on which all concerned parties might agree. Typically these attempts fail to embrace the full concept.[29] Chassin et al.[20] offer a practical distinction between quality assessment and QA.

Quality assessment measures the level of care through the use of outcomes measures. The result can be a series of statements relating to the structure, process, or outcomes of care by a particular physician, hospital, or other segment of the health care system. QA, on the other hand, is the process by which quality assessments are used to improve care that is delivered. An effective QA program uses quality assessments to identify specific weaknesses in care delivery, devise specific interventions to remedy them, followed by a reassessment of intervention effects.

Avedis Donabedian, considered by many as the academic father of quality assessment in health, defined the components of health care delivery to include structure, process, and outcome (Table 1).[5] Structure categorizes the assembled resources that provide health care. Process refers to intermediate products of care. Outcomes are end products of care meaningful to the public.

Three general methods of quality assessment have been used traditionally: implicit review, explicit review, and sentinels. *Implicit review* processes use experts who are qualified to recognize good care when it occurs or, in some cases, groups whose combined knowledge or judgment is thought better than any single individual's. Implicit surveillance methods have focused on peer review functions and are relatively inexpen-

TABLE 1.
Structure, Process, and Outcome

Structure
 1. Mix of health care manpower
 2. The credentials of providers
 3. The facilities
 4. The rules of procedure
Process
 1. Patterns of diagnostic evaluation
 2. Access to care
 3. Rate of utilization
 4. Choice of therapies
Outcomes
 1. Health status
 2. Longevity
 3. Comfort
 4. Satisfaction of clients

sive to administer. These offer several severe disadvantages, including reliability of judgments made. In other words, different reviewers may judge the same cases differently.[30] From the viewpoint of improving provider performance, implicit judgments fail to provide consistent guidance as to why specific encounters may represent poor quality of care.

Explicit review involves specifying criteria for care and review of records or observations to determine if criteria are met.[30] Judgments are reduced and the reviewer tallies appropriate behaviors. Did the physician or chiropractor in his or her history note whether the patient has a past medical history of taking anticoagulants? Did the physician observe and comment on the nature of the patient's elevated body temperature in the report of the physical examination? Was a chest x-ray film performed for the patient with cough, fever, and chest pain? Did the provider coordinate findings and reach a justified diagnosis? Was the treatment plan consistent with the diagnosis?

The explicit assessment of quality care is more complex and difficult than for implicit measures unless high-quality guidelines or treatment protocols are available. Unlike implicit methods, the explicit processes are usually highly specific to an individual clinical or administrative topic. Even for simple conditions, 15 to 20 specific criteria may be necessary.[31–33] Specific criteria lend credibility to the process. More important, they allow collection of specific data that can be used to subsequently improve quality. Results of implicit and explicit review often seem to produce different results.[5] Which method is superior is a matter of continuing debate. Practicing physicians, in general, favor implicit processes, whereas plan managers and regulators favor explicit criteria and scoring systems.

The third method, the *use of sentinels*, advocates use of unacceptable, or "red flag," events. Their appearance triggers detailed investigations of the events using implicit or explicit methods. In the chiropractic profession, sentinel investigations are commonly applied to practice statistics such as visits per claim or total claim costs. Chiropractic providers, when knowledgeable of this surveillance, will change their practice behavior just knowing that they are being observed.[34] Similar behavior has been observed in other industries and is otherwise commonly known as the Hawthorne effect.

The federal government has generated several definitions of quality care. The Congressional Office of Technology Assessment (OTA) adopted the following definition: "The quality of medical care is the degree to which the process of care increases the probability of outcomes desired by the patients and decreases the probability of undesired outcomes, given the state of medical knowledge."[35] A list of quality of care indicators was offered for use in health policy development (Table 2) with good acceptance by consumer and business groups.[30] Caper[36] defined three components of quality: efficacy, appropriateness, and caring. Efficacy is the concern that a diagnostic or therapeutic procedure accomplishes its goal. Appropriateness is the standing of a particular diagnostic or therapeutic course of action that may be indicated after considering the relative costs, risks, and benefits in each phase. The caring function involves the interpersonal, supportive, and psychological aspects of the physician-patient relationship.

TABLE 2.
Summary of Quality of Care Indicators Evaluated by the Office of Technology Assessment*

Hospital mortality rates
Adverse events (include nosocomial infections)
Formal physician disciplinary actions by state medical boards
PRO/Department of Health and Human Services (HHS) sanctions
Malpractice compensation
Physicians' performance evaluations for a specific condition, by a process of outcome measures (e.g., hypertension)
Volume of hospital/physician services
External standards and guidelines, scope of hospital services (e.g., emergency rooms, cancer care, neonatal intensive care units)
Physician specialization
  Specialty board certification
  Practices limited to area of training
Patient satisfaction/care assessment survey

*From US Office of Technology Assessment: *The Quality of Medical Care: Information for Consumers.* Washington, DC, US Government Printing Office, June 1988 (ota-h-386).

Attributes of quality separately have been defined for the primary health care arena (Table 3). Each contributes to the decisions for purchase between health care products or inclusion of health care providers. Attributes are commonly applied by managed care systems and are manifested in QA program tools such as credentialing, utilization management, site visitations, chart reviews, retrospective reviews, and quality improvement (QI) teams. QI teams are typically used to explicitly measure the attributes and monitor their impact on the system.

There has to be a distinction between the science and art of health care. Although application of QM is easier and methodologically sound for the science component, the art of health practice has fuzzier boundaries addressed by customer satisfaction measures. It is common to assess the degree to which the patient perceives that the physician was compassionate, listened carefully to his or her complaints, and explained the reasons why tests were ordered or treatment prescribed.[30] Typically, the narrowly defined applications of quality assessment and QA to individual health care providers tend to favor the practitioner's technical performance.[37] As the definition of quality is broadened in the future, it may include:

- Practitioner management of the personal patient interaction
- Active patient participation in care
- Amenities of the settings in which care is provided
- Ease of access to care
- Social limitations on access (e.g., Medicare/Medicaid)
- Social impact of the health improvements attributable to care

Donabedian's definition of health, as the product of care, broadens beyond physical and physiological function to include the notion of qual-

TABLE 3.
Quality Attributes of Primary Care*

Direct contact
Accessibility
   Availability/attainability
   Acceptability/accommodation
Affordability
Accountability
Continuity of care
Longitudinality
Coordination of care
Comprehensiveness of care
Essential or basic health care
Assessment
Education and counseling
Community involvement

*From Coile RC: *The New Medicine: Reshaping Medical Practice and Health Care Management.* Gaithersburg, Md, Aspen, 1988. Used by permission.

ity of life. This is precisely the emphasis that has evolved from the modern reforms of health delivery and health reimbursement, that is, the expectation for greater quality of life from interventions by health providers. The American health care model has shifted from a physician-centered management to a patient-centered collaboration among purchasing providers and case managers.[38, 39] Unfortunately, it is not yet certain that the objectives of remodeled health care will be met.

Nash and Goldfield[40] highlight major public opinion trends likely to have impact on the quality of health care. The polls point to a national contradiction with an increasing concern about the quality of care in the existing system contrasted with a desire to maintain the status quo for their personal health care choices. Surveys represent data from before 1985 during an era of greater choice among physicians and hospitals. Medical providers had performed dismally in conveying an image of quality. Only one third of the public sampled believed they received high value for their health care dollar in contrast to more than three fourths of physicians who reported that opinion. This disparity has fueled further the current health reform activities.

NATIONAL STANDARDS IN QA

With working definitions of quality applied to the health care setting, the growing trend has been to attempt to manage quality or, in other words, to assure quality. QA and QM "programs and activities are intended to ensure high-quality care in any defined health care setting. The programs must include components intended to identify deficiencies in quality care and to remedy them through educational or policy actions. Instruments include peer or utilization review components, and program self-assessment of its own effectiveness."[34]

Emerging in the health arena is the application of QI principles from industry that are consistent with the new organizational structure of accountable entities units found in health care, including MCOs, public and private sector purchasers, and physician facilities.

QI "is the continuing and systematic effort to improve the level of performance of key process within an industry, such as health care. It involves measuring the level of current performance, finding ways to improve that performance, and implementing new and better methods."[41] QI is also known and referred to as continuous QI and total QM. Health policy organizations such as the Council of the Institute of Medicine have urged health plans and provider groups QA/QM plans to minimize intrusive programs micromanaging care from the outside. External monitoring still will be necessary, however, to ensure the integrity of QM procedures and information and to assess the health status of the population as a whole.[42]

Two national commissions serve this oversight role by awarding certification of accreditation to those facilities or programs that meet standards. Compliance by the chiropractic profession is compelled only by the MCOs and affects only those few providers who are part of their credentialed panels.[3] Ultimately even these organizations must qualify under the oversight rules to obtain contracts for managed care on par with that of other health disciplines. Those chiropractors who are unable to become credentialed under one of these options face a rapidly declining market share for their services. Application of these standards already is impacting doctors, facilities, and medical delivery in many states.

NCQA

As of this writing, the NCQA has had the greatest impact with their standards, now in their fourth iteration.[17] Implementation of quality of care standards is occurring at an increasingly rapid rate affecting hospitals, medical clinics, and private practices. Expanding by the influence of HMO reimbursement and delivery systems, QI teams already use standards to evaluate MCOs in areas listed in Table 4. The guidelines developed by the NCQA were the product of consensus among a broad con-

TABLE 4.
Standards to Evaluate Managed Care Organizations

NCQA[16]	JCAHO[17]
Quality Management and Improvement	Rights, responsibilities, and ethics
Utilization Management	Continuum of care
Credentialing	Education and communication
Preventive health services	Management and human resources
Medical records	Management of information
	Improving network performance

stituency from the managed care industry, health care purchasers, state regulators, and consumers using extensive review and consensus development processes. Compliance with the NCQA standards for accreditation of MCOs is regarded as a badge of honor showing that an MCO is committed to principles of quality and continuous QI. The NCQA system is national in scope with regional assessment teams trained to consistently review HMO and MCO facilities and administration records through site visitations and records review. Contents of the training according to established reviewer guidelines also are available for public inspection, enhancing their credibility and value.

Chiropractic MCOs seeking the financial and social rewards from passing this inspection process have generated QI plans and tools for enhanced compliance, including checklists for facilities inspection and record keeping. Compliance with these standards yields an easier access to the health care market place.[3]

JCAHO

The NCQA's competitor and counterpart for health care institutions is the JCAHO.[18] The JCAHO has its own published standards specifically defining quality parameters for emerging health care networks (see Table 4). Like the NCQA guides, they also focus primarily on the patient or customer and were developed by a consensus from diverse groups. JCAHO has developed a similar list of standards for institutions such as hospitals.[18] As of this writing, the two oversight agencies compete head to head, resorting to intense marketing aimed at the employer-purchaser.[43]

What may not be obvious in this duel is the affinity of NCQA for MCOs vs. the appeal of JCAHO for physicians and hospitals. It is essentially a turf war over the governance of quality in health care.

HEDIS-2.0

In many ways, the thrust of health care policy into QA and continuous QI has been to harvest information. The sheer volume of knowledge about how care is given and profiles on provider behavior and its conversion into meaningful conclusions is a daunting task. The HEDIS-2.0 represents a core set of performance measures developed to respond to a complex but simply defined task.[19] HEDIS empowers large employers to more accurately evaluate and compare health plan performance. Its primary mission is to understand the value of services purchased by the health care dollar and to develop accountability for delivery of health plan promises. HEDIS (like NCQA and JCAHO) guidelines provide a grading system for ranking the quality and cost (i.e., value) of the health care delivery systems.

The main feature of evaluating performance is credibility.[19] For business and industry as purchasers, this amounts to the extent to which employers may rely on health care delivery data collected from past claims experience with an HMO, IPA, or other contracting provider group to predict costs and outcomes. Regardless of whether the health care providers that supply the actual patient services are organized in independent, horizontally or vertically integrated practice styles,[44] the grade to be achieved is dependent on their performance against the selected expectations and standards.

In the field of spine care, current versions of HEDIS focus on the higher cost laminectomy as the benchmark. However, conservative care should not be complacent. The rapid course of health care reform predicts that future editions will expand the benchmark figures to include conservative factors. With the recent action of the Agency for Health Care Policy and Research[16] raising the profile of spinal manipulation and its wide usage, it is reasonable to expect attention to expand in this direction. At this time, there is no representation of the chiropractic profession that sits as a part of the expert panel advising the development of HEDIS criteria.

COUNCIL ON CHIROPRACTIC EDUCATION

The Council on Chiropractic Education (CCE) as an accrediting agency for chiropractic education can be considered to serve also as a defacto oversight organization for definition and recognition of quality attributes in chiropractic practice. Beginning in 1981, the CCE initiated an effort to identify minimal clinical competencies that are requisite to entrance into the profession of chiropractic. On comparison of the competency statement adopted in 1984 with the elements of NCQA and JCAHO guidelines, it is clear that they all define comparable attributes of quality care. Although the CCE advises that the competencies are not to be construed as standards of care, they can serve as yardsticks for delineating quality of care delivered. The modern chiropractor who has graduated from a CCE-accredited chiropractic college has been oriented implicitly to these common expectations, emphasizing the cognitive, affective and psychomotor competencies for each section (Table 5).[45]

Unfortunately, the authority of CCE to implement and enforce is limited only to accredited college settings. The council has no direct impact on the practice of chiropractic with regard to assessing physician behavior and quality of care indicators. National and state trade organizations have, for the most part, distanced themselves from quality of care issues. Despite a recent effort to network licensing authorities and disciplinary boards, resources are inadequate for any global oversight on defining quality of care attributes and implementation of QA for the practice of chiropractic. Compliance with these objectives is based essentially on the intellectual integrity and moral conscience of the individual practitioners and the possibility of being challenged by third-party payer utilization review procedures.

Definitions of quality assessment and applications of QA are developed and implemented largely by public and private sector purchasing authorities with little or no formal guidance by chiropractic providers. With the recent surge in managed care, many chiropractic-owned MCOs are responding to the public mandates for accountability and attention to quality assessment and QA.[3] Measures of quality applied to chiropractic providers in managed care settings have historically included clinical and administrative attributes such as average weeks of care per episode, frequency of multiple diagnostic tests, frequency of second opinions, fre-

TABLE 5.
CCE Index of Clinical Competencies*

Case history
Physical examination
Neuromuscular examination
Roentgenological examination
Clinical laboratory examination
Special studies examinations
Diagnosis or clinical impression
Patient referral
Treatment plan
Spinal adjusting competencies
Extraspinal adjusting competencies
Nonadjustive treatment competencies
Case follow-up and review
Record keeping

*From Clinical Quality Assurance Panel: *Clinical Competency Document.* Phoenix, Council on Chiropractic Education, 1984.

quency of therapeutic interventions, quality of chart notes, radiographic quality, physician compliance to utilization management, clinic facilities, safety, and patient complaints.[46] These measures of quality will continue to be used until more patient-centered assessments of quality are developed and validated.

The Congress of Chiropractic State Associations (COCSA) has launched an effort that has the potential to fill the need for general professional oversight into the arena of quality assessment.[23] Thus far, however, the focused purpose of the Council on Chiropractic Practice is to evaluate and modify existing chiropractic practice parameters. If this organization indeed becomes a reality, the appointed leaders should strategically plan for the organization's function to be responsible for quality of care issues for chiropractic practice and be accountable to the public's trust. The leadership of COCSA should be mindful of the risks to their credibility as a resource to public policy making that can arise if their activities predominate simply as professional advocacy.[25]

Currently, chiropractic authorities for delivery of quality of care are those organizations that have implementation plans for resources like the Mercy document, Agency for Health Care Policy and Research (AHCPR) guidelines, and relevant inventories of quality of care for spine-related disorders.[47] Typically this is manifested as a cohesive managed care entity with strong chiropractic management of quality (e.g., DCs as medical directors, QA committees, QA and QI teams, and DCs serving in multidisciplinary settings like HMOs and vertically integrated centers of care).

Unfortunately, DCs in these capacities are likely either self-trained, on-the-job trained, or self-motivated to learn QA/QI theory and principles on their own. Thus far, formal training in QA/QI is limited in chiropractic education in both the undergraduate and postgraduate levels.[25]

TYPICAL APPLICATIONS OF QA FOR THE CHIROPRACTIC OFFICE

Modern trends in health care delivery are increasingly focusing on applying elements of QA. In this decade of the 1990s, the greatest application of QA is through MCOs. However, with greater public demand, there is increasing legislation for this level of accountability in state health reform movements. Applications of QA can range from superficial acknowledgments by providers or institutions to the more detailed and accountable systems that measure their effectiveness with mathematical arguments. Health care delivery products with the more simplistic and cosmetic applications are easily recognized as such and where they are competing do so mostly as a result of the early emphasis on lower costs. Those delivery systems that provide quality-driven products are not likely the lowest or highest in cost, but they will satisfy the growing public demand for accountable health delivery, which appears to be the current and future focus.

Quality of care indicators have already been identified by the U.S. Congress Office of Technology Assessment, but only a few would aid consumers in determining community quality in health care delivery. The basic elements of these accountable units include physician, economic, facility, and staff credentialing, accessibility, utilization management, continuity of care, and record keeping.

CREDENTIALING OF CHIROPRACTIC DOCTORS

Table 6 lists common credentialing attributes adapted from Kongstvedt[48] to include key issues effective in credentialing chiropractic doctors.[49] Doctor and institutional credentialing should include history of malpractice and discipline activity by professional boards. In credentialing and periodic recredentialing, the doctor or institution needs to acknowledge prior history. Independently, however, the purchasers of provider services verify these histories through a process known as primary source verification. Thus, HMOs and preferred provider organizations (PPOs) make formal contact with boards and malpractice carriers to confirm information submitted for credentialing. Institutions such as hospitals and clinics can be reviewed similarly for accreditation and sanction status, if any.

Organizations such as the National Practitioner Data Bank (NPDB) act similar to that of a consumer credit service in that they accumulate malpractice and disciplinary data on physicians. Data are available to qualified inquirers. Unlike consumer credit, however, errors that arise are not easily corrected by simple correspondence. The clearinghouse for chiropractic disciplinary records (SINBAD) does not as yet have a policy to release this kind of data to organizations outside the state boards. This causes the MCO to seek primary source verification at the level of individual board contact in the states where the applicant may have practiced. Fortunately, malpractice carriers do release information on chiropractors to MCOs with proper notification of permission.

ECONOMIC CREDENTIALING

The health care reimbursement industry has the capacity to collect provider profiles (e.g., hard data about an individual physician's perfor-

TABLE 6.
Credentialing Attributes for Chiropractic Doctors*

Basic Elements of Credentialing	Optional Credentialing Elements for Chiropractors
Professional training	Maintain unrestricted chiropractic license
Specialty board certification	
Current state license	Board certified, board eligible, or enrolled in approved postgraduate program
Hospital/HMO privileges	
Record of continuing education or competencies	
	No history of disciplinary action
Social security number/tax identification number	No unfavorable action by other MCOs
	Utilization statistics and patient complaints
Location and telephone numbers of all offices	
	No history of alcoholism or narcotic addiction
Hours of operation	
Provisions for emergency care	No history of malpractice action
In-office diagnosis capabilities	Professional liability coverage
In-office treatment capabilities	Two continuous years of clinical practice
	Membership fee
	Facilities checklist
	Geographic need

*From McElheran LJ, Sollecito PC: *Top Clin Chiropr* 1:34, 1994. Used by permission.

mance) in a manner to measure the physician's cost efficiency. Hospitals may use economic credentialing to revise the makeup of their physician staffs. Managed care plans credential physicians for the same reason.[7] Practice data collection is not new (Rochester Project) and has been collected for a number of years.[1] Information is proprietary in some cases or available through public domain data bases. Potential networks can access much of these data to examine trends of physician behavior for individuals or groups.

FACILITY AND STAFF CREDENTIALING

Quality attributes for the physician office or clinic setting come from multiple sources, including NCQA, JCAHO, federal agencies (e.g., OSHA and HCFA) and provisions of the Americans with Disabilities Act (1990). The office setting should convey professionalism by maintaining up-to-date equipment and furnishings located in a clean and easily accessed location.[3] Federal and community standards will likely require aids for the physically impaired such as accommodations for wheelchair access and grab bars for toilet areas. Also, strict guidelines for fire, safety, first aid, and blood-borne pathogens require compliance for the safety of patients, employees, and visitors. Loss of credentialed status for otherwise qualified and competent providers has occurred simply for reasons of facility noncompliance. Multiple details of day-to-day operation of a clinic can

STANDARDS:	Meets Requirements	Needs Improvement
1. Facility and Environment		
A. Safety Management		
1. Designated toilet areas serving patients are large enough for independent wheelchair access and are equipped with grab bars.	☐	☐
2. Storage areas, basements, hallways, stairwells and patient areas are clean and uncluttered.	☐	☐
3. Patient files and x-rays are stored neatly, and organized to facilitate tracking and retrieval, with systems in place to maintain patient confidentiality.	☐	☐
4. Floor coverings provide adequate infection control and do not present problems for patients.	☐	☐
5. There is a system for identifying, packaging, handling and disposing of hazardous materials and wastes.	☐	☐
6. There is a system at the site for the safe management of hazardous materials and wastes.	☐	☐
B. Fire Safety		
1. The site has fire safety and other safety systems for the protection of patients, personnel, visitors, and property from fire and combustible products. Lighted exit signs and emergency push bars are recommended.	☐	☐
2. The site has a policy that discourages smoking. No smoking signs are present in the waiting room.	☐	☐

FIGURE 2.
Provider facility assessment. (Courtesy of Network Services, Lynnwood, Wash.)

be affected. Facility requirements stress access and confidentiality of patient records.

Many oversight groups (e.g., MCOs and NCQA) require office policies and posted notices regarding smoking in waiting room areas. Ionizing radiation generators (e.g., x-ray equipment) need to be certified and inspected regularly to ensure radiation protection and exposure reduction. An example of a facilities inspection checklist is provided in Figure 2. With larger MCO, there may be requirement for inspection of the facilities either by live walk throughs on site or by self-administered assessments that are performed by the QA specialists in the physician's office or hospital or clinic.

ACCESSIBILITY

Accessibility is monitored according to factors such as ease for consumers to make appointments, depending on urgency. Managed care networks are striving to have member providers both geographically and temporally accessible, for example, within a 30-minute drive of their insureds. This may be a challenge in rural areas. Provider accessibility is reflected in hours of clinic operation, average number of new patients, and average total patient visits per day. Multiple doctor offices that offer extended hours (early and late) are appealing to MCOs to handle shift workers and people who are products of long work commutes.[49]

Special attention is given to out-of-hours care because of a little recognized benefit. Fewer patients that contact their physicians after hours are admitted to hospitals. More medical practitioners are managing patient issues of after hours calls by telephone. How physicians handle clinical care issues by telephone has not been investigated for the chiropractic profession.[50]

UTILIZATION MANAGEMENT

An aspect of quality care that is becoming an essential component of accountability in managed care is utilization management (UM). Utilization of procedures and technologies can vary significantly in health care practices for all disciplines, including chiropractic.[52] UM is an internal mechanism for MCOs to predict the purchase of necessary care and to prevent purchase of unnecessary care. Utilization management is being applied to most dimensions of health care delivery, especially in the HMO environment. The basic elements of UM are found in Table 7 and typically have a temporal basis to their use. However, the quality and quantity of information obtained and the actions taken at the various levels of management differ greatly.

CONTINUITY OF CARE

Continuity of services refers to an unbroken chain of patient care delivered or coordinated by the practitioner. When a referral is made to other health care providers or agencies, the attending physician maintains an interest and communication in the case, thereby supplying continuity. Implicit in this relationship is the sharing of patient information (with appropriate consents) to reduce duplication of services and unnecessary invasive procedures.[53] Continuity of care has been shown to improve outcomes, including patient compliance, while reducing costs and resulting

TABLE 7.
Utilization Management Definitions*

Prospective review—Method of review that requires each nonemergent hospital admission to be authorized for necessity prior to admittance. Prospective review includes preauthorization or precertification for care based on established criteria. This model of UM can be applied to chiropractic practice.
Concurrent review—The process of monitoring the diagnosis and ensuing care decisions of a plan member while such care is being administered for the purpose of determining or confirming the appropriateness of the care. The objective is to provide optimum quality of care, while avoiding overutilization.
Retrospective review—The examination of patient records and case histories after a care episode has been concluded to determine the appropriateness of the type and amount of care provided. Such procedures serve to identify physician or physicians who are prone to overutilizing certain services.

*From Hansen DT: Quality of care and chiropractic necessity. In Vear H (ed): *Chiropractic Standards of Practice and Quality of Care*. Gaithersburg, Md, Aspen, 275–289, 1992. Used by permission.

in fewer emergency hospital admissions, shorter lengths of stay, and greater patient satisfaction.[50]

RECORD KEEPING

Chiropractors have legal and ethical obligations to maintain complete and accurate records for each patient. The legal basis of these requirements or standards of care come from strong case law and statutory authority.[55] It is not uncommon for a physician to experience difficulty in the adjudication of a patient's claim because the chart is insufficient to justify the billed services. This level of physician responsibility is often the focus of peer review, paper review, and second opinion processes. Where there is dispute over appropriateness or necessity of a procedure, the chart note

---

Chiropractors have the legal and ethical responsibility to maintain complete and accurate records for each patient. Patient files should be stored neatly and organized to facilitate tracking and retrieval, with a system in place to maintain patient confidentiality. The following guidelines are adapted from the 1994 NCQA Guidelines for Medical Record Review.

To be considered complete, chiropractic chart records should include the following features:

Medical Record Overview
1. Chart documentation is organized.
2. The record is legible.
3. If any non-standard abbreviations, codes, or scales are used, a key should be included to allow easy interpretation by any reviewing person.
4. The patient name is prominent on each and every page.
5. The date is noted for each provider contact / office visit / phone call / record review.
6. Entries contain author identification when anyone other than the primary treating doctor makes any entry in the chart record.
7. When there is significant risk of injury from a procedure, there is documentation of informed consent by the patient.

Exam / Intake Records
8. The patient's name / address / age / family status are noted.
9. Past medical / health history are recorded.
10. The list of patient's major problems / diagnosis is prominent, and revised as the patient's condition warrants.
11. Documented examination findings include adequate and appropriate testing for the patient problem.

Daily Chart Records
12. Relevant history / **subjective** findings of the presenting problem noted for each visit.
13. Pertinent **objective** findings noted when there is significant change.
14. **Assessment** / diagnosis noted in encounter entries, corresponding to subjective / objective findings.
15. Treatment **plan** / recommendations noted, corresponding to the patient problem / diagnosis. Return time is noted as weeks, months or PRN.
16. Notation of care prescribed or provided, corresponding to the problem being treated.
17. The care provided appears to be "medically" appropriate.
18. Reports (lab, imaging, second opinion, etc) and correspondence are signed or initialed as reviewed by the provider, significant findings are noted in the record.
19. Notation of patient's response to care.
20. Notation of home exercises / activities / ADLs given.
21. Appropriate diagnostic testing or referral is noted.
22. Notation of review / discussion of specialist findings and further recommendations.
23. All S.O.A.P. areas are updated for each PRN follow-up visit.

FIGURE 3.
Guidelines for chart record content. (From McElheran LJ, Sollecito PC: *Top Clin Chiropr* 1:78, 1994. Used by permission.)

becomes the authoritative witness of the treatment encounter. In court proceedings, the adequacy of the doctor's chart will strengthen his or her testimony, or will result in unfavorable judgment and professional embarrassment.

MCO contracts now require adherence to minimum aspects of quality in record keeping and charting derived from the consensus processes like that for the NCQA standards. Elements of these standards are now being combined with intraprofessional recommendations (e.g., Mercy Center, CCE competencies) and applied in chiropractic-preferred provider programs.[3, 47] According to these standards, the patient's health record should include the features found in the checklist given in Figure 3. Necessary emphasis is placed on requirements for the records to be stored neatly and organized to facilitate tracking and retrieval, with a system in place to ensure patient confidentiality.

QA STAFF POSITION

Coile[51] predicted that practices of the future will gradually shift from solo to group practice styles. Such a shift in practice paradigm facilitates a reduction in costs by sharing of overhead and staff. Opportunity for a new staff position with a unique set of job duties in the administrative maintenance of QA and continuous QI obligations will be afforded. The need for a member of a physician's office to be conversant with QA and QM issues is increasing. Currently, hospitals, clinics, MCOs, and group practice clinics are providing training opportunities as a part of their program orientation for new providers. This specialized staff person oversees all aspects of QM, is accountable to the physician staff, and completes compliance reporting to MCO networks or other credentialing organizations, reducing the burden on the doctor. A sample set of duties is given in Table 8.

TABLE 8.
Suggested Duties for QA Specialist in Chiropractic Office

Trained in quality assessment and QA
Trained in continuous QI
Inspect clinic facilities for safety compliance (OSHA, ADA, local codes)
  X-ray and darkroom
  Diagnosis and treatment equipment (maintenance, calibration)
Manage outcomes instruments
  Instruction to patients
  Assurance of compliance
Oversee records (completeness, confidentiality, storage)
Witness sensitive chiropractor procedures in treatment/examination room
  Informed consent
  Procedures of risk
  Patients at risk
Assist chiropractor in use management for MCOs
Assist in assuring patient compliance with treatment recommendations

The QA specialist also may serve as protection against some risk management issues. For example, staff attendance for sensitive examination and treatment procedures places a witness in the room in the event of a subsequent allegation against the doctor and acknowledges the patient's informed consent. Fundamental training in the areas of quality assessment, QA, QI, safety, regulation and compliance, and legal responsibility is the cornerstone to this position. Hopefully, chiropractic educational institutions will soon begin to meet this challenge.

INFORMED CONSENT

Once a patient has proceeded through the initial consultation and examination procedures, a report of findings with an explanation of the diagnosis and treatment plan helps establish realistic expectations regarding length of treatment, the patient's active involvement, and probable outcome. Explanation of alternative treatment and possible risks involved with the chiropractic procedures planned and written and signed informed consent[54] are strong risk management procedures. Some offices may choose to have patients simply read and sign an informed consent document when they are completing the entrance questionnaires. The timing and format may be optional as long as required information is provided and the patient is given a chance to have his or her questions answered before treatment begins.[3]

OTHER APPLICATIONS IN THE CHIROPRACTIC OFFICE

QA procedures in the chiropractic office may also be useful in the evaluation of diagnostic testing and patient treatment to monitor provider profiles and compliance with managed care expectations.

QA IN CHIROPRACTIC DIAGNOSIS

The use of high-technology assessment methods has grown rapidly. More facts can be acquired on patient anatomy and function than can possibly be assimilated into meaningful information with respect to the diagnosis or treatment of the patient's problem. For care givers who are unfamiliar with the technical and ethical issues of instrumentation use, the barrage of new technical data rapidly can become misleading. What should be measured vs. what can be measured? When should specialty testing be invoked?

Protocols, sometimes called critical pathways of care, focus on decision making of this type, as well as treatment recommendations. Current recommended policy[16] strongly urges that specialty testing, including most radiography, generally is unnecessary in acute low back pain, for example. Evidence has failed to show significant benefits to patient treatment and recovery, especially within the first 30 days of care. Patients with the following historical or physical examination features warrant specialty testing and should not wait:

1. History of significant trauma
2. Man more than age 50 with acute back pain

3. Age 70 or older
4. History of cancer
5. Evidence of infection

Once a patient's response to care has proved disappointing, an appropriate step may be to conduct additional testing to reassess therapy. Often several options are available. For example, a patient with persistent sacroiliac pain may have degenerative joint disease, ankylosing spondylitis, or tumor.[56] Plain radiography may be of limited value, whereas hematogenous testing (antinuclear antibodies, HLA-B27), magnetic resonance imaging (early joint inflammation), diagnostic joint injection, and computed tomography (degenerative disease, tumor) may be of diagnostic value. The final determination may require evaluation of the clinical manifestation and response to therapy, followed by the use of the single-most effective test procedure. Alternatively, it may require a sequence of tests. The task of choosing can be simplified by understanding the principles underlying selection of appropriate tests.[13, 16] The following guidelines list the salient features important to test selection:

1. Test results have been compared to the best available gold standard.
2. Behavior of the test across a spectrum of the target condition is known.
3. Precision and observer variation are known.
4. Behavior of the results from sensibly defined normal subjects is available.
5. Test protocols are standardized.
6. Utility of the test has been determined using widely accepted standards.

Each contributes to the central purpose of testing summarized as (1) reducing physician uncertainty with respect to diagnosis and (2) providing a basis for establishing a new treatment plan to address the nonresponsive condition. In the final analysis, the patient should be demonstrably better off because the test was performed than if it had not been.

Diagnostic imaging uses QA to accentuate accuracy of information obtained on radiographs and other imaging. Poor quality from technique, equipment, or darkroom can result in inadequate information gleaned from the studies to come to a diagnostic conclusion and determine course of management. Quality issues for imaging also include patient selection, selection choice of views, and patient and operator protection.[57, 58]

Critical care pathways or algorithms are becoming more abundant in the chiropractic literature. Clinical flow charts assist the practitioner in diagnostic decision making for common and less common patient complaints (Table 9). Where appropriate, case management according to these algorithms may reduce diagnostic uncertainty and ultimately reduce variations in practice.[59]

QA IN CHIROPRACTIC TREATMENT

Attitudes of the public and of policy makers toward our health care system and its providers have evolved over the past 40 years. They are flavored by the combined effects of increasing technological dependence,

TABLE 9.
Diagnostic Algorithms in Chiropractic Literature

Algorithm	Literature Source
Subluxation	Faucret B, Mao W, Nakagawa T, et al: Determination of bony subluxations by clinical, neurological and chiropractic procedures. *J Manipulative Physiol Ther* 3:165–116, 1980.
Vascular accidents	Henderson DJ: Vertebral artery syndrome. In Vear H (ed): *Chiropractic Standards of Practice and Quality of Care.* Gaithersburg, Md, Aspen, 1992.
Headache	Nelson C, Boline P: A consensus on the assessment and treatment of headache. *J Chiropr Technique* 3:151–168, 1991.
Fatigue	Bowers LJ: Fatigue: Narrowing the differential. *Top Clin Chiropr* 1:73–74, 1994.
Back pain	McCarthy KA. Improving the clinician's use of orthopedic testing: An application to low back pain. *Top Clin Chiropr* 1:78–80, 1994.
Somatization	Milas TB: Psychological considerations in chiropractic practice. *Top Clin Chiropr* 1:70–72, 1994.
Chest/abdominal pain	Souza TA: Back to basics: Differentiating mechanical pain from visceral pain. *Top Clin Chiropr* 1:67–69, 1994.
Soft tissue pain	Henninger R: Back to basics: Evaluation of soft tissue pain. *Top Clin Chiropr* 1:77, 1994.
Upper abdominal pain	Jackson S: Diagnostic screening of patients with upper abdominal pain. *Top Clin Chiropr* 2:89, 1995.
Fever	Evans R: Diagnosis of acute and low grade fever in the adult. *Top Clin Chiropr* 2:91, 1995.

*Adapted from Hansen DT, Mootz RD: *Top Clin Chiropr* 1:46, 1994.

dynamic variations in practice behavior, and increasing costs without a commensurate demonstration of effective outcome from treatment. As a result, doctors and their aides have undergone increasing regulation through QA and QM mechanisms.

The influence of these methods on enhancing the value of services thus far has been equivocal. A principal reason for their failure to successfully reduce costs and maintain quality of service is that none of these procedures result in reasoned and persistent change in provider behavior[21, 60, 61] or the guild mentality of the professional associations. Decisions in health care should be based on the strongest evidence available to support a plan of treatment. Where evidence is lacking, professional expert consensus and experience must suffice as guiding factors.

The QA process uses formal criteria to evaluate and update the care administered to patients. The effect on day-to-day practice is to add, as yet, another layer of expectations on provider performance. These are annually updated and enforced through the certification and recertification processes by which physicians, including chiropractors, are permitted to continue participation in access to patient material. Considerable effort is being expended to set out protocols and guidelines[15, 16] by which individual providers are expected to adhere. Departures from the basic protocols need to be rationally defined based on accepted foundations for which complications are commonly encountered. Such complications or mitigating factors must be adequately defined and action steps taken by the physician to offset or correct them documented in the patient chart. Guidelines and treatment criteria are not new. However, the political inclination for widespread enforcement has been scattered until the advent of health reform, underscored by the premise of provider accountability.

Monitoring of treatment provides this accountability and is not new either. Large computerized data bases (e.g., MEDSTAT),[62] prospective studies,[63-66] and provider profiles[1] harvested from claims data form a basis for evaluating care administered. The critical assumption is that treatment that supplies value causes a change in the clinical status of the patient at a rate equal to or in advance of the natural history.

It should not be surprising that the implementation of a process of accountability has raised concern on the part of health professionals. Debate continues from private office conversation to the professional meetings as to the fairness and appropriateness of guideline and protocol recommendations. Much of the consternation comes from a lack of clarity in understanding the definitions and applications of guidelines, as well as the inappropriate applications made of them by the utilization review process. Several specific issues commonly arise: frequency and duration of passive care, management of the chronic case, and use of instrumentation/imaging in diagnosis and treatment planning.

Benchmarking of care for quality evaluation is based on both economic and clinical data. What follows is a discussion of how these benchmarks can be applied in the daily practice settings by payers and credentialing committees for managed care networks.

Passive Care

The evaluation of treatment, whether by manipulation, exercise, medication, or surgery, should be made in context of the therapeutic objectives, which, in turn, should reflect realistic expectations. Those expectations are dictated by the factors affecting clinical status (Table 10) and the stage of treatment (Table 11) at the time it is implemented. Passive treatment is defined as care administered by a provider that requires no active participation on the part of the patient. Manipulation, physical agents (e.g., ultrasound), and medicines all represent forms of passive care. Studies[16, 62, 63] suggest that passive care plays an important role in case management in the early aspects of treatment of a symptomatic episode. The principal outcomes that should be evident within the first 2 to 6 weeks is a reduction in pain and increase in function. From the perspective of accountability, treatment of the uncomplicated case by passive methods as the primary mechanism should not persist beyond the time frame observed in reports of recovery in untreated cases.[67, 68] Continued reliance on passive modes of care in the small percentage of cases that tend to be

TABLE 10.
Factors Contributing to Clinical Status

Age and gender	Financial status
Comorbidity	Culture and ethnicity
Diagnosis	Patient attitudes
Condition severity	Psychosocial functioning
Chronicity	Lifestyle
Clinical stability	

prolonged in recovery can promote chronicity and physician dependence. In contrast, rapid shift of focus from pain severity as a limiting or indicating factor for treatment to one that emphasizes function and performance is believed to minimize chronic disability.

Use of natural history as a criteria for evaluating treatment outcomes requires attention to the proper fit between the case being evaluated and the type of condition for which the natural history is known. First, all natural history data are based on the response in an episode of pain. Nothing is known about the effects of any treatment over the long term or lifetime course of spine disorders. As a result, it is important that caregivers and policy makers recognize the onset and expected end of independent episodes. At the same time, mitigating factors (see Table 10) must be factored in fairly as assessment of treatment effects are made.

Similarly, the principal diagnosis must be considered. For example, there is good reason to believe that cervical and lumbar spine disorders are likely to have qualitative responses to treatment that are analogous,[69] but there are important differences as well. Recent evidence[70-72] demon-

TABLE 11.
Stages of Treatment: Goals and Objectives

I. Passive care
  A. Acute intervention
    1. Anatomical rest
    2. Reduce spasm
    3. Reduce inflammation
    4. Alleviate pain
II. Active care
  A. Remobilization
    1. Enhance pain free range of motion
    2. Guard against deconditioning
  B. Rehabilitation
    1. Restore strength and endurance
    2. Increase work capacity
  C. Lifestyle modification
    1. Minimize recurrence
    2. Cope with continued impairment

strates an unexpected rate of chronicity in patients with neck complaints over those with lower back pain, for example. The fact that the generic musculoskeletal response to treatment between the two conditions are parallel, the proportion of cases that remain symptomatic is several times higher for the cervical spine.

Chronic Care and Rehabilitation

Much of the debate over guidelines with respect to frequency and duration of care revolves around the concerns for the appropriate management of chronic cases. Some of this controversy arises from failure to apply the definitions of episodic care appropriately. This can be on the part of the provider or the payer. The episodic nature of spine disorders and the fact that they may be periodic are well known. Providers who maintain poor records and who fail to account for this periodicity or payers who ignore it, lumping all care under a diagnosis regardless of episode, do a disservice to the patient or health plan subscriber.

Much has been written and reviewed about the risk for conditions becoming chronic. One breakdown for these factors is:

- Somatic pain nonresponsive to treatment for 2–3 weeks
- Clinical signs of persistent apprehension or anxiety
- Persistent disability
- Persistent drug use (therapeutic or recreational)
- Family disruption
- Job dissatisfaction

Even under circumstances of preexisting subacute and chronic complaints, a limited term of passive treatment can be useful for pain control and restoration of function limited by the pain.[16, 64] It would be expected, however, to see a rapid shift in emphasis toward goal-directed rehabilitation and self-reliance (home care and patient education) to manage residual symptoms. Under these conditions, limiting passive treatment to manage exacerbations or recurrent severe pain often accompanying active rehabilitation will allow the patient to remain in the program and enhance his or her gains.[44]

Rehabilitation may also be appropriate for patients returning to highly exertional job tasks (lifting, pushing, pulling) after having had activity limitation for 30 days or more. More than 40% of these patients are likely to undergo deconditioning and have increased risk for reinjury.[73] No data have been accumulated; however, experience suggests that few patients require ongoing passive treatment for chronic and incurable disorders. When clinical evidence suggests that there is no physician dependence, and trials of therapeutic withdrawal demonstrate regression in clinical status, ongoing supportive care may be appropriate for the chronic patient.[15]

As discussed with diagnostic procedures and methods, there are also critical care pathways and clinical algorithms in the literature for chiropractic and multidisciplinary management of common and uncommon patient manifestations (Table 12). Where appropriate, case management according to these algorithms may reduce diagnostic uncertainty and ultimately reduce variations in practice.[38]

TABLE 12.
Management Algorithms in Chiropractic Literature*

Algorithm	Literature Source
Scoliosis	Nykoliation JS, Cassidy JD, Arthur BE, et al: An algorithm for the management of scoliosis. *J Manipulative Physiol Ther* 9:1–14, 1986.
	Souza TA: Decision making with scoliosis management. *Top Clin Chiropr* 1:75–77, 1994.
Low back pain	Aker PD, Thiel HW, Kirkaldy-Willis WH: Low back pain: Pathogenesis, diagnosis and management. *Am J Chiropr Med* 3:19–24, 1990.
Industrial back pain	Mootz RD, Waldorf VT: Chiropractic care parameters for common industrial low back conditions. *J Chiropr Technique* 5:119–125, 1993.
Exercise	Cook RD, Mootz RD: Determining appropriateness of exercise and rehabilitation for chiropractic patients. *Top Clin Chiropr* 1:75–77, 1994.
Back pain	McCarthy KA: Improving the clinician's use of orthopedic testing: An application to low back pain. *Top Clin Chiropr* 1:78–80, 1994.
	Zografos PT, Thompson J, Gienapp T, et al: Portal of entry management of low back pain in adults. *Top Clin Chiropr* (in press).
Calf/heel pain	Souza TA: Conservative management of orthopedic conditions of the lower leg, foot and ankle. *Top Clin Chiropr* 1:82–83, 1994.
Knee/ankle pain	Souza TA: Conservative management of orthopedic conditions of the lower leg, foot, and ankle. *Top Clin Chiropr* 1:82–83, 1994.
Lower extremity soft tissue	Mullen D, Bowers LJ: Myofascial pain syndromes. A look at the lower extremity. *Top Clin Chiropr* 1:81, 1994.
Frequency/duration	Hansen DT: Back to basics: Determining how much care to give and reporting patient progress. *Top Clin Chiropr* 1:74–75, 1994.
Hypertension	Goertz C, Mootz R: A review of chiropractic management strategies in the care of hypertensive patients. *J Neuromusculoskeletal System* 1:91–108, 1993.
	Mootz RD: Conservative management of hypertension. *Top Clin Chiropr* 2:93, 1995.
Cough	Mootz RD, Frischer AA, Adams AH: Evaluation and management of acute and chronic cough. *Top Clin Chiropr* 2:87–88, 1995.
Gastroesophageal reflux	Jackson S: Management of gastroesophageal reflux disease. *Top Clin Chiropr* 2:90, 1995.

*Adapted from Hansen DT, Mootz RD: *Top Clin Chiropr* 1:46, 1994.

QA AND OUTCOMES

CLINICAL OUTCOMES

Recently policy makers have given much attention to the measurement of quality of care by focusing on the outcomes of that care. An extreme argument in favor of looking only at outcomes is that it does not matter what care was given if the outcomes are uniformly good. The converse is implied, that if the outcomes are poor, the patient must have received poor quality care. Neither of these generalizations stands up to close scrutiny, but they do convey the powerful enticement associated with outcome as a measure of quality.

Health delivery systems will benefit from outcome measures because they really matter to patients and physicians alike. However, Chassin et al.[30] offer three cautions to their exclusive use: specific outcomes are difficult to attribute to specific episodes of care, only a few outcomes are easy to measure, and outcome measures do not identify what went wrong during case management.[30]

Outcome measures have the greatest chance of assessing quality of care when they represent the average response over a sample population and are combined or correlated to some aspect of clinical process or management. For example, time loss days can be used as one outcome measure in the management of acute low back pain and can then be correlated to diagnostic criteria that segregates true radicular complications of low back pain from the less complicated "referred pain syndromes." A chart of significant differences meaningful to future clinical decision making likely would be developed. The current literature would suggest that the total time loss days for uncomplicated back pain (referred pain patterns) would be significantly less than for cases with true radicular complications from herniated nucleus pulposus or lateral stenosis.

With coordination of clinical data and QA processes, outcomes management becomes a system that encourages doctors to follow a set of guidelines (practice parameters or clinical paths) by showing them how their clinical performance ranks with that of their colleagues. Eventually public policy may combine physicians' outcome record with their cost and QM profiles and made public to help consumers make informed decisions about quality care.[7]

The growing field of outcomes research is attempting to determine which treatment procedures get the best clinical results. The goal is to ensure predictable, desired outcomes from delivery of health services. The Agency for Health Care Policy and Research (U.S. Public Health Service) recent release of guidelines on acute low back pain in adults,[16] chronic pain, and benign prostatic hypertrophy are examples of this effort to combine the best available evidence with outcomes research.

Outcomes research and consensus guidelines processes are fledgling fields for the chiropractic profession. Early applications of outcomes management were especially for low back pain,[74, 75] neck pain, and headache.[76] Investigation continues to expand clinical outcomes studies (WSCC, LACC, etc.). Little dissemination of outcomes management technology into clinical practice, however, has occurred.

The Mercy guidelines approached the concept of outcomes in practice and generated a list of procedures and devices by a consensus of members broadly representing the various facets and schools of thought within the profession that have attained some general professional acceptance (Table 13).[15] For many of these procedures to survive the consensus process, evidence of "responsiveness" was necessary. Many physical, functional, and symptomatic measures generally are appropriate for certain patient manifestations. However, what remains for further study are many of the basic chiropractic procedures used to determine the subluxation lesion and its concurrent effects.

The diminutive status of chiropractic outcome measures for treatment of the subluxation and its comorbid conditions quickly establishes a research agenda. Today's emphasis on credibility and accountability gives priority to provider groups and public policy that follow recognized processes of evidence synthesis and testing. Leadership within the chiropractic research community (e.g., the Consortium for Chiropractic Research, National Institute of Chiropractic Research, and the Foundation for Chiropractic Research) has recognized the need for quality of life measures as they relate to technology assessment and responses to treatment. The Council on Health Care Technology[77] has issued authoritative recommen-

TABLE 13.
List of Meaningful Outcomes for Chiropractic Case Management*†

Functional outcome assessments by questionnaire (10.1.1)
   Oswestry pain questionnaire
   Roland-Morris disability questionnaire
   Neck disability index
Pain perception outcome assessments (10.2.1)
   Visual analog scales
   McGill/Melzak pain questionnaire
Patient satisfaction questionnaires (10.2.2)
   Patient satisfaction questionnaire
   Visit-specific questionnaire
General health outcome assessments (10.3.1)
   Sickness impact profile
   SF-36 (medical outcomes study)
   Dartmouth COOP charts
Physiological outcomes
   Range of motion (10.4.1)
   Muscle function (10.4.3)
   Postural evaluations (10.4.5)
Subluxation syndrome
   Vertebral position assessed radiographically (10.5.1)
   Abnormal segmental motion/lack of joint end-play on palpation (10.5.2)
   Soft tissue compliance and tenderness (10.5.4)

*From Hansen DT: *Top Clin Chiropr* 1:7, 1994. Used by permission.
†Mercy recommendation number is in parentheses.

TABLE 14.
Practice Monitoring Outcomes

Utilization	Quality	Costs
Number of services per occurrence	Patient satisfaction	Charges per occurrence
Treatment days/weeks per occurrence	Customer complaints	Charges for services
Utilization of imaging technology	File review	Disability compensation
Interdisciplinary referrals	Utilization management "flags"	
Hospital admissions		

dations concerning the appropriate applications and for cooperative research. The opportunities for chiropractic scientists to engage in collaborative outcomes research is greater than at any time in professional history. Participation offers a chance to elevate the credibility and legitimacy of clinical claims of benefit from chiropractic services, a chance the profession can ill afford to miss.

PRACTICE MONITORING OF OUTCOMES

Beyond the clinical outcomes, health plan managers and administrators also track individual practice monitoring outcomes as a part of their provider profiles. Sophisticated software programs are available to monitor various indices of physician practice and hospital usage. This technology heralds the implementation of the parameters that have been discussed earlier in this chapter. Future theory of health care reform discussions are now facts of daily practice life as managed care expands across the geography of North America (Table 14).

HEALTH STATUS AND HEALTH POLICY

There is real foundation for skepticism toward governmental initiatives in health reform. In the interim political struggle, the health service purchasers consisting of insurance companies, local and state governments, and employers are quietly and independently implementing their visions, focusing on costs and quality. Gone are the days of medicine's dominating influence over development of policy issues. Operating in public forums, health care providers, administrators, and public (consumer) members have made determinations on health planning, certificates of need for hospitals, and expensive technologies. Except for the cooperative HMOs like Kaiser and Group Health Cooperative of Puget Sound, these health service panels have been the first formal effort to integrate public opinion into health policy at the local level. Community panels have had chiropractic delegates, likely representing the first formal inclusion of chiropractic doctors in the arena of health policy deliberation.

The field of health policy has developed quickly as a discipline being supported in academic and research centers since. Health policy involves the values of the society or community in terms of how and to whom health resources are allocated. Besides requirement for acknowledgment of public opinion, health policy specialists concern themselves with economic, cultural, and sociological issues, public health concerns, and the scientific and technological effects of health care delivery. "Best interest" issues and the social values assigned to them have shifted from the physician-centered domain to that of being patient centered, motivating the outcomes management, customer satisfaction, appropriateness research, and technology assessment. Public acceptance of a medical device or procedure is no longer dependent solely on the prevailing opinions of medical experts. The public is asking, "What is your science telling you?," "How good is your science?," and "What are the economic and health risk involved compared to the benefit?"

The evolution of reform concepts has emerged from the dominance of cost containment as the sole focus to one that is more rational: the value of service. Acknowledging the concerns for quality of health care delivery, the idea of value seeks to answer the questions on effects of reform on quality of service. Value of service can be represented by the following relationship:

$$Value = (Quality/Cost)$$

Quite simply, the value of health care is enhanced with higher quality at lower cost. McNerney[78] emphasizes, "The bottom-line issue is value, not price alone. Saving expenditures at the expense of quality is not only unprofessional, it's poor management and poor public policy."

FUTURE CONSIDERATIONS

Health-related industries are struggling with society's demands for change. Efforts are coordinated and funded by government private foundations using accepted structure and process. The chiropractic profession is a participant in but a few instances. Indeed, most of health policy as it relates to benefits and reimbursement for chiropractic patients originates in public-funded entitlements (Medicare/Medicaid) and the dominant, private sector managed care organizations. The number of chiropractor representatives are far less proportionately than the number of American citizens seeking chiropractic care. Although the chiropractic profession is now the third largest health discipline, the interests of its patients are significantly underrepresented in health policy making nationwide.

Career opportunities for chiropractic doctors in health policy and administration are opening faster than the availability of qualified applicants. The undergraduate and postgraduate chiropractic curricula ignore the changing complexions of quality-focused health care and the dynamic health care delivery "culture."[23, 25] This cavalier attitude of the official agents of the profession is puzzling in view of the favorable results experienced when qualified chiropractic candidates participate.[3, 16, 25]

The chiropractic discipline must rise to meet the social challenges of accountability and credibility. Given the limited professional resources, one solution may be to develop a "think tank," a center of excellence holding as its central emphasis the research and development of issues related to public health policy. An integral activity of such an organization would be the collaboration with other academic, political, and health policy organizations to organize experience and training in health policy functions on behalf of the profession. Without the political, academic, research, and clinical practice commitment to centralize and sponsor health policy functions, outside institutions will continue to determine health policy as it relates to the delivery of chiropractic service.

For the limited conditions of which there is sufficient scientific evidence, the data on effectiveness of manipulation—the core treatment used by chiropractors—has afforded the opportunity for chiropractors to participate at the inception of policy making. Expansion of that role to encompass the breadth of influence of interest to the profession will require the commitment to society's concerns on their terms. The health discipline able to supply the evidence of value for their services will be rewarded. Are chiropractic, its leadership and its practitioners, ready to serve its patients' interests in this way?

REFERENCES

1. Weiss KD, Skelton WK, Black ER, et al: *Creating a Community-Based Ambulatory Network in Rochester, NY*. University of Rochester, Rochester, NY, 1993.
2. Goldfield N, Nash DB: *Providing Quality Care: The Challenge to Clinicians*. Philadelphia, American College of Physicians, p 3, 1989.
3. McElheran LJ, Sollecito PC: Delivering quality chiropractic care in a managed care setting. *Top Clin Chiropr* 1:30–40, 1994.
4. Relman AS: Assessment and accountability: The third revolution in medical care. *N Engl J Med* 19:1220–1222, 1988.
5. Berwick DM, Knapp MG. Theory and practice for measuring health care quality. *Health Care Financing Rev* (suppl):49, 1987.
6. McCutcheon JC, Schumacher DN: Health care transformation and the case for a community-wide health information managed environment. *Quality Manage Health Care* 2:1–17, 1994.
7. Coile RC: *Revolution: The New Health Care System Takes Shape*. Knoxville, Tenn, Whittle Books, 1994.
8. Iglehart JK: Foreword, In Goldfield N, Nash DB: *Providing Quality Care: The Challenge to Clinicians*. Philadelphia, American College of Physicians, pp 1–2, 1989.
9. Wolinski H, Brune T: *The Serpent and the Staff—Unhealthy Politics of the American Medical Association*. New York, GP Putnam, pp 1–15, 1994.
10. Starr P: *The Social Transformation of American Medicine*. New York, Basic Books, 1982.
11. Meisinger SR: The Americans with Disabilities Act of 1990: A new challenge for human resource managers [legal report]. *Society of Human Resources*, pp 1–16, Winter, 1990.
12. Postol LP: An employer's guide to the Americans with Disabilities Act: From job qualifications to reasonable accommodations. *John Marshall Law Rev*, pp 1–68, August 1991.
13. Sackett DL, Hayes RG, Guyatt GH, et al: *Clinical Epidemiology—A Basic Science for Clinical Medicine*, ed 2. Boston, Little, Brown, pp 51–68, 187–284, 1985.

14. North American Spine Society Ad Hoc Committee on Diagnostic and Therapeutic Procedures: Committee report on diagnostic and therapeutic procedures. *Spine* 16:1161–1167, 1991.
15. Haldeman S, Chapman-Smith D, Petersen D: *Guidelines for Chiropractic Quality Assurance and Practice Parameters.* Gaithersburg, Md, Aspen, 1992.
16. Bigos S, Bowyer O, Braen G, et al: *Acute Low Back Problems in Adults.* Clinical Practice Guideline No 14, AHCPR Publication No 95–0642. Rockville, Md, Agency for Health Care Policy and Research, Public Health Service, US Department of Health and Human Services, December 1994.
17. O'Kane M: *1994 Standards for the Accreditation of Managed Care Organizations,* Washington, DC, National Commission on Quality Assurance, June 1994.
18. Joint Commission on Accreditation of Healthcare Organizations: *1994 Accreditation Manual for Health Care Networks.* Oakbrook Terrace, Ill, Joint Commission on Accreditation of Healthcare Organizations, vol 1, 1994.
19. *Health Plan Employer Data and Information Set and User's Manual, Version 2.0.* Washington, DC, National Committee for Quality Assurance, 1993.
20. Jonsen AR: *The New Medicine and the Old Ethics.* Cambridge, Mass, Harvard University Press, 1990.
21. Eisenberg JM: *Doctor's Decisions and the Cost of Medical Care.* Ann Arbor, Mich, Health Administration Press, 1986.
22. Wennberg J, Gittelsohn A: Small area variations in health care delivery. *Science* 182:11102–11108, 1973.
23. Hansen DT: Prospects for the future of chiropractic guidelines. In Lawrence D (ed): *Advances in Chiropractic.* Chicago, Mosby, vol 1, 1994.
24. Zalta E: Provider selection standards as a quality indicator. *Managed Care Q* 1:53–61, 1993.
25. Mootz RD, Shekelle PG, Hansen DT: The politics of policy and research. *Top Clin Chiropr* (in press).
26. Audet AM, Greenfield S, Field M: Medical practice guidelines: Current activities and future directions. *Ann Intern Med* 113:709–714, 1990.
27. Hough DE, Balagot MM: *Assessing Your Practice in an Age of Reform.* Chicago, American Medical Association, 1993.
28. Kenen J: Doctors seeking to develop own HMOs and networks. *Reuter's News Service.* Washington, DC, 1995.
29. Steffen GE: Quality medical care: A definition. *JAMA* 260:56–61, 1988.
30. Chassin MR, Kosecoff J, Dubois R: *Health Care Quality Assessment.* Chicago, Midwest Business Group on Health, 1992.
31. Souza TA: Decision making with scoliosis management. *Top Clin Chiropr* 1:75–77, 1994.
32. Mootz RD, Frischer AA, Adams AH: Evaluation and management of acute and chronic cough. *Top Clin Chiropr* 2:87–88, 1995.
33. Mootz RD: Conservative management of hypertension. *Top Clin Chiropr* 2:93, 1995.
34. Hansen DT: Quality of care and chiropractic necessity. In Vear HJ: *Chiropractic Standards of Practice and Quality of Care.* Gaithersburg, Md: Aspen, 1992.
35. US Office of Technology Assessment: *The Quality of Medical Care: Information for Consumers.* Washington, DC, US Government Printing Office (OTA-h-386), June 1988.
36. Caper P: Defining quality in medical care. *Health Aff (Millwood)* 7:49–61, 1988.
37. Donabedian A: Commentary on some studies of the quality of care. *Health Care Financing Rev* (suppl):75, 1987.
38. Hansen DT, Mootz RD: Understanding, developing, and utilizing clinical algorithms. *Top Clin Chiropr* 1:46, 1994.

39. Mould JW, Blake GH, Becker LA: Goal oriented medical care. *Fam Med* 23:46–51, 1991.
40. Nash DB, Goldfield N: Information needs of purchasers. In Goldfield N, Nash DB (eds): *Providing Quality Care: The Challenge to Physicians*. Philadelphia, American College of Physicians, p 8, 1989.
41. Berwick DM, Godfrey AB, Roessner J: *Curing Health Care: New Strategies for Quality Improvement*. San Francisco, Jossey-Bass, p 43, 1990.
42. Council of Institute of Medicine: *Quality Considerations Important to U.S. Health Care Reform*. National Institutes of Health, Institute of Medicine, Washington, DC, 1994.
43. Defino T: JCAHO stokes up fiery competition with NCQA. *Managed Heathcare* 5:24–29, 1995.
44. Triano JJ, Raley B: Chiropractic in the interdisciplinary team practice. *Top Clin Chiropr* 1:58–66, 1994.
45. Clinical Quality Assurance Panel: *Clinical Competency Document*. Phoenix, Council on Chiropractic Education, Oct 1, 1984.
46. Hansen DT: Back to basics: Determining how much care to give and reporting patient progress. *Top Clin Chiropr* 1:2, 1994.
47. Chiropractic Network Services: *Quality Assurance Manual*. Lynnwood, Wash, Chiropractic Network Services, 1993.
48. Kongstvedt PR: Primary care in open panels. In Kongstvedt PR: *The Managed Health Care Handbook*, ed 2. Gaithersburg, Md, Aspen, p 50, 1993.
49. Hansen DT, White LB, Ayres JR, et al: Credentialing of chiropractic providers in a managed care setting: A case study. Paper presented at the Proceedings of the Chiropractic Forum, American Public Health Association, Atlanta, 1991.
50. Bowers LJ, Mootz RD: The nature of primary care: The chiropractor's role. *Top Clin Chiropr* 2:66–84, 1995.
51. Coile RC: *The New Medicine: Reshaping Medical Practice and Health Care Management*. Gaithersburg, Md, Aspen, 1988.
52. Hansen DT: Back to basics: Determining how much care to give and reporting patient progress. *Top Clin Chiropr* 1:1–8, 1994.
53. Kranz K: An overview of primary care concepts. *Top Clin Chiropr* 2:55–65, 1995.
54. Campbell L, Ladenheim CJ, Sherman R, et al: Informed consent: A search for protection. *Top Clin Chiropr* 1:55–63, 1994.
55. Haldeman S, Chapman-Smith D, Petersen D: *Guidelines for Chiropractic Quality Assurance and Practice Parameters*. Gaithersburg, Md, Aspen, 1992.
56. Bernard T, Cassidy D: In Frymoyer J (ed): *The Adult Spine Principles and Practice*. New York, Raven Press, vol 2, pp 2107–2130, 1991.
57. Scuderi DJ: Minimizing patient radiation exposure during radiographic examinations. *Top Clin Chiropr* 1:33–38, 1994.
58. Taylor JAM, Lawson DM: Quality assurance in chiropractic radiology. *Top Clin Chiropr* 1:67–71, 1994.
59. Hansen DT: Understanding, developing, and utilizing clinical algorithms. *Top Clin Chiropr* 1:44–57, 1994.
60. Goldman L: Changing physicians' behavior: The pot and the kettle. *N Engl J Med* 322:1524, 1990.
61. Lomas JM, Enken GM, Anderson GM, et al. Opinion leaders vs. audit and feedback to implement practice guidelines: Delivery after previous cesarean section. *JAMA* 265:2202–2207, 1991.
62. Stano M: A comparison of health care costs from chiropractic and medical patients. *J Manipulative Physiol Ther* 16:291–299, 1993.
63. Triano JJ, Hondras M, McGregor M: Differences in treatment history with ma-

nipulation for acute, subacute, chronic and recurrent spine pain. *J Manipulative Physiol Ther* 15:24–30, 1992.
64. Triano JJ, McGregor M, Hondras M, et al: Manipulation therapy vs. education programs in chronic low back pain. *Spine* (in press).
65. Roland M, Morris R: A study of the natural history of back pain: Development of a reliable and sensitive measure in low back pain. *Spine* 8:141–144, 1983.
66. Roland M, Morris R: A study of the natural history of back pain: Development of a reliable and sensitive measure in low back pain. *Spine* 8:141–144, 1983.
67. Triano JJ: Chiropractic rehabilitation. In Hochschuler S, Cotler H, Guyer R (eds): *Rehabilitation of the Spine: Science and Practice*. St Louis, Mosby, pp 635–645, 1993.
68. Hansen DT (ed): *Chiropractic Standards and Utilization Guidelines in the Care and Treatment of Injured Workers*. Olympia, Washington, Chiropractic Advisory Committee, Department of Labor and Industries, 1988.
69. Triano JJ: Standards of care: Manipulative procedures. In White A, Anderson R (eds): *Conservative Care of Low Back Pain*. Baltimore, Williams & Wilkins, pp 151–168, 1991.
70. Ameis A: Cervical whiplash: Considerations in the rehabilitation of cervical myofascial injury. *Can Fam Physician* 32:1871–1876, 1986.
71. Dartigues J, Henry P, Puymirat E, et al: Prevalence and risk factors of recurrent cervical pain syndrome in a working population. *Neuroepidemiology* 7:99–105, 1988.
72. Deans GT, McGallairard JN, Tutherford WH: Incidence and duration of neck pain among patients injured in car accidents. *BMJ* 292:94–95, 1986.
73. Mayer T, Gatchel R: *Functional Restoration for Spinal Disorders: A Sports Medicine Approach*. Philadelphia, Lea & Febiger, 1988.
74. Hseih CJ, Phillips RB, Adams AH, et al: Functional outcomes of low back pain. *J Manipulative Physiol Ther* 15:4–9, 1992.
75. Hansen DT, Ayres JR: Chiropractic outcome measures. *J Chiropr Technique* 3:63–64, 1991.
76. Vernon H, Mior S: The neck disability index: A study of reliability and validity. *J Manipulative Physiol Ther* 14:409–415, 1991.
77. Council on Health Care Technology: *Quality of Life and Technology Assessment*. National Institutes of Health, Institute of Medicine, Washington, DC, 1989.
78. Shine KI, McNeil BJ, Aiken LK, et al: *America's Health in Transition: Protecting and Improving the Quality of Health and Health Care*. Washington, DC, Institute of Medicine, 1994.

Index

A

Abdominal pain, 657
Abduction, 195
Abnormalities, congenital, see Spinal stenosis
Abortion, spontaneous (miscarriage), 106
Abruptio placentae, 107
Abstracts and indexes, 571–573
Acceleration/deceleration injuries, 1–37
   biomechanics, 3–10
   description, classification, 1–3
   physical and individual factors, 15–21
   sequence of events in injuries, 10–14
   types of injuries and pain, 21–28
Accessibility of health care, 652
Accidents, traffic, 1–37
   back pain after, 24–26
   biomechanics of whiplash, 3–10
   occupant position and whiplash injuries, 21
   personal factors affecting injuries, 18–21
   preparedness for collision impact, 4, 5, 9–10, 18, 21
   rear-impact collisions, 3–7, 10–14, 15–17
   safety devices and injuries, 3, 9, 15–17, 24–26
   second collisions, 15, 17
   sequence of events in whiplash, 10–14
   type of collision and back pain, 25
   type of collision in acceleration/deceleration trauma, 2
   vehicle size and injuries, 5, 17
Accreditation
   activator technique, 473
   chiropractic education, 381, 389
   managed care, 646
Achilles tendinitis, 136, 229, 230
Acromegaly, 56
Acromioclavicular joint
   description, 280
   injuries, 298–302
   shear test, 289–290
Activator adjusting instrument
   definition, 473
   dynamic mechanical properties of spine, 495–500
   history and development, 472, 473
   studies of, reports on, 486–493
   training in use, 513
Activator technique, 471–520
   accredited colleges, instructional offerings, 473
   clinical studies, 486–493
   efficacy and evaluation, 475, 478
   most commonly used techniques, 472
   research on effectiveness, 502
   sciatica and, 487, 488–489
   seminar program, 474, 475, 476, 477
   use of, 453, 454
Adducto varus, 208–209
Adherence to treatment, see Patient compliance
Adjustment
   Activator adjusting instrument, 472, 473
   Activator Method Chiropractic Technique, 513–515
   chiropractors' attitudes toward, 444–445
   definitions, 418, 466–467
   dynamic mechanical stimuli, 498–500
   effects of therapy, 423–428
   localization, 421
   mechanical force manually assisted procedures, 471, 486–493, 502
   patient positioning, 421–423
   techniques, mechanics, 418–421
   vertebral forces and movements, 494–495
Adson's maneuver (shoulder), 294, 296
Advertising, 568–569
Affect, 266–267, 269–270
Age
   low back pain during pregnancy, 98
   onset of spinal stenosis, 59
   whiplash injury factors, 18, 19, 20, 21
Alcoholism, 273
Allen's test (shoulder), 294, 296

Allodynia, 185, 189
Ambulatory care
  AmbuQual quality management system, 527–563
  quality assurance in chiropractic offices, 649
  quality management, 521–563
  quality parameters, 527–528, 532, 541
AmbuQual quality management system, 527–563
  indicator implementation chart, 530–531
  program implementation, 528–532, 543
  qualitative scoring form, 433
  quality improvement plan (QIP), 531, 534
  scoring, 541, 542–543
American Back Society, 377
American Chiropractic Association, 381
American Medical Association, 382
American Psychiatric Association, diagnostic and statistical manuals, 256–259
Analysis of variance, 579
Anatomicophysiological technique, *see* Chiropractic technique
Anesthesia, 380
Anisomelia (anatomically short leg), 476, 477–480
Ankle
  dancer evaluation, 228–229
  dorsiflexion, plantarflexion, 195
  examination in runners, 131
  muscular control in running, 123–124
  pain management algorithms (quality assurance), 661
  rehabilitation (runners), 137–140
Ankylosing spondylitis, 57, 352–353
Ankylosis, 353
Ankylosis, fibrous, 172–173
Anorexia nervosa, 274
Anterior drawer test (shoulder), 285–286
Anterior impingement syndrome, 228, 229
Anterior instability test (shoulder), 286
Antitrust, 373
Apophyseal joints
  growth centers (ossicles of Oppenheimer), 342–343, 345
  lumbopelvic dysfunction and, 225
  psoas insufficiency syndrome, 332
Appearance, 269
Attitude, 266, 269
Apprehension (crank) test for anterior should dislocation, 286

Arm
  muscles, 298
  pain, after crashes, 26
  pain relief, 192
  reflex sympathetic dystrophy, 185
  throwing injuries, 304–309
Armed forces, commissions for chiropractors, 375
Arthralgia, patellofemoral, 134–135
Arthritis, juvenile rheumatoid, 353
Arthritis, rheumatoid, 57, 198, 353
Arthrography, shoulder, 325
Arthrosis, facetal, *see* Osteoarthritis
Article analysis, *see* Journals
Articular functional units, 467
Articular procedures, 452
Athletes, *see* Sports
Atlas inversion, 567
Auditory disturbances, 27
Australia
  chiropractic education, 389
  chiropractic faculty, 403
Automobile accidents, *see* Accidents, traffic
Axillary artery, 282, 311

B

Back, *see* Back muscle injury; Back pain; Spine
Back muscle injury, in dancers, 212
Back pain
  cervical acceleration/deceleration syndrome, 24–26
  characteristics of chiropractic users and nonusers, 376–377
  diagnostic algorithms (quality assurance), 657
  "double-flexion" injury, 26
  education classes, 111–113
  literature assessment (example), 565–566, 580–593
  lower, and Activator adjustment, 487, 491–492
  lower, and anisomelia, 477–480
  lower, and facet tropism, 339
  lower, and pregnancy, 97–120
  lower, management algorithms (quality assurance), 661
  management algorithms (quality assurance), 661
  MRI use, 71
  patient satisfaction with treatment, 378, 379, 428
  postpartum, 99, 116–117

response to treatment, 659–660
risk factors during pregnancy, 98–99
spinal stenosis and, 60
structure vs. function, 450
Barré-Liéou syndrome, 27
Baseball
acceptance of chiropractic, 377
throwing (pitching) injuries, 304–309
β-adrenergic receptors, reflex sympathetic dystrophy, 188–190
Bewegungssegment (term), 463
Biceps, 290, 292, 293
Biomechanics
back pain during pregnancy, 99–100
normal and pathological spine, 517–520
pregnancy and, 98
rear-impact collisions, 3–15
running, 122–123, 132–133
shoulder, 283
throwing, 306–307
whiplash (acceleration/deceleration) injuries, 3–10
Bipolar disorder, 272
Blood pressure, 487
Blue Cross/Blue Shield, 381
Body height, *see* Height
Bone
hyperostosis, 356, 357, 358
resorption (facet joints), 355
scans, reflex sympathetic dystrophy, 187
weakening, contraindications to temporomandibular joint manipulation, 172
Bulimia, 274
Bumpers, *see* Safety devices
Bunions, 229
Bursitis, 281

C

Calcaneal-cuboid joint
calcaneal-navicular coalition, 199, 200
Charcot's joint disease, 198
degenerative joint disease, 201
pronation, 195, 229
Calcaneus, 197, 229
Calcification, 51–53
Calcium crystal deposition disease, 52
Calcium pyrophosphate dihydrate deposition disease, 52
Calf pain, 661
Calluses, 208
Canadian Memorial Chiropractic College, 389
Capsulitis, 167–168, 173–174

Carbon dioxide, 425
Cauda equina, 39, 54, 103
Causalgia, 183, 184
Cavitation, 423, 425, 426
Cervical acceleration/deceleration
injuries, 1–37
syndrome, 22, 23–28
temporomandibular injury, 175–176
terminology, 1
Cervical myelopathy, 51–52, 58
Cervical radiculopathy, 58
Cervical spine
acceleration/deceleration injuries, 1–37, 175–176
articular processes, 337
bilateral facet dislocation, 347–349
burners, 311–312
chronic complaints, 659–660
classification of acceleration/ deceleration, 1, 2
congenital blocking of facets, 342
delayed facet dislocation, 349–350
discogenic spondylosis, 45
experimental auto-crash results, 3–10
facet dislocation, 347–350
facet fractures, 350
facet fusion, hypoplasia, 342, 343
facet joint instability, 360–361
facets and facet joints, 331–335, 343–350
hyperostosis, 358
isolation and pressure test procedures, 484
manipulation loads, 495
naked facet sign, 352
nerve roots, 53, 293, 298
notching, gouge defect, 337
perched facets, 349
personal factors affecting injuries, 18–21
posture and temporomandibular joint problems, 154–155
rotation adjustment, 515
sequence of events in crashes, 10–14
stenosis, 49, 58
trauma and facet disorders, 343–350
Charcot's joint disease, 198
Charts, *see* Medical records
Chemonucleolysis, 53, 54
Chest pain, 657
Chi-square, 579
Children
clavicular physis injuries, 313
dancers, 214

CHIROLARS, 572
Chiropractic, see also Chiropractic education; Chiropractic technique; Managed care; Outcome assessment; headings beginning with Quality; Research
   acceptance, current problems, 373–386
   art, science, philosophy, 437–438
   barriers to emergence of science, 443–444
   chronic care and rehabilitation, 660–661
   college and faculty issues, 383–384
   credentialing, 474, 649–651
   definition of legitimate technique, 445–446
   diversity within, 440–446
   doctor of chiropractic medicine degree, 374
   effect of marginalization, 441
   entrepreneurial practice builders, 383
   future considerations, 665–666
   future path, acceptance as limited medical profession, 384–385
   generalist claims, 443
   health care system reform, 380–381
   hospital staff appointments, 379–380
   ideological confrontations and controversies among chiropractors, 438–439
   insurance reimbursement, 380
   licensure, 375
   management algorithms (quality assurance), 661
   manual therapy, 417–420
   market penetration, 441–442
   marketing plausibility studies, 446
   media portrayal of, 373, 377
   medical resistance to (scientific legitimation), 382, 385
   military commissions, 375
   neurophysiological research needs, 385
   outcomes research and guidelines, 662–663
   pain and decision to treat, 420
   passive care evaluation, 658–660
   patient interactions, 595–633
   patient psychology, 427–428
   peer review, 638–639
   practice characteristics, favored techniques, 452–455
   practice parameters, guidelines and standards of care, 452–455
   primary care providers, 373–375
   principles ("philosophy"), 375
   professional associations and issues, 380–385
   provider profiles, 640
   public acceptance, 376–377
   referrals from physicians, 380
   relations with dentistry, 143–144
   satisfaction of back pain patients, 378, 379
   scientific content and empathy, 387–388
   scientism, 446
   scope of practice, 373, 381–382
   second opinions, 638
   specialist definition, 374
   sports acceptance of, 377
   straights and mixers (traditionalists vs. progressives), 381
   treatment patterns by type of practitioner, 413–414
Chiropractic education, 387–411
   accreditation, 381, 389
   assessment, 399–402
   Australia, 389, 403
   colleges and technique, 447–448
   competency-based, 391–394
   computers and interactive multimedia, 396
   curriculum variations, 382
   distance education, 396–397
   emphases of various colleges, 388–389
   inquiry-based, 398
   interactive videodisk patient simulation, 401
   issues for colleges, 383–384
   mechanistic and holistic paradigms, 389–391, 403–404
   models (constructivism and critical multiplism), 404–405
   outcomes assessment, 389, 390–391, 405–406
   patient management and, 392, 394, 395
   patient simulators and standardized patients, 395–396
   problem solving and problem-based, 392–394, 395, 398
   recent textbooks, 447–448
   staff (faculty) appraisal, 402–403
   students' medical interaction and experience, 383–384
   teaching of techniques, 428–432
   teaching strategies, 394–397

trends, 405–406
trends toward science and medical model, 387–388
Chiropractic literature, see Journals
Chiropractic technique, see also Outcome assessment; headings beginning with Quality; Research
  Activator Methods, 471–520
  Activator Methods Chiropractic Technique summary, 513–515
  anatomicophysiological vs. reflex, 450–451
  categorization of, 451, 452
  categorized by velocity and amplitude, 451
  classification, 448–454
  consensus process, 455
  curriculum in colleges, 447–448
  evaluation (Kaminski protocol), 454, 455
  evaluation, testing, classification, 428, 432
  forceful vs. light-force and non-force techniques, 451
  high-velocity, low-amplitude thrust, 419
  ideological confrontations and controversies, 438–439
  legitimate, 445–446
  manual therapy, 417–420
  misalignment vs. fixation, 449–450
  most common, 472
  overview, 413–435
  patient positioning, 421–423
  practice parameters, 452–455
  primary approach used by chiropractors, 452
  proprietary, 442, 443
  proprietary, allure, 444–445
  proprietary, partial list, 439
  pseudoscientific, 446–447
  psychomotor component, 438
  segmentalism vs. posturalism, 449
  structure vs. function, 450
  system proliferation, 439–446
  systems, contemporary approach, 437–459
  teaching, 428–432
  various forms and developers listed, 429–431
Chondrocalcinosis, 52
Chondrodystrophic spinal stenoses, 40, 41, 43–44
Chondromalacia facetae, 360
Claudication, neurogenic, 60–61

Clavicle
  acromioclavicular joint injuries, 299–300
  fractures, 315, 317–318, 320–321
  osteolysis, 313
  rotation, 283
Clinical trials, see Randomized clinical trials
Clunk test (shoulder), 287, 288
Cognition, 269, 271
Communication, see Physician-patient relationship
Compliance, see Patient compliance
Computed tomography
  facet joints, 332
  fracture detection, 326
  spinal stenosis, 39, 49, 53, 66, 67–72
Computers
  CHIROLARS (chiropractic literature index), 572
  chiropractic education and interactive multimedia, 396
  example of literature search, 586–593
  interactive videodisk patient simulation, 401
  manipulation assisted by, 500–501
Concurrent review, 652
Condyle, mandibular
  articular disk and, 169, 170
  compression, 165, 166
  repositioning, 177, 178, 179
Confidentiality, in quality assurance programs, 554–555
Congress of Chiropractic State Associations, 648
Connective tissue, 426
Constructivism (chiropractic educational model), 404–405
Consumers, see also Physician-patient relationship; Patients
  choice, 441–442
  value for health care dollars, 644
Continuity of care, 652–653
Continuous quality improvement, 522
Cooperation, see Patient compliance
Corpuscular mechanoreceptors, 427
Cortical somatosensory evoked potentials, see Evoked potentials
Corticosteroids, 56, 308–309
Costoclavicular test, 295–296
Cough, 661
Council on Chiropractic Education
  accreditation activities, 381, 382
  index of clinical competencies, 647, 648
  quality assurance activities, 647–648

Cox's technique, 454
Cranial nerves, examination, 165
Credentialing, 474, 649–651
Creep, see Spine
Crepitus, 172
Critical multiplism (chiropractic educational model), 404–405
Cryotherapy, 73
Crystal deposition disease, 353
CT, see Computed tomography

D

Dance, 211–253
   athletic tape, 234
   cause of injury, 212
   equilibrium, 238, 239
   history form and personal information, 214–215, 216
   injuries and faulty technique, 249–250
   injuries and videotaping, 246–249
   injury history, 215, 216
   injury treatment, rehabilitation, 233–249
   joint function and soft tissue, 225
   occupational factors in injuries, 221–223
   orthotics, 234
   postural examination, 223–225
   "pull up," 225, 226
   rotator disks, 241, 242
   schools and young dancers, 249
   screening examination, 213–230
   shoe design, 234–235
   spine evaluation, 225–226
   techniques, 215–221
     arabesque, 218, 220
     demipointe, 230
     developpé, 226, 232
     extension, 220–221, 222, 235
     faulty, 249–250
     Pilates' technique, 244–246, 247
     plié, 217–218, 219
     pointe, 230
     "pull up," 225, 226
     relevé, 230
     "rolling in, out," "sickling," 224, 228
     turnout, 215, 217, 225, 226, 231–232
   tilt (wabble) board, 241–243
   workouts, strengthening and stretching, 230, 233–234, 235
   young dancers, 214
Dartmouth COOP charts, 663
Data interpretation, 577–579
Deceleration injuries, see Acceleration/deceleration injuries

Deep venous thrombosis, 107–108
Degenerative diseases
   facets, 354–358
   intervertebral disk, 341
   joint disease, 201
   spondylolisthesis (pseudospondylolisthesis), 50–51, 360–365
   spondylosis, 48
Dentistry
   bruxing (grinding), 176–177
   dental splint, 176–179
   knowledge of temporomandibular locomotor apparatus, 174–175
   relations with chiropractic, 143–144
Depression, 260–264, 272
Depressive disorders, 255–278
   alcoholism and, 273
   diagnostic and statistical manuals, 256–259
   historical attitudes, 255–256
   medications and, 273
   mood disorder categories, 260
   mood disorder detection, diagnosis, 264–273
   nonpsychiatric medical conditions and, 273–274
   treatment plan, 275–276
Dermotomal somatosensory evoked potentials, see Evoked potentials
Diagnosis, and quality assurance, 655–656, 657
Diagnostic and Statistical Manual of Mental Disorders, 256–259
Diagnostic imaging, see Arthrography; Computed tomography; Electromyography; Magnetic resonance imaging; Myelography; Radiography; Scintigraphy; Sonography
Diffuse idiopathic skeletal hyperostosis, 41, 57
Digastric muscle, 163
DISH disease, 41, 57
Disk, intervertebral, see Intervertebral disk
Diversified technique, 454, 472
Dizziness, and cervical acceleration/deceleration, 26–27
Dorsiflexion, 195, 219, 228, 229
"Double-flexion" injury, 26
Drop arm test (shoulder), 290, 291
DSM-I, -III, IV, 256–259
Dysphagia, 27–28
Dysthymic disorder, 263–264, 272

E

Eating disorders, 274–275
Eclampsia, 107
Economic credentialing, 649–650
Ectopic pregnancy, 106
Education, see Chiropractic education, Patient education
Education, medical, 388
Effectiveness (research results), 578, 583
Efficacy (research results), 578, 583
Electromyography (spinal stenosis diagnosis), 63
Embolism, pulmonary, 107–108
Employer health plans, 646–647
Equinus, 198
Ethics, models of physician behavior (paternalistic, informative, interpretive, deliberative), 601–604
Eversion, 195
Evoked potentials (spinal stenosis diagnosis), 63–64
Exercise
    contraindications, warning signs in pregnancy listed, 114, 115
    dance workouts, strengthening and stretching, 230, 233–234, 235
    foot-ankle rehabilitation, strengthening, 137–140
    low back pain and pregnancy, 108–116
    management algorithms (quality assurance), 661
    postpartum, 117
    pregnant athletes, 115–116
    running injuries, 121–142
    shoulder treatment and rehabilitation, 319–326
    stretching, warmup for runners, 125–126

F

Face
    pain and cervical acceleration/deceleration, 28
    temporomandibular joint examination, 153
Facetal arthrosis, see Osteoarthritis
Facets and facet joints, 331–372
    agenesis, 341
    anatomy, nerve supply, 332–333
    articular cartilage breakdown, 355
    articular pillar angles, 334, 336, 337
    articular pillar fusion, 352, 353
    articular pillars, 341
    articular processes, 337, 343, 346
    asymmetry, 338–341
    bilateral dislocation, 347–349
    capsules, 333, 350, 354
    cervical spine trauma, 343–350
    chondromalacia facetae, 360
    congenital blocking, 341, 342
    degeneration (stages of), 354–358
    degenerative ossicles, 358
    delayed dislocation, 349–350
    developmental variations, 334–335
    Ferguson's sacral base angle, 366, 367
    fibrous invaginations, 333
    fractures, 350, 353
    Hadley's S curve, 363, 365–366
    hyperostosis, 356
    hypertrophy, 356, 357
    hypoplasia or hyperplasia, 341–342, 343, 344, 345
    imbrication (shakelike, overlapping, or telescoping), 362–365
    impingement syndrome, 225
    inflammatory spondyloarthropathy, 352–353
    instability, 358, 359, 360–361
    intra-articular fusion, 359–360
    locked articular processes, 343, 346
    lumbosacral disk angle, 365, 367
    MacNab's line (posterior joint body line), 364, 366–367
    naked facet sign, 351, 352
    normal facet pedicle angle, 362
    notching, gouge defect, 337–338, 339
    ossicles of Oppenheimer, 342–343, 345
    osteoarthritis (facetal arthrosis), 353–354, 355, 356
    perched facets, 349
    "railroad track sign," 352
    role, function, 333–334
    sacral base angle, 366, 367
    segmental instability, 358, 359
    shingling, 351, 352
    spaces (articular process), 333
    spinographic measurements, 365–367
    subarticular bone erosion, 355
    synovial cysts, 358–360
    synovial folds, 333
    synovial hyperplasia, 358
    "trolley track sign," 353
    tropism, 338–341
    unilateral dislocation, 343–344, 346, 347
    ununited apophyseal growth centers, 342–343, 345
    vacuum phenomenon, 358
    visualization, imaging, 331–332

Familial spinal stenosis, 41–42
Fast Fourier transformation, 496, 498
Fatigue, diagnostic algorithms (quality assurance), 657
Feagin test (shoulder), 289, 290
Federation of Straight Chiropractic Organizations, 375, 381
Femur, anteversion and retroversion in dancers, 224, 226
Ferguson's sacral base angle, 366, 367
Fetus, see Pregnancy
Fever, 657
Fibrosis, 54
Fibrous ankylosis of articular disk, 172–173
Fibula stress fractures, 228, 229
Fitness, see Exercise
Fixation, 449–450
Flatfoot, 197–198
   flexible, 198–199
   rigid, 199–200
   runners and, 131, 137
Flexion distraction technique, 472
Flexor hallucis longus tendinitis, 229
Fluoride intoxication, 57
Foot, see also Toes
   dance shoes, 234–235
   dancer evaluation, 229–230
   drop, 116
   examination in runners, 131
   flatfoot, 131, 137, 197–198, 198–199, 199–200
   forefoot valgus, 197
   muscle function, 196–197
   pronation, 195–209
   rearfoot valgus, 197
   rearfoot varus, 197
   rehabilitation (runners), 137–140
Football injuries, 311–312
Footwear, see Shoes
Foramen of Weitbrecht, 281
Forefoot, see Foot
Forestier's disease, 57
Foundation for Chiropractic Education and Research, 383
Fractures, see under parts of body, e.g. Shoulder
Fulcrum test (shoulder), 286, 287
Functional short leg, see Pelvic deficiency

G

Gait analysis, 493
Gait cycle, 122, 124
Gait phases (pronation), 196

Ganglion cysts, 359
Garlic tablets, 568–569
Gastrocnemius muscles, 139
Gastroesophageal reflux, 661
Genu valgus, 197
Gilchrest sign (shoulder), 293
Glenohumeral joint, 280–281, 310
Glenohumeral ligaments, 281, 309
Glenoid labrum, 281, 287, 288
Gluteal tendinitis, 226
Golgi's tendon organs, see Proprioception
Gonstead technique, 454, 472
Gout, 353
Gravitational line of L-3, 367
Guanethidine, 187

H

Hadley's S curve, 363, 365–366
Hallux limitus, 205–207
Hallux rigidus, 205–207
Hallux valgus, 204–205
Halstead's maneuver (shoulder), 294–295, 297
Hammertoes, 207–209, 229
Hamstring, 138–139
Hawkins-Kennedy impingement test (shoulder), 293
Head
   acceleration/deceleration forces in auto crashes, 4, 6,7–15
   pain, screening for temporomandibular joint disorder, 146–152
   posture (temporomandibular joint disorders), 146–150
   restraints in crashes, 15, 16
   sequence of events in whiplash, 10–14
   temporomandibular joint examination, 153
Headache, 24, 657
Health care quality, see headings beginning with Quality
Health care system
   accessibility of services, 652
   chiropractic market penetration, 441–442
   facility credentialing, accessibility, 649–652
   limited or closed panels, 637, 640
   value of services, 644, 665
Health care system reform
   current issues, 380–381
   managed care and, 455–456
   quality assurance and, 639–640, 664–665

Health maintenance organizations, 381
Health Plan Employer Data and Information Set version 2.0, 639, 646–647
Health policy, 664–666
Health reform, *see* Health care system reform
Hearing disturbances, and cervical acceleration/deceleration, 27
HEDIS-2.0, 639, 646–647
Heel
    pain (plantar fasciitis), 136–137
    pain management algorithms (quality assurance), 661
    pronation, 195–209
    strike, 122
Height (whiplash injury factors), 18, 20, 21
Hemorrhage, 569
Heuter's sign (shoulder), 293
Hill-Sachs deformities, 321
Hip
    extension technique in dance, 220–221, 222
    flexion in auto crashes, 6
    grinding, popping, snapping sounds, 235
    osteoarthritis, 54–55
    psoas muscle effects on, 231
    rotation in dancers, 225, 226, 228
    rotation in runners, 130
    sartorius tendinitis, 226
    turnout technique in dance, 217
    uneven levels and temporomandibular joint problems, 155
History taking
    dancers, 214, 215, 216
    patient-centered interview, 604–607, 610, 628–629
    pregnant patients, 100–103
    shoulder injuries, 279–280
    temporomandibular joint patients, 153–166
Hoarseness, and cervical acceleration/deceleration, 27–28
Holistic health, and chiropractic education, 389–391, 397, 399–400, 403–404
Hormones, changes during pregnancy, 97–98
Hospitals
    chiropractors on staff, 379–380
    quality assurance, 523
    quality assurance and, 637–638
Humerus fractures, 315, 316, 318
Hyaline cartilage, 333
Hydroxyapatite deposition disease, 52
Hyperalgesia, 185
Hyperasthesia, 186
Hyperkeratosis, plantar, 208
Hyperlordosis, 224
Hyperostosis, 356, 357, 358
Hyperostosis, diffuse idiopathic skeletal, 41, 57
Hyperpathia, 185
Hypersomnia, 261, 263
Hypertension
    management algorithms (quality assurance), 661
    pregnancy-induced, 107
Hypochondroplasia, 43
Hypophosphatemia vitamin D-resistant rickets, 43
Hypothyroidism, cervical acceleration/deceleration and, 28

I

Iliotibial band syndromes, 135, 227
Impedance, 496–500, 501, 519–520
Impingement test (shoulder), 292–293
Independent chiropractic examiners, 638
Independent medical examiners, 638
Indexes and abstracts, 571–573
Inflammation, in spondyloarthropathy, 352
Informed consent, 610–611, 655
Infraspinatus muscle, 281–282, 314–315
Insight, 269, 271
Insomnia, 261, 263
Insurance
    chiropractic reimbursement, 380
    health plan performance measurement (HEDIS-2.0), 646–647
Insurance review mechanisms, *see* Outcome assessment; headings beginning with Quality
International Chiropractors Association, 381
International Classification of Diseases, 259
Interscapular pain, 24
Intervertebral disk
    abnormalities in asymptomatic people, 71
    deformation (creep), 518
    degeneration and facet tropism, 341
    fragment, 47
    herniation, 46, 48, 72, 341
    herniation and low back pain during pregnancy, 103–104
    model of, 519
    resorption, 45, 48

Isolation test
  definition, 473
  leg alignment reactivity, 480–481, 484

J

JCAHO, see Joint Commission on the Accreditation of Healthcare Organizations
Jerk test (shoulder), 288
Jogging, 125
Joint Commission on the Accreditation of Healthcare Organizations, 645, 646
Joints
  adjustment techniques, mechanics, 418–421
  assessment process, PARTS (pain/tenderness, asymmetry/alignment, range of motion abnormality, tissue tone, texture, temperature abnormality, special tests), 416
  cracking sound ("cavitation"), 423, 425, 426
  distraction, configuration, movement, 420–423
  dysfunction evaluation and detection, 415–416
  effects of adjustive therapy, 423–428
  mechanism for dysfunction, 423–424
  three-joint complex (unit of spinal motion), 462–463
  treatment patterns by type of practitioner, 414, 415
Journals
  abstracts of articles, 572–573
  assessing research materials, 565–594
  evaluating articles for usefulness, 572–579
  example of literature search, 586–593
  indexes, 571–572
  peer review, 571
  selecting and reading relevant literature, 570–572, 593
Judgment, 269, 271
Juvenile rheumatoid arthritis, 353

K

Kaminski protocol (technique evaluation), 454, 455
Kinematics
  normal and pathological spine, 517–520
  role in manipulation/adjustment, 493–494
Kinetic chains, 312

Knee
  dancer evaluation, 226–228
  genu valgus, 197
  hyperextension, genu recurvatum, 224
  iliotibial band syndrome, 135
  isolation and pressure test procedures, 484
  pain, 226
  pain management algorithms (quality assurance), 661
  patellofemoral arthralgia, 134–135
  rehabilitation (runners), 138–140
  rolling in, 224, 226–227
  screwing, 227–228

L

Labor, preterm, 106–107
Laminectomy (postoperative spinal stenosis), 53, 54, 55
Language function, 267–268, 271
Latissimus dorsi tendinitis, 313–314
Learning
  competency-based education, 391–394
  mechanistic and holistic paradigms, 389–391
  models (constructivism and critical multiplism), 404–405
  preferences, 397–399
  problem solving and problem-based, 392–394, 395
  self-directed, 398–399
Leg, see also Ankle; Foot; Heel; Knee; Toe
  alignment reactivity, 473, 479–480
  anatomical faults and conditions, 134–137
  bowlegs, genu varum, 224
  cramps during pregnancy, 104–105
  examination of alignments, 131
  gait cycle in running, 122
  length deficiency/discrepancy, 473, 476, 481–484
  length inequality, 130–131, 133, 198
  muscle stretching for runners, 126
  muscular control of ankle in running, 123–124
  myofascial pain syndromes, management algorithms (quality assurance), 661
  pain, after crashes, 26
  pain and spinal stenosis, 60
  posterior tibial syndrome ("shin splints"), 135–136
  stress fractures in runners, 132
Leg, functional short, see Pelvic deficiency

Leg, reactive, *see* Pelvic deficiency
Legislation (chiropractic scope of practice), 373–375
Levator scapulae muscle, 282, 313
Licensure, 375
Ligamentum flavum
　calcification, ossification, 52–53
　facets and, 333, 348
　postoperative ossification or hypertrophy, 54
　spinal stenosis and, 46, 48, 50
Lightheadedness, *see* Dizziness
Line of drive, definition, 473
Lippman test (shoulder), 293
Literature assessment, *see* Journals
Litigation, following whiplash injuries, 3–5, 21
Lordosis
　cervical curve, 335–336
　dancers, 219–220, 225
　hyperlordosis, 224
　pregnancy and, 98, 99–100
Los Angeles College of Chiropractic, 388
Ludington's test (shoulder), 290, 292
Lumbar corset, 113
Lumbar spine
　Activator Methods Chiropractic Technique, 514
　assisted and resisted positioning, 422–423
　back pain after crashes, 24–26
　congenital and developmental stenosis, 40–44
　dancers, 225
　degenerative spondylolisthesis (pseudospondylolisthesis), 50- 51, 360–365
　disk herniation, 487
　facet joint disorders, 331–332, 334, 338, 340, 341
　familial stenosis, 41–42
　gravitational line of L-3, 367
　impedance and stiffness, 498, 501
　intraspinal synovial cysts, 53
　isolation and pressure test procedures, 484
　lordosis, 98, 99
　manipulation loads, 495
　postoperative stenosis, 53–55
　response to treatment, 659–660
　rotational adjustment, 514
　spondylolytic spondylolisthesis, 50
　stenosis, 48, 58, 59
　Tarlov's cyst, 358–359
　tropism, 338, 340
　ununited apophyseal growth centers, 342–343, 345
　weight bearing, 367
Lumbar vertebrae, *see* Lumbar spine
Lumbosacral disk angle, 365, 367
Lumbosacral junction
　facet angle, 332
　facet hypoplasia, 341, 343
　facet tropism, 341
　plane of orientation, 334
　weakness, 338–339
Lumbosacral plexus, 116

M

MacNab's line (posterior joint body line), 364, 366–367
Magnetic resonance imaging
　facet joints, 332
　shoulder, 326
　spinal stenosis, 39, 49, 66, 67–72
Major depressive disorder, 259–263, 271–275
Malocclusion, 174–175
Managed care
　accreditation, 646
　chiropractic credentialing, 649–651
　chiropractic treatments and, 455–456
　current trends, 381
　evaluation standards, 645
　record keeping, 653–654
　quality assurance, 639
　standardization of care, 474
　utilization management, 652
Mandible
　manipulation, 172
　mobility disorders, 168–171
　postural rest position (temporomandibular joint disorders), 150–151
Mandibular condyle
　articular disk and, 169, 170
　compression, 165, 166
　repositioning, 177, 178, 179
Mania, 262, 263, 272
Manipulation
　chiropractic technique overview, 413–435
　classifications, 417–419
　computer-assisted, 500–501
　definitions, 418, 466, 467
　goals, 424–425
　low back pain and pregnancy, 108
　magnitude and frequency content, 499

Manipulation (cont.)
  postpartum period, 117
  randomized clinical trials, 437–438
  spinal stenosis treatment, 73
  temporomandibular joint, 171–172
  under anesthesia, 380
  vertebral forces and movements, 494–495
Manual therapy
  categorization, 452
  definitions, 418, 466, 467
Marathon runners, 125, 128–129
Mass media, 373, 377
Masseter muscle, 162–163
Masticatory muscles, 168
McGill/Melzak pain questionnaire, 663
Mechanical impedance, see Impedance
Mechanistic paradigm, 389–391
Mechanoreceptors, 427
Median nerve, 293
Medical education, 388
Medical history taking, see History taking
Medical records, 259, 653–654
Meniscoid entrapment, 425
Meniscus, 359–360
Mental disorders, see Depressive disorders
Mental status examination (MSE), 255, 265–271
Meralgia paresthetica, 105
Meric procedure, 486–487
Metatarsal bones
  fifth, fracture, 229
  first, 204
  stress fractures, 229
Metatarsophalangeal joint, 205–207, 229
Metatarsus adductus, 197
Midtarsal joint, see Calcaneal-cuboid joint; Talonavicular joint
Military commissions, for chiropractors, 375
Misalignment, 449–450, 451, 463
Miscarriage, 106
Mobilization
  definitions, 418, 466, 467
  vertebral forces and movements, 494–495
Mood, 266, 269–270
Mood disorders, see Depressive disorders
Morquio's mucopolysaccharidosis, 43
Morton's foot, 131
Motion, range of, see Range of motion
Motion segment (term), 463, 467
Motor unit (term), 463
Motor vehicle accidents, see Accidents, traffic

Mouth examination (temporomandibular joint problems), 165–166
MRI, see Magnetic resonance imaging
Mucopolysaccharidosis, Morquio's, 43
Multiple sclerosis, and pregnancy, 105–106
Muscle fibrosis, 174
Muscle splinting, 172
Muscles
  control of ankle in running, 123–124
  dance workouts, stretching, 230, 233–234, 235
  effects of adjustive therapy, 426
  foot, 196–197
  function, outcomes assessment, 663
  palpation and temporomandibular joint problems, 156–158
  stretching for runners, 126
  temporomandibular joint problems, 162–163, 168, 172
Myelography
  comparison with CT for spinal stenosis, 69
  spinal stenosis, 66–67, 68
Myofascial pain disorders, 23, 26, 103
Myofibrotic contracture, 174

N
Narrative history, see History taking
National Academy of Manipulative Medicine, 377
National Association of Chiropractic Medicine, 381–382
National College Chiropractic Clinics, AmbuQual quality management system, 527–563
National Commission on Quality Assurance, 645–646
NCQA, see National Commission on Quality Assurance
Neck, see also Cervical spine
  acceleration/deceleration forces in auto crashes, 4, 6, 7–15
  disability index, 663
  flexion injury, 312
  hyperextension, 1–3
  injuries and seat belts, 15–17
  muscle hyperflexion-hyperextension and temporomandibular injury, 175–176
  pain, 23
  pain screening for temporomandibular joint disorder, 146–152
  personal factors affecting injuries, 18–21

sequence of events in whiplash, 10–14
stiffness, 23
temporomandibular joint examination,
    154–155
whiplash (acceleration/deceleration)
    injuries, 1–37
Nerves, spinal, see Spinal nerves
Nervous system
  dysfunction and disease relationship,
    414
  effects of adjustive therapy, 427
  facet joints, 333
  nerve roots, 53, 293–294, 298
  neuropathy ("nerve interference"), 444
Neural blockade testing, 187–188
Neural canal (neuroforamen), 39, 46, 47, 62
Neurogenic claudication, 60–61
Neurological diseases, pregnancy and,
    105–106
Neuromusculoskeletal system, 414, 424
Nomenclature
  consensus process, 461, 467–468
  quality, review definitions, 521,
    640–644, 652
  subluxation terminology, 461–469
  treatment definitions, 418, 445–446,
    466, 467, 473
Noncompliance, see Patient compliance
Norwood stress test for posterior
    instability (shoulder), 287–288
Nucleus pulposus, hereditary, 59–60
Nursing, quality assurance, 526
Nystagmus, 27

O

Observed Sequential Competency
    Examination (OSCE), 400–402
Occupational health, among dancers,
    211–253
Ocular dysfunction, see Vision
Orthopractic Manipulative Society of
    North America, 382
Orthotics, 207
Oscillation, 519–520
Osgood-Schlatter disease, 132
Ossicles, degenerative, 358
Ossicles of Oppenheimer, 342–343, 345
Ossification
  ligamentum flavum, 52–53
  posterior longitudinal ligament, 51–52
Osteitis pubis, 104
Osteoarthritis
  facet joints, 346, 353–354
  postoperative spinal stenosis, 54–55

Osteochondritis dissecans, 312
Osteoid osteomas, 321
Osteolysis, 313
Osteopathy, 419
Osteophytes, 65, 66
Osteoporosis
  idiopathic, of pregnancy, 105
  scoliosis and, 51
  spinal stenosis secondary to, 56
Osteosarcoma, 306
Oswestry pain questionnaire, 663
Outcome assessment
  cautions in use, 662
  chiropractic case management, 663
  chiropractic education, 389, 390–391,
    405–406
  measurements (research studies),
    575–576, 589, 591, 592
  quality assurance and, 662–664
  structure vs. function, 450

P

P value, 579
Pacinian corpuscles, see Proprioception
Paget's disease, 56–57, 73
Pain, see also under names of parts of the
    body
  chronic, in health care literature,
    580–581, 586
  control for chronic conditions, 660
  decision to treat and, 420
  diagnostic algorithms (quality
    assurance), 657
  effectiveness of chiropractic therapy, 437
  patient loss of routine functions, 598, 599
  perception, 663
  referred, 465
  reflex sympathetic dystrophy, 183–194
  relief, psychological aspects, 428
  role in treatment decisions, 427
  sensory symptoms of reflex sympathetic
    dystrophy, 185–186
  suffering by patients, 598
  sympathetically maintained syndromes,
    183, 184–186
Palmer, B.J., 375
Palmer College of Chiropractic, 388–389
Palpation
  motion, 449, 450
  reflex sympathetic dystrophy, 187
  temporomandibular joint, 155–158
Panic disorder, 274
Paresthesia, 26
Patella, 227

Patellofemoral arthralgia, 134–135
Patellofemoral dysfunction, 227
Patient compliance, 595–633
   adherence to treatment, 596
   autonomy and dependence in, 599–601
   cooperation compared with, 597, 611–612, 615
   cooperative interaction models (prisoner's dilemma), 618–624, 625
   effect of physician-patient relationship on, 596–597
   family context of, 606–607
   functional concerns of physicians and patients compared, 597–601
   involvement of patient in treatment regimen, 611
   percentages of noncompliance, 595
   relapse after treatment completion, 596–597
   self-reliance and self-esteem, 599, 600, 601
   sick role, 598
   skills promoting cooperation, 625–632
   suffering and loss of routine functions, 598, 599
   treatment success and drop-outs, 600
   values considered in treatment 601–607
Patient education, low back pain and pregnancy, 108–113
Patient management curriculum, 392, 394, 395
Patient relations, *see* Physician-patient relationship
Patient satisfaction
   acknowledgment vs. disqualification, 625–626
   audit, 536, 538–542
   audit questions listed, 561–563
   back pain treatment, 378, 379
   outcomes assessment, 663, 664
Patients, *see also* Physician-patient relationship
   characteristics of chiropractic users and nonusers, 376–377
   interview, 604–605, 610, 628–629
   reports of pain relief, 428
   runners' identification with running, 128–129
Pectoralis major contracture test, 293, 294
Peer review
   chiropractic, 638–639
   physician performance audit, 533, 535, 536, 544
   research articles, 571

Peer review organizations, 638, 639
Pelvic deficiency, 473, 475–477
Pelvic nerves, 116
Pelvis
   dancer problems, 225
   isolation and pressure test procedures, 484
   manipulation loads, 495
   pain, and pregnancy, 99
   pelvic pattern and pubic bone adjustment, 513–514
   tilt, 480
Perception, 268, 271
Performance audit, *see* Quality management
Peripheral nervous system, reflex sympathetic dystrophy, 188–190
Peripheral neuropathy, 62
Peroneal tendinitis, 228
Peroneus brevis muscle, 124
Peroneus longus, 197
Personality disorders, 257–258, 275
Pes cavus, 131, 137
Pes planus, *see* Flatfoot
Phentolamine, 188
Physical fitness, *see* Exercise
Physician-patient relationship, 595–633
   acceptance vs. approval/disapproval, 626–628
   acknowledgment vs. disqualification, 625–626
   coercion, 630, 631
   communication aspects, 608–609
   competition in, 618–624
   complementary interactional sequences, 612–618
   cooperative interaction models (prisoner's dilemma), 618–624, 625
   defections in, 618–624
   definition of, by each party, 609–611
   dimensions of care, 624–625
   empathy vs. reassurance, 629–630
   empowered caring, 603, 614–615
   ethic of care and ethic of rights, 603–604
   flexibility vs. defensiveness, 631–632
   future vs. immediate payoffs, 621–622
   models (paternalistic, informative, interpretive, deliberative), 601–604
   paradoxical interactional sequences, 612, 616–618
   patient-centered care, 625
   patient's story and its context, 604–607, 628–629

physician authority and patient
  dependence (autonomy), 599- 601,
  609, 613
respect vs. advice, 630–631
retelling of medical narrative to patient,
  606
skills promoting cooperation, 625–632
structures in, interactional sequences of,
  612–618
symmetrical interactional sequences,
  612, 614–618
therapeutic value of, 607–612
understanding vs. probing, 628–629
Physicians, see also Physician-patient
  relationship
  burnout, 603, 614
  models of behavior, 601–604
  provider profiles, 640
  quality assurance and, 637–638
Piriformis tendinitis, 226
Pitching, see Throwing injuries
Placenta previa, 107
Plantar fascia, 229
Plantar fasciitis, 136–137, 202–203
Plantar hyperkeratoses, 208
Popliteal tendinitis, 136
Population (research studies), 574, 588,
  590
Positioning, 421–423
Postconcussion syndrome, 22–23
Posterior apprehension test (shoulder),
  289
Posterior drawer test (shoulder), 287
Posterior impingement, 229
Posterior tibial syndrome, 135–136
Posterior tibial tendinitis, 229
Postoperative spinal stenosis, 53–55
Postpartum back pain, see Pregnancy
Posturalism, 449
Posture
  back pain during pregnancy, 99–100
  dancers, 223–225
  evaluation, 663
  temporomandibular joint examination,
    154–155
Postzygapophyses, 332
Practice guidelines and parameters,
  452–455
Preeclampsia-eclampsia, 107
Preferred provider organizations, 474
Pregnancy
  athletes', 115–116
  complications, 106–108
  ectopic, 106

exercise during, 110, 111, 112, 114, 115
history taking and physical examination,
  100–103
low back pain and, 97–120
management of low back pain, 108–116
neurological conditions and, 105–106
postpartum back pain, 99, 116–117
postpartum exercise, 117
preterm labor, 106–107
Pressure test
  definition, 473
  leg alignment reactivity, 480–481, 484
Prezygapophyses, 332
Primary care
  chiropractic, 373–375
  quality attributes, 644
Problem solving, see Learning
Program quality index, 527, 542, 543
Pronation, 195–209
  description, 195–198
  measurement, 131–132
  shoe evaluation, 133
Prone leg check, 485
Proprioception
  dancer rehabilitation, 235–245
  neuromuscular facilitation, 235
  progressive rehabilitation, 237
  receptor injuries, 236–237
  rehabilitative equipment, 240–243
  runner rehabilitation, 137–138
  testing, 237–240, 241
  videotaping and, 246–249
Prospective research studies, 576–577,
  583–584, 589, 591
Prospective review, 652
Protzman's test for anterior stability
  (shoulder), 286
Provider profiles, 640
Provocation elevation test (shoulder),
  298
Pseudospondylolisthesis, 50–51
Pseudospondylolisthesis, degenerative,
  360–365
Psoas muscles
  insufficiency, 235
  insufficiency syndrome, 230–233
  short, 226
Psychiatry, 440
Psychology, 427–428
Psychomotor activity
  component of chiropractic technique,
    438
  depressive disorders and, 261, 266, 269
Psychosocial problems, 258

Pterygoid muscles
  palpation and temporomandibular joint
      problems, 157
  testing, 162, 163
Pubic bone, 513–514
Pubic pain, 104
Public opinion
  acceptance of chiropractic, 376–377
  media portrayal of chiropractic, 373, 377
  value for health care dollars, 644
Pulmonary embolism, 107–108
Push pull test (shoulder), 288–289

Q

Q angle, 130
Quadriceps muscle, 139, 220–221, 222
Quadrilateral space syndrome, 311
Quality assessment, 641–642
Quality assurance, 635–669, see also
    Quality improvement; Quality
    management
  chiropractic diagnosis, 655–656, 657
  chiropractic office applications, 649
  chiropractic organizations and activities,
      647–648
  chiropractic study, 525–526
  chiropractic treatment, 656–661
  committee, 528, 529, 530, 531, 552–553
  compared with quality management, 524
  concurrent review (definition), 652
  confidentiality, 554–555
  coordinator, 531, 550–551, 557–559
  Council on Chiropractic Education,
      647–648
  defining quality, 640–644
  definition of, 521
  effectiveness, 553–554
  future considerations, 665–666
  health reform and, 664–665
  historical and social perspectives,
      521–525, 636–640
  methods of assessment (implicit review,
      explicit review, sentinels), 641–642
  national standards, 644–648
  outcomes and, 662–664
  plan, 528, 544
  plan, National College Chiropractic
      Clinics, 549–555
  process, 641–644
  prospective review (definition), 652
  recent trends, 635–636
  record keeping, 555, 653–654
  retrospective review (definition), 652
  second opinions, 638

  staff specialist, 654–655
  utilization review, 637
  various projects and studies, 525–526
Quality control, see Quality management
Quality improvement see also Quality
    assurance; Quality management
  continuous, 522
  description of, 523–524, 645
  managed care, 646
  plan, 531, 534, 553, 554
Quality management, 521–563, see also
    Quality assurance; Quality
    improvement
  ambulatory care parameters, 527–528,
      532, 541
  AmbuQual system, 527–544
  compared with quality assurance, 524
  customer-driven, 639
  definition, 521
  group, 528, 529, 531, 551–552
  patient satisfaction audit, 536, 538–542,
      561–563
  physician (practitioner) performance
      audit, 532–536, 537–538, 539, 544,
      557–559
  program quality index, 527, 542, 543
  programs, 636
  quality control and, 523
  total, 645
Quality of health care
  attributes of primary care, 644
  defining, 640–644
  description, components of, 522
  indicators, 643
Quality planning, 523
Questionnaires, outcome assessment, 663

R

Radiography
  facet disorders, 358
  quality assurance in chiropractic
      diagnosis, 655–656
  running injuries, 132
  shoulder injuries, 320–321
  spinal stenosis, 64–66
  vertebral position in subluxation
      syndrome, 663
Randomization (research studies), 577
Randomized clinical trials
  activator technique, 486–487
  spinal manipulation, 437–438
  use in research, 577–578
Range of motion
  dancers, 214

dancers' screening examination, 223
knee, 139
mandible, 161–162
metatarsophalangeal joint, 205–207
outcomes assessment, 663
reflex sympathetic dystrophy diagnosis, 187
runners, 129–130
shoulder, 283–285, 298
Reactive leg, see Pelvic deficiency
Reading, see Journals
Referral, physician, to chiropractors, 380
Reflex sympathetic dystrophy, 183–194
definitions, 183–184
diagnosis, 187–188
features, clinical course, 184–187
theories, 188–191
therapy, 191–193
Reflex technique, 450–451
Rehabilitation
foot, ankle, 137–140
quality assurance, 660–661
shoulder, 319–326
Relaxin, 97–98, 99, 117
Research
activator technique, 486–493, 502
Activator Method, 474, 475, 478
assessing material, 565–594
components of studies described (population, sample, assessment, time, treatment, analysis), 573–579, 581–593
design of studies, 582–583, 585, 587, 592–593
education and, 405
issues in chiropractic, 383
literature searches (example), 586–593
quality issues, 592
randomized clinical trials in, 577–578
reading relevant literature, 570–572, 593
results addressing efficacy or effectiveness, 578
studies of chiropractic technique, 443–444, 446–447
Retrospective research studies, 576–577, 583, 589, 591
Retrospective review, 652
Retrozygapophyses, 332
Return to work, 592
Review mechanisms in health care, see headings beginning with Quality
Rheumatoid arthritis, 57, 198, 353
Rhomboid muscles, 282
Ribs, 514–515

Rickets, Vitamin D-resistant, 43
Rockwood test for anterior instability (shoulder), 286
Roland-Morris disability questionnaire, 663
Roos' test (shoulder), 296–297
Rotator cuff
impingement, 308
inflammation, 305
injuries, 302–304
muscles described, 281–282
sonography, 321, 325
tear, 290, 291, 304
tendinitis, 303, 304
Rowe test
anterior instability (shoulder), 286
multidirectional instability (shoulder), 289
Running injuries, 121–142
anatomical faults and conditions, 134–137
biomechanics, 122–123
categories of runners, 124, 125
education on prevention, 122
evaluation, diagnosis, 128–133
incidence, 121
marathon runners, 125, 128–129
pronation and, 126–127
rehabilitation, 137–140
return to running after, 138–140
running as part of runners' identities, 128–129
shoe choice, fit, 126–128
stretching and warmup, 125–126
surfaces for running, 125
training errors, 124–127

S

Sacral base
angle, 366, 367
gravitational line of L-3, 367
Sacroiliac belt, 113
Sacroiliac joint
dancers' problems, 225
low back pain during pregnancy, 98–99, 101–102
syndrome, 102, 487, 490–492
Safety devices
auto, and neck or spine injuries, 3
back pain after crashes, 24–26
minor injuries and, 15–17
rear-impact collisions and, 15–17
seat belt retractors, 9
shock-attenuating bumper systems, 17
Salter-Harris fractures, 318

Sample (research studies), 574–575, 588, 590
Sartorius tendinitis, 226
Scapula
    fractures, 315
    interscapular pain, 24
Scapulothoracic articulation, 281
Sciatica
    Activator adjustments, 487, 488–489
    cervical acceleration/deceleration injuries, 26
    dancers, 226
    facet tropism and, 339
    hereditary nucleus pulposus and spinal stenosis, 59–60
    MRI use, 71
Scintigraphy, reflex sympathetic dystrophy, 187
Scoliosis
    causes of spinal stenosis, 51
    dancers' 224, 232
    management algorithms (quality assurance), 661
Seat belts, see Safety devices
Second opinions, see Quality assurance
Segment motion, 493–494
Segmentalism, 449
Self-esteem/self-reliance, see Patient compliance
Serratus anterior muscle, 282
Severity of injury, cervical acceleration/deceleration trauma classifications, 2
SF-36 (medical outcomes study), 663
Shin splints, 135–136, 229
Shoes
    dance, 234–235
    evaluation, 132–133
    runners' training errors, 126–128
    wear patterns and running injuries, 133
Shoulder
    acceleration/deceleration forces in auto crashes, 4, 6, 7–15
    acromioclavicular joint injuries, 298–302
    anterior instability, 284, 285–287, 309–311
    athlete injuries, 279–329
    biomechanics (elevation, rotation, flexion, extension), 283, 284
    blood vessels, 282–283
    bursae, 281
    cervical burners, 311–312
    clavicular physis injuries, 313
    diagnostic imaging, 320–321, 325–326
    dislocation, 309–311
    fractures, 315–319
    inferior instability, 284, 289
    joints described, 280–281
    latissimus dorsi tendinitis, 313–314
    levator scapulae syndrome, 313
    multidirectional instability, 284, 289
    muscle testing, 290, 291, 292–293, 298
    muscles, 281–282, 284
    muscles and throwing injuries, 305
    neurovascular injuries, 311
    orthopedic examination, 283–298
    osteochondritis dissecans, 312
    osteolysis of distal clavicle, 313
    pain, 24
    patient history, 279–280
    posterior instability, 284, 287–289
    rotator cuff, 281–282, 290, 291, 302–304, 315
    throwing injuries, 304–309
    treatment and rehabilitation, 319–326
    wheelchair athletes, 315
Shoulder harnesses, see Safety devices
Sick role, 598
Sickness impact profile, 663
SINBAD, 649
Sinus tarsitis, 203–204
Social environment, 258
Soft tissue
    effects of adjustive therapy, 426
    injuries, 21–23
    pain, diagnostic algorithms (quality assurance), 657
Somatization disorder, 275, 657
Somatosensory evoked potentials, see Evoked potentials
Sonography, shoulder, 321, 325
Specialists, chiropractors as, 374
Speech, 268, 271
Speed's test (shoulder), 290
Spinal canal
    lateral recesses (stenosis), 49
    narrowing (stenosis), 39
    normal and trefoil shapes depicted, 42
    radiography, 64–66
Spinal cord
    compression, 46
    injuries and bilateral facet dislocation, 348–349
Spinal manipulation, see Manipulation
Spinal motion segment (term), 463, 467
Spinal nerves
    facet joints, 333
    pain in spinal stenosis, 62

root compression, 46, 53
root injuries during obstetric delivery, 116–117
root pain, 60–61
roots, 39, 58, 293, 298
Spinal osteophytosis, see Spondylosis
Spinal stenosis, 39–96
   acquired, 44–53
   age of onset, 59
   asymptomatic, 72–73
   chondrodystrophic, 40, 41, 43–44
   congenital and developmental, 40–44
   diagnosis, 59–72
   diagnostic imaging, 64–72
   electrodiagnosis, 63–64
   familial, 41–42
   idiopathic, 40–43
   major causes of, 41
   neurogenic and vascular claudication, 60–62
   pain management, 73, 75
   postoperative, 53–55
   posttraumatic, 55–56
   surgery, 73–74
   tandem (cervical and lumbar), 58–59
   term described, 39
   treatment, 72–74
   trefoil configuration in idiopathic stenosis, 40–41, 42
Spinal subluxation, see Subluxation
Spine, see also Cervical spine; Facets and facet joints; Lumbar spine; Thoracic spine
   creep, 518
   dancer evaluation, 225–226
   dynamic mechanical properties, 495–500
   facet joints, 331–372
   functional unit definition, 462–463
   Hadley's S curve, 363, 365–366
   lordosis, 98–100, 219–220, 225, 335–336
   movement (spinal motion segment), 415
   response to oscillation (vibration), 519–520
   segment motion patterns (kinematics), 493–494
   spinographic measurements, 365–367
   vertebral displacement forces, 494–495
Splint, dental, see Dentistry
Spondylitis, ankylosing, 57, 352–353
Spondylolisthesis
   dancers, 225
   degenerative pseudospondylolisthesis, 360–365
   facet degeneration, 359
   forms of and descriptions of, 49–51
Spondylolysis, 50, 225
Spondylosis
   acquired spinal stenosis, 44–49
   degenerative, 48
   discogenic, 45
Sports
   acceptance of chiropractic, 377
   categories of runners, 125
   dance and chiropractic medicine, 211–253
   pregnant athletes, 115–116
   runners' identification with running, 128–129
   running injuries, 121–142
   shoulder injury management, 279–329
   wheelchair athletes, 315
Sprains, acromioclavicular, 299, 300–301
Stance phase (in running), 123
Standards of care, 455
State government, and chiropractic scope of practice, 373–375
Statistical analysis, 578–579
Stenosis, spinal, see Spinal stenosis
Sternoclavicular joint, 280
Stirrup muscle, 229
Stretching, see Dance
Students, see also Chiropractic education
   learning preference, 397–399
   self-direction, 398–399
Subluxation
   complex, 467
   contraindications, 464
   definitions, 467, 473
   diagnostic algorithms (quality assurance), 657
   functional short leg, 473, 475–477
   manipulable, 464, 467
   misalignment vs. fixation, 449–450
   reflex sympathetic dystrophy, 190
   related dysfunction, 464–465
   segmentalism vs. posturalism, 449
   technique, 444–445, 448–449
   terminology and usage, 461–469
Subluxation syndrome, 465, 467, 663
Subscapularis muscle, 282
Subtalar joint
   pronation, 195, 196, 197
   pronation during relevé and plié, 224
   rheumatoid arthritis, 198
   rolling in and, 228

Subtalar joint *(cont.)*
   tarsal coalition, 199–200
   tibialis posterior rupture, 201
Sudden infant death syndrome, 567
Sudeck's atrophy, 187
Suffering, *see* Pain
Suicide, 265
Sulcus sign (shoulder), 289
Supraspinatus muscle
   description of, 281
   overuse injuries, 292–293
   synchronization, 308
   tendinitis, 293
   tendon, muscle tears, 291, 292
Surgery
   acromioclavicular joint treatment, 301–302
   contraindications to temporomandibular joint manipulation, 172
   correction of hallux limitus and hallux rigidus, 207
   postoperative spinal stenosis, 53–55
   spinal stenosis, 73–74
Swallowing, 163–164
Swimming, and shoulder stress, 307, 308
Swing phase (in running), 123
Sympathetic nervous system
   ganglion block (neural blockade testing), 187–188
   reflex sympathetic dystrophy, 183–194
Sympathicotonia, 184, 191
Symphysis pubis diastasis, 104
Synovial cysts, 53, 358–360
Synovial folds, 333, 425
Synovial hyperplasia, 358
Synoviochondrometaplasia, 315
Synovitis
   facet joints, 354
   strain injuries, 102
   temporomandibular joint disorders, 167–168

T

T test, 579
Talonavicular joint
   Charcot's joint disease, 198
   coalition, 199–200
   dancer injuries, 229
   degenerative joint disease, 201
   pronation, 195
Tarlov's cyst, 358–359
Tarsal coalition, 198, 199–200
Tarsal tunnel syndrome, 106
Teaching
   chiropractic educational strategies, 394–397
   chiropractic technique, 428–432
   faculty appraisal, 402–403
Temporalis muscle, 162–163
Temporomandibular joint, 143–181
   adjustive procedures, 171–172
   articular disk fibrous ankylosis, adhesion, 172–173
   articular disk problems, 168–171
   articular disk "stickiness," adhesion, 171–172
   auscultation, 159–160
   compression/distraction test, 164, 165
   contraindications to manipulation, 172
   counterirritant test, 163, 164
   dental splint, 176–179
   disk compression/distraction test, 164–165, 166
   disorder signs and symptoms, 167
   disorder treatments, 171–172
   history taking, examination, 153–166
   injury and inflammatory cascade, 172–173
   injury in crashes, 11–12, 23, 27
   injury mechanisms, 175–176
   muscle testing, 162–163
   neck muscle hyperflexion-hyperextension, 175–176
   neurological tests, 165–166
   opening, 160–161
   pain, 172
   palpation, 155–156
   range of motion of mandible, 161–162
   referrals, 147
   role of chiropractors, 143–146
   screening procedures, 146–152
   screening questionnaire, 151–152
   swallowing test, 163–164
   treatment success, techniques and instrumentation, 174
Tendinitis
   Achilles, 136, 229, 230
   flexor hallucis longus, 229
   gluteal, 226
   latissimus dorsi, 313–314
   peroneal, 228
   piriformis, 226
   popliteal, 136
   posterior tibial, 135–136, 229
   rotator cuff, 303, 304
   sartorius, 226
   supraspinatus, 293
Tennis, shoulder stress, 307, 308

Tenosynovitis, 199, 200–201
Teres minor muscle, 282
Terminology, see Nomenclature
Textbooks, 569–570
Thecal sac, 71, 75
Thermography
　arm pain relief, 192
　shoulder, 326
Thompson technique, 454
Thoracic outlet syndrome
　acceleration/deceleration injuries, 23, 26
　shoulder injuries in athletes, 294–298, 311
Thoracic spine
　Activator adjustments, 487
　adjustive techniques, 420–421
　facet joints, 331, 333–334
　fractures, 350
　impedance and stiffness, 498, 501
　isolation and pressure test procedures, 484
　manipulation loads, 495
　rotatory adjustment, 514–515
　spondylolisthesis, 359
　tropism, 338
Thoracolumbar junction, 350–352
Thought content and processing, 268, 271
Thrombosis, 311
Thrombosis, deep venous, 107–108
Throwing injuries, 304–309
Tibia, 135
Tibia varum, 197
Tibialis anterior, 217–218, 219
Tibialis posterior
　muscle, 123–124
　rupture and tenosynovitis, 200–202
　tendon, 135, 197–198, 229
Tinel's sign (shoulder), 293–294
Tinnitus, 27
Toe
　adducto varus, 208–209
　great, lateral deviation (hallux valgus), 204–205
　hammertoes, 207–209, 229
　trigger toe, 229
Tomography, osteoid osteomas of shoulder, 321
Tooth percussion, 158–159
Total quality management, 522
Traffic accidents, see Accidents, traffic
Trapezius muscle, 282
Trochanteric belt, 113
Trochanteric bursitis, 226

U

Upper limb tension test, 293, 295
Utilization management, 652
Utilization review, 637

V

Vacuum phenomenon (facet joints), 358
Value of health services, 644, 665
Vascular claudication, 61–62
Vasoconstriction, 189
Vastus medialis muscle, 227
Vastus medialis oblique muscle, 134
Venous thrombosis, 107–108
Vertebrae, see Cervical spine; Facets and facet joints; Lumbar spine; Spine; Thoracic spine
Vertebral artery syndrome, 657
Vertebral misalignment, see Misalignment
Vertigo, 26, 27
Vibration, 519–520
Videotaping, evaluation of dancers, 246–249
Vision, and cervical acceleration/deceleration, 27
Visual analog scales, 663
Vitamin D-resistant rickets, 43

W

Weight bearing, 367
Weight loss, 261
Western States Chiropractic College, 388
Wheelchair athletes, 315
Whiplash, see also Acceleration/deceleration injuries
　neck injuries, 1–37
　syndrome, 492–493
　temporomandibular injury, 175–176
Wilk et al. vs. AMA et al., 373
Women
　cervical acceleration/deceleration trauma, 9
　degenerative spondylolisthesis (pseudospondylolisthesis), 50-51
　whiplash injuries, 18, 21
Work, return to, 592
Wright's test (shoulder), 294

X

X-rays, see Radiography

Y

Yergason's test (shoulder), 290

Z

Zygapophyseal joint, 344
Zygapophyses, 332